MODERATE TO SEVERE PSORIASIS

MODERATE TO SEVERE PSORIASIS

FOURTH EDITION

Edited by

John Y. M. Koo, MD
Department of Dermatology, University of California at San Francisco

Ethan C. Levin, MD
Department of Dermatology, University of California at San Francisco

Argentina Leon, MD
Department of Dermatology, University of California at San Francisco

Jashin J. Wu, MD, FAAD
Department of Dermatology, Kaiser Permanente Medical Center, Los Angeles

Alice B. Gottlieb, MD, PhD
Department of Dermatology, Tufts Medical Center, Tufts University School of Medicine, Boston

CRC Press
Taylor & Francis Group
Boca Raton London New York

CRC Press is an imprint of the
Taylor & Francis Group, an **informa** business

CRC Press
Taylor & Francis Group
6000 Broken Sound Parkway NW, Suite 300
Boca Raton, FL 33487-2742

Printed on acid-free paper
Version Date: 20140131

International Standard Book Number-13: 978-1-4822-1516-8 (Hardback)

Library of Congress Cataloging-in-Publication Data

Moderate to severe psoriasis / edited by John Y. M. Koo, Ethan C. Levin, Argentina Leon, Jashin J. Wu, Alice B. Gottlieb. -- Fourth edition.
p. ; cm.
Includes bibliographical references and index.
ISBN 978-1-4822-1516-8 (hardcover : alk. paper)
I. Koo, John Y. M., editor of compilation. II. Levin, Ethan, editor of compilation. III. Leon, Argentina, editor of compilation. IV. Wu, Jashin J., editor of compilation. V. Gottlieb, Alice B., editor of compilation.
[DNLM: 1. Psoriasis--therapy. 2. Dermatologic Agents--therapeutic use. WR 205]

RL321
616.5'2606--dc23 2013045002

Visit the Taylor & Francis Web site at
http://www.taylorandfrancis.com

and the CRC Press Web site at
http://www.crcpress.com

CONTENTS

CONTRIBUTORS

Lauren Becker
Departments of Dermatology and Pediatrics
Feinberg School of Medicine
Northwestern University
Chicago, Illinois

Tina Bhutani
Department of Dermatology
University of California, San Francisco
San Francisco, California

Andrew Blauvelt
Oregon Medical Research Center
Portland, Oregon

Daniel C. Butler
University of Arizona College of Medicine
Tucscon, Arizona

Anne L. S. Chang
Department of Dermatology
Stanford University School of Medicine
Redwood City, California

Kelly M. Cordoro
Departments of Dermatology and Pediatrics
University of California, San Francisco
San Francisco, California

Maya G. Debbaneh
University of California Irvine School of Medicine
Irvine, California

Rosemary deShazo
University of Utah Health Sciences Center
Salt Lake City, Utah

Kristina Callis Duffin
University of Utah Health Sciences Center
Salt Lake City, Utah

Charles N. Ellis
Department of Dermatology
University of Michigan Medical School
Ann Arbor, Michigan

Jason Emer
Mount Sinai School of Medicine
New York, New York

Shannon Famenini
David Geffen School of Medicine at UCLA
Los Angeles, California

Whitney A. Fisk
University of California Davis School of Medicine
Sacramento, California

Dafna D. Gladman
Toronto Western Research Institute
University of Toronto
and
Toronto Western Hospital
Toronto, Ontario, Canada

Alice B. Gottlieb
Department of Dermatology
Tufts Medical Center
Tufts University School of Medicine
Boston, Massachusetts

Rishu Gupta
Keck School of Medicine of University of Southern California
Los Angeles, California

Judith Hong
Department of Dermatology
University of California, San Francisco
San Francisco, California

Monica Huynh
Chicago College of Osteopathic Medicine
Chicago, Illinois

Edward W. B. Jeffes III
Department of Dermatology
University of California
Irvine, California

Faranak Kamangar
Department of Dermatology
University of California, Davis
Sacramento, California

John Y. M. Koo
Department of Dermatology
Psoriasis and Skin Treatment Center
University of California
San Francisco Medical Center
San Francisco, California

Jonathan W. Kowalski
Global Health Outcomes Research
Allergan Inc.
Irvine, California

Chris M. Kozma
University of South Carolina
Columbia, South Carolina

Gerald G. Krueger
University of Utah Health Sciences Center
Salt Lake City, Utah

Mark G. Lebwohl
Department of Dermatology
Mount Sinai School of Medicine
New York, New York

Argentina Leon
Department of Dermatology
Psoriasis and Skin Treatment Center
University of California
San Francisco Medical Center
San Francisco, California

Ethan C. Levin
Department of Dermatology
Psoriasis and Skin Treatment Center
University of California
San Francisco Medical Center
San Francisco, California

Wilson Liao
Department of Dermatology
University of California, San Francisco
San Francisco, California

M. Alan Menter
Division of Dermatology and Psoriasis Research Institute
Baylor University Medical Center
Dallas, Texas

Warwick L. Morison
Johns Hopkins University School of Medicine
Baltimore, Maryland

Amy S. Paller
Departments of Dermatology and Pediatrics
Feinberg School of Medicine
Northwestern University
Chicago, Illinois

Elisabeth G. Richard
Johns Hopkins University School of Medicine
Baltimore, Maryland

Eric Y. Sako
David Geffen School of Medicine at UCLA
Los Angeles, California

Eva Wang
University of South Alabama School of Medicine
Mobile, Alabama

Gerald D. Weinstein
Department of Dermatology
University of California
Irvine, California

Jashin J. Wu
Department of Dermatology
Kaiser Permanente Los Angeles Medical Center
Los Angeles, California

Chapter 1

An Overview of Psoriasis

M. Alan Menter

INTRODUCTION

Psoriasis has historically been considered an inflammatory skin disorder of unknown etiology producing red scaly patches of mere cosmetic nuisance to patients. However, with knowledge gleaned over the past decade on the immunopathogenesis and genetics of psoriasis together with what may be termed the biological revolution in therapy, all of which will be discussed in later chapters, psoriasis is presently considered a dynamic, genetic, immune-mediated, systemic disorder manifesting on the body surface as well as in the joints in approximately 30% of patients. Patients and dermatologists alike thus need to shift their focus from considering psoriasis as a mere skin disease likely to be controlled with topical therapy to a condition no different from other immune-mediated disorders such as Crohn's disease, rheumatoid arthritis, and lupus erythematosus, all of which have a wide range of clinical manifestations with significant comorbidities. Just as the complete spectrum of these disorders needs to be carefully considered, so too does psoriasis need a careful clinical evaluation, taking into account the extent and the form of the disease, quality-of-life issues, and comorbidities such as obesity and the full spectrum of the metabolic syndrome as well as the potential for coexistent psoriatic joint disease. All of this, particularly on an initial patient visit, will not be accomplished in a traditional five- to ten-minute patient encounter. It will require time and dedication from the physician and his or her support staff to improve patient adherence to therapy as well as the depression and the "disappointment factor" frequently noted in the psoriatic population. Never has psoriasis been so much at the forefront; the buzz among researchers, immunologists, clinicians, and indeed patients with the advent of our understanding of the immunopathogenesis and comorbidities (such as cardiac disease), together with multiple new therapies, is palpable. It behooves us as dermatologists to rise to the challenge, to refocus our energies and thought processes on the treatment of this most prevalent of all immune-mediated diseases, and to take our place with our rheumatology and gastroenterology colleagues in target-based biological therapeutics. A significant portion of the psoriatic population will require a more intensive workup and innovative therapies. The explosion of this new knowledge, and with it new therapeutics, will enable patients and physicians alike to tailor therapy to individual forms of psoriasis as well as to individual patient needs and hence improve significantly the quality of life of all our patients with this distressing lifelong disorder.

CLINICAL MANIFESTATIONS

Psoriasis is defined by the Committee on Guidelines of Care and the Task Force on Psoriasis of the American Academy of Dermatology as follows: "A chronic skin disease that is classically characterized by thickened, red areas of skin covered with silvery scales" [1]. The extent of skin involvement can range from discrete, localized areas to generalized body involvement. The joints, nails, as well as, frequently, mucous membranes may also be affected by the disease. "Psoriasis has a significant phenotypic variability," with a range of clinical manifestations from mild disease with a few isolated plaques to multiple different morphological variants including guttate, discoid, annular, rupoid, and erythrodermic forms, with or without psoriatic joint disease. Psoriasis may be symptomatic throughout one's lifetime, may progress with age, or may wax and wane in severity. The disease is frequently readily apparent to others and is associated with functional impairment, disfigurement, and emotional distress out of proportion to the actual extent of clinical disease. When severe, in the judgment of the patient, the effects of psoriasis can have a deleterious impact on work performance, on social performance and acceptability, on sexual function, and on mental health. The diagnosis of psoriasis is normally straightforward, although conditions such as cutaneous T-cell lymphoma, pityriasis rubra pilaris, eczema, tinea infections, and secondary syphilis may on occasion cause confusion and should be considered in the differential diagnosis, particularly when patients fail to respond to traditional antipsoriatic therapy. A full medical, family, and personal history are likewise important (Table 1.1) [2]. The classic morphological variants are noted in Table 1.2 [2,3].

Although psoriasis normally remains true to form during one's lifetime—with discoid plaques predominating—the whole range of morphological subtypes may present in an individual patient either simultaneously or progressively with increasing age. Thus, patients with palmar–plantar psoriasis may have no other clinical evidence of psoriasis, may have coexistent flexural psoriasis, or may have classic discoid plaque psoriasis involving a few anatomical sites or major portions of the body surface area (BSA). In addition, erythrodermic psoriasis also classically shows significant palmar–plantar involvement, frequently causing difficulty in distinguishing psoriasis from Sezary's disease. It is likely that as we unravel the complex genetics of psoriasis, this clinical range will be

TABLE 1.1 Important Factors in Patient's History

Medical history
Chronic scaling of the ears
Coexistent or previously diagnosed immune-mediated diseases
Long-standing "dandruff"
Atopy
Pruritus ani or vulvae
Associated joint problems
Family history
Psoriasis
Rheumatological disorders
Comorbidities including the Metabolic Syndrome 5 components
Precipitating factors
Antecedent infections, particularly streptococcal
Stress (physical, emotional, or metabolic)
Medications (see Table 1.7)

Source: Menter A et al., *Lancet* 338, 231–234, 1991.

shown to have a genotypic basis. The recognition that psoriasis is a condition of wide clinical variability, just like lupus erythematosus, will make evident that what we call "psoriasis" is in reality an umbrella term for more than one disease with a similar histopathological picture of a hyperplastic epithelium, and an inflammatory cell infiltrate in both the epidermis and the dermis consisting predominantly of T lymphocytes. Before considering the various clinical forms and manifestations of psoriasis more specifically, it is worthwhile to review definitions of mild, moderate, and severe psoriasis.

Psoriasis has traditionally been classified purely on the basis of BSA: mild corresponding to less than 5% BSA, moderate psoriasis 5% to 10% or 15% BSA, and severe psoriasis affecting over 10%–15% BSA. Krueger et al. [4] attempted to revise these definitions to include not only BSA involvement but also quality-of-life issues as well as the patient's perception and his or her ability to withstand as well as deal with side effects relating to their individual treatments (Table 1.3) [3].

TABLE 1.2 Morphological Variants of Psoriasis

Discoid
Elephantine
Erythrodermic
Flexural
Guttate
Palmar–plantar
Pustular
Localized
Generalized

Source: Menter A et al., *Lancet* 338, 231–234, 1991.

TABLE 1.3 Classification of Psoriasis

Mild psoriasis	Disease does not alter the patient's quality of life. Patients can minimize the impact of disease and may not require treatment.
	Treatments have no known serious risks (e.g., class 5 topical steroids).
	Generally less than 5% of BSA is involved with disease.
Moderate psoriasis	Disease does alter the patient's quality of life.
	The patient expects therapy will improve quality of life.
	Therapies used for moderate disease have minimal risks (i.e., although these therapies may be inconvenient, expensive, time-consuming, and less than totally effective, they are not recognized as having the potential for altering short- or long-term health).
	Generally between 2% and 20% of BSA is involved with disease.
Severe psoriasis	Disease alters the patient's quality of life.
	Disease does not have a satisfactory response to treatments that have minimal risks.
	Patients are willing to accept life-altering side effects to achieve less disease or no disease.
	Generally more than 10% of BSA is involved with disease.
	Other factors
	Patient's attitude about disease
	Location of disease (e.g., face, hands, fingernails, feet, genitals)
	Symptoms (e.g., pain, tightness, bleeding, or severe itching) Arthralgias, Arthritis

Source: Adapted from Griffiths CE et al., *Br J Dermatol* 156, 258–262, 2007.

THE GENETICS OF PSORIASIS

Psoriasis Relating to Age of Onset

Traditionally, two distinct forms of psoriasis have been noted: type I disease with early onset (before age of 40), likely genetic in origin, and type II late onset (older than 40 years), less likely to be genetic. In a clinical and epidemiological study from Spain [5], 1774 patients were studied. In this population, the disease started at a wide range of ages, with a mean age of onset of 29.1 years, with a slight female preponderance for earlier age of onset. In accordance with other studies, more than 60% of patients experienced their psoriasis before the age of 30. As in similar prior studies, this large cohort of patients confirmed the association of a positive family history (in up to 40% of patients) with early onset psoriasis, showing an increasing family history of disease. From a morphological point of view, the only significant relationship between the age of onset and clinical forms of the disease related to guttate psoriasis (more frequently seen in patients with early-onset psoriasis) and palmar–plantar pustular psoriasis (more prevalent in late-onset psoriasis). In addition, patients with the early-onset form tended to have more extensive disease and a more severe clinical course.

In a large series of patients followed at the University of Kiel, Germany, a bimodal age of onset of psoriasis was noted with one peak occurring in young patients and a second peak occurring in older patients (mean age 57–60 years) [6], which are similar findings to the Spanish study. The features of psoriasis in these two patient groups, type I and type II disease, are summarized in Table 1.4 [5].

In the Kiel population, type I psoriasis had a strong association with a human leukocyte antigen (HLA-)Cw6 genotype with 85% having this gene compared to 15% of type II psoriatics. Overall, approximately 70% of psoriatics were classified as having type I disease, with the clinical course of type I psoriasis tending toward more severe involvement.

The genetic influence on psoriasis is best illustrated in twin studies comparing the development of this disorder in monozygotic and dizygotic twin pairs [7]. In dizygotic (not genetically identical) twins, psoriasis was found in both individuals in about one-fourth of the pairs, whereas in monozygotic (genetically identical twins), psoriasis was found in both individuals in about two-thirds of the pairs. The significantly higher prevalence of psoriasis in identical twins strongly suggests a genetic component to its development. However, in one-third of identical twin pairs only one individual developed psoriasis, thus suggesting an epigenetic influence on its expression. The genetic transmission of psoriasis

TABLE 1.4 Characteristics of Type I and Type II Psoriasis

Characteristics	Type I	Type II
Age at onset	Peak around age 20	Peak around age 60
Family history	Common	Rare
HLA association	Cw6 definite, B13 and B17 probable	Rare
Clinical course	Tends toward more generalized refractory or severe disease	Milder

Source: Adapted from Ferrandiz C et al., *J Am Acad Dermatol* 46, 867–873, 2002.

has been evaluated in some families in which this trait occurs in a higher percentage of individuals [8]. Its transmission in some of these families suggests that a dominant gene is responsible, but that, as in the twin studies, acquiring the gene does not always produce the condition (variable genetic penetrance). In large population studies, a clear grouping of psoriasis in families has been confirmed, but the transmission has not followed simple autosomal dominant or recessive patterns. It has thus been proposed that its inheritance in the broad population is multifactorial, combining a genetic component and an environment influence.

Update in Genetic Research

Let us now consider recent research relating to the genetics of psoriasis. It has been known for years that there is a significant association between HLA and psoriasis, specifically, class I antigens HLA-B57, B13, Cw6, and Cw7, with HLA-Cw6 appearing to confer the highest risk. The first susceptibility locus at the distal end of chromosome 17 was described in 1994 in *Science* [9]. This came about as a result of research at the National Psoriasis Tissue Bank based in Dallas, TX, at Baylor University Medical Center and sponsored by the National Psoriasis Foundation. In 1997, the Michigan-Kiel Group confirmed this susceptibility locus [10]. In this study of 224 sib-pairs, Nair and colleagues found linkages in the HLA region as well as additional loci on chromosome 16q and chromosome 20p. Of interest was the overlap in the 16q region with a previously described locus for Crohn's disease; psoriasis appears more commonly in patients with Crohn's disease. Furthermore, an Italian group has shown a locus in chromosome 1, that is, 1q21 [11]. Bowcock (the co-discoverer, with the author, of the original 17q locus) and Bhalerao in 1999 also confirmed this Italian finding [12]. Recently, after 18 years of research on this locus, the relationship between this 17q locus, CARD14, and NF-κ has been confirmed [13].

The majority of interest and work in this field of psoriasis genetics has been confined to Psorsl on chromosome 6p21.3, which is considered the most important locus for psoriasis susceptibility in the majority of populations studied. Fortunately in 1999, the full sequence and gene map of the human major histocompatibility complex was described [14]. In a study from the United Kingdom published in *Lancet* in 1999 [15], the polymorphic *S* gene ("S for skin") which lies 160 kb telomeric of HLA-C showed significant evidence for gene linkage and disease association, thus supporting evidence that the *S* gene plays a major role in psoriasis susceptibility. This *S* gene encodes the corneodesmosin (CDSN) gene protein, which plays a role in epidermal differentiation as well as in the adhesion of the stratum corneum. It was the authors' conclusion that the *S* gene was a more attractive potential candidate gene than HLA-C itself. Subsequently, other genes in this region including the coiled-coil α-helical rod protein 1 (CCHCR1, or the *HCR* gene) have been considered to play a role in the pathogenesis of psoriasis. Despite intensive investigation within and around this HLA-Cw6 region, the definitive candidate gene in this area has hitherto not been conclusively identified. More recent evidence suggests that the *S* gene (or *CDSN* gene) may not appear to account for disease susceptibility any better than HLA-Cw6 itself, as underscored by a paper in 2000 from the Michigan-Kiel group [16]. In this paper, Nair and coworkers defined the psoriasis susceptibility gene as a 60-kb region between HLA-C and HCR, suggesting that this region is the region most likely to carry the disease allele at the 6p 21 locus.

Recently, 15 new psoriasis susceptibility loci were identified on a longitudinal study using a meta-analysis of three genome-wide association studies (GWAS) and two independent data sets genotyped on the Immunochip, including 10,558 cases and 22,806 controls [17]. A number of these new loci were shared with other autoimmune diseases, particularly relating to innate host defense. They also encoded several proteins engaged in the important tumor necrosis factor (TNF), interleukin-23 (Il-23), and IL-17 signaling pathways central to psoriasis and targeted by our current and future biological therapies.

In summary, the identification of the specific gene(s) for psoriasis has shown that multiple loci are implicated. Once a specific candidate gene on chromosome 6p21.3 (Psors1) is identified, potential interactions (epistasis) between this gene and other psoriatic loci previously and recently discovered appear likely to be confirmed. The collaboration between molecular geneticists around the world certainly is bearing fruit, and the potential exists for the exact molecular defect underlying psoriasis susceptibility being discovered in the not too distant future.

PATHOPHYSIOLOGY OF PSORIASIS

Epidermal Hyperproliferation

The histopathology of the psoriatic epidermis was always noted to consist of many mitoses. In 1963, Van Scott determined that there was a marked increase in mitoses/surface of psoriasis in comparison to the normal epidermis. He developed the concept called the hyperplasia of psoriasis [18]. This information was then expanded in a series of studies using radioactive isotopic techniques to examine static and dynamic aspects of psoriatic epidermal hyperproliferation. The data showed that the transit time of psoriatic basal cells moving upward to the beginning of the stratum corneum took only two days in comparison to the normal epidermis, which had a slower upward movement of about 12 days through a much thinner epidermis [19]. Further studies using tritiated thymidine injected *in vivo* into psoriatic skin determined a cell cycle of approximately 37 hours compared to approximately 300 hours in normal skin [20]. Although finding that psoriatic cells were hyperproliferative, it did not reveal the mechanism(s) by which the skin would change its pattern of proliferation and conversion into the phenotype of psoriasis. However, it did suggest at least one reason why a drug such as methotrexate might be active in the treatment of this disease. Additional studies indicate that lymphocytes are more sensitive to methotrexate than epidermal cells, suggesting that methotrexate may affect at least two different cellular components of psoriatic tissue [21].

Immunology of Psoriasis

Since the early 1980s, evidence has shown that there is a strong immunological component to the pathogenesis of psoriasis. This concept was initiated by the serendipitous observation in 1979 that a patient receiving the immunosuppressive drug cyclosporine found that his or her coexistent psoriasis improved dramatically. This is not unlike a similar serendipitous observation in 1951 that the folic acid antagonist, aminopterin (later replaced by methotrexate), produced clearing of psoriasis. The immunological milieu of psoriatic skin includes the presence of many T lymphocytes, particularly CD4+ (helper) and CD8+ (suppressor/cytotoxic) cells. Thus, many cytokines have been discovered that influence the inflammatory aspects of psoriasis and trigger, directly or indirectly, the hyperproliferation of psoriatic keratinocytes. The most important discovery in the last decade has been the finding of a new subset of T cells, such as Th17, with appropriate understanding of its relationship with a host of cytokines including IL17 and TNF-α [22].

The science of immunology (as it pertains to many diseases) is now being used to develop new therapeutic approaches to illnesses including psoriasis, rheumatoid arthritis, psoriatic arthritis, multiple sclerosis, Crohn's disease, and others. From research on the immunopathogenesis of psoriasis, these findings are creating an extensive pipeline of new drugs described in this book [23–26] (Chapters 13 and 16) with a significant amount of emphasis currently being placed on new large, as well as, small molecular therapeutic agents with significant clinical efficacy.

CLINICAL MANIFESTATIONS

Scalp Psoriasis

The majority of patients with psoriasis will show evidence of scalp involvement. Despite the full range of therapeutic modalities now available, including topicals, light treatments, systemic therapies, and biological agents, psoriasis of the scalp remains one of the most difficult to control. Classically, psoriasis is a highly symmetrical disease, but lesions on the scalp are frequently asymmetrical, almost certainly related to the inevitable koebnerization of scalp psoriasis due to the patient's picking, scratching, and harsh shampooing. This leads to lichenified plaques with involvement usually on the posterior scalp or above either ear (i.e., areas of easy accessibility). When scalp psoriasis predominates with or without associated facial involvement, overlap with seborrheic dermatitis may produce the clinical variant known as sebopsoriasis.

Guttate Psoriasis

This form is well known to most dermatologists, often presenting in young adults or children with a prior history of a streptococcal throat infection. Numerous other trigger factors, such as viral infections, medications, major stress episodes, and rapid discontinuation of systemic therapy (steroids, methotrexate, or cyclosporine) may also produce this inflammatory, papular form of psoriasis. In addition, patients with previous stable plaque psoriasis may experience, at intervals, guttate flares, either related to the aforementioned trigger factors or spontaneously. It is fortunate that pure guttate psoriasis is amenable to treatment with phototherapy and, if necessary with culture-proven streptococcal infection, concomitant antibiotics. Parents of children presenting with guttate psoriasis as a first indication of the condition should be counseled about the likelihood of more classic discoid-type psoriasis in young adult life as well as the need to interact with their pediatrician for future interventions with further upper respiratory infections, particularly of the streptococcal variety.

Discoid Plaque Psoriasis

This most common form of the disease classically presents symmetrically, ranging in size from small coin-sized plaques to larger plaques that may coalesce to form large geographic areas (Figure 1.1). As discussed in the definitions of mild, moderate, and severe disease, it is essential to do a full-body evaluation of the patient's plaque involvement to ascertain whether

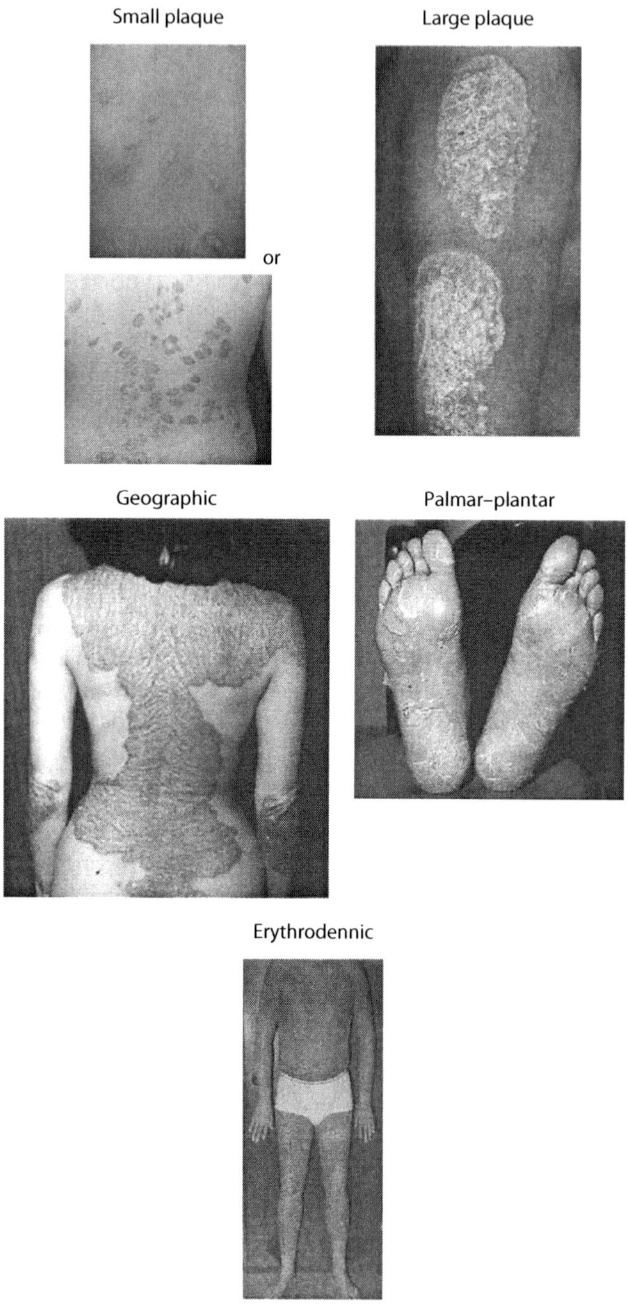

FIGURE 1.1 (See color insert.) Morphological variants of psoriasis: Is this one disease?

topical therapy, for instance, is likely to be both of value and appropriate for each individual's needs and for potential long-term adherence to topical therapy.

Erythrodermic Psoriasis

This inflammatory and severe form of psoriasis (fortunately affecting only a minority of patients) is frequently precipitated by trigger factors such as infections, inappropriate systemic steroid usage, or burns incurred during phototherapy. Other trigger factors may relate to abrupt discontinuation of systemic therapy, particularly methotrexate and cyclosporine. It is important to differentiate other forms of erythroderma, particularly in patients with no known prior history of stable, chronic plaque psoriasis. Thus, eczema of all forms, particularly atopic in nature, the Sézary form of cutaneous T-cell lymphoma, pityriasis rubra pilaris, and drug-related causes may all need to be considered. Despite the continued decrease in hospitalization of psoriasis patients, erythrodermic psoriasis is the one form of the disease that frequently necessitates inpatient therapy. In our experience, it is critical to rule out systemic sepsis prior to initiating specific antipsoriatic therapy because a certain proportion of patients will have staphylococcal sepsis. In fact, a recent referral to our clinic in Dallas was a young patient with prior stable plaque psoriasis well controlled on cyclosporin who experienced sudden worsening and increased inflammation. The dosage of cyclosporin was increased by his referring dermatologist to 5 mg/kg/day, despite which his psoriasis continued to worsen. Coagulase-positive *Staphylococcus* was cultured in his blood, and appropriate systemic antibiotic therapy was initiated resulting in a dramatic improvement in his psoriasis with no further need for antipsoriatic therapy. Likewise, it is important to observe these patients for evidence of cardiac and renal failure, particularly elderly patients in whom these organ systems may already be compromised. A certain proportion of these patients do respond to hospitalization and conservative treatment with wet compresses, dilute topical steroids with or without occlusion, and supportive therapy, such as fluid balance control [27].

Flexural Psoriasis

This form of psoriasis, like scalp psoriasis, is frequently resistant to traditional forms of therapy. In obese patients, areas such as breast folds, as well as groin and abdominal folds, may frequently be complicated with secondary candidiasis necessitating specific anti-*Candida* therapy. In addition to standard antipsoriatic therapy, such as dilute topical steroids, the newer nonsteroidal calcineurin inhibitor topical agents, tacrolimus and pimecrolimus, are effective in this location as compared to their poor effect in other cutaneous sites, except for the face.

Palmar–Plantar Psoriasis

This is classically divided into the hyperkeratotic form and the pustular form. In many instances, there is an overlap between these two polar types with fissuring, erythema, crusting, and pustules coexisting in individual patients, with or without evidence of psoriasis on other anatomical sites. Intensive topical therapy is indicated with remissions, unfortunately, usually short-lived. This leads to major problems in quality of life in a significant proportion of patients, particularly relating to day-to-day life, including ambulation, and manual activities. Many patients with this form of psoriasis will therefore require systemic/biologic therapy and/or phototherapy either singularly or in combination [28].

Psoriatic Arthritis

Why is it so important that dermatologists understand this condition? It is now recognized that psoriatic arthritis is far more common than the previously considered number of 10% of patients with psoriasis (29). Thus, up to one-third of all psoriasis patients are likely to develop joint tenderness and psoriatic arthritis. Psoriatic arthritis is often considered a relatively benign arthropathy associated with cutaneous psoriasis, with skin manifestations likely to precede joint complaints by up to 10 years in the majority of patients. However, it can frequently be debilitating and disabling and, like rheumatoid arthritis, is frequently progressive, leading to disability and eventual need for surgical intervention. Five clinical patterns of psoriatic arthritis have been recognized that can coexist with overlapping clinical expressions. A more recent classification [30] has expanded this concept (Tables 1.5 and 1.6).

Patients with distal interphalangeal (DIP) disease are likely to have psoriatic nail changes, and thus, it is imperative that—at all clinic visits—the dermatologist closely examines the nails in addition to inquiring whether the patient has early morning stiffness and/or joint pain, tenderness, or swelling involving small and large joints (Table 1.7). Removing the patient's shoes is essential at each and every visit as dactylitis of the toes (Figure 1.2a) is as common there as in fingers. Palpation of the Achilles tendon (Figure 1.2b), as well as the plantar fascia (extension of the Achilles tendon beyond the talus) is important to assess for enthesitis.

Dermatologists are frequently the portal of entry for psoriatic patients, and thus, referral to our rheumatology colleagues is essential to prevent further disability and progression of the

TABLE 1.5 Classification of Psoriatic Arthritis: Types and Incidence

Type	Key Clinical Features	Incidence (%)
Asymmetrical polyarthritis or oligoarthritis	Morning stiffness, distal (DIP) and proximal interphalangeal (PIP) involvement, nail disease, ≤4 joints involved	>47
Symmetrical polyarthritis	Simultaneous development of psoriasis and arthritis	25
Ankylosing spondylitis	Progressive low back pain, morning stiffness, sacroiliac, and axial joint involvement	23
DIP joint disease	Nail and joint involvement (DIP) predominate	Rare
Arthritis mutilans	Destructive form of arthritis, telescoping, joint lysis, typically in phalanges, and metacarpals	Rare

Source: Courtesy of Amgen Corporation.

TABLE 1.6 Classification of Psoriatic Arthritis: CASPAR[a] Study Group 2006

At least three of five:

1. Evidence of current psoriasis, personal or family history of psoriasis
2. Typical psoriatic nail dystrophy: onycholysis, pitting, and hyperkeratosis
3. Negative RF
4. Current or history of dactylitis
5. Radiographic evidence of juxta-articular new bone formation (excluding osteophytes)

Source: Taylor WJ, et al., *Arthritis Rheum* 54, 2665–2673, 2006.

[a] CASPAR = ClASsification criteria for Psoriatic ARhritis.

TABLE 1.7 What Is the Role of the Dermatologist in Identifying Psoriatic Arthritis?

No one expects dermatologists to be rheumatologists.	
However, dermatologists should be aware of and vigilant for the arthritic component of psoriasis and refer as needed	
Dermatologists should:	
Examine for	*Ask about*
PIP and DIP involvement	Morning stiffness
Tender and/or swollen joints	Persistent joint pain or other arthritic symptoms
Nail involvement	Fluctuations of joint pain with exacerbations of psoriasis
	Family history of psoriatic arthritis

Source: Courtesy of Amgen Corporation.

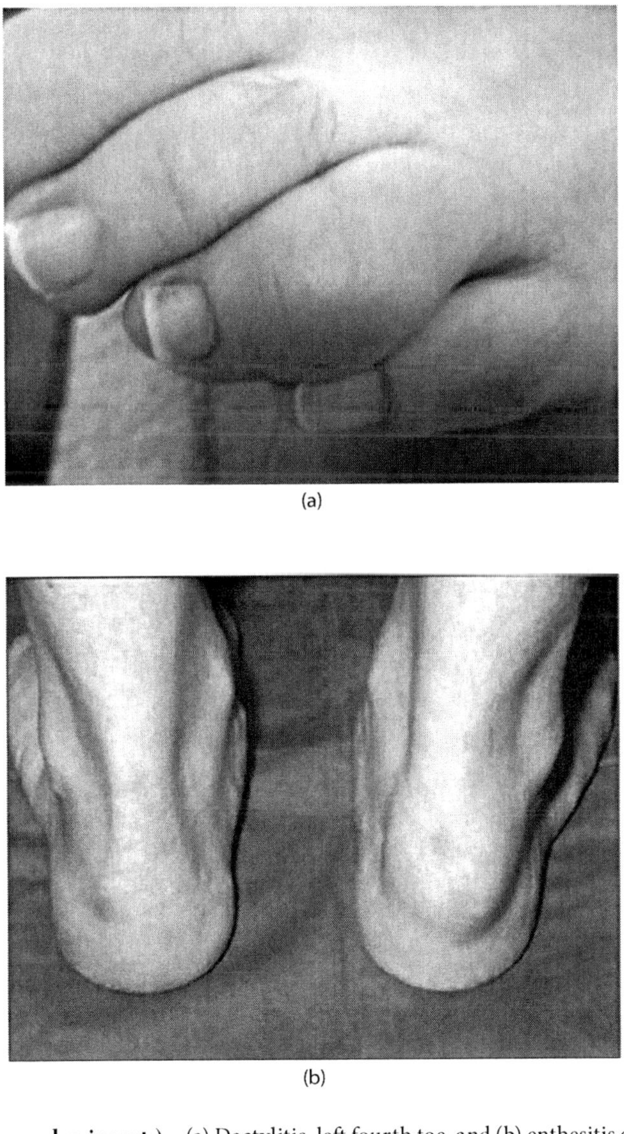

(a)

(b)

FIGURE 1.2 (See color insert.) (a) Dactylitis, left fourth toe, and (b) enthesitis of achilles tendon.

disease. This is especially important with the array of systemic biologic medications currently available, which have been shown to prevent further joint damage.

ITCHING IN PSORIASIS

Most major texts state that itching of psoriasis, although present in a fairly significant proportion, is frequently mild in nature. Prevalence and degree of severity are frequently higher in patients with more severe disease. In this regard, a study of 200 psoriasis patients found that 92% had pruritus at some time [31]. In a study of patients from a psoriasis outpatient clinic with significant plaque involvement, pruritus was a feature in 84% of 108 patients, being daily in 77% of patients, weekly in 18% of patients, and less frequently in 5%. All body sites were affected, with the back, legs, and arms the most commonly involved. The face and neck were less commonly involved [32]. Important in this study was the fact that the pruritus in the majority of patients was unresponsive to treatment with traditional antipruritics. Phototherapy also did not significantly relieve the itch. Thus, itching is a symptom (like many other symptoms of psoriasis) that has a negative impact on the response to therapy and on the quality of life in the majority of patients with psoriasis. This will be discussed in more detail subsequently.

FACTORS AFFECTING REMISSIONS AND FLARES

Because psoriasis is a chronic condition that often waxes and wanes in severity, it is clearly desirable to identify factors that can worsen disease activity or that can prolong the duration of therapy-induced remission. Much more is known about circumstances under which psoriasis worsens than about favorable conditions or treatments that will significantly extend a period of remission or of low-level disease activity. Presently, many psoriatic patients are continued on standard therapeutic agents following clinical clearing of their disease in order to suppress recurrences (maintenance therapy). Other than maintenance therapy, there are no specific treatments for extending remission periods, except through efforts made to avoid skin injury or drugs for other therapies that will lead to worsening of psoriasis. Warm weather, summertime, and rest and relaxation in beach-type vacation environments may provide significant periods of improvement without accompanying medical treatments. The relaxation component may be the most significant part of the improvement in a stress-prone patient. Factors that have been shown to exacerbate psoriasis are summarized in Table 1.8.

Expression of active, lesional psoriasis is linked to mitotic and biochemical activation of keratinocytes and immunological cells within a localized area of skin. Because both sets of cells are functionally activated by common cytokines, it is not surprising that psoriasis can be triggered by a variety of different stimuli that activate either epidermal keratinocytes or lymphocytes locally in skin. Any form of injury to the epidermis that triggers resting keratinocytes into a wound repair pathway can also trigger psoriasis in susceptible (Koebner-responsive) patients. Thus tape stripping, superficial or deep abrasions, lacerations, thermal burns, sunburns, or other physical injury can locally trigger psoriasis [33]. In normal individuals, each of these forms of injury would lead to a transient period of altered epidermal activity (termed regenerative epidermal maturation) or an alternative pathway of keratinocyte differentiation that would repair the injury. In this regard, the difference between Koebner-responsive psoriatics

TABLE 1.8 Factors That Can Induce or Exacerbate Psoriasis in Susceptible Individuals

Physical trauma to skin
Superficial abrasion
Blister
Laceration/incision
Thermal burn
Phototoxic reactions
Solar
Ultraviolet B
PUVA induced
Activation of local cellular immunity
Contact allergens
Immunizations in skin
Infections in skin (bacterial or viral)
Systemic immunological activation or alteration
Hypersensitivity to drug or other antigen
Group A streptococcal infections
HIV infection
Systemic drugs (probable action through pharmacological properties of the agent)
Corticosteroids
Interferons
Lithium
Antimalarials (chloroquine, hydroxychloroquine, quinacrine, quinidine)
β-Blockers (adrenergic receptor antagonists: many different agents both selective and nonselective)
Nonsteroidal anti-inflammatory drugs
Angiotensin-converting enzyme inhibitors
Gemfibrozil and a number of other drugs in case reports
Emotional stress

and nonresponsive individuals is probably the ability to turn off or to downregulate a physiologically relevant cell growth pathway. Another physiological cell-activation process that can occur locally in skin is delayed-type hypersensitivity, local T-cell activation via antigen presentation by epidermal Langerhans cells. The most common expression of this pathway in skin is contact allergy to an external substance, but local immunity can also be triggered by focal skin infections, vaccinations, or reactions to systemic medications. Each of these conditions that activates cellular immunity has also been shown to cause a flare of psoriasis in some susceptible individuals. Flares of guttate psoriasis, especially in adolescents, are often attributed to antecedent pharyngeal infections with group A streptococci. Although the skin is not directly infected with this organism, systemic immunological activation may lead to increased T-cell activation in skin as the initiating reaction in a guttate flare. It should also be emphasized that widespread systemic immune dysfunction induced by human immunodeficiency virus (HIV) sometimes leads to a form of psoriasis that, paradoxically, worsens with decreasing T-cell counts [34].

Psoriasis can be exacerbated or induced in some susceptible individuals by a number of systemic drugs [35,36]. These include lithium, betablockers (β), receptor blockers, antimalarials, nonsteroidal anti-inflammatory drugs, angiotensin-converting enzyme inhibitors, gemfibrozil, and corticosteroids (Table 1.8). In individuals with demonstrated or suspected worsening of psoriasis due to one of these agents, it is desirable to discontinue the suspected drug or to try an unrelated alternative if the patient's medical condition permits and if other therapeutic options are available. Although systemic corticosteroids are not infrequently and erroneously used to treat psoriasis, the response in this regard is limited by significant exacerbation of baseline disease activity (termed rebound or flaring), including induction of pustular flares, following their discontinuation. Thus, unless a concurrent medical condition dictates the need for systemic corticosteroids, their use in the treatment for psoriasis should be avoided. In a study of 103 patients with generalized pustular psoriasis, more than 30% had previously received treatment with oral steroids [37]. Such exacerbations of psoriasis have also been seen after extensive use of topical corticosteroids, particularly when they are applied under occlusion. Rebound and flaring of psoriasis following discontinuation of systemic corticosteroids are probably not obligate consequences of systemic immunological suppression, because psoriasis recurs without rebound or pustular flares less frequently following discontinuation of cyclosporine therapy.

STRATEGY OF THERAPY

The strategy of therapy starts with an educational process that informs the patient as to the nature of psoriasis, the potential comorbidities, and the therapeutic capabilities available for the type and extent of disease in each individual patient. The initial visit with a patient must include consideration of topics that pertain to the current disease manifestations, interpersonal relationships, exacerbating factors, familial hereditary concerns, and psychological factors (Table 1.9). The discussion should conclude with the important goal of improving the patient's quality of life without producing undue harm medically or fiscally, although improving the patient's emotional outlook and status. The physician is challenged with presenting to the patient a realistic but, hopefully, optimistic "big picture" of therapy, keeping in mind the chronicity of this disease, as well as its comorbidities [38].

Today, the therapeutic approaches to psoriasis include topical or local medications, phototherapeutic modalities, systemic drugs, and biological agents. The simplest and safest treatments are topical agents used primarily in patients with localized and limited amounts of skin involvement. There is no precise definition of limited (or mild) disease. My definition is that the location and amount of BSA affected can be effectively treated

TABLE 1.9 Doctor–Patient Discussion of Psoriasis

Lesions/symptoms/diagnosis
Hereditary aspects
Systemic manifestations: arthritis
Exacerbating and favorable factors
Response to past treatments
Range of therapeutic options
Chronic long-term disease
Psychological ramifications
Optimism for tomorrow, new therapies in the pipeline

with topical medications (single or in combination) with good patient long-term maintenance of therapy (adherence).

Quality of life comes into this consideration: smaller, more localized areas of involvement but in critical areas (such as for employment or social appearance) may override consideration of a simple BSA calculation [4]. Topical therapy in patients with a BSA greater than 10% requires large quantities of medications with commensurate higher costs. The amount of time necessary for applications leads to an inevitable poor adherence to therapy and inconvenience depending on the choice of drug and vehicle. Currently available topical therapy does not usually produce long-term clinical improvement. Patients with more limited disease undergo repeated trials of different medications frequently accumulating a medicine chest filled with topical preparations. At some point, however, those frustrated patients with more substantial disease (i.e., 10% or more BSA), or those unresponsive to topical therapy, become frustrated and hence become candidates for more "aggressive" forms of therapy, such as phototherapy and/or systemic/biological drugs that are, fortunately, now available.

In 1993, a survey of American Academy of Dermatology members revealed that there were approximately 2.4 million visits annually to dermatologists by psoriatic patients, with each dermatologist seeing an average of 28 patients with psoriasis/month. Using a working definition of mild psoriasis as a patient being treated with topical therapy, 77% were estimated to have mild (limited) disease. The remainder of the patients received phototherapy or systemic treatment and were considered to have moderate to severe disease. Other criteria frequently used to define moderate to severe disease are listed in Table 1.10.

In patients receiving topical therapy, corticosteroids, particularly in the United States, are the choice of 85% of physicians. The remaining patients receive either topical calcipotriene, topical tazarotene, or combinations of each with corticosteroids. Within the steroid selection category, class I to II (potent-superpotent) steroids were chosen by 62% of the dermatologists, and 37% selected the midpotency compounds. Potent steroids generally produce good to excellent results, but the major problem is that these results do not persist for long periods of time. Whether this is truly secondary to resistance (tachyphylaxis) or to a lack of adherence to therapy is debatable. Survey information also indicates that by three months after maximal improvement with steroids, relapse of disease is seen in approximately 50% of patients, even with continuing use of medication. Older therapies—tars and anthralin—are less effective than the potent steroids, are less aesthetic, and hence are used less frequently today.

TABLE 1.10 Working Definitions of Moderate to Severe Psoriasis

Greater than 20% of BSA involved
Psoriasis not responsive to topical therapy
Extensive disease not economically feasible to treat topically
Psychologically stressful disease
Gainful employment prevented
Pustular or erythrodermic psoriasis

In summary, although the potent topical steroids may be reasonably effective for the treatment of psoriasis, their value is limited by lack of long-term remission and maintenance. The frequency with which patients carry bags of different topical medications, often half used, into their physician's office testifies to this frustrating dilemma. As of 2013, there still is a paucity of new topical drug modalities for the approximately 70% of psoriatic patients who only have mild or minimal psoriasis and hence do not require phototherapy and systemic or biologic medications.

The moderate to severe psoriatic patient presents an interesting, satisfying, and valuable therapeutic challenge. There is no other extensive (noninfectious) dermatological disease that has available to it such an armamentarium of effective therapeutic approaches. There are at least seven groups of psoriasis therapy (Table 1.11) for which extensive information has been acquired. These treatments are discussed fully in this book.

It is interesting to consider that approximately half of all the new medications that have ever been developed for our most common dermatological diseases (including the advances in therapy of psoriasis) have taken place in the last 50 years (Table 1.12). The use of systemic steroids in our psoriasis population has certainly increased the number of patients presenting with pustular or inflammatory psoriasis.

In treating patients with a chronic disease such as psoriasis, treatment effectiveness, duration of effectiveness, and safety are integral components of a treatment plan. As indicated

TABLE 1.11 Therapeutic Approaches to Moderate to Severe Psoriasis

Phototherapy: UVB with or without tar and narrowband UVB
Photochemotherapy (PUVA)
Methotrexate
Acitretin
Cyclosporine
Isotretinoin (pustular psoriasis)
Immunomodulatory drugs (biologicals)

TABLE 1.12 Major Dermatology Drug Discoveries since the 1940s

Pre-1950	**Tar/UVB**; penicillin, antibiotic era begins
1950s	**Corticosteroid** era begins, **methotrexate**, griseofulvin, antifungals, antihistamines
1960s	5-Fluorouracil, topical retinoids
1970s	Retinoids (isotretinoin), **PUVA**, acyclovir
1980s	**Retinoids (etretinate, acitretin)**
1990s	**Cyclosporine, topical calcipotriene, topical tazarotene**
2000s	Tacrolimus
	Pimecrolimus
	Calcipotriene-steroid topical combinations
	Immunomodulatory drugs (biologic agents)

Note: Bold names indicate psoriasis therapies. These therapies used for psoriasis represent half of the therapeutic medical advances in dermatology.

earlier, topical steroids may have good short-term effects but maintenance of long-term lesion clearance is far from satisfactory, leading to significant quality-of-life concerns.

Surveyed dermatologists were asked for their perception of the effectiveness of topical therapy for mild psoriasis in comparison to the effectiveness of phototherapy or systemic treatments for more extensive psoriasis. The criteria for judgment included quality and duration of improvement. Each of the phototherapy or systemic treatments was perceived to work *better* than topical steroids (Figure 1.3) [34]. One might conclude that the available topical forms of therapy are not yet as effective for psoriasis, lesion for lesion, as the photo/systemic/biological modalities. Subsequent chapters in this book will describe in detail the quality and duration of improvement achieved by these treatments.

With moderate to severe psoriasis, the assumption must be made that this disease will generally remain active in some form for much of the patient's future. Therapeutic planning must consider that the currently available treatments will be used for many years. Thus, they must be used in a manner that will minimize long-term toxicity so that they can be safely used intermittently for possibly the remainder of the patient's life. For two of our major treatments, ultraviolet B (UVB) with tar and methotrexate, we have clinical experience for 70 and 50 years, respectively. Long-term experience with psoralen ultraviolet A (PUVA) and the oral retinoids, etretinate and acitretin, has also been accumulated, although cyclosporine experience in the treatment of psoriasis is approximately 25 years old. We now have approximately 10 years of experience with the new biologic agents. Fortunately, more than three million patients with all forms of immune mediated diseases (rheumatoid arthritis and inflammatory bowel disease) have been treated with the three TNF-inhibiting agents, giving

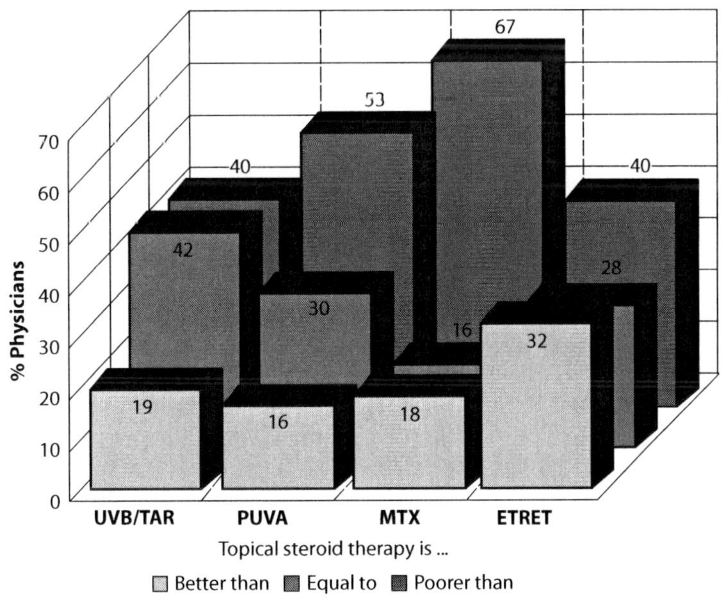

FIGURE 1.3 Comparison of topical steroid therapy efficacy for mild psoriasis using photo/systemic therapy for widespread disease (in the opinion of physicians surveyed). (From Kaplan MH et al., *J Am Acad Dermatol* 16, 485–506, 1987.)

TABLE 1.13 Mean Annual Costs of Psoriasis Care

Treatment	Total ($)	Laboratory Work	Drug
Outpatient Goeckerman (day-care setting)	3914	0	0
PUVA	2604	138	473
Outpatient UVB (3 times/week)	1966	0	0
Methotrexate	1381	470	458
Etretinate	1995	465	1267
Cyclosporine	6648	1021	4119

Source: Baker H, Ryan T, *Br J Dermatol* 80, 771–773, 1968.

those of us in the psoriasis field a great deal of safety data to share with our patients. However, the presence of multiple comorbidities in our psoriasis population, such as metabolic syndrome, makes long-term safety data for these agents essential to our psoriasis patients. The therapeutic indices do suggest that benefits significantly outweigh risks in long-term maintenance therapy. Risk factors appear to accumulate with continuing therapy, as seen, for example, in the liver changes accompanying large cumulative dosages of methotrexate or in skin cancers following hundreds of PUVA treatments. The prior "rotation regimen" (i.e., one year each on a number of various modalities) has been superseded by long-term (i.e., five years of therapy with a single agent, e.g., a biologic drug or methotrexate) without evidence of significant toxicity.

Today, more than ever, the economics of long-term disease therapy must be considered. Recent reports detail the annual therapy costs for moderate to severe psoriasis [39,40]. Costs for outpatient forms of therapy range from $1400 to $6600 (Table 1.13) [37]. Inpatient therapy, which is generally a modified form of the Goeckerman regimen, is substantially more expensive and is now used very infrequently because of economic changes relating to hospitalization and to length of stay issues. Psoriasis, especially in those patients with moderate to severe disease, should not be viewed as a minor cosmetic problem. With the advent of biologic therapy in our psoriasis population over the past decade, these costs have inevitably, considerably increased.

It is highly likely that over the following decade these costs will be reduced by the introduction of biosimilar agents as alternatives to our current biologic agents [41]. Two biosimilar Infliximab agents were approved by EMA (European Medicine Agency) in September 2013.

COUNSELING AND EDUCATION

As dermatologists, we are faced with the very difficult and sensitive responsibility of discussing a chronically discomforting, cosmetically disfiguring disease with multiple comorbidities with our psoriasis patients. The physically discomforting problems of itching, dryness, irritation, fissuring, and a host of other symptoms are the more immediate difficulties. The issue of cosmesis may be more distressing than anything else, leading to psychological difficulties from an altered self-image. With new patients, particularly young adults who are socially distressed, it has always been of value to spend time discussing the emotional aspects of the disease. This often allows the patient to vent many pent-up feelings and frustrations to which the sympathetic physician can respond and offer encouragement. The availability of local support groups for psoriasis, particularly the National Psoriasis

Foundation, is very helpful in this regard. The patient needs optimism and education. Both of these needs can be discussed in terms of the considerable amount of research being done on psoriasis. This research has led to the development of several new therapies in the past 30 years, including PUVA, oral retinoids, cyclosporine, and the full range of biologic agents. As dermatologists accumulate more experience with each of the therapeutic modalities, additional patients with borderline severe disease should be included in the treatment groups for some of the drugs described in this book. With the basic mystery of psoriasis continuing to unravel and with more emphasis on immunological mechanisms, new therapies are being developed that will more specifically impact immunological pathways affecting the skin.

PSYCHOLOGICAL INTERVENTION

The physician's role is, and always has been, very much that of educator and psychotherapist. To know how to induce peace of mind in the patient and to enhance his or her faith in the healing powers of the health-care provider requires psychological knowledge and skills [42,43]. The practitioner's sensitivity to changes in body image and to fears of social rejection, and a physician's willingness to listen to and understand the familial, social, and sexual impact of the disorder aid in the recovery of the whole person. Within this supportive context, encouragement is more readily received.

The relationship between stress and psoriasis has been investigated by Baughman and Sobel [44] and by Arnetz et al. [45] among others. Cognitive interpretation (how stressful life events are perceived by each individual) may be a crucial factor in what constitutes that which we call stress [46]. Cognitive interpretation, as an intervening variable that mediates between stressful life events and somatic reactivity, may explain why some patients with psoriasis believe their disorder is caused by or exacerbated by stress although others do not. Thus, patients in Baughman and Sobel's sample are described as stress reactors and nonstress reactors. In contrast, the Arnetz et al. study suggests that, during stressor exposure, the psoriatic group reported significantly higher strain levels "accompanied by higher levels of urinary adrenaline and lower levels of plasma cortisol." No psycho-endocrine differences were found during resting conditions between the two groups.

The continuing "stress and psoriasis" controversy makes research into treatment programs that combine state-of-the-art dermatological therapy with psychological intervention worth investigating. Yet self-control strategies and/or psychotherapy are not generally incorporated into treatment. Relaxation training and psoriasis-specific guided imagery as adjuvant treatment to dermatological therapy have been investigated in a study of 25 subjects with severe psoriasis [47]. The results of this study do suggest a useful place for adjuvant psychological intervention in the management of severe psoriasis. There is a strong need for further research in this area.

REFERENCES

1. Drake LA, Ceilley RI, Cornelison RL, et al. Guidelines of care for psoriasis. *J Am Acad Dermatol* 1993; 28: 632–637.
2. Menter A, Barker J, Fonelli WN. Psoriasis in practice. *Lancet* 1991; 338: 231–234.

3. Griffiths CE, Christophers E, Barker JN, et al. A classification of psoriasis vulgaris according to phenotype. *Br J Dermatol* 2007; 156: 258–262.
4. Krueger GG, Feldman SR, Camisa C, et al. Two considerations for patients with psoriasis and their clinicians: what defines mild, moderate, and severe psoriasis? What constitutes a clinically significant improvement when treating psoriasis? *J Am Acad Dermatol* 2000; 43: 281–285.
5. Ferrandiz C, Pujol RM, Garcia-Patos V, et al. Psoriasis of early and late onset: a clinical and epidemiologic study from Spain. *J Am Acad Dermatol* 2002; 46: 867–873.
6. Henseler T, Christophers E. Psoriasis of early and late onset: characteristics of two types of psoriasis vulgaris. *J Am Acad Dermatol* 1985; 13: 450–456.
7. Farber EM, Nall ML. Epidemiology: natural history and genetics. In: Roenigk HHJ, Maibach HI, eds. *Psoriasis*, 2nd ed. New York: Marcel Dekker; 1991, 209–253.
8. Farber EM, Nall ML. Genetics of psoriasis: twin study. In: Farber EM, Cox AJ, eds. *Psoriasis—Proceedings of the International Symposium*. Stanford, CA: Stanford University Press; 1971, 7–13.
9. Tomfohrde J, Silverman A, Barnes R, et al. Gene for familial psoriasis susceptibility mapped to the distal end of chromosome 17q. *Science* 1994; 264: 1141–1145.
10. Nair RP, Henseler T, Jenisch S, et al. Evidence for two psoriasis susceptibility loci (HLA and 17q) in two novel candidate regions (16q and 20p) by genome-wide scan. *Hum Mol Genet* 1997; 6: 1349–1356.
11. Capon F, Novelli G, Semperini S, et al. Searching for psoriasis susceptibility genes in Italy: genome scan and evidence for a new locus to chromosome 1q. *J Invest Dermatol* 1999; 112: 32–35.
12. Bhalerao J, Bowcock A. The genetics of psoriasis: a complex disorder of the skin and immune system. *Hum Mol Genet* 1999; 7: 1537–1545.
13. Jordan CT, Cao L, Roberson ED, et al. Rare and common variants in *CARD14*, encoding an epidermal regulator of NF-kappaB, in psoriasis. *Am J Hum Genet* 2012; 90: 796–808.
14. Beck S, Geraghty D, Inoko H. Complete sequence and gene map of a human major histocompatibility complex. *Macher* 1999; 401: 921–923.
15. Allen MH, Veal C, Faassen A, et al. A non-HLA gene within the MHC in psoriasis. *Lancet* 1999; 353: 1589–1590.
16. Nair RP, Stuart P, Henseler T, et al. Localization of psoriasis susceptibility locus. PSORS 1 to a 60 kilobase interval telomeric 2 HLA-C. *Am J Hum Genet* 2000; 66: 1833–1844.
17. Tsoi LC, Spain SL, Knight J, et al. Identification of 15 new psoriasis susceptibility loci highlights the role of innate immunity. *Nat Genet* 2012; 44: 1341–1348.
18. Van Scott EJ, Ekel TM. Kinetics of hyperplasia in psoriasis. *Arch Dermatol* 1963; 88: 373–381.
19. Weinstein GD, Van Scott EJ. Turnover time of human normal and psoriatic epidermis by autoradiographic analysis. *J Invest Dermatol* 1966; 45: 561–567.
20. Weinstein GD, McCullough JM, Ross PA. Cell kinetic basis for the pathophysiology of psoriasis. *J Invest Dermatol* 1985; 85: 579–583.
21. Jeffes EWB, III, McCullough JL, Pittelkow MR, et al. Methotrexate therapy of psoriasis: differential sensitivity of proliferating lymphoid and epithelial cells to the cytotoxic and growth-inhibitory effects of methotrexate. *J Invest Dermatol* 1995; 104: 183–188.
22. Nestle FO, Kaplan DH, Barker J. Psoriasis. *N Engl J Med* 2009; 361: 496–509.
23. Nickoloff BJ. The immunologic and genetic basis of psoriasis. *Arch Dermatol* 1999; 135: 1104–1110.
24. Gottlieb AB. Psoriasis: immunopathology and immunomodulation. *Dermatol Clin* 2001; 19: 649–657.
25. Lowes MA, Bowcock AM, Krueger JG. Pathogenesis and therapy of psoriasis. *Nature* 2007; 445: 866–873.
26. Liu Y, Helms C, Liao W, et al. A genome-wide association study of psoriasis and psoriatic arthritis identifies new disease loci. *PLoS Genet* 2008; 4: e1000041.
27. Boyd AS, Menter A. Erythrodermic psoriasis. Precipitating factors, course, and prognosis in 50 patients. *J Am Acad Dermatol* 1989; 21: 985–991.
28. Farley E, Masrour S, McKey J, et al. Palmoplantar psoriasis: a phenotypical and clinical review with introduction of a new quality-of-life assessment tool. *J Am Acad Dermatol* 2009; 60: 1024–1031.
29. Gladman DD, Farewell VT, Nadeau C. Clinical indications of progression in psoriatic arthritis: multivariate relative risk model. *J Rheumatol* 1995; 22: 675–679.
30. Taylor W, Gladman D, Helliwell P, et al. Classification criteria for psoriatic arthritis: development of new criteria from a large international study. *Arthritis Rheum* 2006; 54: 2665–2673.

31. Newbold PCH. Pruritus in psoriasis. In: Farber EM, Cox AJ, eds. *Proceedings of the Second International Symposium*. New York: Yorke Medical Books; 1977, 334–336.
32. Yosip OV, Itca G, Goon A, et al. The prevalence and clinical characteristics of pruritus among patients with extensive psoriasis. *Br J Dermatol* 2000; 143: 969–973.
33. Eyre RW, Krueger GG. Response to injury of skin involved and uninvolved with psoriasis, and its relation to disease activity: Koebner and "reverse" Koebner reactions. *Br J Dermatol* 1982; 106: 153–159.
34. Kaplan MH, Sadick N, McNutt NS. Dermatologic findings and manifestations of acquired immunodeficiency syndrome (AIDS). *J Am Acad Dermatol* 1987; 16: 485–506.
35. Able EA, DiCicco LM, Orenberg EK, et al. Drugs in exacerbation of psoriasis. *J Am Acad Dermatol* 1986; 15: 1007–1022.
36. Gilleaudeau P, Vallat VP, Carter DM. Arniotensim converting enzyme inhibitor as possible exacerbating drugs in psoriasis. *J Am Acad Dermatol* 1993; 28: 490–492.
37. Baker H, Ryan T. Generalized pustular psoriasis: a clinical and epidemiological study of 103 cases. *Br J Dermatol* 1968; 80: 771–773.
38. Weinstein GD, White GM. An approach to the treatment of moderate to severe psoriasis with rotational therapy. *J Am Acad Dermatol* 1993; 28(3): 454–459.
39. Sander HM, Morris LF, Phillips CM, et al. The annual cost of psoriasis. *J Am Acad Dermatol* 1993; 28(3): 422–425.
40. Lee GC, Weinstein GD. Comparative cost effectiveness of different treatments for psoriasis. In: Rajagopalan R, Sherertz EF, Aderson RT, eds. *Care and Management of Skin Diseases: Life Quality and Economic Impact*. New York: Marcel Dekker, 21, pp. 269–298.
41. Strober BE, Armour K, Romiti R, et al. Biopharmaceuticals and biosimilars in psoriasis: what the dermatologist needs to know. *J Am Acad Dermatol* 2012; 66: 317–322.
42. Section contributed by Marcia Z. Weinstein, Ph.D.
43. Engel GL. The need for a new medical model: a challenge for biomedicine. *Science* 1977; 196: 4286.
44. Baugham R, Sobel R. Psoriasis, stress, and strain. *Arch Dermatol* 1971; 103: 599–605.
45. Arnetz BB, Fjellner B, Eneroth P, et al. Stress and psoriasis: psychoendocrine and metabolic reactions in psoriatic patients during standardized stressor exposure. *Psychosom Med* 1985; 47: 528–541.
46. Lazarus RS. *Psychological Stress and the Coping Process*. New York: McGraw Hill; 1966.
47. Weinstein MZ. Psoriasis-specific relaxation training/guided imagery as adjuvant treatment for intractable psoriasis. Doctoral dissertation, Nova University, 1988.

Chapter 2

Evaluating Psoriasis in Patients

John Y. M. Koo, Jonathan W. Kowalski, Mark G. Lebwohl, Chris M. Kozma, M. Alan Menter, and Charles N. Ellis

INTRODUCTION

According to a National Psoriasis Foundation survey, 78% of members with severe psoriasis reported frustration with the efficacy of their current treatment, and 32% indicated that the treatment they are receiving was not aggressive enough [1]. In addition, 87% of all psoriasis patients were receiving only topical medication for their psoriasis, and only 26% of patients were very satisfied with their treatment regimens.

Several highly effective systemic therapies already exist for psoriasis, and other potential new systemic therapies are in development for patients with psoriasis. The majority opinion is that a greater percentage of the total psoriasis population can benefit from the use of systemic agents. However, what may be needed is an instrument to assist in the critical decision of whether more aggressive therapy is necessary or not.

There has been no convenient tool that can assist dermatologists in identifying patients who would benefit from systemic therapy for psoriasis and, at the same time, justify these decisions to third-party payers. However, tools such as these exist for other chronic diseases treated by rheumatologists (e.g., rheumatoid arthritis) and urologists (e.g., benign prostatic hyperplasia). Such a tool for psoriasis would need to incorporate the assessments of health-related quality of life and the other measures of disease severity and associated joint disorder [2].

The Koo–Menter Psoriasis Instrument (KMPI) has been designed to be a practical assessment tool, which dermatologists can quickly and easily use in their daily practice to help guide them in identifying patients with psoriasis who may be candidates for systemic therapy. In addition to assessing who should receive systemic therapies, methods to monitor patients' responses to therapies are also important. Although valuable for patient selection and for insurance reimbursement, the KMPI does not change substantially during therapy. Instead, rating scales such as those used in clinical trials may be used to monitor patients during treatment. Unfortunately, many of these scales are complex. These will be discussed later in this chapter.

OVERVIEW

The KMPI is a two-page questionnaire on a single sheet (Figures 2.1 and 2.2). On the front page, the patient completes three brief sections while awaiting evaluation by the physician. The topics of these sections include validated psoriasis-specific quality of life, parts of body currently affected by psoriasis, and psoriatic arthritis/joint symptomatology.

The physician then completes the reverse side of the instrument during the physical examination. The quality-of-life score is easily totaled from the front page; body surface area (BSA)

Koo-Menter Psoriasis Instrument

Patient Self-Assessment **Name:** ______________________ **Date:** __________

Part 1: Quality of Life—Please answer each of the following questions as they pertain to your Psoriasis <u>during the past month</u>. (Circle on number per question)

	Not at All				***Somewhat***						***Very Much***
1. How self-conscious do you feel with regard to your psoriasis?	0	1	2	3	4	5	6	7	8	9	10
2. How helpless do you feel with regard to your psoriasis?	0	1	2	3	4	5	6	7	8	9	10
3. How embarrassed do you feel with regard to your psoriasis?	0	1	2	3	4	5	6	7	8	9	10
4. How angry or frustrated do you feel with regard to your psoriasis?	0	1	2	3	4	5	6	7	8	9	10
5. To what extent does your psoriasis make your appearance unsightly?	0	1	2	3	4	5	6	7	8	9	10
6. How disfiguring is your psoriasis?	0	1	2	3	4	5	6	7	8	9	10
7. How much does your psoriasis impact your overall emotional well-being?	0	1	2	3	4	5	6	7	8	9	10
8. Overall, to what extent does your psoriasis interfere with your capacity to enjoy live?	0	1	2	3	4	5	6	7	8	9	10

How much have each of the following been affected by your psoriasis <u>during the past month?</u> (Circle on number per question)

	Not at All				***Somewhat***						***Very Much***
9. Itching?	0	1	2	3	4	5	6	7	8	9	10
10. Physical irritation?	0	1	2	3	4	5	6	7	8	9	10
11. Physical pain or soreness?	0	1	2	3	4	5	6	7	8	9	10
12. Choice of clothing to conceal psoriasis?	0	1	2	3	4	5	6	7	8	9	10

Total Quality-of-Life Score (0 - 120) ☐☐☐
*** (Medical staff to calculate)**

Part 2:

A. Using the figures below, place an "X" on the parts of your body that <u>currently</u> have psoriasis.

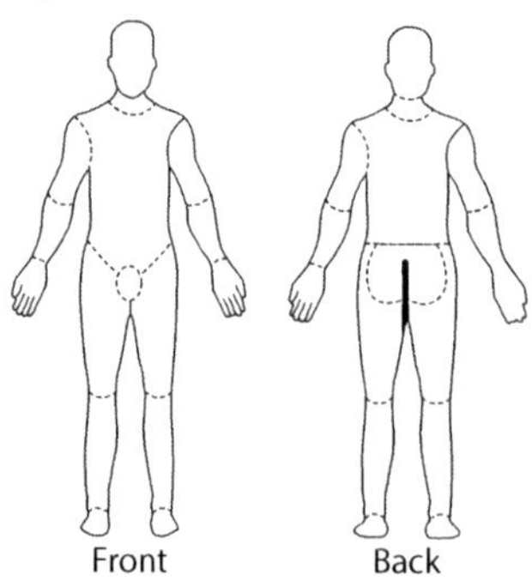

Part 3:

A. Have you ever been diagnosed with psoriatic arthritis?

Yes ☐ No ☐

B. Do you have swollen, tender, or stiff joints (e.g., hands, feet, hips, back)?

Yes ☐ No ☐

If yes, how many joints are affected? (Check on box)

1 ☐ 2 ☐ 3 ☐ More than 4 ☐

If yes, how much have your joint symptoms affected your daily activities?

Not at all ☐ A little ☐ A lot ☐ Very much ☐

STOP Once completed, please return to medical staff

FIGURE 2.1 Koo–Menter psoriasis instrument: patient self-assessment.

Koo–Menter Psoriasis Instrument

Physician Assessment **Name:** ______________________ **Date:** ____________

Part 1: Total Quality-of-Life assessment score (from part 1 of previous page)	⟹	☐☐☐

Part 2: Area of total body involvement: % BSA (body surface area)

Head	☐ %	Head up to 9% of total BSA	
Anterior Trank	☐☐ %	Anterior Trunk up to 18%	Note: Patient's open hand (from wrist to tips of fingers) with fingers tucked together and thumb tucked to the side equals approximately 1% body surface area
Posterior Trunk	☐☐ %	Posteror Trunk up to 18%	
Right Leg	☐☐ %	Right Leg: up to 18% (includes buttock)	
Left Leg	☐☐ %	Left Leg: up to 18% (includes buttock)	
Both Arms	☐☐ %	Both Arms: up to 18%	
Genitalia	☐ %	Genitalia: 1%	
Total BSA	☐☐☐ %		

Part 3: In terms of psoriasis severity, does the patient have:	**Check Answer**	
Plaque, erythrodermic, or pustular psoriasis with >10% BSA involvement?	Yes	No
Persistent guttate psoriasis?	Yes	No
Localized (<10% BSA) psoriasis but resistant to optimized attempts at topical therapy or physically disabling (e.g., palmar and/or plantar psoriasis)?	Yes	No
Localized (<10% BSA) but serious subtype with possibility of progression (e.g., pustular or pre-erythrodermic psoriasis)?	Yes	No
Psoriatic arthritis that affects daily activities (arthritis based on prior diagnosis or Part 3 of patient self-assessment and physician clinical assessment)?	Yes	No
Substantial psychosocial or quality-of-life impact documented by patient Quality-of-Life self-assessment score of ≥50?	Yes	No
Part 4: Is phototherapy an option?	**Check Answer**	
Is a suitable phototherapy unit readily accessible to the patient?	Yes	No
Does the anatomical location or form of psoriasis (e.g., scalp, inverse, erythrodermic) preclude phototherapy?	Yes	No
Does the patient have the dedication, time, stamina, or transportation for phototherapy?	Yes	No
Has phototherapy, as monotherapy, failed in the past?	Yes	No
Is phototherapy contraindicated (e.g., photosensitive drugs, history of multiple skin cancers)?	Yes	No
In your clinical judgement, is phototherapy likely to yield substantial improvement to justify its use before systemic therapy?	Yes	No

Physician/Nurse comments: ____

If at least one of the shaded boxes in both Part 3 and Part 4 above are checked, then the patient is a candidate for systemic therapy.

CONCLUSION: The patient is a candidate for systemic therapy	**Yes**	**No**

FIGURE 2.2 Koo–Menter psoriasis instrument: physician assessment.

involvement is assessed using the "rule of nines," and a series of simple "yes" or "no" questions allows the physician to quickly characterize the patient's disease and treatment history. The physician uses the psoriasis-specific quality-of-life score, the total percentage of BSA involvement, and the overall clinical assessment of the patient's psoriasis to determine the need for systemic therapy.

COMPONENTS OF THE KMPI

Patient Self-Assessment

Part 1: Health-Related Quality of Life The patient completes the 12-item psoriasis quality-of-life questionnaire (PQOL-12). Developed from the original 41-item PQOL (which was created a decade ago based on literature review, patient focus groups, and pilot testing in 505 patients with psoriasis), the items from the PQOL-12 were identified using new data from 474 patients with psoriasis and were determined to be valid and reliable in assessing the impact of psoriasis on patients across the spectrum of psoriasis severity. In addition, the items of the PQOL-12 are responsive and sensitive in measuring clinically meaningful change and improvement following treatment.

The PQOL-12 was chosen as the quality-of-life measure for the KMPI because of its brevity, broad applicability across disease severity, the rigor of its development and psychometric validation, and its psoriasis-specific focus. The validation data for PQOL-12 will be described later in this chapter under the section "Background on the 12-item PQOL-12."

Part 2: Patient Indication of Psoriasis Sites The patient indicates the location of his or her psoriatic lesions by placing "Xs" on figures illustrating the front and back of the human body. The patient's indication of psoriasis sites helps facilitate the physician's evaluation of the area of psoriatic involvement in the patient.

Part 3: Joint Symptoms The patient answers four questions about joint symptoms and psoriatic arthritis. These items, developed based on feedback from leading arthritis experts, are included to facilitate early detection of this important associated condition while ensuring that the decision for systemic therapy is also based on joint symptomatology.

Physician Assessment

Part 1: Total Quality-of-Life Assessment Score The physician totals the patient's quality-of-life score from the front page.

Part 2: Area of Involvement The physician calculates the patient's BSA involvement using the rule of nines or by estimation (using the area of open hand as approximately 1% of the total body surface).

Part 3: Assessment of Psoriasis Severity The following severity criteria are then assessed by the physician using simple "yes" or "no" options:

- Plaque, erythrodermic, or pustular psoriasis with more than 10% BSA involvement
- Guttate psoriasis

- Localized psoriasis (less than 10% BSA involvement) that is resistant to topical therapy or is disabling (e.g., palmar–plantar psoriasis)
- One of the serious subtypes of localized psoriasis (less than 10% BSA involvement) that has a possibility of progression (e.g., generalized pustular or erythrodermic psoriasis)
- Clinical evidence of psoriatic joint disease as assessed by the patient and physician

Part 4: Feasibility of Phototherapy Lastly, the feasibility and clinical appropriateness of phototherapy are rapidly evaluated in six simple questions.

Determination of Candidacy for Systemic Therapy

Using the responses to the "yes" or "no" questions in Part 3 and Part 4 of the physician assessment, the candidacy for systemic therapy is determined.

If the physician has checked at least one of the shaded boxes in Part 3 and Part 4, then the patient is a candidate for systemic therapy.

BACKGROUND ON THE PQOL-12 QUESTIONNAIRE

The PQOL-12 is a valid and reliable subset of the original PQOL, a 41-item, self-administered, disease-specific questionnaire initially developed in 1991 by John Koo [3–5]. The questionnaire items were generated through focus groups in which patients discussed their experiences with psoriasis. A nationwide, population-based, demographically balanced sample of 50,000 households was then used to identify 599 psoriasis patients in the United States for item testing. The 41-item PQOL was qualitatively divided into two domains: psychosocial and physical. The psychosocial domain consisted of 22 items requiring patients to characterize the impact of psoriasis on their interactions with friends and family and on their feelings and self-perception. The physical domain consisted of 19 items requesting that patients rate the impact of their psoriasis symptoms on their daily activities. PQOL items were rated on an 11-point Likert-type scale where 0 = "not at all," 5 = "somewhat," and 10 = "very much."

APPLICATION OF THE ORIGINAL PQOL QUESTIONNAIRE

The 41-item PQOL was used in a clinical study of 71 patients with stable plaque psoriasis on up to 20% of their total BSA, and plaque elevation of at least moderate severity [6]. Psychometric analysis of the 41-item PQOL showed satisfactory reliability, validity, and responsiveness to change [3]. Items within each domain had approximately equal variances and contributed equally to the total score; they were, therefore, summed without weighting. The 41-item PQOL was scored by computing the mean score for each domain, on a 0–10 scale.

DEVELOPMENT OF THE PQOL-12 QUESTIONNAIRE

The 41-item PQOL was too lengthy for frequent use in clinical practice, and the assumption of two domains (psychosocial and physical) was not entirely appropriate because analyses following its development had shown overlap among these domains. A shorter instrument measuring unique constructs was needed for clinicians and researchers who were interested in assessing psoriasis-specific health-related quality of life (HRQOL) in clinical research or daily practice. Factor analysis techniques were used to refine the 41-item PQOL. The resulting questionnaire (PQOL-12) consisted of 12 items measured on one domain. Psychometric properties of the PQOL-12 were assessed using data from a multicentered office-based study (Study 1) and a randomized clinical trial (Study 2).

STUDY 1: MULTICENTERED OFFICE-BASED STUDY

Item Reduction

The PQOL was refined and reduced to a 12-item instrument using data from an office-based study of 483 patients stratified by physician-rated psoriasis severity at three U.S. psoriasis centers from October 2001 to May 2002 [7,8]. Severity was assessed by the investigator at the time of enrollment and included a psoriasis area and severity index (PASI) evaluation. Physicians completed several different symptom severity assessment questionnaires: global assessment of severity ranging from mild, moderate, and severe based on the BSA affected; PASI; overall lesional assessment (OLA); and severity of symptoms experienced by patients. In addition, each patient was asked to complete a demographic questionnaire: the PQOL, the dermatology life quality index (DLQI), and a disease severity assessment. Patient-rated severity was defined as mild, moderate, or severe with the question "How would you rate the overall severity of your psoriasis, during the past month?"

For this study, one compound question from the 41-item PQOL (i.e., item #22: How much does your psoriasis interfere with making social contacts and relationships?) in the psychosocial domain was divided into two questions, creating a 42-item instrument. A combination of qualitative review and factor analysis was used to refine the questionnaire. Observations were randomly assigned to an exploratory or confirmatory dataset. The exploratory dataset (n = 301) was used to reduce and refine the existing PQOL instrument, and the confirmatory dataset (n = 182) was used to test the reliability of the findings from the exploratory analysis. Each PQOL item was evaluated for missing values, mean scores, floor/ceiling effects, reading level, translatability, and applicability to all patients. Qualitative criteria were applied by assessing items for redundancy, wording, and meaning/conceptual characteristics. Factor analysis was used to assess the factor structure and item loadings on factors. An item-retention grid consisting of all analytical parameters was created to evaluate all item parameter estimates simultaneously and to facilitate the item-reduction decision process. Once reduced, all analyses performed on the exploratory dataset (i.e., descriptive and factor analysis) were repeated on the revised questionnaire (i.e., PQOL-12) using the confirmatory dataset. The confirmatory analyses yielded results consistent with the exploratory analyses.

Validity and Reliability

Following the confirmatory analysis, the psychometric properties of the PQOL-12 were assessed using Multitrait Analysis Program-Revised for Windows® PC-SAS®–based software 7 [9] and the pooled dataset (n = 482). The PQOL-12 demonstrated desirable psychometric properties. Ninety-nine percent of respondents completed the survey providing evidence of appropriate item responses of the PQOL-12. The PQOL-12 also exhibited support for the assumptions of summated scales. The PQOL-12 items had approximately equal variances (so they could be summed) and contributed equally to total score (i.e., no weighting needed). All items demonstrated desirable item internal consistency by exceeding the criteria of 0.40 correlation with the total score. The instrument therefore demonstrated good potential for responsiveness. Cronbach's-α was 0.95 and the mean inter-item correlation was 0.62, providing evidence of reliability (Tables 2.1 and 2.2). Although the questionnaire could have been reduced even further, some questions that have been deemed important in clinical practice were retained. Investigation of construct validity indicated that the mean PQOL-12 score was moderately correlated with clinical measures and highly correlated with patient-rated psoriasis severity ($r = 0.61$) and with the DLQI ($r = 0.78$) (Table 2.3).

Individual item correlations with overall patient-rated severity ranged from 0.40 ("How helpless do you feel with regard to your psoriasis?") to 0.61 (physical irritation). There were low-to-moderate correlations with physician-rated severity. A probable explanation for the more

TABLE 2.1 Item Descriptive Statistics for the PQOL-12 from an Office-Based Study (Study 1) and the Clinical Trial at Baseline (Study 2)

	Study 1 (*n* = 482)			**Study 2 (*n* = 71)**		
Item	**Mean**	**SD**	**Range**	**Mean**	**SD**	**Range**
Over the past month ...						
How self-conscious do you feel with regard to your psoriasis?	6.10	3.28	0–10	6.56	2.71	0–10
How helpless do you feel with regard to your psoriasis?	5.60	3.39	0–10	6.51	2.97	0–10
How embarrassed do you feel with regard to your psoriasis?	5.76	3.45	0–10	6.42	3.03	0–10
How angry or frustrated do you feel with regard to your psoriasis?	5.93	3.48	0–10	5.99	2.91	0–10
To what extent does your psoriasis make your appearance unsightly?	5.09	3.25	0–10	5.31	2.71	0–10
How disfiguring is your psoriasis?	4.24	3.25	0–10	4.21	2.95	0–10
How much does your psoriasis impact your overall emotional well-being?	4.39	3.29	0–10	4.07	3.11	0–10
Overall, to what extent does your psoriasis interfere with your capacity to enjoy life?	4.11	3.39	0–10	3.63	3.21	0–9
During the past month, how much have each of the following been affected by your psoriasis?						
Itching?	5.32	3.41	0–10	6.58	2.76	0–10
Physical irritation?	4.98	3.40	0–10	5.77	3.07	0–10
Physical pain or soreness?	3.84	3.40	0–10	4.23	3.40	0–10
Choice of clothing to conceal psoriasis?	5.04	3.84	0–10	6.15	3.48	0–10
Mean PQOL-12 Score	5.03	2.76	0–10	5.45	2.13	0.58–9.42

Note: PQOL-12, 12-item psoriasis quality-of-life questionnaire; SD, standard deviation.

TABLE 2.2 Summary of the Psychometric Properties of the 12-Item PQOL in Two Studies

Property	Description/Rationale (Criterion)	Study 1 ($n = 483$)	Study 2 ($n = 71$)
Reliability			
Internal item consistency	Extent to which each item correlates with the total score (≤0.40; ≥0.30 if domain contains many items)	Correlations ranged from 0.70–0.83	Correlations ranged from 0.42–0.78
Internal item consistency reliability	Homogeneity of a domain and extent to which domain is free of random error (Cronbach's $\alpha = 0.70–0.95$)	Cronbach's $\alpha = 0.95$	Cronbach's $\alpha = 0.91$
Validity			
Item means and variances	Interchangeability of items within each domain (similar means variances, so scores can be summed without adjustment)	Means of the items were 3.84–6.10 (SD, 3.25–3.84)	Means of the items were 3.63–6.58 (SD, 2.71–3.48)
Construct validity	Relationship of item to domain, assessed by item/domain correlations corrected for overlap (similar, moderate item/domain correlations. Items should contribute equally to domain score so that item weighting is unnecessary)	Correlation of items with total score ranged from 0.70–0.83	Correlation of items with total score ranged from 0.42–0.78
External validity	Relationship of items to external, often clinical, endpoints (at least moderate Spearman correlations)	PQOL-12 score at baseline correlated significantly ($p < 0.05$) with physician-rated severity (0.38), patient-rated severity (0.61), overall lesional assessment (0.38), BSA (0.33), PASI (0.36), and the DLQI (0.78)	PQOL-12 score at baseline correlated significantly ($p < 0.05$) with overall discomfort (0.49), percent BSA affected (0.42), pruritus (0.41), and overall disease severity (0.34); PQOL-12 was not significantly correlated with physician assessment of plaque elevation, scaling, or erythema

Responsiveness			
Distribution of responses	Item acceptability and comprehension of meaning by respondents (responses should span the majority of the scale)	Mean PQOL-12 total score = 5.03, SD = 2.76, range = 0–10	Mean PQOL-12 total score = 5.45, SD = 2.13, range = 0.58–9.42
Lack of floor or ceiling effects	Position of initial score (initial scores should not be too close to the minimum or maximum values; scales should have sufficient range on either side of the initial score to show improvement or deterioration)	No significant floor (1.5%) or ceiling (1.0%) effects	No significant floor (0.0%) or ceiling (0.0%) effects
Responsive to disease severity	Scores should vary systematically across disease severity categories so that milder severity is associated with lower scores than more severe disease	For physician ratings of severity, mean PQOL-12 scores were 3.9 for mild, 5.0 for moderate, and 6.4 for severe disease; pairwise comparisons of PQOL-12 means by physician-rated severity groups were significantly different (p 0.0002)	For physician ratings of severity, there was 1 to 1.5 point difference in scores between mild and severe ($p = 0.009$), mild and moderate, ($p = 0.08$) moderate and severe disease ($p = 0.08$) categories at baseline
		For patient-rated severity, mean PQOL-12 scores were 3.2 for mild, 5.2 for moderate, and 7.6 for severe disease; pairwise comparisons were statistically significant ($p < 0.0001$)	For patient-rated severity, there was 1 to 3 point difference in mean PQOL-12 scores between mild and moderate ($p = 0.003$), mild and severe ($p = 0.001$) and moderate and severe ($p = 0.03$) at baseline
Responsive to treatment	Scores change due to treatment-related improvement	Not assessed	Within group change from baseline scores was significantly different with treatment ($p < 0.001$)

(Continued)

TABLE 2.2 (*Continued*) Summary of the Psychometric Properties of the 12-Item PQOL in Two Studies

Property	Description/Rationale (Criterion)	Study 1 (n = 483)	Study 2 (n = 71)
Minimally important difference			
Difference in scores between improvers vs. those who did not change on measures of severity	The MID defined as the difference in mean change from baseline PQOL-12 score for patients who improved by at least one point on the patient- or physician-rated severity scale vs. the mean change from baseline for those who showed no change	Not assessed	Difference for improvers vs. those who showed no change was 1.24 ($p < 0.05$) on the patient-rated severity scale and 0.39 ($p = 0.45$) on the physician-rated severity scale
Difference in scores between improvers vs. those who did not change on global evaluation of response to treatment	The MID defined as the difference in mean change from baseline PQOL-12 score for patients who showed at least moderate response to treatment vs. the mean change from baseline for those who showed only slight response (some improvement—about 25%; however, significant evidence of study condition remains) or no response to treatment (study condition has not changed)	Not assessed	Difference for those who showed moderate improvement vs. those who showed no change or only slight improvement on the physicians' assessment of the global response to treatment was 1.14 ($p = 0.18$)

Note: PQOL-12, 12-item psoriasis quality-of-life questionnaire; BSA, body surface area; MID, minimally important difference; SD, standard deviation; SE, standard error; DLQI, dermatology life quality index; PASI, psoriasis area and severity index.

TABLE 2.3 Correlations[a] between Final PQOL-12 and Clinical or Other Patient-Reported Measures (Study 1)

Question	Physician (*n* = 474)	Patient (*n* = 481)	OLA (*n* = 480)	BSA (*n* = 481)	PASI (*n* = 482)	DLQI (*n* = 482)
In the past four weeks ...						
How self-conscious do you feel with regard to your psoriasis?	0.26	0.48	0.25	0.20	0.22	0.64
How helpless do you feel with regard to your psoriasis?	0.20	0.40	0.26	0.20	0.22	0.50
How embarrassed do you feel with regard to your psoriasis?	0.23	0.44	0.23	0.20	0.22	0.64
How angry or frustrated do you feel with regard to your psoriasis?	0.25	0.46	0.29	0.21	0.24	0.58
To what extent does your psoriasis make your appearance unsightly?	0.35	0.51	0.28	0.30	0.30	0.66
How disfiguring is your psoriasis?	0.41	0.54	0.36	0.38	0.40	0.66
How much does your psoriasis impact your overall emotional well-being?	0.26	0.44	0.23	0.26	0.26	0.64
Overall, to what extent does your psoriasis interfere with your capacity to enjoy life?	0.27	0.42	0.25	0.25	0.26	0.69
During the past four weeks, how much have each of the following been affected by your psoriasis?						
Itching?	0.35	0.58	0.41	0.32	0.36	0.62
Physical irritation?	0.40	0.61	0.44	0.34	0.38	0.65
Physical pain or soreness?	0.33	0.57	0.40	0.31	0.36	0.66
Choice of clothing to conceal psoriasis?	0.37	0.49	0.33	0.29	0.32	0.68
Mean PQOL-12 score	0.38	0.61	0.38	0.33	0.36	0.78

Note: PQOL-12, 12-item psoriasis quality-of-life questionnaire; BSA, body surface area; DLQI, dermatology life quality index; OLA, overall lesional assessment; RS, rated severity; PASI, psoriasis area and severity index.

[a] Spearman correlations for ordinal measurement scales (physician- and patient-rated severity) and Pearson correlations for interval measurement scales (OLA, BSA, PASI, DLQI).

TABLE 2.4 Mean PQOL-12 Scores at Baseline and End-of-Treatment, by Physician- and Patient-Rated Severity

		Office-Based Study (Study 1)		Clinical Trial (Study 2)			
				Baseline		End of Treatment	
Rater	**Severity**	***n***	**Mean (SD)**	***n***	**Mean (SD)**	***n***	**Mean (SD)**
Physician	Cleared	0	NA	0	0 (0)	8	3.35 (1.92)
	Mild	168	3.9 (2.6)	7	3.90 (2.19)	38	3.13 (2.21)
	Moderate	151	5.0 (2.8)	47	5.36 (1.89)	24	4.89 (2.72)
	Severe	155	6.4 (2.3)	17	6.36 (2.41)	1	8.00 (NA)
Patient	Cleared	0	NA	0	0 (0)	1	2.25 (NA)
	Mild	185	3.2 (2.3)	17	3.59 (1.42)	26	2.38 (1.42)
	Moderate	178	5.2 (2.3)	35	5.64 (1.99)	15	4.74 (2.26)
	Severe	118	7.6 (1.8)	18	6.80 (1.81)	5	6.18 (2.35)

Note: Total $n < 483$ (office-based study) or < 71 (clinical trial) due to missing physician- or patient-rated severity data.

modest correlations with physician-rated severity was that physicians based their severity assessment on BSA using an ordinal scale (mild <5%, moderate 5%–10%, and severe >10%) and lesion morphology that focused strictly on physical characteristics of the patient's condition. The correlations between individual PQOL-12 items and the DLQI items ranged from 0.50 to 0.69. The total PQOL-12 score was moderately correlated with OLA (0.38), BSA (0.33), and the PASI (0.36), providing evidence of convergent instrument and construct validity.

Mean PQOL-12 scores were calculated for each disease severity level by patients and physicians (Table 2.4). All pairwise comparisons of PQOL-12 means for physician and patient ratings of severity in the office-based study were statistically significant ($p < 0.001$), providing evidence of discriminant validity.

Responsiveness

The potential for responsiveness was assessed in this office-based cross-sectional study (Study 1) using the PQOL-12. The mean score for the PQOL-12 was 5.03 (SD = 2.76). Only 1.5% of the responses were at the floor and 1% of responses were at the ceiling, indicating that the scale has the capability to assess both extremes and that the instrument would be capable of detecting changes during a clinical trial. Responsiveness was further assessed with the following clinical trial data (Study 2).

STUDY 2: USING DATA FROM THE RANDOMIZED CLINICAL TRIAL

In Study 2, data from the clinical trial on the 41-item PQOL was used to evaluate psychometric properties of the PQOL-12. Disease severity was measured from physician and patient perspectives. Physicians were asked to evaluate overall patient discomfort; overall disease severity, defined as mild, moderate, or severe; percentage of BSA involvement; signs and symptoms of disease (e.g., pruritus); and overall response to treatment. Patients were asked to complete the 41-item PQOL and an overall evaluation of their disease severity. Patient severity was defined as cleared, mild (trace, mild), moderate (moderate), or severe (severe, very severe) with the question "How would you rate the overall severity of your psoriasis at this time?"

The 12 items of the PQOL were used to retrospectively assess validity, reliability, responsiveness, and the minimally important difference (MID) [10] (i.e., a change in the PQOL-12 questionnaire that would indicate the need for a change in therapy). The PQOL-12 demonstrated validity and reliability. Item-to-total correlations were moderate to high, and Cronbach's-α was 0.91. Correlations of the total PQOL-12 score and the individual PQOL-12 items with the clinical measures were moderate for all measures (Table 2.5). The PQOL-12 also discriminated among physician- and patient-rated severity at baseline and at end of treatment (Table 2.4).

Responsiveness

In Study 2 (using the clinical trial data retrospectively), the responsiveness assessment included examination of floor and ceiling effects, differences in severity levels, and treatment effects. There were no floor or ceiling effects observed for the PQOL-12, indicating that it has

TABLE 2.5 Spearman Correlations between PQOL-12 Items and Clinical Measures (Study 2)

Question	Disease Discomfort	Disease Severity	Percentage BSA	Pruritus
In the past four weeks ...				
How self-conscious do you feel with regard to your psoriasis?	0.34[a]	0.29[a]	0.43[a]	0.30[a]
How helpless do you feel with regard to your psoriasis?	0.32[a]	0.14	0.25[a]	0.25[a]
How embarrassed do you feel with regard to your psoriasis?	0.35[a]	0.13	0.30[a]	0.25[a]
How angry or frustrated do you feel with regard to your psoriasis?	0.44[a]	0.19	0.28[a]	0.28[a]
To what extent does your psoriasis make your appearance unsightly?	0.37[a]	0.36[a]	0.36[a]	0.22
How disfiguring is your psoriasis?	0.31[a]	0.34[a]	0.59[a]	0.18
How much does your psoriasis impact your overall emotional well-being	0.50[a]	0.32[a]	0.29[a]	0.22
Overall, to what extent does your psoriasis interfere with your capacity to enjoy life?	0.31[a]	0.23	0.28[a]	0.04
During the past four weeks, how much have each of the following been affected by your psoriasis?				
Itching?	0.38[a]	0.22	0.16	0.67[a]
Physical irritation?	0.36[a]	0.31[a]	0.25[a]	0.60[a]
Physical pain or soreness?	0.31[a]	0.28[a]	0.17	0.33[a]
Choice of clothing to conceal psoriasis?	0.22	0.15	0.35[a]	0.22
Mean PQOL-12 score	0.49[a]	0.34[a]	0.42[a]	0.41[a]

Note: PQOL-12, 12-item psoriasis quality-of-life questionnaire; BSA, body surface area.
[a] Significant at the ex = 0.05 level.

the capability to detect improvement and decline in this patient population. Mean PQOL-12 scores were calculated for each disease severity level by patients and physicians. At the baseline and at the end of treatment, differences between severity levels were generally one or two points for physician and patient ratings (Table 2.4).

MINIMALLY IMPORTANT DIFFERENCE

The MID was assessed using an anchor-based approach. The MID is the smallest (or minimal) change in an HRQOL measure that is considered meaningful (or important) by either a clinician or a patient [8]. A technique adapted from Juniper et al. was used to calculate the MID using data from Study 2 [8]. Three anchors or measures of improvement were investigated including patient-rated disease severity, physician-rated disease severity, and physician-evaluated global response to treatment. A difference of 1.24 points was observed between those who improved and those who reported no change in the patient-rated severity. The difference in the means of these two groups was statistically significant, indicating an important and statistically significant difference between these two groups. Difference between those who improved and those who did not experience a change was calculated as 1.14 using the physician rating of global response to treatment, although the means were not statistically significant between these two groups. In contrast, differences between physician ratings of severity were smaller (0.39) and the means of improvers and patients who did not experience change were not statistically significant. This finding suggests that a 0.4-point change may be sufficient to distinguish these groups on this measure. In summary, these results suggest that the MID for PQOL-12 score is about 1 point, although it may be as low as 0.4 points.

TEST–RETEST RELIABILITY OF THE PQOL-12 QUESTIONNAIRE

Although the earlier study designs precluded assessment of the test–retest reliability of PQOL-12, preliminary analyses from subsequent research indicate that the test–retest correlation of PQOL-12 exceeds 0.80 when conducted over a period of 2–30 days.

CALCULATING THE PQOL-12 QUESTIONNAIRE SCORE WITHIN THE KMPI

To be consistent with the desire for the KMPI to be a simple and easily used tool within clinical practice, the calculation of the PQOL-12 score for use within the KMPI differs from how the PQOL-12 score is reported earlier. Whereas the PQOL-12 score alone ranges from 0 (best) to 10 (worst) and is calculated by taking the mean of the item scores, the scoring for the PQOL-12 within the KMPI does not involve calculating mean item score but rather uses a simple sum of the item scores for a score that ranges from 0 (best) to 120 (worst).

Because the burden of psoriasis on a patient's health-related and psoriasis-specific quality of life is determined by a range of variables unique to each patient's disease symptoms and life circumstances, a comprehensive and practical approach was employed to determine a PQOL-12 score criterion for use within Part 3 of the KMPI. Qualitative review of the data from Study 1 and Study 2 along with quantitative analyses (i.e., exploratory cluster analysis) was conducted to identify if there was a natural "cut-point" between patients with mild and moderate psoriasis that was relatively stable over the various patient- and physician-rated severity measures. In addition, we sought to balance this with a cutoff point where a therapeutic intervention might be expected to have an impact on psoriasis-specific quality of life—while also accounting for the minimum important difference on the PQOL-12, which is approximately one to two points. Analysis results indicated that such a cutoff point might be as low as a score of 25 using the scoring method for the PQOL-12 within the KMPI; however, clinical opinion suggested the use of a more conservative 50 points for the final instrument. Further research is needed to better understand the minimum point where treatment might positively impact psoriasis patients based on their PQOL-12 score.

DISCUSSION OF KMPI

The KMPI provides a quick and easy way to identify and document patients with psoriasis who require systemic therapy.

The KMPI is short enough to be completed during a routine visit to a dermatologist. It takes approximately five minutes for the patient to complete the front page of the instrument while waiting in the reception area or in the examination room prior to being seen by the physician. Similarly, the physician assessment takes approximately five to seven minutes to complete, and the resulting instrument can become part of the patient's medical record for reference at subsequent patient visits.

The KMPI is unique in providing a complete evaluation of the patient's disease status—incorporating assessments of psoriasis-specific quality of life with a validated questionnaire (PQOL-12), psoriasis severity, and psoriatic joint disease.

The KMPI alerts the physician and patient of the need to assess health-related quality of life and joint-related symptoms in the clinical evaluation of psoriasis and determines the suitability (or not) for systemic therapy in individual patients.

The KMPI has the potential to improve physician–patient communication by involving the patient in characterizing their disease and its impact on their lives.

MONITORING PSORIASIS SEVERITY

The KMPI is typically used at the initial visit and when needed for insurance purposes. Yet at each office visit, the severity of the patient's psoriasis is assessed. For the most part, physicians use a gestalt method for evaluating psoriasis severity in clinical practice. Most practitioners have their own thresholds for labeling their patients' psoriasis as mild, moderate, or severe. In addition, practitioners may remember patients from visit to visit, and thus be able to determine if the patient is improving. Also, patients or their family members may be asked if the patient is doing better. In addition, a more static approach involves looking at the patient and determining what type of therapy is to be prescribed at the current visit based on physician and patient assessment of severity, along with patient and physician preferences for various treatments.

There is no widely accepted tool for assessing psoriasis severity in clinical practice. The PASI is a term recognized by most practitioners because many psoriasis therapies have received FDA approval based on clinical trials that demonstrated that the therapy causes an improvement in the PASI. However, most practitioners have never performed a PASI score on their patients. Indeed, it is a time-consuming method and subject to significant variability, particularly if the physician has limited experience with its use.

Naldi et al. [11] reviewed clinical trials for the treatment of psoriasis from 1997 to 2000 and determined that more than 40 different methods of determining severity were used in the 171 randomized clinical trials. Thus, there has been little consensus on what system to use. The PASI, which was first published in 1978 as part of a clinical trial [12], became a frequently used method. Surprisingly, it was not until 2004 that the PASI was validated for the first time [13]. Even though there were little data on the reproducibility of the PASI, it did form the basis of the approval of many therapies, particularly the biologics. More recently, however, the FDA has discarded the PASI for determining the effectiveness of therapies for which approval is sought. Instead, various forms of a physician's global assessment have been used.

The physician's global assessment, sometimes called investigator's global assessment (IGA) or psoriasis global assessment (PGA), is a nonstandard approach to assessing psoriasis using various terminologies; one example is shown in Table 2.6 [13]. Attempts have been made to standardize the PGA, which has led to the development of the Lattice System–Physician's Global Assessment (LS-PGA, www.ls-pga.com) and the Copenhagen Psoriasis Severity Index (CoPSI) [13,14]. Standardizing the PGA is desirable to reduce the gestalt elements involved in the PGA and to yield more consistency among investigators; these measures have proved successful in validation trials [13–15]. Whether a standardized approach or less reproducible approaches such as the original PGA will supplant the "gestalt" method in the practitioner's office will depend on the ease of use and the value to the patient and physician of a more careful assessment of psoriasis severity.

Naturally, the patient's opinion is important. Some measures of severity have focused on the patient's self-evaluation [16] or on a combination of typical physicians' evaluations with elements of the patient's quality-of-life measures [17]. In recent years, quality-of-life evaluations have become of greater interest in evaluating psoriasis patients. There are a number of measures of quality of life; one of the most frequently used is the DLQI [18]. There are also measures of the disability caused by psoriasis such as the psoriasis disability index (PDI) [18]. A simple way to track activity of psoriatic arthritis is to ask patients how many minutes of morning stiffness they have.

TABLE 2.6 A Physician's Global Assessment

Severe	Very marked plaque elevation, scaling, and/or erythema
Moderate to severe	Marked plaque elevation, scaling, and/or erythema
Moderate	Moderate plaque elevation, scaling, and/or erythema
Mild to moderate	Intermediate between moderate and mild
Mild	Slight scaling plaque elevation, scaling, and/or erythema
Almost clear	Intermediate between mild and clear
Clear	No signs of psoriasis (postinflammatory hyperpigmentation may be present)

Although some of the instruments that measure quality of life are rather short (e.g., the DLQI has only 10 questions), the use of these questionnaires is uncommon in clinical practice; asking patients in what way psoriasis is affecting their daily life may be valuable. Useful information may be obtained by simply asking the patient to indicate whether the psoriasis affects any element of their work or personal life and to what degree (e.g., rarely, sometimes, or daily). Just broaching the subject of psoriasis and its impact on quality of life is important to patients.

CONCLUSION

The KMPI is a practical assessment tool that dermatologists can quickly and easily use in their daily practice to help guide them in identifying patients with psoriasis who may be candidates for systemic therapy, as well as to justify these decisions to third-party payers.

REFERENCES

1. Krueger G, Koo J, Lebwohl M, et al. The impact of psoriasis on quality of life: Results of a 1998 National Psoriasis Foundation patient-membership survey. *Arch Dermatol* 2001; 137: 280–284.
2. Krueger GG, Feldman SR, Camisa C, et al. Two considerations for patients with psoriasis and their clinicians: What defines mild, moderate, and severe psoriasis? What constitutes a clinically significant improvement when treating psoriasis? *J Am Acad Dermatol* 2000; 43: 281–285.
3. Koo J, Kozma CM, Reinke K. The development of a disease-specific questionnaire to assess the quality of life for psoriasis patients: An analysis of the reliability, validity, and responsiveness of the psoriasis quality of life questionnaire. *Dermatol Psychosom* 2002; 3: 171–179.
4. Feldman S, Koo J, Menter A, et al. Decision points for the initiation of systemic treatment for psoriasis. *J Am Acad Dermatol* 2005; 53: 101–107.
5. Koo J. Population-based epidemiologic study of psoriasis with emphasis on quality of life assessment. *Dermatol Clin* 1996; 14: 485–496.
6. Koo JY, Martin D. Investigator-masked comparison of tazarotene gel q.d. plus mometasone furoate cream q.d.vs. mometasone furoate cream b.i.d. in the treatment of plaque psoriasis. *Int J Dermatol* 2001; 40: 210–212.
7. Koo J, Menter A, Lebwohl M, et al. The relationship between quality of life and disease severity: Results from a large cohort of mild, moderate, and severe psoriasis patients [abstr]. *Br J Dermatol* 2002; 147: 1078.
8. Koo J, Kozma CM, Menter A, et al. Development of a disease-specific quality of life questionnaire: The 12-item psoriasis quality of life questionnaire (PQOL-12). *61st Annual Meeting of the American Academy of Dermatology*, 2003.
9. Ware JE, Jr, Harris WJ, Gandek B, et al. *MAP-R for Windows: Multitrait/Multi-item Analysis Program—Revised User's Guide*. Boston, MA: Health Assessment Laboratory; 1997.
10. Juniper EF, Guyatt GH, Willan A, et al. Determining a minimal important change in a disease-specific quality of life questionnaire. *J Clin Epidemiol* 1994; 47: 81–87.
11. Naldi L, Svensson A, Diepgen T, et al. Randomized clinical trials for psoriasis 1977–2000: The EDEN survey. *J Invest Dermatol* 2003; 120: 738–741.
12. Fredriksson T, Pettersson U. Severe psoriasis—oral therapy with a new retinoid. *Dermatologica* 1978; 157: 238–244.
13. Langley RG, Ellis CN. Evaluating psoriasis with Psoriasis Area and Severity Index, Psoriasis Global Assessment, and Lattice System Physician's Global Assessment. *J Am Acad Dermatol* 2004; 51: 563–569.
14. Berth-Jones J, Thompson J, Papp K, et al. A study examining inter-rater and intrarater reliability of a novel instrument for assessment of psoriasis: The Copenhagen Psoriasis Severity Index. *Br J Dermatol* 2008; 159: 407–412.
15. Berth-Jones J, Grotzinger K, Rainville C, et al. A study examining inter- and intrarater reliability of three scales for measuring severity of psoriasis: Psoriasis Area and Severity Index, Physician's Global Assessment and Lattice System Physician's Global Assessment. *Br J Dermatol* 2006; 155: 707–713.

16. Louden BA, Pearce DJ, Lang W, et al. A simplified area severity index (SPASI) for rating psoriasis severity in clinic patients. *Dermatol Online J* 2004; 10: 7.
17. Kirby B, Richards HL, Woo P, et al. Physical and psychologic measures are necessary to assess overall psoriasis severity. *J Am Acad Dermatol* 2001; 45: 72–76.
18. Finlay AY, Khan GK, Luscombe DK, Salek MS. Validation of Sickness Impact Profile and Psoriasis Disability Index in Psoriasis. *Br J Dermatol.* 1990 Dec; 123(6): 751–756.

Chapter 3

Topical Agents

Rosemary deShazo, Gerald G. Krueger, and Kristina Callis Duffin

INTRODUCTION

Topical therapies, particularly topical corticosteroids, are considered the most commonly prescribed agents for psoriasis in the United States and Europe [1,2]. Topical corticosteroids are fast-acting, highly effective, easy to administer, and relatively safe, making short-term use acceptable to patients and physicians. However, for patients with moderate to severe disease, topical agents may not be appropriate or acceptable. Application to a large body surface area is time-consuming and expensive, and puts the patient at increased risk for systemic adverse effects. Cutaneous side effects may be intolerable over a large area. Topical agents can be messy and may look or feel unacceptable to the patient. Using quality-of-life parameters, response to treatment has been used to define severity; by this definition, severe psoriasis does not have a satisfactory response to treatments that have minimal risks [3]. Thus, moderate to severe psoriasis may, by definition, be moderate to severe because it does not respond to topical agents.

Despite their limitations, topical therapies have an important role in the treatment of moderate to severe psoriasis. Select patients may be able to clear their psoriasis and sustain the response with the judicious use of topical agents. Occasionally, patients with moderate to severe psoriasis will be unable or unwilling to use systemic agents or phototherapy, even when such treatments may be more appropriate. Side effect profiles, laboratory monitoring, and costs related to systemic agents or phototherapy may be unacceptable to some patients. In these settings, the physician is obliged to develop the most appropriate and efficacious topical regimen (Table 3.1).

More realistically, as highlighted below in the following sections on combinations with systemic agents, the topical therapies in this population are best used as adjuvant therapies to systemic treatments or phototherapy. Although biologic therapies are considered highly efficacious, complete clearance is frequently not achieved. A recent cross-sectional comparative effectiveness study of patients with moderate to severe psoriasis revealed that far fewer patients reach "clear/almost clear" in a real-world setting compared to phase III studies of biologics; furthermore, 60% of these patients reported concomitant use of topical agents [4].

The goal of this chapter is to provide a concise overview of topical agents that are used to treat psoriasis, with special emphasis on how they can be used safely and effectively for patients with moderate to severe disease. The information is designed to assist in

TABLE 3.1 Indications for Use of Topical Therapies in Moderate to Severe Psoriasis

Initial treatment after determining severity, patient's desires (comfort only to complete clearing), ability and willingness to apply medication, and prior response to topical therapies
Maintenance therapy after clearance with topical and/or systemic agents
Combination therapy with oral agents or phototherapy for augmentation of effect, dose-sparing, or treatment of recalcitrant areas
Palliative therapy (i.e., patient comfort while awaiting onset of systemic therapy)
Initial, maintenance, or palliative therapy in patients unable or unwilling to use systemic agents

answering the following questions that arise when topicals are used to treat moderate to severe psoriasis:

1. What are the most effective topical therapies for the treatment of psoriasis?
2. What adverse events are associated with topical treatments?
3. How can topical therapies be combined most safely and effectively?
4. Is there any advantage to combining topical therapy with systemic medications?

CORTICOSTEROIDS

Topical corticosteroids are the cornerstone of most topical psoriasis treatment regimens. Used as single agents, superpotent corticosteroids have the maximum potential to temporarily clear or nearly clear psoriatic plaques more effectively than other topical therapies. However, the potential for adverse effects limits the quantity, duration, and location of their use. This section will present strategies advocated to maximize efficacy and compliance while minimizing risks.

Pharmacology and Mechanism of Action

Corticosteroids act on psoriasis via anti-inflammatory, immunosuppressive, and antiproliferative properties. At the molecular level, corticosteroids act on gene transcription by forming complexes with receptors and by binding to DNA to modulate transcription. Corticosteroids exert their anti-inflammatory actions by inhibiting the movement and function of leukocytes, by reducing dermal edema, and by vascular permeability. T lymphocytes are particularly sensitive to the effects of corticosteroids. Corticosteroids cause reduced total circulating lymphocyte count and cytokine production. In the epidermis and dermis, corticosteroids inhibit the proliferation of keratinocytes and fibroblasts [5–8].

Topical corticosteroids are ranked in the Stoughton–Cornell classification, originally based on an assay of the corticosteroid's ability to cause vasoconstriction [9]. The efficacy of most topical corticosteroids is generally well correlated with the potency [10–12]. Potency of a corticosteroid is associated with its chemical modification, such as the presence of an acetate moiety, its vehicle formulation, the hydration status of the skin, and with occlusion. Penetration is also enhanced in certain sites of application such as the eyelids and face [13].

Efficacy

Corticosteroids as Monotherapy The efficacy of superpotent (class I) corticosteroid ointments in the treatment of plaque-type psoriasis is well established [14–17]. Katz et al. showed that clobetasol-17-propionate and betamethasone dipropionate produced clearance or marked improvement in 75% and 80% of patients, respectively, treated for three weeks [18]. In another study, the onset of the therapeutic effect of halobetasol propionate 0.05% occurred within five days of starting treatment and resulted in clearance or marked improvement in 88% of patients over a four-week period, compared to 64% of patients treated with betamethasone valerate [16]. The use of class II corticosteroids is less impressive: only 10% of patients achieve clearance with an average of 47% of patients achieving 75% improvement [16,19–21].

Newer formulations of corticosteroids have proven efficacious in treating psoriasis, perhaps mostly due to improved acceptance by patients and their resulting compliance. Ease of use contributed in part to the appeal of a product known as Skin Cap, a medicated spray containing zinc pyrithione ultimately found to contain clobetasol propionate, which was available in the United States without a prescription in the 1990s [22]. A small study of 20 patients who sampled corticosteroids in various vehicles also confirmed that patients preferred solutions and foams over gels, creams, and ointments [23]. The spreadability of foams and sprays also was shown to reduce the amount of time it takes to apply these medications [24]. A review of randomized controlled trials using clobetasol propionate in different vehicles for body and scalp psoriasis showed that there is no substantial evidence that ointment vehicles, though considered moisturizing, have better efficacy over non-moisturizing (e.g., foam or spray) vehicles [25]. For these reasons, the location of areas to be treated and patient preference should be strongly considered when determining a choice of agent.

Foam Three corticosteroids are available in the United States as a foam: clobetasol propionate (Olux® and Olux-E®), betamethasone valerate (Luxiq®), and desonide (Verdeso®). Olux and Luxiq both have a thermolabile formulation with ethanol, and cetyl and stearyl alcohol, which allows for rapid drying and no residue after application. Clobetasol foam resulted in clearance or near-clearance of scalp psoriasis in 74% of patients in one study [26] and has also been shown to be efficacious in the treatment of body plaques [27]. A study conducted by Bergstrom et al. showed that clobetasol foam was superior to clobetasol cream and was a solution for treatment of body and scalp plaques by the Psoriasis Area and Severity Index (PASI), quality of life measures, clearance of scalp lesions, and in time of application [24]. Although the foam vehicle is often not prescribed due to its cost, this study showed there were no significant differences in cost after controlling for body surface area. The Olux-E formulation, which primarily differs from Olux by the absence of ethanol and the addition of cyclomethicone and white petrolatum, also has efficacy in plaque psoriasis [28,29]. Betamethasone valerate foam was shown to clear or nearly clear scalp psoriasis in 72% of patients and was preferred by patients over the lotion vehicle [30]. In the United States, desonide foam is indicated for treatment of moderate to severe atopic dermatitis in adults and in children as young as three months of age [31]. It could be considered for off-label use in psoriasis (if a foam vehicle is preferred) when low potency corticosteroid is indicated.

Spray Clobetasol spray was developed to provide an easy-to-use formulation that allows treatment of large or difficult-to-reach areas [32]. In a randomized, double-blind trial of 120 patients with up to 20% body surface area, 82% were clear or almost clear after four weeks of twice-daily application [33]. In order to assess the effectiveness and safety of clobetasol spray in a more real-world setting, a study known as the Clobex® Spray Community-Based Research Assessment (COBRA) was conducted involving 455 community dermatologists and nearly 2500 subjects [34]; 1254 patients received clobetasol spray monotherapy twice daily, and 731 had the spray added to an existing therapeutic regimen twice daily. Data suggested that both regimens were effective and tolerable; the most common adverse events were the typical cutaneous effects seen with corticosteroids, including erythema, scaling, dryness, and stinging. There were no unexpected adverse events noted. Interestingly, the mean body surface area (BSA) of the participants was 11.1%, suggesting that add-on therapy with clobetasol spray is a reasonable option in patients with moderate to severe psoriasis.

Lotion Betamethasone dipropionate lotion and clobetasol lotion (Clobex) have been studied in patients with psoriasis. In one study, 192 patients were randomized using clobetasol lotion, vehicle placebo, or clobetasol cream. Efficacy of the lotion was comparable to the cream at four weeks and was associated with a lower remission rate at four weeks posttreatment [35]. Lotion formulations also have greater patient acceptability compared to thicker emollient preparations [36]. Betamethasone dipropionate lotion has also been compared to clobetasol scalp solution and in one study, it had comparable efficacy but more rapid improvement of induration and scaling [37].

Shampoo Shampoo has the advantage of being convenient, and because it provides only short-contact, there are possible safety advantages. Studies have been conducted using clobetasol shampoo (Clobex shampoo) for scalp psoriasis. After four weeks of daily use, 42.1% and 28.3% achieved a physician global assessment of clear or almost clear in studies A and B, respectively (prescribing information for Clobex shampoo) [38]. When a lower potency steroid is indicated, fluocinolone, available with the indication for seborrheic dermatitis, is available as Capex shampoo.

Tape Applied once daily, flurandrenolide tape (Cordran® tape) has been shown to produce >75% improvement in 64% of patients over four weeks and has been found to be superior to diflorasone diacetate ointment applied twice daily over four weeks [14]. This vehicle is particularly useful in the treatment of more lichenified plaques.

Solution Numerous corticosteroids are available as solutions. Solutions have the advantage of easy spreadability, particularly on the scalp or other hair-bearing surfaces. They are available as generic preparations, limiting the cost to the patient. Just as with some of the foam preparations, solutions often contain alcohol that can lead to stinging or burning. Clobetasol scalp solution has been widely used for scalp psoriasis. In one study, greater than 50% clearance was seen in 81% of patients compared to placebo, with 26% of patients achieving complete clearance [39].

Corticosteroids in Combination with Systemic Agents The efficacy of topical corticosteroids in combination with systemic agents is less well studied, but combined use occurs frequently in clinical practice [1]. As part of the Galderma-sponsored COBRA trial, subjects on existing topicals for at least one month and on existing systemic therapy for at least three months received the addition of clobetasol propionate 0.05% spray for a four-week period. At four weeks, 80% of subjects' target plaques were scored as clear, almost clear, or had improved from baseline severity by at least two points on a six-point scale. In the same time period, the investigators' global assessment of improvement showed 62% of subjects were clear or almost clear. Side effects were infrequent but included erythema, peeling/scaling, dryness, and stinging/burning and pruritus. Less than 1% of patients had telangiectasia, and 1.2% were reported to have the presence of skin atrophy [40]. Similarly, a COBRA substudy including 159 participants on existing biologic therapy added clobetasol propionate 0.05% spray for three months. After the treatment period, 81% of patients with moderate disease at baseline, 79.5% of those with severe disease, and 58.8% of those with very severe disease were clear or almost clear [41].

Studies have also been conducted to determine if addition of topical agents to specific biologics is effective and tolerable. The BELIEVE study, sponsored by Abbott (now Abbvie), compared treatment with adalimumab as monotherapy to daily treatment with adalimumab combined with topical calcipotriol/betamethasone ointment. This study showed that participants receiving the additional topical ointment achieved at least 75% improvement in the PASI score (PASI 75) more readily in four weeks than those receiving adalimumab alone. However, PASI 75 at 12 weeks was the same in both treatment groups [42]. Another study, which randomized patients to either etanercept or etanercept plus option to add clobetasol propionate 0.005% foam at weeks 11 to 12 and at weeks 23 to 24 after starting etanercept, demonstrated similar findings. At 12 weeks, the clobetasol foam plus etanercept group showed significantly better PASI 75, PASI 90, and static physician global assessment scores of clear/almost clear, but week 24 scores were not significantly different [43]. There were no unexpected adverse events related to the addition of topical corticosteroids in these studies. Results suggest that limited use of concomitant topical corticosteroids or of combination topical agents is likely safe and effective for patients who desire more rapid improvement during the initiation phase or for those who suffer from particularly stubborn remaining plaques. One caveat is that addition of topical corticosteroids at the same time as initiation of a system may confound the interpretation of response to a biologic. For corticosteroids in combination with phototherapy, refer to Chapter 11.

Cutaneous Side Effects

The adverse effects of topical corticosteroids are well known and limit the frequency and continuity of treatment (Table 3.2). Cutaneous adverse events are the most common and usually occur when corticosteroids are used with excessive frequency or duration or on steroid-sensitive sites such as the face or intertriginous areas. The same antiproliferative and antimitotic actions of topical corticosteroids that make them effective for psoriasis also contribute to their atrophogenic potential. Early signs of atrophy include visualization of the superficial vascular plexus [44]. With further atrophy of the epidermis and dermis, the skin becomes thin and fragile and is easily lacerated and bruised. Further loss of dermal elements

TABLE 3.2 Adverse Effects of Topical Corticosteroids

Cutaneous	Systemic
Irritation	HPA axis suppression
Burning	Cushing syndrome
Pruritus	Glaucoma
Atrophy of the skin	
Striae	
Telangiectasia	
Acneiform eruption	
Rosacea	
Perioral dermatitis	
Folliculitis	
Infection (bacterial, fungal)	
Contact dermatitis	
Hypopigmentation	
Purpura/ecchymoses	
Folliculitis	
Rebound of psoriasis	
Tachyphylaxis	

leads to vascular dilatation with telangiectasia formation and tearing of dermal connective tissue, causing irreversible, purplish striae. Acneiform eruptions may occur, particularly if high potency agents are used on the face. Irritation may occur as a result of epidermal atrophy or intolerance to components of the vehicle. Allergic contact dermatitis is rare but has been reported [45]. Rebound (the abrupt worsening of psoriasis or the development of pustular psoriasis after discontinuation of topical steroids) has been observed, particularly when agents are applied under occlusion [46–48].

Systemic Side Effects

Although this is rarely clinically evident, topical corticosteroids can cause the same systemic side effects as systemically administered steroids. Hypothalamic–pituitary–adrenal (HPA) axis suppression can be demonstrated on laboratory testing after only one to two weeks of using moderate-to-superpotent corticosteroids, but is rarely clinically significant [49]. Exacerbation of hyperglycemia, glucosuria, and hypertension may be seen. Iatrogenic Cushing syndrome [50] and osteonecrosis of the femoral head [51], both rare side effects of systemic corticosteroid use, have been reported from long-term topical steroid application. By virtue of their body surface involvement, patients with moderate to severe psoriasis require increased vigilance for systemic effects of corticosteroids.

GUIDELINES FOR USING TOPICAL CORTICOSTEROIDS IN PATIENTS WITH MODERATE TO SEVERE PSORIASIS

Although monotherapy with topical corticosteroids as a long-term strategy is not generally considered a viable option for most patients with extensive psoriasis, the rapid onset, efficacy, and safety of corticosteroid monotherapy support their short-term use in patients who may be flaring, who may be starting a new therapy, or who are wary of the potential side effects of systemic agents.

Select the Appropriate Strength for the Body Surface

Superpotent corticosteroids are often the most suitable choice for initial treatment of scalp and body surfaces excluding the face, axilla, groin, and genitals. Less than superpotent steroids are less likely to result in clearance but may be used if relief of symptoms is the treatment goal. For face and body folds, low-potency topical corticosteroids or other topical agents such as calcipotriene or immunomodulators should be chosen for routine use.

Select the Appropriate Vehicle for the Body Surface

Although superpotent corticosteroids in an ointment vehicle have been assumed to be the most efficacious agents for plaque psoriasis, more recent studies have shown that foams, sprays, and lotions are just as efficacious and are often preferred over ointments, creams, and solutions. For example, the spray vehicle is useful for more difficult-to-reach areas, such as on the back. Foams and solutions are more appropriate for the scalp, other hair-bearing areas, or when features of other vehicles such as greasiness or tackiness are bothersome to the patient.

Monitor Frequency and Duration

If used as a single agent, continuous twice-daily application of a superpotent corticosteroid should be limited to a two-week course, in accordance with Food and Drug Administration (FDA) approved package insert. How often these courses can be repeated safely and the length of the intervals between courses has never been clearly established. It is the authors' opinion that twice-daily application to nonintertriginous areas for two months will result in visible atrophy. When used once daily, onset of atrophy is delayed but does occur as early as two to three months. The scalp is more resistant to atrophy but it does occur; frequently, telangiectasia precedes atrophy. Application on one or two consecutive days out of each week, known as pulse therapy, provides adequate maintenance in some patients. However, maintenance therapy in combination with calcipotriene or tazarotene is more efficacious (see sections on these agents that follow).

Prescribe the Appropriate Quantity for the Frequency of Application and Treatment Area

It is very frustrating to the patient when the quantity of a medication prescribed is inadequate for an outlined course of therapy. In general, 1 g of a topical preparation will cover approximately 3% of the BSA. Conversely, limiting quantities and refills may facilitate frequent follow-up and close observation, providing the opportunity to assess adverse effects and to continually educate the patient.

Monitor for Lack of Response and Compliance

One of the most frustrating aspects of treating psoriasis with topical corticosteroids is that over time their effectiveness may wane. This is frequently attributed to the phenomenon of tachyphylaxis, defined as the diminished or lack of response to an agent after repeated

TABLE 3.3 Selection of Topical Corticosteroids

Area of Body	Strength	Examples of Compounds/Vehicles
Trunk and extremities	Class I	Clobetasol propionate ointment or cream 0.05%
		Halobetasol propionate ointment or cream 0.05%
		Betamethasone dipropionate ointment 0.05%
		Diflorasone diacetate ointment 0.05%
Scalp	Class I	Clobetasol propionate solution 0.05%
		Clobetasol propionate foam 0.05%
	Class IV	Betamethasone valerate foam or lotion 0.12%
Face, body folds, axilla, groin, genitals	Class V–VI	Hydrocortisone butyrate cream 0.1%
		Tridesilon cream 0.05%
Lichenified body plaques	Class I	Flurandrenolide tape

applications, which has been observed with corticosteroid application on normal skin [52,53]. However, in a study of 32 patients who applied betamethasone dipropionate twice daily for 12 weeks, tachyphylaxis was not observed [54]. The authors suggested that lack of therapeutic efficacy and poor compliance may be responsible for what is perceived as tachyphylaxis. Carefully reviewing the patient's actual application practice is therefore imperative when evaluating lack of response. If tachyphylaxis is suspected, a break from corticosteroids is warranted. The time needed to recover from what is termed the tachyphylactic state is unknown. Likewise, there is no information as to how likely it is to recur after a break, or if switching to a different steroid in the same class is of benefit (see Table 3.3).

Poor compliance is probably a much more common cause of lack of improvement than tachyphylaxis. Patients often do not comply with therapy for a number of social and medication-related reasons, including adverse effects, fear of adverse effects, frustration due to lack of efficacy, dislike of vehicle, dislike for applying the medication or the time it takes to apply, forgetting to apply or being too busy to apply the medication, being fed up with their disease, cost, and many others. Studies utilizing the medication event monitoring system (MEMS) cap, an electronic cap that records opening of the container, have shown that adherence to medication decreases from time of therapy initiation and increases near time of an appointment [55,56]. Compliance in clinical trials is directly associated with the frequency of visits, the use of reminders and diaries, and incentives such as payment while participating in a trial. Numerous techniques can be employed when trying to improve compliance, including early and frequent follow-up, patient education, keeping treatment regimens simple, selection of the appropriate vehicle, and selecting a therapy that is used daily rather than twice daily.

VITAMIN D ANALOGS

Topical Vitamin D analogs are an established therapy for psoriasis. The mechanism of action is not clear but is thought to be related to the hypoproliferative effect on keratinocytes [57,58]. The topical vitamin D analog class includes calcipotriene (calcipotriol), calcitriol, and tacalcitol. Calcipotriene (Dovonex®, Sorilux®), also known as calcipotriol (Daivonex® or Psorcutan®) outside the United States, is a vitamin D_3 analog that was developed after patients with psoriasis experienced improvement when treated with oral and topical calcitriol (1,25-dihydroxy vitamin D_3). It has been a widely prescribed therapy for psoriasis, in part attributable to its paucity of side effects, aesthetic acceptability, and therapeutic advantages over anthralin and tar. In the United States, calcipotriene is available as a 0.0025% and 0.005% cream, foam, and as a solution for scalp use. Topical calcitriol is available as a 3 mcg/g ointment (Vectical®) and as a gel intended for scalp use. It is considered equally effective as calcipotriene but has been shown to be less irritating in sensitive areas [59,60]. Tacalcitol is not yet available in the United States.

Pharmacology and Mechanism of Action

Calcipotriene is the structural analog of calcitriol (1,25-dihydroxy vitamin D_3). Calcitriol and calcipotriene exhibit similar keratinocyte receptor binding and affinity, but calcipotriene is 100 times less potent in its effects on calcium metabolism. Although its mechanism of action on psoriasis is not completely understood, the beneficial effects of calcipotriene on psoriasis are based on gene-regulatory events. Calcipotriene has been shown to promote terminal differentiation and inhibition of proliferation of keratinocytes [61]. The metabolite of vitamin D_3, 1,25 $(OH)_2$ D_3, may modulate the proliferation of T lymphocytes [62,63].

Calcipotriene is a relatively unstable molecule and is inactivated by an acid pH. It is therefore not compatible in combination with some therapies. It was found to be compatible with halobetasol propionate 0.05% ointment and cream, tazarotene gel, and Estargel *in vitro* [64,65]. Some degradation was found in combination with hydrocortisone-17-valerate 0.2% ointment and ammonium lactate 12% lotion. Mixing with salicylic acid 6% caused rapid degradation of calcipotriene.

Efficacy

Vitamin D Analog Monotherapy As a single agent, calcipotriene ointment is comparable to the efficacy of a class II corticosteroid ointment such as fluocinonide 0.05% [18,19,39–41,66–68]. Calcipotriene cream is less efficacious than ointment and is considered comparable in efficacy to betamethasone valerate and coal tar. Studies have suggested that the cream formulation is a more desirable vehicle for body lesions and that a twice daily regimen of calcipotriol cream in the morning and ointment in the evening is associated with improved compliance [69]. Monotherapy with calcipotriene foam has been shown to be efficacious for scalp psoriasis compared to vehicle foam, and it is the preferred vehicle for scalp or other hair-bearing areas [70]. It is the authors' opinion that topical calcipotriene, as a single agent administered twice daily, is not used by the great majority of patients for months on end. This is because the onset of action is slow and the cost benefit ratio perception by patients is poor. Most who use it successfully do so in combination with other agents as sequential therapy [71].

Vitamin D Analog—Corticosteroid Combination Preparations Numerous strategies have been employed to take advantage of the rapid onset and efficacy of potent topical corticosteroids and the safety of vitamin D analogs. Some dermatologists have advocated mixing or simultaneously applying calcipotriene and superpotent corticosteroids. However, formulations of these agents may not be compatible when applied together or mixed in this fashion [64]. The availability of a stable two-compound ointment has obviated the need for applying two separate agents. The two-compound ointment (in the United States, Taclonex®, and in Europe and Canada, Dovobet®) contains calcipotriene 0.005% (equivalent to calcipotriene 50μg/g) and betamethasone dipropionate 0.064% (equivalent to betamethasone 0.5 mg/g) [72] and is indicated for the treatment of psoriasis in adults for up to four weeks of continuous therapy. Taclonex® is also available as a gel for hair-bearing areas. Douglas et al. showed that the two-compound ointment used twice daily for four weeks was associated with a mean reduction of PASI from a baseline of 74.4%, which was significantly better than betamethasone dipropionate ointment twice daily (mean PASI reduction 61.3%) and calcipotriene ointment alone twice daily for four weeks (mean changes from baseline PASI of 55.3%). Papp et al. had similar results [73]. Studies of daily application of the two-compound ointment produced a mean PASI reduction of 69%–71% over four weeks [74,75] and a mean PASI reduction of 73.1% with daily use over eight weeks [76]. Once daily application has also been associated with greater compliance than twice daily application in two studies [77,78]. These studies suggest that the two-compound ointment, applied daily or b.i.d., has superior efficacy compared to betamethasone dipropionate or calcipotriene monotherapy. However, a head-to-head study of clobetasol propionate spray and once daily two-compound ointment revealed that 74% of clobetasol spray-treated patients obtained clear or almost clear, whereas only 47% of patients applying the two-compound ointment achieved clear/almost clear [79]. Although the two-compound ointment may not be as efficacious as b.i.d. superpotent clobetasol, once daily therapy for many patients may be a more desirable regimen.

Sequential Therapy with Calcipotriene Dermatologists have commonly used vitamin D analogs as part of a strategy known as sequential therapy, where the first or "clearing" phase of treatment involves using a superpotent topical corticosteroid once or twice daily for two weeks, followed by a second phase where topical corticosteroids and vitamin D analogs are applied in a pulse or weekend fashion [71,80]. A third or maintenance phase is then sometimes implemented using calcipotriene as monotherapy. A variety of sequential regimens have been shown to be efficacious. Lehwohl et al. showed that a two-week treatment of morning calcipotriene and evening halobetasol followed by a maintenance regimen of calcipotriene twice daily on weekdays with halobetasol twice daily on weekends provided a six-month remission in 76% of patients, compared to only 40% of patients who used weekend halobetasol and weekday vehicle [80]. Another regimen compared daily augmented betamethasone for four weeks to betamethasone applied daily on weeks 1 and 3, and calcipotriene applied twice daily on weeks 2 and 4. The alternating calcipotriene/betamethasone regimen resulted in clearance or marked improvement in 96% of patients, compared to 40% with the single-agent regimen [81]. One limitation to utilizing these regimens in the United States is that these studies were performed using calcipotriene ointment, which is no longer available. Although calcipotriene cream is available, it is associated with lower efficacy than the ointment; therefore, these studies may not be reproducible. An outline of various treatment regimens is provided in Table 3.4.

TABLE 3.4 Use of Calcipotriene in Moderate to Severe Psoriasis

Prescribe as part of a combination regimen with topical corticosteroids or tazarotene.
Limit application to 100 g/week (this will treat a body surface area of 15% twice daily).
Apply twice daily to body plaques.
Apply once or twice daily to face, axilla, groin, body folds, and genitals.
If facial irritation occurs, reduce frequency of application or discontinue use.
Instruct patient to wash hands after application to other areas to avoid inadvertent contact of medication with face.
Apply with petrolatum jelly to reduce irritation.
Discontinue treatment if lesional or perilesional irritation persists.

Combination with Systemic Agents

Addition of calcipotriene to some systemic agents has been shown in small clinical trials to provide increased efficacy with a lower dosage of the systemic agent. Adding calcipotriene to cyclosporine has been shown to be beneficial and dose sparing [82,83]. In the study by Grossman et al., calcipotriene applied concomitantly with low-dosage oral cyclosporine (2 mg/kg/day) resulted in >90% improvement in 50% of patients compared to 11.8% of patients treated with cyclosporine and vehicle. Calcipotriene and systemic retinoids can also be combined with the similar dose-sparing and efficacy benefits. In one study, the addition of calcipotriene to acitretin therapy resulted in clearance or marked improvement in 67% of patients compared to 41% of patients receiving acitretin and vehicle [84]. Methotrexate has also been studied with calcipotriol. In a study of 97 patients who were randomized to continue or discontinue methotrexate and add either calcipotriol or vehicle, the time to relapse was significantly increased in the calcipotriol group compared to the vehicle group (113 days vs. 35 days); overall, those treated with calcipotriol had lower methotrexate cumulative doses. As referenced here (in the corticosteroid section), topical calcipotriol/betamethasone was studied in combination with adalimumab and showed improved PASI 75% in the first four weeks of therapy [42]. To date, no safety concerns have been raised in studies of combination therapy with calcipotriene.

Combination with Phototherapy

Studies have been performed to evaluate the compatibility and the efficacy of combining calcipotriene with ultraviolet therapy. In order to test compatibility of this combination, Lebwohl et al applied calcipotreine ointment to an area of the skin before ultraviolet B (UVB), PUVA, ultraviolet A (UVA), or sham exposure. After phototherapy, the ointment was collected and a liquid chromatography assay was performed to determine if the phototherapy caused calcipotriene to degrade. This study showed that calcipotriene was unaffected by UVB, but PUVA and UVA caused reduction in the concentration of detectable calcipotriene, suggesting that UVA inactivates this compound. However, a more recent study of six patients who applied vitamin D analogs before or after PUVA or narrowband ultraviolet B (NBUVB) did not detect differences in efficacy [85].

Other studies have shown that adding vitamin D analogs to ultraviolet light has improved time to clearance and reduction of cumulative exposure. A study of 13 patients treated with calcipotriol or placebo twice daily and PUVA revealed that the calcipotriol-treated plaques cleared more rapidly and required a lower UVA dose than those treated with placebo ointment [86]. Topical calcipotriene has also been combined with UVB to improve efficacy and to reduce cumulative exposure. Although one study of 53 patients did not show increased efficacy when calcipotriene was applied twice daily in conjunction with narrowband UVB, a study of broadband UVB twice weekly with calcipotriene cream applied twice daily was shown to be equivalent in efficacy to UVB three times weekly with vehicle, significantly decreasing cumulative UVB exposure [87].

Cutaneous Side Effects

The most common cutaneous side effect associated with calcipotriene monotherapy is skin irritation. This usually presents as lesional or perilesional burning, stinging, erythema, or scaling. Facial irritation is common, either due to intentional application or transfer of the medication from the hands after application elsewhere. Reducing the frequency of application or diluting calcipotriene with petrolatum has been advocated to reduce irritation [88]. The irritative effects sometimes lessen with time.

Treatment with the two-compound ointment has also been well tolerated, with the most common reported events being erythema, burning, and pruritus [89] with generally fewer lesional or perilesional effects than with calcipotriene alone [73–76]. A 52-week study of continuous treatment with the two-compound ointment, used daily as needed, was actually associated with fewer adverse events compared to the four weeks of two-compound ointment therapy followed by calcipotriene monotherapy [89]. Local and systemic adverse events associated with the topical corticosteroid in the two-compound ointment were observed at low rates, the most common being atrophy and folliculitis [76]. Topical calcitriol, although equally effective, has been shown in a multicenter investigator blinded trial to be better tolerated than calcipotriol, particularly in sensitive areas [60].

Systemic Side Effects

Long-term studies of calcipotriene or calcipotriol have demonstrated few significant effects on calcium metabolism. Hypercalcemia has been reported in patients who have applied excessive quantities over large surface areas over a significant amount of time [90,91]. A review by Braun et al. of all reported cases in the literature found that in 90% of the cases, doses exceeded 100 g of calcipotriol/week [92]. Subjects with renal impairment have developed hypercalcemia when 170–180 g/week were applied. Although studies have suggested that minor alterations in calcium metabolism during calcipotriol treatment can be seen, including increased urinary calcium excretion, decreased serum parathyroid hormone levels, and dose-dependent increases in serum calcium and phosphate (within the normal range), it appears that patients with normal renal function who do not exceed recommended weekly doses of vitamin D analog are unlikely to develop hypercalcemia. Hypercalciuria, although clinically insignificant, has been observed in subjects applying 100 g/week for four weeks. No effect on bone metabolism was observed in a study of 34 patients who applied less than 100 g/week for three weeks [93]. Authors have advocated obtaining serum calcium levels at weekly intervals in the first three weeks of therapy in patients who approach the maximum weekly dosage or who have impaired renal function or calcium metabolism because hypercalcemia has been observed in patients as early as the fourth day of treatment [92]. In a study of 253 patients using topical calcitriol 3 mcg/g ointment, five patients had slight hypercalcemia [94].

TAZAROTENE (TAZORAC)

Tazarotene is a topical retinoid that was approved for use in the United States in 1997. It is available as a 0.1% and 0.05% gel and cream. Although this agent is approved in the United States as monotherapy, many patients experience significant local irritation that limits its use. Using it off-label in combination with topical corticosteroids increases efficacy and diminishes irritation, and it can be used as part of a long-term combination maintenance regimen. Tazarotene can also be added to UVB therapy for more rapid improvement, increased efficacy, and cumulative UV dosage reduction.

Pharmacology and Mechanism of Action

Tazarotene is a vitamin A derivative that selectively binds to the γ and β retinoic acid receptors (RAR); *in vivo* it is rapidly converted to its biologically active metabolite, tazarotenic acid [95]. Its mechanism of action in psoriasis may include reduction of number of lymphocytes in the dermis, decreased expression of inflammatory markers such as intracellular adhesion molecule 1 (ICAM-1), and modification of abnormal keratinocyte differentiation and proliferation [96].

Efficacy

Under clinical trial conditions, tazarotene 0.1% gel applied as a single agent once daily resulted in 70% of patients having reached the clinical endpoint of treatment success, with 41% maintaining significant improvement 12 weeks after stopping use of the drug [97]. More rapid improvement, improved efficacy, and decreased irritation have been shown in clinical trials combining tazarotene with intermediate and superpotent corticosteroids [98–100]. A reported additional benefit to concomitant application of retinoids and corticosteroids is the prevention of atrophy [61]. A recent review article by Lebwohl notes unpublished data showing that tazarotene has similar potential to reduce corticosteroid-related atrophy [101].

Tazarotene also appears to be stable *in vitro* when combined with a variety of topical corticosteroids and with calcipotriene, and it does not appear to affect adversely the stability of the other compounds [65]. A left–right comparison study has shown that a two-week course of tazarotene gel 0.1% applied once daily combined with calcipotriene twice daily was comparable to clobetasol dipropionate 0.05% ointment applied twice daily [102].

Administration

Patients using tazarotene as monotherapy should apply the medication once daily, taking care to avoid surrounding unaffected skin. Patients should be warned of the likelihood of irritation, particularly if the agent is used on the face and neck. Intertriginous regions and genitals should be avoided. If significant irritation occurs, the patient may benefit from what is termed a short contact regimen [103]. The patient is instructed to apply the medication for a shortened period of time (5–60 minutes) then to wash off the medication. This can be

TABLE 3.5 Use of Tazarotene in Moderate to Severe Psoriasis

Apply once daily.
If irritation develops, try "short contact" therapy:
Apply tazarotene to plaques for a short period of time. We suggest that the first time be 10 minutes, but therapeutic effect is claimed with as little as 1 minute.
Gradually increase application time by one to five minutes as tolerated.
Wash medication off after prescribed time period and apply an emollient.
In combination with superpotent corticosteroid:
Apply corticosteroid after short contact with tazarotene or apply tazarotene in the morning and the corticosteroid each evening.
Wean superpotent corticosteroid after two weeks to avoid atrophy.
In combination with UVB:
Apply after UV exposure.
If added to an already existing UVB regimen, reduce UV dosage by one-third.

followed by application of an emollient. Utilizing tazarotene every other day or changing to the 0.05% concentration or cream formulation may also help to reduce irritation but may be less effective.

Tazarotene may be most efficacious and best tolerated (therefore improving compliance) when applied in combination with topical corticosteroids. Initial treatment with once-daily application of tazarotene coupled with once-daily application of a superpotent corticosteroid, with subsequent tapering of the frequency of each agent (Table 3.5), is an effective regimen to prolong response.

Phototherapy Combination: UVB and Tazarotene

Tazarotene has been successfully combined with broadband [104,105] and narrowband UVB [106] for more effective and rapid clearing of psoriasis compared with either treatment alone. In a study of 54 patients, tazarotene applied immediately after UVB phototherapy three times weekly achieved initial treatment success in half the time with significantly reduced cumulative UVB exposure and no unusual photosensitivity [105]. Tazarotene applied nightly combined with narrowband UVB five times/week was likewise shown to be more effective than narrowband UVB alone [106]. No unusual photosensitivity has been reported in these studies. Irritation from tazarotene also appears to be reduced when combined with UV therapy. Although no trials have been reported using tazarotene immediately prior to UVB exposure, the compound is stable with UV exposure [107]. To date, no trials have assessed efficacy or safety of tazarotene use prior to UVB exposure. Therefore, if used in combination with UVB, tazarotene should be applied after light treatment. Because tazarotene has been shown to reduce epidermal thickness, concerns have been expressed regarding the increased risk of burning. It has been suggested that the UV dosage be reduced by one-third if tazarotene is added during phototherapy [107] (see Table 3.6).

Side Effects

The most frequently reported side effect at lesional and perilesional application sites is irritation, including itching, burning, stinging, and erythema. Although the medication is not

TABLE 3.6 Combination Regimens for Resistant Lesions and Maintenance after Improvement with Systemic or UV Therapy

Initial Treatment (Phase 1) (Two Weeks)
Superpotent corticosteroid twice daily (b.i.d.)
Calcipotriene (am) + superpotent corticosteroid (pm)
Tazarotene (am) + superpotent corticosteroid (pm)
Tazarotene and calcipotriene (am) + calcipotriene (pm)
Calcipotriene-betamethasone dipropionate two-compound ointment daily (b.i.d.)
Transitional and Maintenance Programs
Calcipotriene b.i.d. weekdays + superpotent corticosteroid b.i.d. weekends
Calcipotriene b.i.d. × one week alternating with superpotent corticosteroid b.i.d. × one week
Calcipotriene-betamethasone dipropionate two-compound ointment daily prn
Short-contact[a] tazarotene, then calcipotriene (pm) + calcipotriene (am) × one week, alternating with short-contact tazarotene then superpotent corticosteroid (pm) + corticosteroid (am)

Note: Patients should be evaluated within four to six weeks after initialing treatment to monitor for efficacy, side effects, compliance, and patient satisfaction. Patients using close to 100 g/week of calcipotriene should have serum calcium levels in the first one to two weeks of therapy. These combinations can be used for patients with moderate to severe psoriasis who cannot use or are fearful of systemic or UV treatment.

[a] 5–30-minute application, then wash off prior to application of second agent.

phototoxic or photoallergenic, the FDA-approved package insert cautions against sunlight and sunlamp exposure. When combined with UVB, thinning of the stratum corneum has been demonstrated, predisposing patients to burn more easily [107]. Tazarotene is potentially teratogenic (pregnancy category X); women of childbearing potential should have a pregnancy test prior to therapy and use adequate contraception during treatment.

TACROLIMUS (PROTOPIC®) AND PIMECROLIMUS (ELIDEL®)

Tacrolimus ointment is the topical formulation of FK 506, an immunomodulatory agent first used as an oral drug in patients undergoing organ transplantation. Oral tacrolimus has been shown to be efficacious in psoriasis [108]. Topical tacrolimus gel and cream have been shown to reduce Ki67-positive cells, human leukocyte antigen DR (HLA-DR) expression, and several T lymphocyte subsets *in vivo*, although not as readily as calcipotriol. The topical ointment (available in 0.03% and 0.1% concentrations) is effective in the treatment of atopic dermatitis but has been less effective for plaque psoriasis [109]. The lack of efficacy on plaques is presumable due to lack of absorption, supported by the fact that topical tacrolimus is effective for psoriasis on the face and intertriginous areas [110,111]. Addition of 6% salicylic acid to tacrolimus 0.1% ointment has been shown to produce greater improvement of plaques than tacrolimus alone [112].

Pimecrolimus 1% cream, an immunomodulatory agent approved for use in atopic dermatitis, has also been used off-label for psoriasis. Like tacrolimus, it also suffers from limited efficacy on plaques unless under occlusion. It has been shown to be effective in small studies evaluating facial and intertriginous psoriasis. An open label study of 20 patients revealed that twice daily application to facial psoriasis for 8–16 weeks produced significant improvement of lesions and was well tolerated [113]. In a study evaluating its efficacy in intertriginous psoriasis, 71% of patients treated with pimecrolimus cream achieved the endpoint of clear/almost clear at eight weeks [114].

Treatment with tacrolimus ointment and pimecrolimus cream is limited by their lack of FDA approval and cutaneous side effects including burning and stinging, particularly for tacrolimus. Anecdotally, application of a low- to mid-potency steroid such as tridesilon cream or hydrocortisone butyrate with tacrolimus ointment reduces the pruritus and burning seen with initial treatment with tacrolimus.

ANTHRALIN

Anthralin, or dithranol, has never been widely used in the United States. Historically, anthralin has been used in the treatment of moderate to severe psoriasis in the hospital or day care setting in combination with ultraviolet therapy, but its use has been superceded by more effective and convenient systemic therapies. Due to its lower efficacy than calcipotriene and its undesirable side effect profile, anthralin's role in moderate to severe psoriasis is reserved for well-motivated patients whose disease has demonstrated intolerance to other agents.

Pharmacology and Mechanism of Action

Anthralin is the synthetic equivalent of chrysarobin, the active component in Goa powder, used since the mid-19th century. Synthetic anthralin has been used since the 1930s when it was successfully substituted for coal tar by Ingram in the Goeckerman regimen. Its exact mechanism of action in psoriasis is unknown. Possible mechanisms include inhibition of DNA synthesis and proliferation [115], generation of free radicals, alteration in the epidermal growth factor receptor pathway, and alterations in mitochondrial respiratory function. Dithranol may suppress the interferon-γ-induced upregulation of cytokeratin 17 as a putative psoriasis autoantigen *in vitro* [116].

In the United States, the only commercially available anthralin is Psoriatec (1% anthralin cream), which is formulated in a temperature-sensitive vehicle that releases active medication when applied to skin [117]. This controlled-release technology may reduce staining of fabrics and hair as long as cool water is used for washing. Anthralin can be compounded by an experienced pharmacist for the desired strength and vehicle.

Efficacy

As a single agent, anthralin appears most effective when given as short contact therapy. Studies have demonstrated clearance in approximately 30% of patients treated for an average of five weeks [118–120]. Twice-daily application of calcipotriol was shown to be superior to short contact anthralin cream with better patient acceptability in one study [66], although a more recent study suggests that there are no statistical differences in quality-of-life measures between twice daily calcipotriol and dithranol [121]. Anthralin has been shown to enhance efficacy of many agents when used in combination; however, the disadvantages frequently outweigh the benefits. It is therefore seldom used in clinical practice in the United States.

TABLE 3.7 Directions for Application of Anthralin

Application
Apply to body plaques for prescribed time period once daily
Avoid face, axilla, intertriginous sites, genitals, and eyes
Use a bland emollient, such as petrolatum jelly, on noninvolved contiguous skin surrounding plaques to prevent contact and irritation
Removal
After allotted time, remove anthralin completely
Medication should be completely washed off so that the skin is dry and completely without medication
Use baby wipes, or baby mineral, or vegetable oil on an old cloth or towel
Shower or bathe with neutral pH soap
Apply an emollient (i.e., Eucerin, Cetaphil, or Aquaphor)
Observation
Patient should observe area over the next 48 hours for erythema
Discontinue treatment if significant erythema or irritation occurs
Stain Prevention
Apply medication with disposable latex gloves
Completely wash and dry area of application prior to dressing
Use an old or disposable cloth or towel for removal and drying
Cleanse tub or shower fixture immediately
If staining to a noncolored surface occurs, remove with household bleach

Note: Patients selected for this treatment should be motivated and able to follow detailed instructions. Patients should carefully adhere to total duration of application prescribed by the dermatologist; duration should begin at 10–30 minutes. Basic application instructions are supplied in this table.

Administration

For motivated patients whose disease has failed to respond to other topical and systemic modalities, short contact anthralin programs can be developed (Table 3.7).

Side Effects

The cutaneous side effects of anthralin include erythema, edema, and staining. Erythema usually occurs within six hours and peaks in 48–72 hours. Allergic contact dermatitis has been reported rarely. Oxidation of anthralin causes staining of the skin, hair (particularly blonde), and clothing or other household fabrics.

SALICYLIC ACID AND EMOLLIENTS

Salicylic Acid

Salicylic acid has been used in the treatment of psoriasis for years. It likely acts on the stratum corneum by disrupting desmosomes and may reduce thickness and scaling. It is available as a 6% gel but is most commonly found in shampoos or compounded with other psoriasis therapies. Salicylic acid enhances penetration and efficacy of corticosteroids [122]. The combination of 5% salicylic acid and 0.1% mometasone furoate ointment has been shown to be more effective than either agent alone [123], but to date there are no commercially available combinations of salicylic acid and high-potency corticosteroids in the United States.

Emollients

Emollients are commonly used and highly recommended as concomitant therapy in the treatment of psoriasis. Use of emollients usually increases comfort by relieving dryness, scaling, and pruritus. The authors recommend frequent application of a cream or ointment (such as Cetaphil, Eucerin, Aquaphor, and petrolatum).

IN THE PIPELINE: JANUS KINASE INHIBITORS

Tofacitinib and Ruxolitinib

Protein tyrosine kinase inhibitors, specifically in the Janus kinase (JAK) family, have shown efficacy in the treatment of psoriasis. Tofacitinib, the most studied in this class for psoriasis, is a selective Janus kinase 3 (Jak3) inhibitor, manufactured in oral and topical forms. Tofacitinib suppresses receptors for interleukin-2 (IL-2), IL-4, IL-9, IL-15, and IL-21 and disrupts activation of helper T and cytotoxic T cells [124]. Ports et al. randomized 71 subjects to tofacitinib 20 mg/g in two different ointment formulations, compared to respective ointment vehicle alone, applied twice daily for four weeks. The two ointment formulations differed by presence or absence of a proprietary penetration enhancer. Target plaque area and itch severity improved with statistical significance in the formulation of tofacitinib with a penetration enhancer but not the other formulations or vehicles. No significant safety or tolerability limitations were identified in the study population [125]. Another JAK inhibitor, ruxolitinib, was studied in 0.5%, 1.0%, and 1.5% concentrations in a blinded comparator trial against vehicle, calcitriol alone, or betamethasone alone over 28 days. Ruxolitinib in concentrations of 1.0% and 1.5% showed improved plaque scores when compared to vehicle. Comparison between ruxolitinib and calcipotriene or betamethasone showed similar improvement, although there were not enough patients to reach statistical significance. Adverse events included redness, stinging, dryness, and irritation at the site treated [126].

TREATMENT OF MODERATE TO SEVERE SCALP PSORIASIS WITH TOPICAL THERAPIES

Scalp psoriasis is the most frequent site of involvement in patients, with 50%–80% of patients reporting either scalp involvement alone or concomitantly with other body lesions [127–129]. Scalp psoriasis often significantly impacts quality of life and psychosocial well-being, given the visibility of the lesions and proximity to the face. Although the treatment of scalp psoriasis traditionally employs shampoos containing tar, salicylic acid, anti-fungals, or topically applied tar, anthralin, corticosteroids, and calcipotriene, there are actually very few placebo-controlled studies that support their use (as reviewed in Papp et al.) [130]. A 2002 meta-analysis showed that, of 42 well-designed published studies, only seven were aimed at treatment of scalp psoriasis and that results were consistent with studies of body lesions—that potent and superpotent corticosteroids, vitamin D analogs, and combinations of the vitamin D analogs and corticosteroids are the most efficacious scalp psoriasis therapies [131].

TABLE 3.8 Aggressive Therapy for Moderate to Severe Scalp Psoriasis

Evening

1. Superpotent corticosteroid (solution or foam vehicle)
2. Calcipotriene solution
3. Tazarotene 0.1% gel
4. Cover with plastic wrap and conform to scalp with thigh section of ladies nylon stocking
5. Leave in place for 8–12 hours

Morning

1. Shampoo with tar-based shampoo (with or without keratolytics)
2. Superpotent corticosteroid (solution or foam vehicle)
3. Calcipotriene solution

Note: Patients are asked to adhere to this regimen for two months. If the patient is compliant but his or disease is not 75% improved, systemic therapy should be considered. To assess improvement, patient should be asked the following question at baseline, at follow-up, and at the end of the two-month trial: "If '1' is equivalent to having no psoriasis, and '10' is equivalent to psoriasis being the worst ever, what is it today?" A score of 3 or less is considered a success.

All of the agents discussed in this chapter can be used on the scalp when prescribed in an acceptable vehicle, such as a solution, foam, lotion, or shampoo. However, patients with moderate to severe psoriasis isolated to the scalp often have tried and failed to respond to topical agents. It is the authors' opinion that moderate to severe psoriasis, even if isolated to the scalp, can (and some would argue should) be treated with systemic agents once topical therapies have been proven ineffective for the individual patient. The challenge to the treating dermatologist is determining treatment failure. It is our assessment that the most common reason for patients declaring that topical treatments do not work for scalp psoriasis is because they have not been compliant and/or have had unreal expectations. Our approach with these patients is to determine if topical therapy has a chance of reaching their expectations. For this, we prescribe the vigorous program outlined in Table 3.8—a combination regimen of superpotent corticosteroids, calcipotriene, and/or tazarotene and occlusion. Patients are asked to adhere to this regimen for two months. We announce to the patient that we have high expectations. If they are compliant and do not gain 75% improvement in two months, we will have to turn to systemic therapy or to adjust topical approaches to achieve less than clearance (i.e., comfort measures). We find that a follow-up in the first two to four weeks is useful for answering questions and to emphasize the need for an assessment of response by the patient (see Table 3.8).

Although not yet available in the United States, the two-compound calcipotriene–betamethasone dipropionate scalp formulation appears effective for scalp psoriasis [132,133]. The larger of the two trials, a randomized, controlled, double-blind trial of 1505 patients, revealed that 71% of patients achieved clear/almost clear after eight weeks of once daily application and it was more effective than either medication alone [133].

REFERENCES

1. Pearce DJ, Stealey KH, Balkrishnan R, Fleischer AB, Jr, Feldman SR. Psoriasis treatment in the United States at the end of the 20th century. *Int J Dermatol* 2006; 45(4): 370–4.
2. Lebwohl M, Ali S. Treatment of psoriasis. Part 1. Topical therapy and phototherapy. *J Am Acad Dermatol* 2001; 45(4): 487–98; quiz 499–502.

3. Krueger GG, Feldman SR, Camisa C, Duvic M, Elder JT, Gottlieb AB, et al. Two considerations for patients with psoriasis and their clinicians: what defines mild, moderate, and severe psoriasis? What constitutes a clinically significant improvement when treating psoriasis? *J Am Acad Dermatol* 2000; 43(2 Pt 1): 281–5.
4. Gelfand JM, Wan J, Callis Duffin K, Krueger GG, Kalb RE, Weisman JD, et al. Comparative effectiveness of commonly used systemic treatments or phototherapy for moderate to severe plaque psoriasis in the clinical practice setting. *Arch Dermatol* 2012; 148(4): 487–94.
5. Kragballe K. Topical corticosteroids: mechanisms of action. *Acta Derm Venereol Suppl* 1989; 151: 7–10; discussion 47–52.
6. Gower WR, Jr. Mechanism of glucocorticoid action. *J Fla Med Assoc* 1993; 80(10): 697–700.
7. Barnes PJ, Adcock I. Anti-inflammatory actions of steroids: molecular mechanisms. *Trends Pharmacol Sci* 1993; 14(12): 436–41.
8. Boumpas DT, Chrousos GP, Wilder RL, Cupps TR, Balow JE. Glucocorticoid therapy for immune-mediated diseases: basic and clinical correlates. *Ann Intern Med* 1993; 119(12): 1198–208.
9. Cornell RC, Stoughton RB. Correlation of the vasoconstriction assay and clinical activity in psoriasis. *Arch Dermatol* 1985; 121(1): 63–7.
10. Barry BW, Fyrand O, Woodford R, Ulshagen K, Hogstad G. Control of the bioavailability of a topical steroid; comparison of desonide creams 0.05% and 0.1% by vasoconstrictor studies and clinical trials. *Clin Exp Dermatol* 1987; 12(6): 406–9.
11. Gibson JR, Kirsch JM, Darley CR, Harvey SG, Burke CA, Hanson ME. An assessment of the relationship between vasoconstrictor assay findings, clinical efficacy and skin thinning effects of a variety of undiluted and diluted corticosteroid preparations. *Br J Dermatol* 1984; 111(Suppl 27): 204–12.
12. Cornell RC. Clinical trials of topical corticosteroids in psoriasis: correlations with the vasoconstrictor assay. *Int J Dermatol* 1992; 31(Suppl 1): 38–40.
13. Feldmann RJ, Maibach HI. Regional variation in percutaneous penetration of 14C cortisol in man. *J Invest Dermatol* 1967; 48(2): 181–3.
14. Krueger GG, O'Reilly MA, Weidner M, Dromgoole SH, Killey FP. Comparative efficacy of once-daily flurandrenolide tape versus twice-daily diflorasone diacetate ointment in the treatment of psoriasis. *J Am Acad Dermatol* 1998; 38(2 Pt 1): 186–90.
15. Katz HI, Gross E, Buxman M, Prawer SE, Schwartzel EH, Gibson JR. A double-blind, vehicle-controlled paired comparison of halobetasol propionate cream on patients with plaque psoriasis. *J Am Acad Dermatol* 1991; 25(6 Pt 2): 1175–8.
16. Blum G, Yawalkar S. A comparative, multicenter, double blind trial of 0.05% halobetasol propionate ointment and 0.1% betamethasone valerate ointment in the treatment of patients with chronic, localized plaque psoriasis. *J Am Acad Dermatol* 1991; 25(6 Pt 2): 1153–6.
17. Goldberg B, Hartdegen R, Presbury D, Smith EH, Yawalkar S. A double-blind, multicenter comparison of 0.05% halobetasol propionate ointment and 0.05% clobetasol propionate ointment in patients with chronic, localized plaque psoriasis. *J Am Acad Dermatol* 1991; 25(6 Pt 2): 1145–8.
18. Katz HI, Hien NT, Prawer SE, Mastbaum LI, Mooney JJ, Samson CR. Superpotent topical steroid treatment of psoriasis vulgaris—clinical efficacy and adrenal function. *J Am Acad Dermatol* 1987; 16(4): 804–11.
19. Bruce S, Epinette WW, Funicella T, Ison A, Jones EL, Loss R, Jr, et al. Comparative study of calcipotriene (MC 903) ointment and fluocinonide ointment in the treatment of psoriasis. *J Am Acad Dermatol* 1994; 31(5 Pt 1): 755–9.
20. Molin L, Cutler TP, Helander I, Nyfors B, Downes N. Comparative efficacy of calcipotriol (MC903) cream and betamethasone 17-valerate cream in the treatment of chronic plaque psoriasis. A randomized, double-blind, parallel group multicentre study. Calcipotriol Study Group. *Br J Dermatol* 1997; 136(1): 89–93.
21. Tristani-Firouzi P, Krueger GG. Efficacy and safety of treatment modalities for psoriasis. *Cutis* 1998; 61(2 Suppl): 11–21.
22. Smith K. Skin cap: what have we learned, and when did we learn it? *Dermatol Online J* 1997; 3(2): 11c.
23. Housman TS, Mellen BG, Rapp SR, Fleischer AB, Jr, Feldman SR. Patients with psoriasis prefer solution and foam vehicles: a quantitative assessment of vehicle preference. *Cutis* 2002; 70(6): 327–32.

24. Bergstrom KG, Arambula K, Kimball AB. Medication formulation affects quality of life: a randomized single-blind study of clobetasol propionate foam 0.05% compared with a combined program of clobetasol cream 0.05% and solution 0.05% for the treatment of psoriasis. *Cutis* 2003; 72(5): 407–11.
25. Warino L, Balkrishnan R, Feldman SR. Clobetasol propionate for psoriasis: are ointments really more potent? *J Drugs Dermatol* 2006; 5(6): 527–32.
26. Melian EB, Spencer CM, Jarvis B. Clobetasol propionate foam, 0.05%. *Am J Clin Dermatol* 2001; 2(2): 89–92; discussion 93.
27. Lebwohl M, Sherer D, Washenik K, Krueger GG, Menter A, Koo J, et al. A randomized, double-blind, placebo-controlled study of clobetasol propionate 0.05% foam in the treatment of nonscalp psoriasis. *Int J Dermatol* 2002; 41(5): 269–74.
28. Olux Prescribing Information. In.
29. Olux-E Prescribing Information. In.
30. Franz TJ, Parsell DA, Halualani RM, Hannigan JF, Kalbach JP, Harkonen WS. Betamethasone valerate foam 0.12%: a novel vehicle with enhanced delivery and efficacy. *Int J Dermatol* 1999; 38(8): 628–32.
31. Verdeso Foam Prescribing Information. In.
32. Beutner K, Chakrabarty A, Lemke S, Yu K. An intra-individual randomized safety and efficacy comparison of clobetasol propionate 0.05% spray and its vehicle in the treatment of plaque psoriasis. *J Drugs Dermatol* 2006; 5(4): 357–60.
33. Clobex Spray Prescribing Information. In.
34. Koo JY. Relevance of the COBRA trial in current psoriasis practice. *Cutis* 2007; 80(5 Suppl): 4–11.
35. Lowe N, Feldman SR, Sherer D, Weiss J, Shavin JS, Lin YL, et al. Clobetasol propionate lotion, an efficient and safe alternative to clobetasol propionate emollient cream in subjects with moderate to severe plaque-type psoriasis. *J Dermatol Treat* 2005; 16(3): 158–64.
36. Decroix J, Pres H, Tsankov N, Poncet M, Arsonnaud S. Clobetasol propionate lotion in the treatment of moderate to severe plaque-type psoriasis. *Cutis* 2004; 74(3): 201–6.
37. Katz HI, Lindholm JS, Weiss JS, Shavin JS, Morman M, Bressinck R, et al. Efficacy and safety of twice-daily augmented betamethasone dipropionate lotion versus clobetasol propionate solution in patients with moderate-to-severe scalp psoriasis. *Clin Ther* 1995; 17(3): 390–401.
38. Jarratt M, Breneman D, Gottlieb AB, Poulin Y, Liu Y, Foley V. Clobetasol propionate shampoo 0.05%: a new option to treat patients with moderate to severe scalp psoriasis. *J Drugs Dermatol* 2004; 3(4): 367–73.
39. Olsen EA, Cram DL, Ellis CN, Hickman JG, Jacobson C, Jenkins EE, et al. A double-blind, vehicle-controlled study of clobetasol propionate 0.05% (Temovate) scalp application in the treatment of moderate to severe scalp psoriasis. *J Am Acad Dermatol* 1991; 24(3): 443–7.
40. Feldman SR. Effectiveness of clobetasol propionate spray 0.05% added to other stable treatments: add-on therapy in the COBRA trial. *Cutis* 2007; 80(5 Suppl): 20–8.
41. Feldman SR, Koo JYM, Johnson LA, Preston NJ. Clobetasol propionate spray 0.05% add-on therapy to a stable regimen of biologic treatment in patients with moderate to very severe plaque psoriasis. *Cutis* 2009; 84(4 Suppl): 25–32.
42. Thaci D, Ortonne JP, Chimenti S, Ghislain PD, Arenberger P, Kragballe K, et al. A phase IIIb, multicentre, randomized, double-blind, vehicle-controlled study of the efficacy and safety of adalimumab with and without calcipotriol/betamethasone topical treatment in patients with moderate to severe psoriasis: the BELIEVE study. *Br J Dermatol* 2010; 163(2): 402–11.
43. Lebwohl MG, Kircik L, Callis Duffin K, Pariser D, Hooper M, Wenkert D, et al. A randomized study to evaluate the efficacy and safety of adding topical therapy to etanercept in patients with moderate to severe plaque psoriasis. *J Am Acad Dermatol* 2013; 69: 385–92.
44. Katz HI, Prawer SE, Mooney JJ, Samson CR. Preatrophy: covert sign of thinned skin. *J Am Acad Dermatol* 1989; 20(5 Pt 1): 731–5.
45. Alani MD, Alani SD. Allergic contact dermatitis to corticosteroids. *Ann Allergy* 1972; 30(4): 181–5.
46. van de Kerkhof PC, Chang A, van der Walle HB, van Vlijmen-Willems I, Boezeman JB, Huigen-Tijdink R. Weekly treatment of psoriasis with a hydrocolloid dressing in combination with triamcinolone acetonide. A controlled comparative study. *Acta Derm Venereol* 1994; 74(2): 143–6.
47. Volden G. Successful treatment of chronic skin diseases with clobetasol propionate and a hydrocolloid occlusive dressing. *Acta Derm Venereol* 1992; 72(1): 69–71.

48. Mommers JM, van Erp PE, van De Kerkhof PC. Clobetasol under hydrocolloid occlusion in psoriasis results in a complete block of proliferation and in a rebound of lesions following discontinuation. *Dermatology* 1999; 199(4): 323–7.
49. Levin C, Maibach HI. Topical corticosteroid-induced adrenocortical insufficiency: clinical implications. *Am J Clin Dermatol* 2002; 3(3): 141–7.
50. Nathan AW, Rose GL. Fatal iatrogenic cushing's syndrome. *Lancet* 1979; 1(8109): 207.
51. Kubo T, Kojima A, Yamazoe S, Ueshima K, Yamamoto T, Hirasawa Y. Osteonecrosis of the femoral head that developed after long-term topical steroid application. *J Orthop Sci* 2001; 6(1): 92–4.
52. du Vivier A. Tachyphylaxis to topically applied steroids. *Arch Dermatol* 1976; 112(9): 1245–8.
53. du Vivier A, Stoughton RB. Tachyphylaxis to the action of topically applied corticosteroids. *Arch Dermatol* 1975; 111(5): 581–3.
54. Miller JJ, Roling D, Margolis D, Guzzo C. Failure to demonstrate therapeutic tachyphylaxis to topically applied steroids in patients with psoriasis. *J Am Acad Dermatol* 1999; 41(4): 546–9.
55. Carroll CL, Feldman SR, Camacho FT, Manuel JC, Balkrishnan R. Adherence to topical therapy decreases during the course of an 8-week psoriasis clinical trial: commonly used methods of measuring adherence to topical therapy overestimate actual use. *J Am Acad Dermatol* 2004; 51(2): 212–16.
56. Feldman SR, Camacho FT, Krejci-Manwaring J, Carroll CL, Balkrishnan R. Adherence to topical therapy increases around the time of office visits. *J Am Acad Dermatol* 2007; 57(1): 81–3.
57. Jensen AM, Llado MB, Skov L, Hansen ER, Larsen JK, Baadsgaard O. Calcipotriol inhibits the proliferation of hyperproliferative CD29 positive keratinocytes in psoriatic epidermis in the absence of an effect on the function and number of antigen-presenting cells. *Br J Dermatol* 1998; 139(6): 984–91.
58. Rizova E, Corroller M. Topical calcitriol—studies on local tolerance and systemic safety. *Br J Dermatol* 2001; 144(Suppl 58): 3–10.
59. Mason AR, Mason J, Cork M, Dooley G, Hancock H. Topical treatments for chronic plaque psoriasis. *Cochrane Database Syst Rev* 2013; 3: CD005028.
60. Ortonne JP, Humbert P, Nicolas JF, Tsankov N, Tonev SD, Janin A, et al. Intra-individual comparison of the cutaneous safety and efficacy of calcitriol 3 microg g(-1) ointment and calcipotriol 50 microg g(-1) ointment on chronic plaque psoriasis localized in facial, hairline, retroauricular or flexural areas. *Br J Dermatol* 2003; 148(2): 326–33.
61. Smith EL, Walworth NC, Holick MF. Effect of 1 alpha, 25-dihydroxyvitamin D3 on the morphologic and biochemical differentiation of cultured human epidermal keratinocytes grown in serum-free conditions. *J Invest Dermatol* 1986; 86(6): 709–14.
62. Lemire JM, Adams JS, Kermani-Arab V, Bakke AC, Sakai R, Jordan SC. 1,25-Dihydroxyvitamin D3 suppresses human T helper/inducer lymphocyte activity *in vitro*. *J Immunol* 1985; 134(5): 3032–5.
63. Tsoukas CD, Provvedini DM, Manolagas SC. 1,25-dihydroxyvitamin D3: a novel immunoregulatory hormone. *Science* 1984; 224(4656): 1438–40.
64. Patel B, Siskin S, Krazmien R, Lebwohl M. Compatibility of calcipotriene with other topical medications. *J Am Acad Dermatol* 1998; 38(6 Pt 1): 1010–11.
65. Hecker D, Worsley J, Yueh G, Lebwohl M. *In vitro* compatibility of tazarotene with other topical treatments of psoriasis. *J Am Acad Dermatol* 2000; 42(6): 1008–11.
66. Berth-Jones J, Chu AC, Dodd WA, Ganpule M, Griffiths WA, Haydey RP, et al. A multicentre, parallel-group comparison of calcipotriol ointment and short-contact dithranol therapy in chronic plaque psoriasis. *Br J Dermatol* 1992; 127(3): 266–71.
67. Cunliffe WJ, Berth-Jones J, Claudy A, Fairiss G, Goldin D, Gratton D, et al. Comparative study of calcipotriol (MC 903) ointment and betamethasone 17-valerate ointment in patients with psoriasis vulgaris. *J Am Acad Dermatol* 1992; 26(5 Pt 1): 736–43.
68. Kragballe K. Calcipotriol for psoriasis. *Lancet* 1991; 337(8751): 1229–30.
69. van de Kerkhof PC, Franssen M, de La Brassine M, Kuipers M. Calcipotriol cream in the morning and ointment in the evening: a novel regimen to improve compliance. *J Dermatol Treat* 2001; 12(2): 75–9.
70. Feldman SR, Mills M, Brundage T, Eastman WJ. A multicenter, randomized, double-blind study of the efficacy and safety of calcipotriene foam, 0.005%, vs vehicle foam in the treatment of plaque-type psoriasis of the scalp. *J Drugs Dermatol* 2013; 12(3): 300–6.
71. Koo J. Systemic sequential therapy of psoriasis: a new paradigm for improved therapeutic results. *J Am Acad Dermatol* 1999; 41(3 Pt 2): S25–8.

72. Traulsen J. Bioavailability of betamethasone dipropionate when combined with calcipotriol. *Int J Dermatol* 2004; 43(8): 611–17.
73. Papp KA, Guenther L, Boyden B, Larsen FG, Harvima RJ, Guilhou JJ, et al. Early onset of action and efficacy of a combination of calcipotriene and betamethasone dipropionate in the treatment of psoriasis. *J Am Acad Dermatol* 2003; 48(1): 48–54.
74. Guenther L, Van de Kerkhof PC, Snellman E, Kragballe K, Chu AC, Tegner E, et al. Efficacy and safety of a new combination of calcipotriol and betamethasone dipropionate (once or twice daily) compared to calcipotriol (twice daily) in the treatment of psoriasis vulgaris: a randomized, double-blind, vehicle-controlled clinical trial. *Br J Dermatol* 2002; 147(2): 316–23.
75. Kaufmann R, Bibby AJ, Bissonnette R, Cambazard F, Chu AC, Decroix J, et al. A new calcipotriol/betamethasone dipropionate formulation (Daivobet) is an effective once-daily treatment for psoriasis vulgaris. *Dermatology* 2002; 205(4): 389–93.
76. Kragballe K, Noerrelund KL, Lui H, Ortonne JP, Wozel G, Uurasmaa T, et al. Efficacy of once-daily treatment regimens with calcipotriol/betamethasone dipropionate ointment and calcipotriol ointment in psoriasis vulgaris. *Br J Dermatol* 2004; 150(6): 1167–73.
77. Douglas WS, Poulin Y, Decroix J, Ortonne JP, Mrowietz U, Gulliver W, et al. A new calcipotriol/betamethasone formulation with rapid onset of action was superior to monotherapy with betamethasone dipropionate or calcipotriol in psoriasis vulgaris. *Acta Derm Venereol* 2002; 82(2): 131–5.
78. Zaghloul SS, Goodfield MJ. Objective assessment of compliance with psoriasis treatment. *Arch Dermatol* 2004; 140(4): 408–14.
79. Menter A, Abramovits W, Colon LE, Johnson LA, Gottschalk RW. Comparing clobetasol propionate 0.05% spray to calcipotriene 0.005% betamethasone dipropionate 0.064% ointment for the treatment of moderate to severe plaque psoriasis. *J Drugs Dermatol* 2009; 8(1): 52–7.
80. Lebwohl M, Yoles A, Lombardi K, Lou W. Calcipotriene ointment and halobetasol ointment in the long-term treatment of psoriasis: effects on the duration of improvement. *J Am Acad Dermatol* 1998; 39(3): 447–50.
81. Singh S, Reddy DC, Pandey SS. Topical therapy for psoriasis with the use of augmented betamethasone and calcipotriene on alternate weeks. *J Am Acad Dermatol* 2000; 43(1 Pt 1): 61–5.
82. Grossman RM, Thivolet J, Claudy A, Souteyrand P, Guilhou JJ, Thomas P, et al. A novel therapeutic approach to psoriasis with combination calcipotriol ointment and very low-dose cyclosporine: results of a multicenter placebo-controlled study. *J Am Acad Dermatol* 1994; 31(1): 68–74.
83. Kokelj F, Lavaroni G, Guadagnini A. UVB versus UVB plus calcipotriol (MC 903) therapy for psoriasis vulgaris. *Acta Derm Venereol* 1995; 75(5): 386–7.
84. van de Kerkhof PC, Cambazard F, Hutchinson PE, Haneke E, Wong E, Souteyrand P, et al. The effect of addition of calcipotriol ointment (50 micrograms/g) to acitretin therapy in psoriasis. *Br J Dermatol* 1998; 138(1): 84–9.
85. Adachi Y, Uchida N, Matsuo T, Horio T. Clinical effect of vitamin D3 analogues is not inactivated by subsequent UV exposure. *Photodermatol Photoimmunol Photomed* 2008; 24(1): 16–18.
86. Speight EL, Farr PM. Calcipotriol improves the response of psoriasis to PUVA. *Br J Dermatol* 1994; 130(1): 79–82.
87. Ramsay CA, Schwartz BE, Lowson D, Papp K, Bolduc A, Gilbert M. Calcipotriol cream combined with twice weekly broad-band UVB phototherapy: a safe, effective and UVB-sparing antipsoriatric combination treatment. The Canadian Calcipotriol and UVB Study Group. *Dermatology* 2000; 200(1): 17–24.
88. Koo J. Diluting dovonex. *Psoriasis Forum* 1995; 1: 6.
89. Kragballe K, Austad J, Barnes L, Bibby A, de la Brassinne M, Cambazard F, et al. A 52-week randomized safety study of a calcipotriol/betamethasone dipropionate two-compound product (Dovobet/Daivobet/Taclonex) in the treatment of psoriasis vulgaris. *Br J Dermatol* 2006; 154(6): 1155–60.
90. Dwyer C, Chapman RS. Calcipotriol and hypercalcaemia. *Lancet* 1991; 338(8769): 764–5.
91. Georgiou S, Tsambaos D. Hypercalcaemia and hypercalciuria after topical treatment of psoriasis with excessive amounts of calcipotriol. *Acta Derm Venereol* 1999; 79(1): 86.
92. Braun GS, Witt M, Mayer V, Schmid H. Hypercalcemia caused by vitamin D3 analogs in psoriasis treatment. *Int J Dermatol* 2007; 46(12): 1315–17.
93. Mortensen L, Kragballe K, Wegmann E, Schifter S, Risteli J, Charles P. Treatment of psoriasis vulgaris with topical calcipotriol has no short-term effect on calcium or bone metabolism. A randomized, double-blind, placebo-controlled study. *Acta Derm Venereol* 1993; 73(4): 300–4.

94. Gerritsen MJ, Van De Kerkhof PC, Langner A. Long-term safety of topical calcitriol 3 microg g(-1) ointment. *Br J Dermatol* 2001; 144(Suppl 58): 17–19.
95. Chandraratna RA. Tazarotene—first of a new generation of receptor-selective retinoids. *Br J Dermatol* 1996; 135(Suppl 49): 18–25.
96. Duvic M, Asano AT, Hager C, Mays S. The pathogenesis of psoriasis and the mechanism of action of tazarotene. *J Am Acad Dermatol* 1998; 39(4 Pt 2): S129–33.
97. Krueger GG, Drake LA, Elias PM, Lowe NJ, Guzzo C, Weinstein GD, et al. The safety and efficacy of tazarotene gel, a topical acetylenic retinoid, in the treatment of psoriasis. *Arch Dermatol* 1998; 134(1): 57–60.
98. Koo JY, Martin D. Investigator-masked comparison of tazarotene gel q.d. plus mometasone furoate cream q.d. vs. mometasone furoate cream b.i.d. in the treatment of plaque psoriasis. *Int J Dermatol* 2001; 40(3): 210–12.
99. Lebwohl M, Poulin Y. Tazarotene in combination with topical corticosteroids. *J Am Acad Dermatol* 1998; 39(4 Pt 2): S139–43.
100. Lesnik RH, Mezick JA, Capetola R, Kligman LH. Topical all-trans-retinoic acid prevents corticosteroid-induced skin atrophy without abrogating the anti-inflammatory effect. *J Am Acad Dermatol* 1989; 21(2 Pt 1): 186–90.
101. Lebwohl M, Lombardi K, Tan MH. Duration of improvement in psoriasis after treatment with tazarotene 0.1% gel plus clobetasol propionate 0.05% ointment: comparison of maintenance treatments. *Int J Dermatol* 2001; 40(1): 64–6.
102. Bowman PH, Maloney JE, Koo JYM. Combination of calcipotriene (Dovonex) ointment and tazarotene (Tazorac) gel versus clobetasol ointment in the treatment of plaque psoriasis: a pilot study. *J Am Acad Dermatol* 2002; 46(6): 907–13.
103. Veraldi S, Caputo R, Pacifico A, Peris K, Soda R, Chimenti S. Short contact therapy with tazarotene in psoriasis vulgaris. *Dermatology*. 2006; 212(3): 235–7.
104. Lowe NJ. Optimizing therapy: tazarotene in combination with phototherapy. *Br J Dermatol* 1999; 140(Suppl 54): 8–11.
105. Koo JY, Lowe NJ, Lew-Kaya DA, Vasilopoulos AI, Lue JC, Sefton J, et al. Tazarotene plus UVB phototherapy in the treatment of psoriasis. *J Am Acad Dermatol* 2000; 43(5 Pt 1): 821–8.
106. Behrens S, Grundmann-Kollmann M, Schiener R, Peter RU, Kerscher M. Combination phototherapy of psoriasis with narrow-band UVB irradiation and topical tazarotene gel. *J Am Acad Dermatol* 2000; 42(3): 493–5.
107. Hecker D, Worsley J, Yueh G, Kuroda K, Lebwohl M. Interactions between tazarotene and ultraviolet light. *J Am Acad Dermatol* 1999; 41(6): 927–30.
108. Systemic tacrolimus (FK 506) is effective for the treatment of psoriasis in a double-blind, placebo-controlled study. The European FK 506 Multicentre Psoriasis Study Group. *Arch Dermatol* 1996; 132(4): 419–23.
109. Zonneveld IM, Rubins A, Jablonska S, Dobozy A, Ruzicka T, Kind P, et al. Topical tacrolimus is not effective in chronic plaque psoriasis. A pilot study. *Arch Dermatol* 1998; 134(9): 1101–2.
110. Lebwohl M, Freeman AK, Chapman MS, Feldman SR, Hartle JE, Henning A. Tacrolimus ointment is effective for facial and intertriginous psoriasis. *J Am Acad Dermatol* 2004; 51(5): 723–30.
111. Yamamoto T, Nishioka K. Topical tacrolimus is effective for facial lesions of psoriasis. *Acta Derm Venereol* 2000; 80(6): 451.
112. Carroll CL, Clarke J, Camacho F, Balkrishnan R, Feldman SR. Topical tacrolimus ointment combined with 6% salicylic acid gel for plaque psoriasis treatment. *Arch Dermatol* 2005; 141(1): 43–6.
113. Jacobi A, Braeutigam M, Mahler V, Schultz E, Hertl M. Pimecrolimus 1% cream in the treatment of facial psoriasis: a 16-week open-label study. *Dermatology* 2008; 216(2): 133–6.
114. Gribetz C, Ling M, Lebwohl M, Pariser D, Draelos Z, Gottlieb AB, et al. Pimecrolimus cream 1% in the treatment of intertriginous psoriasis: a double-blind, randomized study. *J Am Acad Dermatol* 2004; 51(5): 731–8.
115. Klem EB. Effects of antipsoriasis drugs and metabolic inhibitors on the growth of epidermal cells in culture. *J Invest Dermatol* 1978; 70(1): 27–32.
116. Bonnekoh B, Bockelmann R, Ambach A, Gollnick H. Dithranol and dimethylfumarate suppress the interferon-gamma-induced up-regulation of cytokeratin 17 as a putative psoriasis autoantigen *in vitro*. *Skin Pharmacol Appl Skin Physiol* 2001; 14(4): 217–25.
117. Volden G, Bjornberg A, Tegner E, Pedersen NB, Arles UB, Agren S, et al. Short-contact treatment at home with Micanol. *Acta Derm Venereol Suppl* 1992; 172: 20–2.

118. Schaefer H, Farber EM, Goldberg L, Schalla W. Limited application period for dithranol in psoriasis. Preliminary report on penetration and clinical efficacy. *Br J Dermatol* 1980; 102(5): 571–3.
119. Goransson A. Comparison of dithranol and butantrone in short contact therapy of psoriasis. *Acta Derm Venereol* 1987; 67(2): 149–53.
120. Statham BN, Ryatt KS, Rowell NR. Short-contact dithranol therapy—a comparison with the Ingram regime. *Br J Dermatol* 1984; 110(6): 703–8.
121. de Korte J, van der Valk PG, Sprangers MA, Damstra RJ, Kunkeler AC, Lijnen RL, et al. A comparison of twice-daily calcipotriol ointment with once-daily short-contact dithranol cream therapy: quality-of-life outcomes of a randomized controlled trial of supervised treatment of psoriasis in a day-care setting. *Br J Dermatol* 2008; 158(2): 375–81.
122. Krochmal L, Wang JC, Patel B, Rodgers J. Topical corticosteroid compounding: effects on physicochemical stability and skin penetration rate. *J Am Acad Dermatol* 1989; 21(5 Pt 1): 979–84.
123. Koo J, Cuffie CA, Tanner DJ, Bressinck R, Cornell RC, DeVillez RL, et al. Mometasone furoate 0.1%-salicylic acid 5% ointment versus mometasone furoate 0.1% ointment in the treatment of moderate-to-severe psoriasis: a multicenter study. *Clin Ther* 1998; 20(2): 283–91.
124. West K. CP-690550, a JAK3 inhibitor as an immunosuppressant for the treatment of rheumatoid arthritis, transplant rejection, psoriasis and other immune-mediated disorders. *Curr Opin Investig Drugs* 2009; 10(5): 491–504.
125. Ports WC, Khan S, Lan S, Lamba M, Bolduc C, Bissonnette R, et al. A randomised phase 2a efficacy and safety trial of the topical Janus kinase inhibitor tofacitinib in the treatment of chronic plaque psoriasis. *Br J Dermatol* 2013; 169: 137–45.
126. Punwani N, Scherle P, Flores R, Shi J, Liang J, Yeleswaram S, et al. Preliminary clinical activity of a topical JAK1/2 inhibitor in the treatment of psoriasis. *J Am Acad Dermatol* 2012; 67(4): 658–64.
127. van de Kerkhof PC, Franssen ME. Psoriasis of the scalp. Diagnosis and management. *Am J Clin Dermatol* 2001; 2(3): 159–65.
128. Farber EM, Nall L. Natural history and treatment of scalp psoriasis. *Cutis* 1992; 49(6): 396–400.
129. Dawber R, vanNeste D. *Hair and Scalp Disorders. Common Presenting Signs, Differential Diagnosis and Treatment*. Philadelphia, PA: JB Lippincott; 1995.
130. Papp K, Berth-Jones J, Kragballe K, Wozel G, de la Brassinne M. Scalp psoriasis: a review of current topical treatment options. *J Eur Acad Dermatol Venereol* 2007; 21(9): 1151–60.
131. Mason J, Mason AR, Cork MJ. Topical preparations for the treatment of psoriasis. a systematic review. *Br J Dermatol* 2002; 146(3): 351–64.
132. Buckley C, Hoffmann V, Shapiro J, Saari S, Cambazard F, Milsgaard M. Calcipotriol plus betamethasone dipropionate scalp formulation is effective and well tolerated in the treatment of scalp psoriasis: a phase II study. *Dermatology* 2008; 217(2): 107–13.
133. Jemec GB, Ganslandt C, Ortonne JP, Poulin Y, Burden AD, de Unamuno P, et al. A new scalp formulation of calcipotriene plus betamethasone compared with its active ingredients and the vehicle in the treatment of scalp psoriasis: a randomized, double-blind, controlled trial. *J Am Acad Dermatol* 2008; 59(3): 455–63.

Chapter 4

The Art and Practice of UVB Phototherapy and Laser

Monica Huynh, Maya G. Debbaneh,
Ethan C. Levin, and John Y. M. Koo

INTRODUCTION

Ultraviolet B (UVB) is one of the oldest therapeutic modalities for the treatment of psoriasis. Because of its long track record of safety and efficacy, UVB phototherapy continues to enjoy widespread use in spite of the development of many newer modalities for treating psoriasis, including biologic agents. According to available published data, certain forms of UVB phototherapy, such as that used with the traditional Goeckerman regimen, induce a prolonged remission; indeed, Goeckerman treatment is the gold standard against which newer modalities are compared in terms of remission times [1].

This chapter will discuss the entire spectrum of UVB phototherapy. UVB regimens range from simple treatment in a UVB phototherapy box to a much more elaborate and aggressive modality in which the intensity of UVB radiation used varies not only among patients but also according to different anatomical regions within the same patient. Combining UVB phototherapy with various topical and systemic agents can also enhance UVB phototherapy. Even though some of these techniques are discussed in the context of the psoriasis day treatment program, it is important to note that such techniques can be carried out for selected recalcitrant psoriatic lesions in a regular office setting. These techniques will be discussed one by one, starting with the simplest regimen followed by more effective—but also more involved—uses of this modality. We will also discuss new developments in phototherapy including targeted UVB laser therapy and other forms of localized phototherapy.

UVB PHOTOTHERAPY

There are two types of UVB: broadband UVB (BB-UVB), which emits wavelengths between 290 and 320 nm, and narrowband UVB (NB-UVB), which emits wavelengths between 308 and 313 nm. Broadband was the first form of UVB used to treat psoriasis. However, once psoriasis was shown to be most responsive to wavelengths closer to 312 nm, NB-UVB became the standard of care [2]. Another form of generalized phototherapy includes the use of psoralen plus ultraviolet A (PUVA), which is also very effective for the treatment of psoriasis (see Chapter 5).

Even the simplest use of UVB phototherapy requires some commitment, time, and effort from patients. Hence, outpatient UVB phototherapy is usually reserved for patients whose disease does not adequately respond to topical medications such as steroids, calcipotriol, tazarotene, tar, or anthralin. It is also indicated for those patients who initially respond to topical agents but develop tachyphylaxis over time or for patients with such extensive involvement that topical therapy is nearly impossible. For patients with generalized psoriasis, UVB phototherapy is a reasonable first choice among the various available options because of its proven safety profile. Important points to consider when initially discussing UVB phototherapy with a patient are the patient's employment schedule and flexibility, location of the phototherapy unit, transportation, and overall convenience for the patient.

NB-UVB PHOTOTHERAPY

The lamps used in NB-UVB phototherapy are known as "TL-01." These lamps emit a "narrowband" of high-intensity light ranging from 311 to 313 nm, thus eliminating high-energy, shorter wavelengths responsible for burning, premature aging, and increased incidence of skin cancer. During early studies in the 1980s, the authors examined various wavelengths and discovered that 313 nm allowed for the lowest effective dosage of light with the least erythema [3,4]. The particular efficacy of this band of light should not be misinterpreted to mean that other UV wavelengths are not effective, only that UV in the range around 312 nm has the optimal therapeutic effect. Improvement in psoriasis is also seen with a wide range of UVB and UVA wavelengths. NB-UVB has been used extensively throughout Europe and Australia and has now gained popularity in the United States as evidence documenting its effectiveness has continued to accumulate.

Through decades of study and clinical experience, BB-UVB and PUVA have become essential components in the treatment of psoriasis. However, NB-UVB is now used as first-line generalized phototherapy because it seems to be more effective than BB-UVB for psoriasis treatment and more convenient and less carcinogenic than PUVA.

Contraindications

UVB phototherapy is contraindicated in patients who react badly to light, either because of medication they are taking or because of an underlying photosensitive disease. Numerous medications can potentially photosensitize patients, including thiazide diuretics and certain antibiotics such as tetracycline or doxycycline. However, such medications do not always induce photosensitivity. In fact, if phototherapy is strongly indicated, it is frequently possible to go ahead and conduct phototherapy after exposing a selected test area of the skin to UVB light without a reaction. Another option is scheduling phototherapy so that the maximum time elapses between administration of the photosensitizing medication and UVB therapy. This ensures a minimum blood level of the photosensitizing medication at the time of light exposure, thereby minimizing the risk of a phototoxic reaction. In addition, it is imperative that when patients begin new medications, whether for psoriasis or other medical conditions, that such information is communicated to the dermatologist and phototherapy staff. If any new medications are believed to cause photosensitivity, then the phototherapy staff may need to adjust the dosage of UVB light the patient is receiving.

UVB phototherapy is contraindicated in patients with photosensitizing diseases such as systemic lupus erythematosus or polymorphous light eruption, unless the phototherapy is specifically used to harden the skin as a therapeutic strategy in patients with such conditions.

Although much of the published literature regarding this hardening process refers to PUVA, UVB is also effective [5,6]. A discussion of each photosensitizing medication and disease is beyond the scope of this chapter, but detailed references regarding these conditions can be readily found in standard textbooks [7].

Some *in vitro* data suggest that UVB exposure may enhance activation of human immunovirus (HIV) infection [8–11]. However, in practice, UVB therapy is used to treat not only HIV-infected patients with psoriasis but also cases of HIV pruritus and folliculitis, including eosinophilic folliculitis. After almost two decades of use, practitioners have not noticed widespread occurrence of adverse reactions to this therapy in HIV-infected patients. UVB phototherapy is still considered safer, by most practitioners, than other therapeutic alternatives, including PUVA, methotrexate, and cyclosporine, especially in light of published research describing the lack of changes in immune function among HIV-positive patients undergoing UVB phototherapy [12].

Dosage and Administration

There are two ways to determine the initial dose of UVB radiation for any given patient, whether using BB-UVB or NB-UVB. The first method involves formal minimal erythema dose (MED) testing, in which small, defined areas of skin are sequentially exposed to different intensities of UVB radiation (Figure 4.1). The MED is defined as the amount of UVB that produces barely perceptible erythema in noninvolved skin 12–18 hours after exposure. Once the MED for a particular patient has been determined, the initial exposure may range anywhere from 50% (i.e., suberythemogenic) to 100% (i.e., erythemogenic) of the MED,

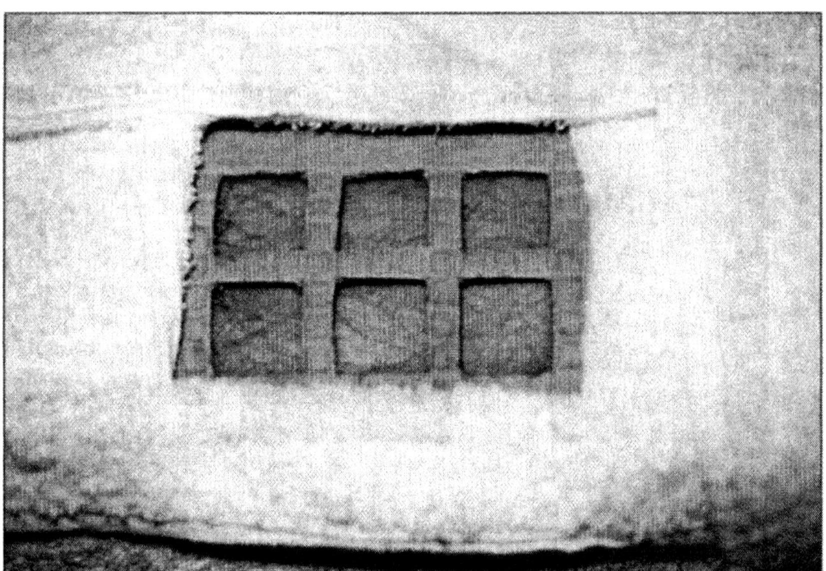

FIGURE 4.1 (See color insert.) When conducting formal MED testing, a different amount of UVB radiation is applied sequentially to each opening in the template, which is made of an opaque material such as a thick piece of cardboard. The increment of UVB exposure is usually 15 or 30 seconds when a UVB box with fluorescent lights is used.

depending on the desired aggressiveness of the dosing schedule. In an erythemogenic schedule, an attempt is made to maintain barely perceptible erythema following each UVB treatment session [13–18]. To compensate for tanning and other forms of tolerance, subsequent dosages of UVB radiation may be increased by 10%–25% of the previously applied dosage, if necessary, to maintain mild, nontender erythema in the noninvolved skin.

The erythemogenic schedule is ideal in theory because UVB phototherapy tends to produce maximal results when used at or near a patient's MED [19–22]. In practice, the erythemogenic dosage schedule is not practical for many patients either because they experience uncomfortable burning sensations at MED or because practitioners do not want to risk burning patients by attempting to maintain MED. The alternative is the suberythemogenic schedule [23]. In this schedule, the initial dosage of UVB radiation is 50% of the MED. If the patient does not improve, the subsequent dose of UVB can be increased. The rationale behind using a less aggressive, suberythemogenic schedule is to minimize the cumulative dosage of UVB radiation and also to minimize the risk of inducing UVB burns. However, patients also tend to respond more slowly when a less aggressive schedule is used. As will be discussed later (in the section on tar), this shortcoming can be largely overcome by using tar preparations concurrently.

In a busy phototherapy practice with a high volume of patients, formal MED testing may be cumbersome because it is labor intensive and potentially disruptive to the natural flow of patients undergoing phototherapy. In our clinic, instead of MED testing, a defined guideline is used to determine the starting dosage for UVB therapy based on patients' skin types (Table 4.1). Subsequent dosing depends on the response of psoriasis and on the presence or absence of phototoxic reactions to previous doses. As illustrated in Table 4.1, a wide range of dosing increases is possible. The underlying principle is to increase UVB gradually either until the psoriasis lesions respond well to phototherapy or until the MED is reached and then to try to maintain the UVB dose just below the MED. This approach eliminates the need for formal MED testing in most patients. It is also simpler and more efficient than methods using incremental dosages calculated as a certain percentage of the previous dosage.

Efficacy

To induce steady improvement of existing psoriatic lesions, outpatient BB-UVB or NB-UVB phototherapy should be performed ideally at least three times per week. If UVB phototherapy is conducted less than three times/week, the rate of clinical improvement may diminish significantly; it is unusual to see significant improvement in clinical status if UVB is conducted less than twice/week. Reduction in scaling may be noted after the first three to six treatments and a significant response seen after six to nine treatments. It generally takes 30–40 UVB treatment sessions (usually three months) to induce significant improvement or clearance in an average patient with scattered plaque-type psoriasis. Once patients have achieved marked improvement of their psoriasis, the number of weekly treatments may be slowly tapered over weeks or months to a single weekly exposure. This once weekly "maintenance" regimen may be continued indefinitely to prevent recurrence of psoriasis [24]. In the author's experience,

TABLE 4.1 University of California San Francisco Psoriasis and Skin Treatment Center UVB Dosing Protocols

Broadband UVB: Initial Dosing Protocol			Missed Dosing Protocol	
Skin Type	BBUVB Dose (mj)	Subsequent Increase (mj)	Missed Visit	Action (for all skin types)
I	10	10–50	1–6 days	Increase dose
II	20	10–50	7 days	Repeat last dose
III	30	10–50	8–14 days	Decrease dose by 25%
IV	40	10–50	15–21 days	Decrease dose by 50%
V	50	10–75	22–30 days	Restart with initial dose
VI	60	10–75		

Narrowband UVB: Initial Dosing Protocol			Missed Dosing Protocol	
Skin Type	NBUVB Dose (mj)	Subsequent Increase (mj)	Missed Visit	Action (for all skin types)
I	130	15–50	1–7 days	Increase dose
II	220	15–75	8–11 days	Hold dose constant
III	260	15–100	12–20 days	Decrease by 25%
IV	330	15–150	21–27 days	Decrease by 50%
V	350	15–200	28 or more days	Restart with initial dose
VI	400	15–200		

Patients with any photosensitizing drug, decrease one skin type when starting light; patients adding photosensitizing drugs during therapy, decrease dose by 50%.

the success rate for basic UVB phototherapy ranges from 50% to 80%, depending on how success is defined. With basic UVB phototherapy, most patients show significant improvement or clearance of trunk lesions. In other words, if one makes an allowance for residual lesions on the extremities—such as on the elbows, knees, and shins—approximately 80% of the patients can be considered successfully treated. However, if one aims to achieve a significant improvement or clearing on both the trunk and the extremities, then a more sophisticated approach involving two- or three-step phototherapy is often necessary in many patients. This may include a process in which the entire body is given light first, followed by covering the face and treating the body and, finally, covering the body and trunk and treating the extremities.

A practical text of broadband and narrowband light treatment protocols for psoriasis and other skin disorders is available [25]. Readers should note that different equipment can dramatically change the required protocol. These are guidelines and should be interpreted with flexibility for each patient's requirements. Adjustments should be made according to each patient's response in conjunction with physician judgment.

Optimizing UVB Exposure

Adequate intensity of UV exposure is a basic requirement to maximize therapeutic benefit from phototherapy. The optimal UVB exposure lies at the MED for most patients with

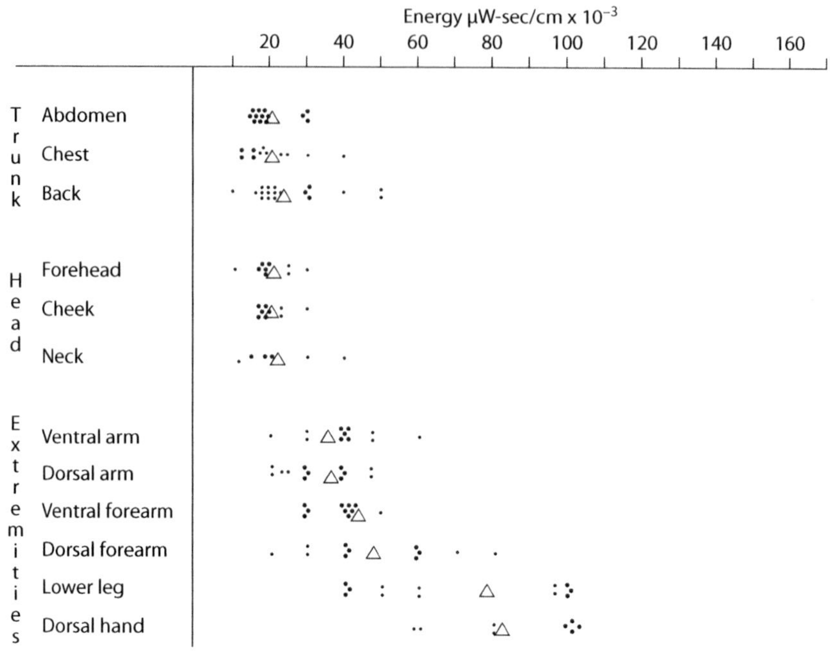

FIGURE 4.2 The MED differs in different parts of the body. (From Olson RL et al., *Arch Dermatol* 93, 211–215, 1996.)

psoriasis [19–22]. However, the task of delivering adequate UVB exposure is complicated by the fact that the MED differs in different anatomical areas (Figure 4.2) [26]. In most patients, the MED assumes its highest value on distal extremities such as elbows and shins; it is lowest in flexural areas including the popliteal and antecubital fossae, face, and anterior chest. The MED usually assumes some midpoint value for the trunk. In fact, the MED for so-called difficult-to-treat areas such as the elbows and shins typically runs two to three times that of the trunk. This is thought to be one explanation for the fact that many patients experience only a partial response to UVB box therapy; they typically improve adequately on their trunk but relatively poorly on their distal extremities.

Rather than declaring these patients UVB-resistant cases, a logical approach is to give extra exposure to those areas that require higher intensity of UVB for optimal therapeutic effect. The simplest way to accomplish this is to practice two-step UVB box phototherapy. The patient goes into a UVB box for overall exposure; the patient comes out of the box to cover areas with a low MED, such as the face (the face should be covered from the start if there are no psoriatic lesions), trunk, and flexural areas; and then the patient goes back into the UVB box for additional exposure to the extremities. One drawback of this method is that the intensity of UVB radiation drops off sharply at the top and bottom of UVB boxes (Figure 4.3) [27]. Ironically, patients end up getting less UVB exposure in precisely the areas that need it most. Because of this, even the two-step approach may not be adequate for optimal UVB exposure to areas such as the shins. A better approach is using equipment such as hot quartz lamps, or Dermalight, that are designed to give intense exposure to localized areas

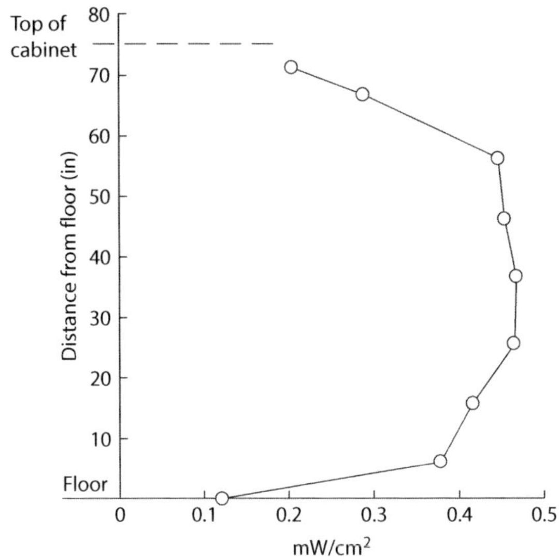

FIGURE 4.3 The intensity of UVB output drops off dramatically at the top and bottom sections of a typical phototherapy box lined with fluorescent lights. (From Chue B et al., *J Am Acad Dermatol* 18, 641–645, 1988.)

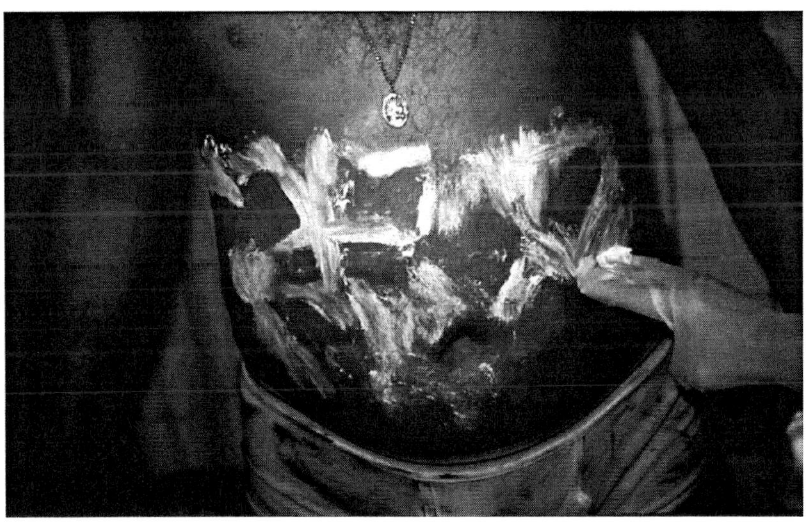

FIGURE 4.4 (See color insert.) Because noninvolved skin burns much more easily than psoriatic plaques, zinc oxide paste is used to protect the noninvolved skin in between the psoriatic plaques before the patient is treated with a high-intensity UVB source such as a hot quartz lamp.

(Figures 4.4 and 4.5). These metal-halide units give off several times the intensity of UVB radiation of traditional fluorescent lamp boxes, and they do not have the fall-off effect characteristic of fluorescent lamps. In short, by exposing different anatomical areas to different intensities of UVB radiation, one can frequently clear lesions that are otherwise resistant to regular UVB box therapy.

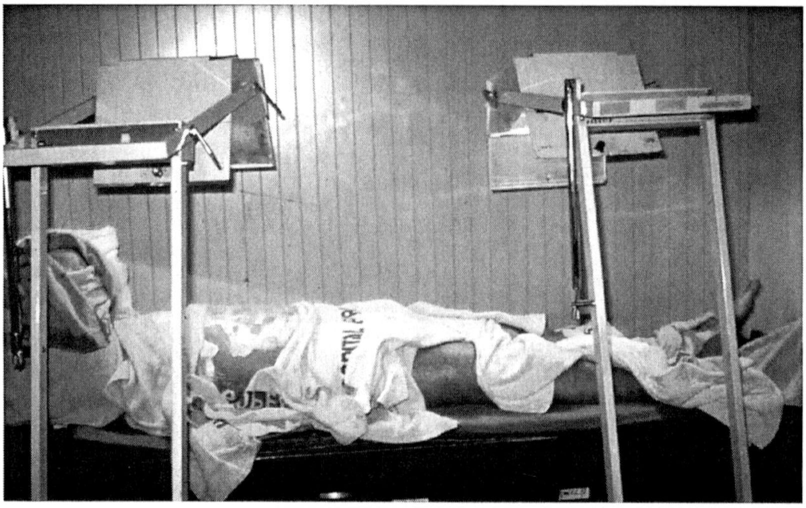

FIGURE 4.5 (See color insert.) Because patients are treated lying down, one advantage of a hot quartz lamp is that it is relatively easy to cover the noninvolved areas with towels to avoid unnecessary exposure to UVB.

NB-UVB Compared to BB-UVB

For the treatment of psoriasis, comparator studies have documented NB-UVB to be more effective than BB-UVB [28–32]. Clearance is more rapid [30,33], requires fewer treatments in some cases, and is preferred by more patients [32,34]. One disadvantage is that NB-UVB requires higher dosages of light to achieve minimal erythema and thus requires longer treatment times than those of BB-UVB [29–34]. This could be difficult for disabled or elderly patients who do not tolerate long periods of standing, and busy clinics may not be able to accommodate large volumes of patients.

To compensate for higher required dosages of light, several options are available. NB-UVB boxes are sold containing 24–48 bulbs, whereas standard UVB boxes typically contain 8–16 bulbs. More bulbs correspond to shorter treatment times. Several reports indicate that psoriasis does clear with less aggressive NB regimens that do not lead to erythema [3,35–37]. Therefore, treatment times may be shortened without sacrificing efficacy. Finally, as discussed earlier, combination therapy should be considered as a way to shorten treatment times. Each method of treatment may not clear psoriasis completely but when used in combination may produce results better than either modality used alone. NB-UVB is no exception to this rule. Combination therapy can reduce light treatment times and light dosing requirements. Studies demonstrate that combining NB-UVB with tazarotene gel, anthralin, or calcipotriol can provide faster, more effective clearance with less irradiation and fewer treatments [38–40].

Remission Rates with NB-UVB

Few data are available comparing remission rates of NB-UVB and BB-UVB. In one study, the authors reported a stark difference in remission rates favoring NB-UVB [33]. Thirty-eight percent of the NB-UVB group was still in remission one year after cessation of therapy.

The average time to relapse was three months for the remaining 62%. Only 5% of BB-UVB patients in a different study conducted by the same investigators were still in remission one year after treatment. Time to relapse was not mentioned for this group. This comparison may be flawed because the BB-UVB group was much smaller than the NB-UVB group, the studies were conducted at different times, and the BB-UVB therapy may have been suboptimal as evidenced by the high burning rates even with a regimen of only twice-weekly therapy. However, in another 52-patient cohort study, Psoriasis Area and Severity Index (PASI) 50 was retained in 56% of the patients for at least one year after a four-week course of NB-UVB phototherapy, demonstrating its long-term efficacy [41].

NB-UVB Compared to PUVA

There are several factors to consider when comparing NB-UVB to PUVA including efficacy, carcinogenesis, remission rates, and ease of administration. The first investigations comparing the efficacy of PUVA and NB-UVB were conducted in 1990 using bilateral comparison methods in patients with widespread psoriasis [42]. Although the two treatments were found to be equally effective, more patients preferred NB-UVB. Looking more closely at the data revealed that PUVA was actually more effective in clearing extremities, and NB-UVB was more effective in clearing trunk psoriasis. These findings indicated that PUVA might be better for clearing lesions that are more recalcitrant to therapy, such as those usually found on the extremities. Other studies have reported similar findings [36,43]. The most recent study done in 2006 showed that, of 71 patients with skin types I to IV, 84% cleared on PUVA while 65% cleared on NB-UVB. Patients had cleared on PUVA with a significantly lower average number of sessions and with a larger mean reduction in PASI scores compared to NB-UVB. Sixty-eight percent of patients that cleared on PUVA were still clear of their psoriasis at six months while 35% of patients cleared on NB-UVB were still clear at six months. Clearance rates did not vary with severity. The largest study comparing NB-UVB to PUVA involved 100 patients and demonstrated that given twice weekly PUVA is more effective than NB-UVB with significantly fewer treatments and almost three times the remission rate at six months after treatment [44]. PUVA is well known to induce remission rates of four to six months or even longer, a definite advantage over NB-UVB. For palmoplantar psoriasis, PUVA may be a more efficacious option as well. In a study of 21 patients treated with PUVA on one hand and NB-UVB on the other, an average improvement of 85% was seen in PUVA-treated hands while an improvement of 61% was seen on NB-UVB–treated hands. NB-UVB may not penetrate the skin as effectively as PUVA [45].

One major disadvantage associated with long-term PUVA is the risk of skin cancer, especially in fair-skinned Caucasian patients [46]. In contrast, there is no reliable association between skin cancer and long-term UVB phototherapy. Most of the epidemiological studies in which patients on long-term UVB therapies were followed for up to two decades in the United States and Europe failed to show any increase in skin cancer rates when compared to the general population [47]. Further, NB-UVB offers some major logistical advantages over PUVA that may be important when choosing therapy for an individual patient. It is less time-consuming and easier to perform, and does not require concomitant administration of a photosensitizer (i.e., psoralen) that may cause nausea, cataracts, phototoxic reactions, and unwanted drug reactions. Other advantages also include safe use in pregnant women and children and no drug costs.

NB-UVB for the Treatment of Other Skin Diseases

Although NB-UVB is promoted for the treatment of psoriasis, it may prove to be beneficial for other recalcitrant skin diseases. As any dermatologist knows, management of atopic dermatitis can be challenging and often unsatisfactory. Current methods of treatment can result in severe cutaneous and systemic side effects. Over the past 10 years, several studies have shown NB-UVB to be a hopeful option for patients with atopic dermatitis [48–51]. Seborrheic dermatitis is another persistent skin disease affecting 2%–10% of the adult population. One study has shown the effectiveness of NB-UVB in seborrheic dermatitis [52]. NB-UVB is also a suitable alternative for treating photodermatoses and may be especially useful for UVA-sensitive patients: those with actinic prurigo, hydroa vacciniforme, idiopathic solar urticaria, polymorphic light eruption, pityriasis lichenoides, and nodular prurigo [53–57]. In these patients, NB-UVB produces a hardening photoprotective effect while avoiding the risk of provocation by UVA wavelengths. NB-UVB treatment has been shown to be promising for treatment of vitiligo [58,59] and to be safe and effective in childhood vitiligo, significantly improving patients' quality of life [60].

Side Effects of NB-UVB

Similar to other phototherapies, the side effects of NB-UVB include erythema and blistering, but they may be more severe. Compared to PUVA, a greater proportion of patients treated with NB-UVB develop erythema, but PUVA-treated patients are more likely to miss treatments due to burning, which is a reflection of the long-lasting nature of PUVA erythema [44]. Data on the incidence and severity of burning when compared to BB-UVB are controversial. Burning episodes with NB-UVB have been reported as fewer than [32,33], equal to [31], and more [30,61] than those with BB-UVB. Tissue biopsies obtained from 1.0 to 2.0 MED sites reveal that the frequency of sunburn cells is similar at 1.0 MED but 10–12 times greater in NB-UVB than BB-UVB at 2.0 MED [30]. In addition, these cells are more widely distributed throughout the epidermis in NB-UVB-treated skin. These findings suggest more damaging potential of NB-UVB when 1.0 MED is exceeded. Animal studies similarly demonstrated more severe and persistent burning [62].

With NB-UVB therapy, there have also been some reports of rare blistering strictly at the site of psoriatic lesions while the surrounding normal skin remains completely unaffected [43,63,64]. Some have speculated that due to the rapid clearance by NB-UVB, the psoriatic plaques may not gain the same photoprotection as the surrounding normal skin, thus exposing them to a burning dose midway through treatment [63]. Other authors similarly concluded after histological examination that blisters result from quick reduction of acanthosis and desquamation before the development of tolerance, which results from an increase in pigmentation and stratum corneum thickness [64].

Safety of NB-UVB

In patients treated for many years with conventional BB-UVB, there is little or no increased risk of skin cancer [65]. In a large retrospective study involving 2886 NB-UVB-treated patients, the number of cases of basal cell carcinomas (BCC), squamous cell carcinomas (SCC), and melanomas was comparable to the matched populations [66]. Only patients that were receiving both NB-UVB and PUVA had a higher incidence of BCC than the expected incidence in the general population.

In a follow-up study involving 195 patients who received either BB- or NB-UVB treatment for psoriasis, one patient developed melanoma *in situ*. The diagnosis was made during the same year phototherapy was instituted. Thus, the development of melanoma may have been unrelated to the limited number of UVB exposure [67]. Another study followed patients who had long-term NB-UVB treatment with an average duration of four years of therapy. The study found no incidence of melanoma or squamous cell carcinoma (SCC) [68]. Ten patients developed basal carcinoma mostly on the face as compared to the expected incidence of 4.7 in the matched population. The predilection of BCC for the face may be due to increase in solar exposure because patients with psoriasis often engage in this self-treatment, whereas office-based phototherapy typically entails covering the patient's face during whole-body UVB (or PUVA) irradiation.

AGGRESSIVE UVB THERAPY

There are many different ways to enhance UVB phototherapy. Generally, the strategies for enhancement fall into three different categories: optimizing UVB exposure (discussed earlier), combining UVB phototherapy with topical agents, and combining UVB phototherapy with systemic agents. These three strategies are not mutually exclusive. For a physician faced with a truly recalcitrant case, it is often possible to prevail by combining all three approaches because they generally work synergistically. By using these strategies, it is possible to make UVB therapy nearly as therapeutically efficacious as PUVA therapy or as systemic agents. The newest form of UVB phototherapy, excimer laser therapy, is also an aggressive and effective form of therapy for recalcitrant psoriatic plaques.

Enhancing UVB Phototherapy with Topical Agents

Keratolytics Thick, micaceous psoriatic scales scatter light, and any light that is not absorbed into the skin is wasted. Using keratolytic agents to remove as much scale as possible diminishes this problem and enhances the therapeutic effect of phototherapy. This measure is especially important in UVB phototherapy because UVB rays cannot penetrate the skin as deeply as UVA rays. Keralyt Gel is a topical salicylic acid preparation frequently used for this purpose. For thicker and more resistant lesions, pharmacists can compound higher concentrations of salicylic acid in liquor carbonis detergens (LCD) or in crude coal tar for use under occlusion for maximal keratolytic effect. At the University of California San Francisco (UCSF) Medical Center, 10% crude coal tar (black tar, Koppers Company, Pittsburgh, PA) with up to 10% salicylic acid (Spectrum Chemical Manufacturing, Gardena, CA) in petrolatum is often used for extremely hyperkeratotic lesions on the palms, soles, elbows, and shins under plastic wrap, gloves, or shower cap occlusion. Shower caps work well for occluding the soles when held in place with a sock. If the patient cannot tolerate salicylic acid, topical lactic acid preparations up to prescription strength can be used in place of salicylic acid. Ideally, psoriatic lesions should be kept relatively free of scaling during UVB phototherapy. In a minority of cases where these measures are still not adequate, low-dosage acitretin can be used to minimize hyperkeratosis and induration. At some phototherapy units, mineral oil or clear emollients are applied prior to light therapy; these agents do not block UVB light penetration and are thus acceptable to use before phototherapy [69].

Tar There are many commercially available tar preparations, including creams, shampoos, and soaks. High concentrations of tar can be compounded to enhance the therapeutic effect. If the pharmacist has the right equipment, LCD can be compounded up to 20% concentration in Aquaphor®, and the original black tar can be compounded up to 10% concentration in petrolatum. It is generally accepted by dermatologists who run day treatment programs that black tar holds a significant therapeutic advantage over LCD or other refined tar products. Several studies suggest that when the MED is reached in UVB therapy, tar may not add much benefit for most patients with psoriasis [19–22]. As mentioned earlier, in practice, it is frequently not feasible to attain minimal erythema because patients often complain of burning, stinging, and other uncomfortable symptoms. On the other hand, when the intensity of the UVB therapy is titrated to a *sub*erythemogenic level, tar preparations provide additional therapeutic benefit [15]. In practice, if patients are willing, *sub*erythemogenic doses of UVB are used together with tar preparations.

At our UCSF Psoriasis Treatment Center, patients admitted for all day Goeckerman therapy have previously failed to respond to outpatient regimens using 20% LCD in Aquaphor and intense UVB exposure, yet their skin routinely clears with the use of true black tar supplemented with UVB phototherapy. Although this may represent greater efficacy of black tar over other tar preparations, it may also reflect the difficulty to comply with tar products in the home setting.

In the day treatment setting, 10% crude coal tar with up to 10% salicylic acid in petrolatum is typically the strongest regimen used. This preparation is very difficult to use at home because of its messiness. However, if patients are highly motivated, it is possible to prescribe this formulation for home use to localized resistant areas such as shins and elbows. Many patients with truly recalcitrant and indurated lesions find that they can apply this under plastic wrap occlusion overnight without experiencing irritation or folliculitis.

Anthralin Ingram therapy consists of the combined used of anthralin and UVB phototherapy. Anthralin powder (Paddock Labs, Minneapolis, MN) is available commercially, and can be compounded up to 10% concentration. Compounded anthralin can be prepared in a cream base with salicylic acid in concentrations of 3%, 5%, or 10%. Salicylic acid functions both as the preservative for anthralin and as a keratolytic agent. Higher concentrations of anthralin should be used only on patients who can tolerate 1% anthralin (Psoriatec, Sirius Laboratories, Sweden) without irritation. Compounded anthralin is most often used as a short contact agent and applied to the skin for at least 30–60 minutes once daily. Some patients with recalcitrant, indurated psoriatic plaques can tolerate even higher concentrations of anthralin under plastic wrap occlusion overnight.

The use of compounded anthralin and black tar is not mutually exclusive. In fact, some have suggested that patients would experience less irritation from anthralin if black tar were used concurrently. It has been shown that adding crude coal tar to anthralin reduces skin irritation without compromising antipsoriatic efficacy [70]. At our clinic, the most common use of compounded anthralin in an outpatient setting is a short contact application in the evening to be washed off at bedtime and followed by tar. If the patient tolerates prolonged applications of compounded anthralin, the tar is then simply applied over the anthralin at bedtime, and they are both washed off in the morning. In this way, both anthralin and tar can be used to enhance UVB phototherapy. In patients with both large plaques and scattered small plaques, anthralin can be used on the larger lesions although tar may be used on the scattered lesions that are less amenable to the careful application of anthralin.

COMBINATION USE OF UVB PHOTOTHERAPY AND CALCIPOTRIENE OR TAZAROTENE

A number of calcipotriene and UVB regimens have been studied [71]. Twice-weekly UVB with twice-daily calcipotriol cream proves to be just as effective as UVB three times/week with only vehicle cream applied twice daily [72]. This equivalent therapeutic result was obtained with less than one-third the cumulative UVB exposure in the calcipotriol cream group compared to the vehicle cream group. This finding is important because there are many patients who are simply too busy to do UVB phototherapy three times/week, but can do it twice/week. For patients who have copayments for visits, cutting down on the number of UVB visits/week is ideal. Due to rare reports of an immediate burning sensation when calcipotriol is applied around the same time as UVB phototherapy, it should not be applied within two to three hours prior to exposure.

Tazarotene also enhances UVB phototherapy significantly, even if phototherapy is conducted aggressively three times/week [73]. In a multicenter study headed by Koo et al., tazarotene 0.1% gel applied only three times/week was found to enhance aggressive UVB phototherapy regimens significantly. A statistically significant difference was noted between active agent and UVB phototherapy compared to UVB alone or UVB plus vehicle in the number of patients who achieved marked improvement (i.e., 75% or better improvement). The cumulative UVB exposure for the group receiving tazarotene three times/week plus UVB phototherapy was less than one-quarter the UVB exposure required in the other two groups to reach a threshold of 50% improvement in their lesional scores. No unusual photosensitivity from tazarotene was noted in the entire clinical trial. Because tazarotene was only applied three times/week after UVB phototherapy, whether or not photosensitivity would have occurred if tazarotene were applied daily or just prior to UVB exposure is unknown.

COMBINATION THERAPY WITH PUVA PHOTOTHERAPY

UVB therapy and PUVA therapy can be combined for an additive effect. This combination is especially useful for those patients who experience a flare of their psoriasis despite the use of their home UVB light box. In theory, PUVA and UVB can be combined as long as each session is separated by at least 24 hours to ensure that the blood level of psoralen

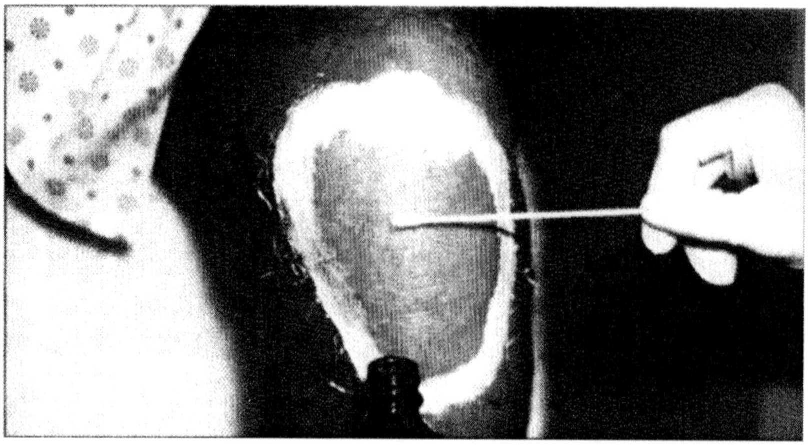

FIGURE 4.6 (See color insert.) The application of topical "paint" PUVA therapy to selected, resistant psoriatic plaque. Zinc oxide paste is sometimes used to prevent inadvertent application of 0.1% Oxsoralen solution to the noninvolved skin.

reaches zero before the patient is exposed to UVB. This so-called washout time is critical because many UVB boxes also emit some UVA radiation leading to overexposure if treatments were conducted without adequate time between them. There are many patients whose skin clears adequately when PUVA therapy is based on the above schedule, even though these patients fail to respond adequately to PUVA or UVB alone. For patients who are using home UVB and yet experience a gradual flare, twice-weekly supplementation with PUVA frequently allows their psoriatic lesions to clear. Also, patients undergoing UVB therapy who are left with a few truly resistant lesions in areas such as elbows and shins can often clear with topical paint PUVA therapy. Oxsoralen® solution or ointment is applied selectively to the resistant plaques followed in 30 minutes by exposure to UVA radiation (Figure 4.6).

DAY TREATMENT PROGRAM

Day treatment programs can be viewed as the ultimate attempt short of hospitalization to maximize the efficacy of UVB phototherapy. This regimen was developed mainly to minimize the cost of treatment from inpatient hospitalization because patients with severe, generalized psoriasis often require a treatment period of four to six weeks to clear their psoriasis completely. Traditionally, day treatment programs can be classified into two main types: Goeckerman therapy and Ingram therapy. However, with enough attention to detail, it is possible to use tar and anthralin simultaneously. Topical PUVA can also be conducted simultaneously with UVB phototherapy. At the UCSF Medical Center, the main treatment modality in the day treatment program is Goeckerman therapy, which combines crude coal tar with UVB phototherapy. If a patient proves to have a truly recalcitrant case of psoriasis, therapy can be escalated to combine Goeckerman, Ingram, and bath PUVA, while supplementing with oral retinoids, calcipotriol, and/or tazarotene. (See Chapter 6 for further information on the Goeckerman day treatment program.)

COMBINATION THERAPY WITH SYSTEMIC AGENTS

Retinoids

In many ways, retinoids such as acitretin are better suited for use in low dosages to enhance phototherapy than in high dosages as monotherapy (see Chapter 8, Systemic Retinoids). Acitretin has been shown to enhance efficacy of UVB phototherapy. In an eight-week, randomized, comparator study, more than twice the number of patients in the combined BB-UVB and acitretin cohort reached PASI 75 as compared to the BB-UVB only cohort [74]. When acitretin is used to enhance PUVA or UVB phototherapy, the dosage required often ranges from 25 mg every other day up to 50 mg/day. Sometimes as little as 10 mg/day may be adequate to enhance phototherapy. Acitretin is especially useful for patients with extremely indurated and hyperkeratotic lesions into which UVB radiation may not penetrate adequately unless the lesion is thinned by keratolytic agents (as described earlier) or by retinoids. Lastly, if a female patient of childbearing age requires retinoid supplementation, isotretinoin in a similar dosage can be used to enhance phototherapy. This agent is also teratogenic but has a shorter half-life.

There are two approaches when using acitretin to enhance UVB phototherapy. The first is to start the patient on acitretin approximately two weeks before starting phototherapy in order to prepare the skin for phototherapy. The second is to reserve low-dosage acitretin as a supplement after attempted UVB phototherapy alone proves unsatisfactory. Many patients who are motivated to commit the time and effort required for phototherapy prefer the latter approach to avoid the use of systemic agents. On the other hand, adding low-dosage acitretin to established UVB phototherapy increases the possibility of developing delayed photosensitivity. The phenomenon "delayed retinoid burn" was first reported in the medical literature when a psoriasis patient experienced a severe phototoxic reaction as a result of adding acitretin 25 mg daily to a previously tolerated UVB dose. Because acitretin induces cell differentiation and leads to sloughing of keratinocytes from psoriatic plaques, this leads to excessive light penetration and results in phototoxicity. To prevent this adverse event, the authors suggest reducing the UV dose by 50% if a concomitant oral retinoid therapy is started [75].

Hydroxyurea

Hydroxyurea (Hydrea®) is another systemic agent that can be used to enhance UVB or PUVA phototherapy. The usual dosage for a healthy, average-sized adult is 500 mg orally twice daily. Although hydroxyurea is certainly not as effective as methotrexate, similar to low-dosage acitretin, it is well suited for long-term enhancement of phototherapy in patients who experience a partial but less than adequate response to phototherapy alone. One of the main advantages of hydroxyurea is the minimal risk of hepatotoxicity associated with its long-term use. Hydroxyurea can be an alternative for a patient who is a candidate for methotrexate but refuses to consider the possibility of undergoing a liver biopsy. Another advantage is that hydroxyurea used to enhance UVB phototherapy does not increase the risk of photosensitivity. However, hydroxyurea has a narrow therapeutic index and can be associated with bone marrow suppression and nephrotoxicity. Therefore, complete blood count (CBC), liver function tests (LFT), and measurements of blood urea nitrogen (BUN) and creatinine should be periodically followed while using this agent.

Almost every patient who is on long-term treatment with hydroxyurea develops macrocytosis. Because it is usually not associated with anemia, the clinical relevance is questionable. Taking 1 mg/day folic acid minimizes the risk of macrocytic anemia. Although hydroxyurea is well described in the medical literature with respect to its use in psoriasis therapy, this drug is not approved by the U.S. Food and Drug Administration (FDA) for the treatment of psoriasis.

Methotrexate

Methotrexate can be used in conjunction with UVB phototherapy but with extreme caution due to the rare risk of acute photosensitivity (see Chapter 9 on methotrexate) [76]. There are at least three settings in which methotrexate may be combined with phototherapy or used prior to the initiation of phototherapy:

1. Methotrexate is used to control widespread inflammation in a patient presenting with intense erythroderma prior to starting UVB phototherapy. This is especially useful if the patient is not a candidate for cyclosporine or is unable to participate in day treatment.
2. Methotrexate is used in the short term while initiating UVB phototherapy as an initial push to the therapeutic process.
3. Methotrexate is used to enhance phototherapy when a patient's response to UVB phototherapy plateaus. In this situation, hydroxyurea or acitretin can also be used to accomplish the same result. A decision to use methotrexate depends on factors such as the patient's prior response to methotrexate, intolerance to other agents, or, in the case of acitretin, their reproductive status.

Because of the aforementioned risk of acute photosensitivity induced by methotrexate, it is critical that the patient not be exposed to phototherapy for 48–72 hours during and following methotrexate treatment. For example, a patient undergoing UVB phototherapy on Mondays, Wednesdays, and Fridays may start a weekly dose of methotrexate on Friday morning right after receiving phototherapy. By the time he or she returns for UVB phototherapy on Monday, the risk of methotrexate photosensitivity is negligible. By using this combination, one can minimize the cumulative methotrexate needed to clear the psoriasis. Once the psoriasis clears completely, methotrexate can be discontinued altogether and the patient's disease can usually be controlled with UVB phototherapy alone.

In addition, some patients are referred to outpatient UVB therapy or to the day treatment program for the specific purpose of tapering off methotrexate. These are generally patients who have already received a high cumulative dosage of methotrexate. The same precautions regarding acute photosensitivity must be observed while initiating UVB phototherapy.

In a study comparing sequential treatment of methotrexate with NB-UVB to NB-UVB phototherapy alone, 24 patients with more than or equal to 20% body surface area (BSA) affected by plaque psoriasis were randomly assigned to receive methotrexate 15 mg/week or placebo 15 mg/week for three weeks, prior to starting a standard phototherapy regimen [77].

Patients received NB-UVB phototherapy three times/week with initial dosage of UVB at 70% of the patient's MED, and dosages were increased by 20%, 10%, or 0% depending on the patient's reaction to light. UVB dose was increased in an incremental fashion until the patient achieved clearance defined as a 90% reduction in the PASI score, or at 24 weeks, whichever came first. In patients receiving methotrexate and NB-UVB, the median PASI score at the end of the treatment period was 0.15, as compared to 3.15 in the placebo–NB-UVB group. In the methotrexate–NB-UVB group, 10 of 11 (90.9%) patients achieved clearance, again defined as a reduction in the PASI score by 90%, as compared to 5 of 13 (38.5%) patients in the placebo–NB-UVB group. When comparing mean cumulative UVB dose in each treatment arm, patients who achieved clearance in the methotrexate–NB-UVB arm received 26.92 J/cm^2 as compared to 59.25 J/cm^2 for patients in the placebo group. For those patients receiving methotrexate, median time until clearance was approximately four weeks. In general, both treatment regimens were well tolerated; adverse events included two episodes of erythema in each group and generalized hyperpigmentation in all patients. Another study reported that the combination of methotrexate and NB-UVB phototherapy provided more rapid clinical improvement (compared with NB-UVB monotherapy) in the treatment of chronic plaque-type psoriasis. There were greater reports of increased itching and erythema in those patients receiving NB-UVB; nausea was the one adverse event that was only reported by those patients receiving methotrexate and NB-UVB [78]. Thus, combination therapy of methotrexate with NB-UVB phototherapy may be efficacious in the treatment of plaque-type psoriasis, but further randomized, controlled clinical trials with larger patient populations should be done to study the safety and efficacy of this combination.

Cyclosporine

In theory, the combination of cyclosporine and phototherapy (especially PUVA therapy) can increase the risk of skin cancer in Caucasian patients. Long-term use of cyclosporine with phototherapeutic modalities is not currently recommended [79]. However, there is one frequently encountered group in which cyclosporine can be of great assistance in conducting phototherapy—patients with widespread, highly inflammatory lesions. Controlling inflammation is critical in setting the stage for initiating phototherapy. Erythrodermic patients have a great risk of developing a paradoxical reaction with either UVB or PUVA therapy; their skin becomes more inflamed if phototherapy is initiated. Therefore, adequate control of the inflammatory state is critical before these patients can be safely started on a phototherapy regimen.

For many decades, this process of cooling down was accomplished in an inpatient setting with topical steroids, cool compresses, and soothing baths. More recently, limited reimbursement has led to new approaches such as short-term oral cyclosporine (3–5 mg/kg divided twice daily), which can be extremely effective in controlling erythema and inflammation (Figure 4.7) (see Chapter 10 on cyclosporine). One can conceivably use methotrexate or acitretin for controlling erythroderma; however, cyclosporine has a faster onset of action, no required test dose, and it more reliably controls widespread inflammation. Once the skin is no longer severely erythematous, phototherapy with UVB or PUVA can be initiated

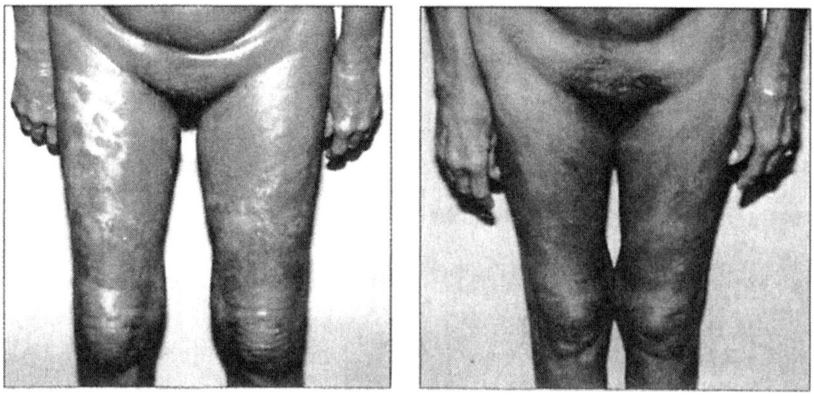

(a) (b)

FIGURE 4.7 (See color insert.) Erythrodermic patient with psoriasis and intense leg edema (a) before and (b) after short-term cyclosporine followed by long-term UVB phototherapy. This therapeutic regimen makes use of the powerful anti-inflammatory property of cyclosporine while minimizing the risk of systemic effects, which may be associated with long-term use of cyclosporine.

and the cyclosporine dosage tapered down to 3 mg/kg/day. It can be gradually tapered off altogether once phototherapy is optimized and the patient's erythroderma has resolved. Using cyclosporine for short periods of time (three months or less) decreases the risk of side effects such as nephrotoxicity. Hypertension may be encountered but is readily reversible with initiation of an antihypertensive agent or by adjusting the dosage of cyclosporine. Moreover, the theoretical increased risk of malignancy can also be minimized by short-term use [80,81].

In a 2003 study, sequential therapy with cyclosporine and NB-UVB was compared to therapy with NB-UVB alone [82]. In this study, 30 patients with severe psoriasis received 3 mg/kg/day of cyclosporine for four weeks, followed by phototherapy with NB-UVB three times/week. The dose of cyclosporine was reduced by 1 mg/kg/week until discontinuation. The other treatment arm consisted of 30 patients receiving NB-UVB three times weekly with no systemic medication. In both groups, phototherapy was continued until a patient had a PASI score of 0 or until the patient had the same PASI score in two subsequent weekly evaluations. In both treatment groups, there was an effective reduction in the PASI score. In the group receiving sequential therapy of cyclosporine and NB-UVB, the mean baseline PASI score was 28.58. After four weeks of treatment, these patients had an average PASI score of 12.38 and a mean PASI score of 1.95 at the end of the treatment cycle. In the group receiving phototherapy alone, the mean baseline PASI score was 26.69, with an average PASI score of 14.38 after four weeks of therapy and a mean PASI score of 2.37 at the end of the treatment cycle. The difference in final mean PASI scores, favoring the cyclosporine treatment arm, may be attributed to better control of psoriatic lesions in areas that are completely or almost completely UV shielded, such as the armpits and inner thighs. When comparing the total number of NB-UVB exposures and cumulative dosages of light therapy, the sequential therapy group had an average of 12.11 NB-UVB exposures as compared to 19.59 exposures in group receiving phototherapy alone. In addition, the cyclosporine treatment arm received less cumulative dosage of UVB light at 8.94 J/cm^2 as compared to 18.34 J/cm^2 in the group receiving phototherapy alone. Overall, patients receiving sequential therapy with cyclosporine and NB-UVB and those receiving NB-UVB alone achieved marked improvement in their PASI scores, and treatment regimens were well tolerated in both study arms. However, in patients receiving four weeks of cyclosporine treatment, the number of NB-UVB exposures and cumulative dosage of UVB light was decreased. This may be a significant factor to consider for patients who live far from a phototherapy facility or whose busy schedule makes numerous phototherapy sessions difficult to comply with.

Biologic Agents

Narrowband UVB phototherapy was combined with the biologic agent etanercept (ENBREL®) in the Utilization of Narrowband UVB Phototherapy and Etanercept for the Treatment of Psoriasis (UNITE) study [83]. Patients with moderate to severe plaque psoriasis were eligible for the study if they met the following criteria: PASI score of more than or equal to 15, body surface area (BSA) involvement of more than or equal to 5%, and at least 25% of plaques considered severe [83]. Patients who had received previous or current anti-tumor necrosis factor-alpha (TNF-α) therapy were excluded. The study was a 12-week, single-arm, open-label study with 86 patients participating in 14 sites. Patients received 50 mg etanercept biweekly as subcutaneous injections and NB-UVB treatment three times/week. For the NB-UVB regimen, the dosage was escalated at 10%–15% of the preceding dose, with initial dosage determined by the patient's Fitzpatrick skin type.

The majority of patients in this clinical trial had severe psoriasis at baseline, with an average of 28% BSA affected [83]. After 12 weeks of combination therapy, 85% of patients achieved a PASI 75 response and 58% of patients achieved a PASI 90 response. At week 12, 26% of patients achieved PASI 100, or complete clearing of their psoriasis. When looking at length of time to achieve a response, 50% of patients achieved PASI 75 after 57 days and 75% of patients achieved a PASI 75 response after 84 days of combination therapy. In addition, improvement was seen in the patient-reported Dermatology Life Quality Index with a mean improvement from baseline of 84.4%.

The most common adverse events experienced with combination NB-UVB and etanercept included UVB-induced skin injury (62.8% of patients), injection-site reactions (20.9%), nasopharyngitis (5.8%), and upper respiratory tract infections (3.5%) [83]. Overall, the combination of NB-UVB with etanercept was well tolerated and very efficacious in the treatment of moderate to severe plaque psoriasis in adults.

Economics of NB-UVB

Starting an NB-UVB practice or adding it to an existing one is costly, due to the requirements for equipment, replacement parts, bulbs, staff training, and the increased overhead expense. Currently, reimbursement for NB-UVB is no different than that for UVB; a separate, current procedural terminology billing code has not yet been established. Many options are available when purchasing a NB-UVB unit. As of this writing, units with 48 bulbs range in cost from US$16,000 to 21,500. Units with fewer bulbs are cost effective. The best unit for a busy practice is one with the most bulbs so that clinics are not slowed and patients are not forced to stand for long periods of time due to longer treatments. Combination boxes provide less intense NB-UVB light and thus require longer treatment times, which is a disadvantage in a busy phototherapy practice. For small phototherapy practices, cheaper options include units without fans, standing platforms, built-in dosimetry and protocols, or panel units. Panel units are typically used for home NB-UVB therapy but are sometimes sold to clinics as well. NB-UVB phototherapy is also available in hand and foot units or in handheld units for localized areas, hard-to-reach places, and the scalp, to be used with a removable comb attachment.

Available since 1989, NB-UVB bulbs (TL-01 fluorescent lamps) are manufactured by the Phillips Company in Holland. They are sold in four sizes: 6 ft bulbs, 2 ft bulbs, 22 in. twin tubes, and 7 in. twin tubes. The need for more bulbs with NB-UVB as compared to BB-UVB translates to higher relamping costs. Bulb prices are shown in Tables 4.2 and 4.3. At this writing, National Biologic sells 6 ft NB-UVB bulbs for $125 ($25 more than BB-UVB bulbs of the same size). Daavlin offers the two products each for $105. The Psoralite Corporation offers the 6 ft bulbs for $105. The running life span of the TL-01 has not yet been well quantified, and estimates vary from 300 to 500 hours. In practice, the bulb life expectancy seems to be shorter than that of BB-UVB or UVA bulbs, thus requiring more frequent replacements, which also increases the cost of NB-UVB versus BB-UVB.

Measuring light output is an important part of safe and effective phototherapy. Some machines are sold with built-in dosimetry meters so that output is machine-monitored and calibration needs to be done only once yearly. Daavlin offers a meter for UVA, BB-UVB,

TABLE 4.2 NB-UVB Options and Prices Offered by Psoralite Corporation

Unit	Number of Lamps	Price (US$)
Model 57000–44 NB	44	15,595
Model 57000–36 NB	36	13,995
Model 57000–24 NB	24	11,995

TABLE 4.3 NB-UVB Options and Prices Offered by Daavlin Corporation

Unit	Number of Lamps	Price (US$)
Spectra 311-48	48	21,500
Spectra 311-24	24	18,000
Spectra 311-350	24 NB/24 UVA	20,500
Theraflex 311-48	4	16,090
Theraflex 311-24	24	14,000
Theraflex 311-350	24 NB 24 BB	16,250
Theraflex 311-305	36 NB 12 BB	17,500
UVA 6-ft lamp	Single bulb	20
NB-UVB 6-ft lamp	Single bulb	105
BB-UVB 6-ft lamp	Single bulb	105
UVA 2-ft lamp	Single bulb	22
NB-UVB 2-ft lamp	Single bulb	75
BB-UVB 2-ft lamp	Single bulb	75

and NB-UVB, for $2400 or a three-year plan in which maintenance personnel perform the measurement for a package price of $1500. National Biologic offers UVB meters for $690. It has been common practice to use a BB-UVB meter device for both BB-UVB and NB-UVB although Daavlin now offers a device specifically for NB-UVB for $1400. Manufacturers recommend replacing the bulbs when energy output drops to 0.75 mW/cm^2. However, because energy output decreases with the continuous usage of the bulb, patients must remain in the light box for longer periods of time in order to receive the adequate dose. In a high-volume practice, it is more cost-effective to replace bulbs promptly and to maintain short patient visits; however, in a low-volume practice, it is more cost-effective to replace bulbs less frequently thereby requiring longer patient visits.

LOCALIZED PHOTOTHERAPY FOR PSORIASIS

As discussed earlier, UVB is an effective treatment for patients with severe generalized psoriasis. Because long-term follow-up studies detect no increased risk of skin cancer following UVB phototherapy, it probably offers among the best risk/benefit ratios of any of the treatments for generalized psoriasis. In a review by Lee et al., 10 out of the 11 studies showed no increased skin cancer risk with UVB phototherapy [84]. Although there are few head-to-head trials comparing different treatments, the clearance rate reported for UVB is quite respectable [85].

Most patients with psoriasis, however, have relatively localized disease treated primarily with topical agents. Although topical agents are generally more convenient than phototherapy and systemic therapy, they are also considerably less so for generalized psoriasis patients. Moreover, although patients with generalized disease are often quite satisfied with a reduction in the disease and associated symptoms, patients who present for treatment with very localized disease are often unsatisfied unless full clearance of the lesions is achieved.

The use of UVB phototherapy on a localized basis offers the potential of a more effective option for localized plaques refractory to topicals alone. Although localized phototherapy can be achieved with the use of standard phototherapy equipment and careful blocking of surrounding skin, the use of a UVB laser makes this procedure better suited for a clinical practice. This modality is also a potential treatment option for specific, perhaps more resistant, lesions in patients with more extensive disease.

Unmet Need for Localized Psoriasis Treatment

Patients with psoriasis desire a treatment that provides high efficacy, including clearance of the lesions, and a long-term, treatment-free remission of the disease [86]. Patients also seek therapies that are safe, convenient, and inexpensive. Compared to topical therapies, localized UV therapy meets many of these goals except, perhaps, that of low cost.

Ultraviolet Laser Therapy

One of the newest advances in phototherapy is targeted UVB excimer laser therapy. The excimer laser device is a major technical achievement and is manufactured by multiple companies. The authors are most familiar with the manufacturer PhotoMedex and use the

PhotoMedex XTRAC® Ultra and newer XTRAC® Velocity laser machines. Targeted UVB laser therapy is one of the newest and most efficacious treatments for psoriasis. This laser is based on a xenon-chloride lasing medium, which produces UV light at a wavelength of 308 nm. At high fluences, 308 nm light can be used to ablate tissue, such as cornea or atherosclerotic plaque, or other materials [87,88]. At the relatively low fluences used to treat psoriatic plaques, the laser does not destroy tissue but rather acts as a form of localized UVB phototherapy. The excimer laser is 308 nm (0.1 angstroms wide), and this narrowband is near the optimal peak of the psoriasis action spectrum. Excimer laser phototherapy is narrower than NB-UVB, which ranges from 308 to 313 nm in wavelength. Perhaps due to the coherence of laser light, this may provide some benefit over traditional forms of UV phototherapy [89].

The excimer laser device requires an optically pure fiber optic cable to deliver the monochromatic 308 nm UV light. Currently, the excimer laser has been used in more than 400,000 treatments, where approximately 80% were for patients with psoriasis. Laser phototherapy offers several benefits in that localized laser phototherapy is often quicker and more convenient than other forms of UV phototherapy, due to the fact that fewer treatments are generally required because higher dosages of UV light can be administered to the plaques. In targeted laser phototherapy, normal skin, which would not tolerate the higher dosages tolerated by psoriatic plaques, is not exposed to UV light.

Earlier, excimer laser therapy was considered a treatment for cases of localized, resistant psoriasis. The machine XTRAC Ultra has an average power of 1–2 W and generally has been used in treating mild to moderate psoriasis. PhotoMedex has now developed a newer excimer laser machine, the XTRAC Velocity, which is 300%–400% more powerful than the previous XTRAC Ultra machine. With the newer XTRAC Velocity, the standard dosing protocol (Table 4.4) is similar, but the time required for administration is significantly decreased. This allows physicians to consider using laser therapy as part of the treatment regimen for patients with generalized psoriasis, with 10%–20% total BSA involvement.

Ultraviolet Laser Dosage and Administration

The XTRAC laser excimer machine delivers monochromatic 308 nm light as a uniform square beam measuring 2 cm × 2 cm, or 4 cm^2. The excimer laser may be used in either paint or tile mode. In paint mode, monochromatic UV light is delivered continuously as the handpiece is moved over the plaques. In tile mode, the handpiece is held in place, a predetermined amount of UV light is given, and the handpiece is then moved to an adjacent area of the plaque. Tile mode is generally preferred in the research setting because it is more reproducible, and it allows better standardization between operators and centers. In clinical practice, many physicians use paint mode because it is more rapid and convenient.

Administration of excimer laser therapy is usually conducted biweekly for a series of 10 treatments to start. Treatment times vary depending on the extent or number of plaques a patient has. There should be a minimum of 48 hours between treatments. Patients are encouraged not to miss sessions and to stick to the therapy schedule as closely as possible.

TABLE 4.4 XTRAC Ultra and XTRAC Velocity Excimer Laser Protocol

(A) Determining dose for first treatment of psoriasis

		Fitzpatrick Skin Type	
Plaque thickness	**Induration score**	**1–3 (mJ/cm²)**	**4–6 (mJ/cm²)**
Mild	1	300	400
Moderate	2	500	600
Severe	3	700	900

(B) Determining dose for subsequent treatments of psoriasis

Clinical observation

No Effect	Minimal Effect	Good Effect	Considerable Improvement	Moderate/Severe Erythema
No erythema at 12–24 hours and no plaque improvement	Slight erythema at 12–24 hours but no significant improvement	Mild to moderate erythema response at 12–24 hours	Significant improvement with plaque thinning or reduced scaliness or pigmentation occurred	With or without blistering
No erythema at 12–24 hours and no plaque improvement	Slight erythema at 12–24 hours but no significant improvement	Mild to moderate erythema response at 12–24 hours	Significant improvement with plaque thinning or reduced scaliness or pigmentation occurred	With or without blistering
Typical dosing change from prior treatment dose				
Increase dose by 25%	Increase dose by 15%	Maintain dose	Maintain dose or reduce dose by 15% (reduction intended to minimize hyperpigmentation effect and/or to avoid increased erythema)	Reduce dose by 25% (treat around any blistered area; do not treat blistered area until healed with crust disappeared)

Source: XTRAC® clinical reference guide: Dosing guideline for targeted UVB phototherapy of psoriasis. XTRAC treatment guidelines. 12-95359-01 Rev. C.

Note: This dosing guideline is provided for guidance purposes only. Each patient may react differently; therefore, the physician should determine the actual treatment regimens based on patient history and their own clinical experience and expertise.

Patients may see a response after as few as four to six treatment sessions, and some patients may notice marked reduction in pruritus after 24 hours. Plaque thickness does vary from patient to patient, and larger plaques with more induration may be more difficult to treat. The outer active border of plaques tends to be one of the last areas to clear, compared to the center of plaques.

When determining the dosage for laser phototherapy administration, there is a standard protocol card that physicians can follow, which is included with XTRAC laser machines (Table 4.4). Historically, physicians initiated treatment at one to three times the MED, and based the administration of UV light on a patient's noninvolved tissue. However, psoriatic tissue has a much higher tolerance for blistering and erythema as compared to healthy tissue. Some physicians found an optimal dosage by gradually increasing the amount of UV light until either the psoriasis improved significantly or the patient experienced blistering of the skin. Earlier, two specific protocols were provided with the XTRAC excimer laser—one MED-based protocol and another based on induration of the psoriatic lesion. However, the current standard protocol is based on induration rather than MED and uses the actual dose of light therapy as measured in millijoules, rather than adjusting dosimetry by multiples of MED. This protocol was established by PhotoMedex after reviewing more than 30 clinical trials testing localized laser therapy in the treatment of psoriasis. Notably, various other excimer laser machines may have differing protocol regimens to follow; the protocol table included is an example of an induration-based protocol, which is used for the Photomedex XTRAC Ultra and XTRAC Velocity machines.

As patients are treated, psoriatic plaques become acclimated to previous dosages and may require a higher dose of laser treatment for further improvement in the plaque [90]. In addition, as lesions show improvement, physicians must be careful to ensure that thinning lesions do not receive an excessively high dose that results in blistering or erythema, even though the same dose was tolerated previously when the plaques were thicker. The standard induration-based protocol, with incremental dosing changes, takes these factors into account. Another advantage in targeted UVB phototherapy is that different regions of the body can have differing optimal therapeutic doses of UV light. Therapy can be tailored to a patient's anatomical variance in dosage, and higher doses can be used to target thicker plaques.

A commonly held misconception may be that patients with high MED thresholds are not necessarily good candidates for excimer laser therapy, but patients with higher Fitzpatrick skin types and higher MED thresholds may still benefit provided that appropriately aggressive dosimetry is used. Of course, skin type and sensitivity are important in determination of dosage, and thus skin type is factored into both protocols.

Ultraviolet Laser Efficacy

The efficacy of the 308 nm excimer UVB laser was tested in several studies [91–95] and is approved by the FDA for mild, moderate, and severe psoriasis. Initial promising case reports were followed by a multicenter study [96]. One-hundred and twenty-four patients with stable plaque psoriasis covering less than 10% BSA were enrolled and 80 completed the study. Seventy-two percent of patients achieved at least 75% clearing in an average of 6.2 treatments. Thirty-five percent achieved 90% clearing in an average of 7.5 treatments. In a follow-up study of subjects in this multicenter trial, 25% of subjects reported that the laser treatment was better than any other treatment they had tried; 55% reported overall satisfaction with the treatments. The most common side effects were erythema, blisters, hyperpigmentation, and superficial erosion, and these were well tolerated. The most common reason for not completing the study was noncompliance with treatment. Another open prospective study of 102 patients showed at least 90% clearance in 85% of the subjects under a protocol in which the dosage was determined by a standard MED of noninvolved skin, although in a comparable group of 43 patients, clearance was shown in 84% under a different protocol in which dosage was determined by an MED of the involved skin only (MED-I), which is dependent on plaque thickness. The second protocol was justified by the tendency for psoriatic lesions to withstand a higher MED than normal skin. The second group on average required a smaller number of treatments (7.07 treatments vs. 13 treatments) and a lower cumulative dose (6.25 J cm^{-2} vs. 11.25 J cm^{-2}) [97]. Because involved skin could tolerate a higher dose initially, it was more useful to determine treatment dosage based on plaque thickness to achieve similar results with less treatment sessions.

Laser has also been shown to be effective for palmoplantar psoriasis in some studies; however, it was shown to have similar efficacy as topical PUVA treatment [98–101]. Scalp psoriasis can also be treated with the excimer laser as demonstrated by two studies in which the hair was parted manually to deliver the pulses [102,103].

Traditional light box and systemic therapy may be more practical for patients with extensive disease, whereas the excimer laser has been more commonly used in patients with localized resistant psoriasis. In clinical practice, there are no hard guidelines on how much area is appropriate to treat. The excimer laser is used more commonly in patients with less than 10% BSA; however, the authors have documented its effective use in patients with up to 20% BSA, which may take up to 20 minutes/treatment session. In a pilot study by Gattu et al., 13 patients with greater than 10% but less than 30% involvement received twice-weekly laser treatments for 12 weeks. Overall, 54% reached PASI 75 by week 12. However, when inappropriate candidates for laser therapy (Fitzpatrick skin type I [$n = 2$] or unusually hyperkeratotic plaques [$n = 1$]) were excluded from the analysis, 77% (7/9) of subjects achieved a PASI 75 by week 12 [104].

In the future, the time it takes to treat the patient with the excimer laser is expected to diminish with availability of more powerful machines. Treating larger BSA may be associated with a higher possibility of skin irritation. In clinical practice, it seems sensible to use the excimer laser in combination with one or more of these topical therapies to achieve faster and more extensive clearing, although more studies are required to determine the effectiveness of combination therapy. A recent blinded study comparing the use of a combination of flumetasone ointment and excimer laser therapy to laser monotherapy showed no significant difference in PASI scores by the end of five weeks. However, the group receiving the combination therapy required less cumulative laser dosage during treatment, resulting in fewer side effects. In addition, when the excimer laser was used in combination with PUVA ($n = 272$), there was no improvement in efficacy but patients went into remission in half the treatment time and with half the cumulative UVA dose compared to PUVA alone [105,106].

Ultraviolet Laser Safety

The most common side effects of the excimer laser include erythema, blistering, and hyperpigmentation. It has been the authors' experience that much of the hyperpigmentation is tanning and will fade over time. These laser side effects are limited to localized areas (in contrast to large areas seen with full body treatments using traditional phototherapy). In addition, patients may use topical steroids to minimize these side effects. As of the summer of 2008, there were 400,000 psoriasis treatments with the XTRAC laser and no incidence of skin cancer was reported in association with laser treatment.

Other Lasers

The use of the pulsed-dye laser for treatment of psoriasis was reported in 1996 [107], and long-term remission of disease was reported. In a small study of eight patients, a 5 mm spot diameter delivered at a fluency of 8.5 J cm^{-2} proved to be optimal. Four patients had reached clearance with the pulsed-dye laser just eight weeks after their last laser treatment [108]. Some patients reported pain following treatment, for which cooling procedures such as ice packs were employed. Nevertheless, widespread use of the pulsed-dye laser did not materialize. Limitations of pulsed-dye laser treatment included pain with treatment, small treatment spot size, and high cost, which made its use seem impractical. Furthermore, multiple treatments may be required, and complete clearing is not always achieved [109].

Coding for and Regulation of Laser Treatment for Psoriasis

Excimer laser therapy has been approved by the FDA for mild, moderate, and severe psoriasis. Many guidelines suggest that laser therapy can be used for patients with 10% or less BSA affected because it would take an unreasonable amount of time to treat patients with more extensive psoriasis. However, guidelines may change with the advent of the more powerful XTRAC Velocity machine. The current procedural terminology codes for laser treatment for inflammatory skin diseases are as follows: 96920 for BSA up to 250 ft^2, 96921 for BSA from 250 to 500 ft^2, and 96922 for BSA greater than 500 ft^2. The use of medical lasers is regulated on a state-by-state basis. Some states require laser treatments to be delivered by a physician. Physicians should consult with their state medical board to determine their local regulations.

LIMITATIONS OF UVB PHOTOTHERAPY

Despite many recent advancements in psoriasis treatments, UVB phototherapy remains among the safest, very effective, and versatile treatments for psoriasis. Nevertheless, the limitations of phototherapy need to be recognized. The most limiting feature of UV phototherapy is inconvenience. There is time spent in the office preparing for and undergoing the phototherapy treatment, as well as travel time and expected time lost from work. Even though phototherapy is one of the most cost-effective treatments for psoriasis, the cost of phototherapy to the patient is not inconsequential. Under some forms of insurance, patients are required to pay a copayment at each visit. The disincentive for patients may account in part for the less frequent use of phototherapy in the United States [110]. For some patients, the inconvenience of phototherapy (and the cost as well) may be ameliorated through the use of home UVB phototherapy. If office UVB phototherapy is not available, tanning bed treatments may be beneficial for some patients [111]. As with all other forms of psoriasis therapy, it is essential to consider the impact of the treatment on the patient's lifestyle when selecting the treatment plan.

PRACTICAL RESOURCES

A number of practical resources are available to support physicians interested in providing phototherapy to their patients. The National Psoriasis Foundation (NPF, www.psoriasis.org) provides very helpful patient-oriented materials, including a specific brochure on phototherapy. Providing a patient with this brochure not only educates the patient on the benefits and risks of (and alternatives to) phototherapy but also provides the physician a ready way to document that this information has been provided in writing. Through the NPF's *Psoriasis Forum*, physicians can gain access to sample letters that may be used to help patients gain insurance coverage for phototherapy. The NPF has also produced and distributed an educational resource for insurers to increase their understanding of psoriasis as a disease and of the treatments that fall within the standard of care. The NPF will even assist individual patients with difficulties they may encounter in finding a phototherapy center or in obtaining coverage from their insurer. Another valuable NPF service is its course, "Phototherapy from the Ground Up: How to Give Light Treatment Correctly." This is a two-and-a-half-day course that offers training and tips to help nurses and phototherapy technicians. It is held three times a year, and participants receive educational credits (through the American Nurses Association) for their attendance. A practical textbook of phototherapy is also available that provides detailed protocols, flow sheets, and consent forms [84].

REFERENCES

1. Koo J, Lebwohl M. Duration of remission of psoriasis therapies. *J Am Acad Dermatol* 1999; 41: 51–59.
2. Parrish JA, Jaenicke KF. Action spectrum for phototherapy of psoriasis. *J Invest Dermatol* 1981; 76: 359–362.
3. Diffey BL, Farr PM. An appraisal of ultraviolet lamps used for the phototherapy of psoriasis. *Br J Dermatol* 1987; 117: 49–56.
4. Van Weelden H, Young E, van der Leun JC. Therapy of psoriasis: comparison of photochemotherapy and several variants of phototherapy. *Br J Dermatol* 1980; 103: 1 9.
5. Birt AR, Davis RA. Hereditary polymorphic light eruption of American Indians. *Int J Dermatol* 1975; 14: 105–111.
6. Gshnait G, Honigsmann H, Brenner W, et al. Induction of UV light tolerance by PUVA in patients with polymorphous light eruption. *Br J Dermatol* 1978; 99: 293–295.
7. Elmets CA. Drug-induced photoallergy. *Dermatol Clin* 1986; 4: 231–241.
8. Valerie K, Delers A, Bruck C, et al. Activation of human immunodeficiency virus type 1 by DNA damage in human cells. *Nature* 1988; 333: 78–81.
9. Stein B, Kramer M, Rahmsdorf HJ, et al. UV-induced transcription from the human immunodeficiency virus type 1 (HIV-1) transcription in nonirradiated cells. *J Virol* 1989; 63: 4540–4544.
10. Legrand-Poels S, Vaira D, Pincemil J, et al. Activation of human immunodeficiency virus type 1 by oxidative stress. *AIDS Res Hum Retroviruses* 1990; 6: 1389–1397.
11. Osborn L, Kunkel S, Nabel GJ. Tumor necrosis and interleukin 1 stimulate the human immunodeficiency virus enhancer by activation of the nuclear factor kB. *Proc Natl Acad Sci U S A* 1989; 86: 2336–2340.
12. Meola T, Soter NA, Ostreicher R, et al. The safety of UVB phototherapy in patients with HIV infection. *J Am Acad Dermatol* 1993; 29: 216–220.
13. Adrian RM, LeVine MJ, Parrish JA. Treatment frequency for outpatient phototherapy of psoriasis. A comparative study. *Arch Dermatol* 1981; 117: 623–626.
14. LeVine MJ, Parrish JA. Outpatient phototherapy of psoriasis. *Arch Dermatol* 1980; 116: 552–554.
15. Menkes A, Stern RS, Arndt KA. Psoriasis treatment with suberythemogenic ultraviolet B radiation and a coal tar extract. *J Am Acad Dermatol* 1984; 12: 21–25.

16. Morison WL. *Phototherapy and Photochemotherapy of Skin Disease*, 2nd ed. New York: Raven Press; 1991, p. 80.
17. Petrozzi JW. Updating the Goeckerman regimen for psoriasis. *Br J Dermatol* 1987; 98: 437–444.
18. Stern RS. Effect of continued ultraviolet B phototherapy on the duration of remission of psoriasis: a randomized study. *J Am Acad Dermatol* 1986; 15: 546–552.
19. Lowe NJ, Wortzman MS, Breeding J, et al. Coal tar phototherapy for psoriasis reevaluated: erythematous versus suberythemogenic ultraviolet with a tar extract in oil and crude coal tar. *J Am Acad Dermatol* 1983; 8: 781–789.
20. Belsito DV, Kechijian P. The role of tar in Goeckerman therapy. *Arch Dermatol* 1982; 118: 319–321.
21. Petrozzi JW, De los Reyes O. Ultraviolet phototherapy in psoriasis with hydrophilic ointment alone or with crude coal tar. *Arch Dermatol Res* 1982; 272: 257–262.
22. LeVine M, White HAD, Parrish JA. Components of the Goeckerman therapy. *J Invest Dermatol* 1979; 73: 170–173.
23. Frost P. Tar gel-phototherapy for psoriasis. *Arch Dermatol* 1979; 115: 840–846.
24. Do AN, Koo JYM. Initiating narrow-band UVB for the treatment of psoriasis. *Psoriasis Forum* 2004; 10: 1–6.
25. Zanolli MD, Clark AR, Feldman SR, et al. *Phototherapy Treatment Protocols: For Psoriasis and other Phototherapy Responsive Dermatoses*. New York: CRC Press- Parthenon Publishing; 2000.
26. Olson RL, Sayre RM, Everett MA. Effect of anatomic location and time on ultraviolet erythema. *Arch Dermatol* 1996; 93: 211–215.
27. Chue B, Borok M, Lowe NJ. Phototherapy units; comparison of fluorescent ultraviolet B and ultraviolet A units with a high-pressure mercury system. *J Am Acad Dermatol* 1988; 18: 641–645.
28. Van Weelden H, van der Leun JC. Improving the effectiveness of phototherapy for psoriasis [abstract]. *Br J Dermatol* 1984; 111: 484.
29. Van Weelden H, Baart de la Faille H, Young E, et al. A new development in UVB phototherapy of psoriasis. *Br J Dermatol* 1988; 119: 11–19.
30. Coven TR, Burack LH, Gilleaudeau P, et al. Narrow band UV-B produces superior clinical and histopathological resolution of moderate-to-severe psoriasis in patients compared with broadband UV-B. *Arch Dermatol* 1997; 133: 1514–1522.
31. Karvonen J, Kokkonen EL, Ruotsalainen E. 311 nm UVB lamps in the treatment of psoriasis with the Ingram regimen. *Acta Derm Venereol (Stockh)* 1989; 69: 82–85.
32. Picot E, Meunier L, Picot-Debeze MC. Treatment of psoriasis with a 311-nm UVB lamp. *Br J Dermatol* 1992; 127: 509–512.
33. Green C, Ferguson J, Lakshmipathi T, et al. 311 nm UVB phototherapy – an effective treatment for psoriasis. *Br J Dermatol* 1988; 119: 691–696.
34. Larko O. Treatment of psoriasis with a new UVB-lamp. *Acta Derm Veneorol (Stockh)* 1989; 69: 357–359.
35. Fischer T, Alsins J, Berne B. Ultraviolet action spectrum and evaluation of ultraviolet lamps for psoriasis healing. *Int J Dermatol* 1984; 23: 633–637.
36. Hofer A, Fink-Puches R, Kerl H, et al. Comparison of phototherapy with near vs. far erythemogenic doses of narrow-band ultraviolet B in patients with psoriasis. *Br J Dermatol* 1998; 138: 96–100.
37. Walters IB, Burack LH, Coven TR, et al. Suberythemogenic narrow-band UVB is markedly more effective than conventional UVB in treatment of psoriasis vulgaris. *J Am Acad Dermatol* 1999; 40: 893-900.
38. Behrens S, Grundmann-Kollmann M, Schiener R, et al. Combination phototherapy of psoriasis with narrow-band UVB irradiation and topical tazarotene gel. *J Am Acad Dermatol* 2000; 42: 493–495.
39. Carrozza P, Hausermann P, Nestle FO, et al. Clinical efficacy of narrow-band UVB (311 nm) combined with dithranol in psoriasis. *Dermatology* 2000; 200: 35–39.
40. Kerscher M, Volkenandt M, Plewig G, et al. Combination phototherapy of psoriasis with calcipotriol and narrow-band UVB [letter]. *Lancet* 1993; 342: 923.
41. Karakawa M, Komine M, Takekoshi T, et al. Duration of remission period of narrowband ultraviolet B therapy on psoriasis vulgaris. *J Dermatol* 2011; 38: 655–660.
42. Van Weelden H, Baart De La Faille H, Young E, et al. Comparison of narrow-band UV-B phototherapy and PUVA photochemotherapy in the treatment of psoriasis. *Acta Derm Venereol (Stockh)* 1990; 70: 212–215.

43. Tanew A, Radakovic-Fijan S, Schemper M, et al. Narrow-band UV-B phototherapy vs photochemotherapy in the treatment of chronic plaque-type psoriasis: a paired comparison study. *Arch Dermatol* 1999; 135: 519–524.
44. Gordon PM, Diffey BL, Matthews JNS, et al. A randomized comparison of narrow-band TL-01 phototherapy and PUVA photochemotherapy for psoriasis. *J Am Acad Dermatol* 1999; 41: 728–732.
45. Sezer E, Erbil AH, Kurumlu Z, et al. Comparison of the efficacy of local narrowband ultraviolet B (NB-UVB) phototherapy versus psoralen plus ultraviolet A (PUVA) paint for palmoplantar psoriasis. *J Dermatol* 2007; 34: 435–440.
46. Stern RS, Laird N. The carcinogenic risk of treatments for severe psoriasis. *Cancer* 1994; 73: 2759–2764.
47. Larko O, Swanbeck KG. Is UVB treatment in psoriasis safe? A study of exclusively UVB-treated psoriasis patients compared with a matched control group. *Acta Derm Venereol (Stockh)* 1982; 62: 507–512.
48. George SA, Bilsland DJ, Johnson BE, et al. Narrow-band (TL-01) UVB air- conditioned phototherapy for chronic sever adult atopic dermatitis. *Br J Dermatol* 1993; 128: 49–56.
49. Grundmann-Kollmann M, Behrens S, Podda M, et al. Phototherapy for atopic eczema with narrow-band UVB. *J Am Acad Dermatol* 1999; 40: 995–997.
50. Hudson-Peacock MJ, Diffey BL, Farr PM. Narrow-band UVB phototherapy for severe atopic dermatitis. *Br J Dermatol* 1996; 135: 330–345.
51. Reynolds NJ, Franklin V, Gray JC, et al. Narrow-band ultraviolet B and broad-band ultraviolet A phototherapy in adult atopic eczema: a randomized controlled trial. *Lancet* 2001; 357: 2012–2016.
52. Pikhammer D, Seeber A, Honigsmann H, et al. Narrow-band ultraviolet B (TL-01) phototherapy is an effective and safe treatment option for patients with severe seborrhoeic dermatitis. *Br J Dermatol* 2000; 143: 964–968.
53. Bilsland D, George SA, Gibbs NK, et al. A comparison of narrow band phototherapy (TL 01) and photochemotherapy (PUVA) in the management of polymorphic light eruption. *Br J Dermatol* 1993; 129: 708–712.
54. Collins P, Ferguson J. Narrow-band UVB (TL-01) phototherapy: an effective preventative treatment for the photodermatoses. *Br J Dermatol* 1995; 132: 956–963.
55. Gupta G, Man I, Kemmett D. Hydroa vacciniforme: a clinical and follow-up study of 17 cases. *J Am Acad Dermatol* 2000; 42: 208–213.
56. Aydogan K, Saricaoglu H, Turan H. Narrowband UVB (311 nm, TL01) phototherapy for pityriasis lichenoides. *Photodermatol Photoimmunol Photomed* 2008; 24: 128–133.
57. Tamagawa-Mineoka R, Katoh N, Ueda E, et al. Narrow-band ultraviolet B phototherapy in patients with recalcitrant nodular prurigo. *J Dermatol* 2007; 34: 691–695.
58. Westerhof W, Nieuweboer-Krobotova L. Treatment of vitiligo with UV-B radiation vs topical psoralen plus UV-A. *Arch Dermatol* 1997; 133: 1525–1528.
59. Scherschun L, Kim JJ, Lim HW. Narrow-band ultraviolet B is a useful and well-tolerated treatment for vitiligo. *J Am Acad Dermatol* 2001; 44: 999–1003.
60. Njoo MD, Bos JD, Westerhof W. Treatment of generalized vitiligo in children with narrow-band (TL-01) UVB radiation therapy. *J Am Acad Dermatol* 2000; 42: 245–253.
61. Alora MBT, Taylor CR. Narrow-band (311) UVB phototherapy: an audit of the first year's experience at the Massachusetts General Hospital. *Photodermatol Photoimmunol Photomed* 1997; 13: 82–84.
62. Wulf HC, Hansen AB, Bech-Thomsen N. Differences in narrow-band ultraviolet B and broad-spectrum ultraviolet photocarcinogenesis in lightly pigmented hairless mice. *Photodermatol Photoimmunol Photomed* 1994; 10: 192–197.
63. George SA, Ferguson J. Lesional blistering following narrow-band (TL-01) UVB phototherapy for psoriasis: a report of four cases. *Br J Dermatol* 1992; 127: 445–446.
64. Calzavara-Pinton PG, Zane C, Candiago E, et al. Blisters on psoriatic lesions treated with TL-01 lamps. *Dermatol* 2000; 200: 115–119.
65. Freeman RG. Data on the action spectrum for ultraviolet carcinogenesis. *J Natl Caner Inst* 1975; 55: 1119–1122.
66. Weischer M, Blum A, Eberhard F, et al. No evidence for increased skin cancer risk in psoriasis patients treated with broadband or narrowband UVB phototherapy: a first retrospective study. *Acta Derm Venereol* 2004; 84: 370–374.

67. Man I, Crombie IK, Dawe RS, et al. The photocarcinogenic risk of narrowband UVB (TL-01) phototherapy: early follow-up data. *Br J Dermatol* 2005; 152: 755–757.
68. Nguyen T, Koo J. Ultraviolet therapy for psoriasis. Advances in Psoriasis. *Adv Dermatol.* 1997; 12: 47–72; discussion 73.
69. Lebwohl M, Martinez J, Weber P, et al. Effects of topical preparations on the erythemogenicity of UVB: implications for psoriasis phototherapy. *J Am Acad Dermatol* 1995; 32: 469–471.
70. Schulze H-J, Schauer S, Mahrle G, et al. Combined tar-anthralin versus anthralin treatment lowers irritancy with unchanged antipsoriatic efficacy: modifications of short-contact therapy and Ingram therapy. *J Am Acad Dermatol* 1987; 17: 19–24.
71. Kokelj S, Lavaroni G, Guadagnini A. UVB versus UVB plus calcipotriol therapy for psoriasis vulgaris. *Acta Derm Venereol (Stockh)* 1995; 75: 386–387.
72. Ramsay CA, Schwartz BE, Lowson D, et al. Calcipotriol cream combined with twice weekly broad-band UVB phototherapy: a safe, effective and UVB-sparing antipsoriatric combination treatment. The Canadian Calcipotriol and UVB Study Group. *Dermatology* 2000; 200: 17–24.
73. Koo J, Lowe N, Lew-Kaya D, et al. *Tazarotene plus UVB phototherapy in the treatment of psoriasis. J Am Acad Dermatol* 2000; 43: 821–828.
74. Ruzicka T, Sommerburg C, Braun-Falco O, et al. Efficiency of acitretin in combination with UV-B in the treatment of severe psoriasis. *Arch Dermatol* 1990; 12: 482–486.
75. Busse K, Koo J. Introducing the delayed retinoid burn: a case report and discussion of this potential risk of retinoid-phototherapy combination management. *J Am Acad Dermatol* 2011; 64: 1011–1012.
76. Paul BS, Momtaz K, Stern RS, et al. Combined methotrexate–ultraviolet B therapy in treatment of psoriasis. *J Am Acad Dermatol* 1982; 7: 758–762.
77. Asawanonda P, Nateetongrungsak Y. Methotrexate plus narrowband UVB phototherapy versus narrowband UVB phototherapy alone in the treatment of plaque-type psoriasis: a randomized, placebo-controlled study. *J Am Acad Dermatol* 2006; 54: 1013–1018.
78. Mahajan R, Kaur I, Kanwar AJ. Methotrexate/narrowband UVB phototherapy combination vs. narrowband UVB phototherapy in the treatment of chronic plaque-type psoriasis—a randomized single-blinded placebo-controlled study. *J Eur Acad Dermatol Venereol* 2010; 24: 595–600.
79. Oxholm A, Thomsen K, Menne T. Squamous cell carcinomas in relation to cyclosporin therapy of non-malignant skin disorders. *Acta Derm Venereol (Stockh)* 1989; 69: 89–90.
80. Krupp P, Monka C. Side-effect profile of cyclosporin A in patients treated for psoriasis. *Br J Dermatol* 1990; 122: 47–56.
81. Penn I. Cancers following cyclosporin therapy. *Transplantation* 1987; 43: 32–35.
82. Calzavara-Pinton P, Leone G, Venturini M, et al. A comparative non randomized study of narrow-band UVB phototherapy versus sequential therapy with oral administration of low-dose Cyclosporin A and NB-UVB phototherapy in patients with severe psoriasis vulgaris. *Eur J Dermatol* 2005; 15: 470–473.
83. Kircik L, Bagel J, Korman N, et al. Utilization of narrow-band ultraviolet light B therapy and etanercept for the treatment of psoriasis (UNITE): efficacy, safety, and patient-reported outcomes. *J Drugs Dermatol* 2008; 7: 245–253.
84. Lee E, Koo J, Berger T. UVB phototherapy and skin cancer risk: a review of the literature. *Int J Dermatol* 2005; 44: 355–360.
85. Al Suwaidan SN, Feldman SR. Clearance is not a realistic expectation of psoriasis treatment. *J Am Acad Dermatol* 2000; 42: 796–802.
86. Rapp SR, Exum ML, Reboussin DM, et al. The physical, psychological and social impact of psoriasis. *J Health Psychol* 1997; 2: 525–537.
87. Avrillier S, Ollivier JP, Gandjbakhch I, et al. XeCl excimer laser coronary angioplasty: a convergence of favourable factors. *J Photochem Photobiol* 1990; 6: 249–257.
88. Muller-Stolzenburg N, Muller GJ. Transmission of 308 nm excimer laser radiation for ophthalmic microsurgery—medical, technical and safety aspects. *Biomed Tech (Berl)* 1989; 34: 131–138.
89. Novak Z, Bonis B, Baltas E, et al. Xenon chloride ultraviolet B laser is more effective in treating psoriasis and in inducing T cell apoptosis than narrow-band ultraviolet B. *J Photochem Photobiol B* 2002; 67: 32–38.
90. Taneja A, Trehan M, Taylor C. 308-nm excimer laser for the treatment of psoriasis—induration based dosimetry. *Arch Dermatol* 2003; 139: 759–764.
91. Bonis B, Kemeny L, Dobozy A, et al. 308 nm UVB excimer laser for psoriasis [letter]. *Lancet* 1997; 350: 1522.

92. Asawanonda P, Anderson RR, Chang Y, et al. 308-nm excimer laser for the treatment of psoriasis: a dose-response study. *Arch Dermatol* 2000; 136: 619–624.
93. Kemeny L, Bonis B, Dobozy A, et al. 308-nm excimer laser therapy for psoriasis. *Arch Dermatol* 2001; 137: 95–96.
94. Housman TS, Pearce DJ, Feldman SR. Case report: efficacy of 308 nm excimer laser therapy for psoriasis. *Cosmet Dermatol* 2001; 14: 17–20.
95. Trehan M, Taylor CR. High-dose 308-nm excimer laser for the treatment of psoriasis. *J Am Acad Dermatol* 2002; 46: 732–737.
96. Feldman SR, Mellen BG, Housman TS, et al. Efficacy of the 308-nm excimer laser for treatment of psoriasis: results of a multicenter study. *J Am Acad Dermatol* 2002; 46: 900–906.
97. Gerber W, Arheilger B, Ha TA, et al. Ultraviolet B 308-nm excimer laser treatment of psoriasis: a new phototherapeutic approach. *Br J Dermatol* 2003; 149: 1250–1258.
98. Al-Mutairi N, Al-Haddad A. Targeted phototherapy using 308 nm Xecl monochromatic excimer laser for psoriasis at difficult to treat sites. *Lasers Med Sci* 2013; 28: 1119–24.
99. Goldberg DJ, Chwalek J, Hussain M. 308-nm excimer laser treatment of palmoplantar psoriasis. *J Cosmet Laser Ther* 2011; 13: 47–49.
100. Neumann NJ, Mahnke N, Korpusik D, et al. Treatment of palmoplantar psoriasis with monochromatic excimer light (308-nm) versus cream PUVA. *Acta Derm Venereol* 2006; 86: 22–24.
101. Nistico SP, Saraceno R, Stefanescu S, et al. A 308-nm monochromatic excimer light in the treatment of palmoplantar psoriasis. *J Eur Acad Dermatol Venereol* 2006; 20: 523–526.
102. Morison WL, Atkinson DF, Werthman L. Effective treatment of scalp psoriasis using the excimer (308 nm) laser. *Photodermatol Photoimmunol Photomed* 2006; 22: 181–183.
103. Taylor CR, Racette AL. A 308-nm excimer laser for the treatment of scalp psoriasis. *Lasers Surg Med* 2004; 34: 136–140.
104. Gattu S, Pang ML, Pugashetti R, et al. Pilot evaluation of supra-erythemogenic phototherapy with excimer laser in the treatment of patients with moderate to severe plaque psoriasis. *J Dermatol Treat* 2010; 21: 54–60.
105. Dong J, He Y, Zhang X, et al. Clinical efficacy of flumetasone/salicylic acid ointment combined with 308-nm excimer laser for treatment of psoriasis vulgaris. *Photodermatol Photoimmunol Photomed* 2012; 28: 133–136.
106. Trott J, Gerber W, Hammes S, et al. The effectiveness of PUVA treatment in severe psoriasis is significantly increased by additional UV 308-nm excimer laser sessions. *Eur J Dermatol* 2008; 18: 55–60.
107. Zelickson BD, Mehregan DA, Wendelschfer-Crabb G, et al. Clinical and histologic evaluation of psoriatic plaques treated with a flashlamp pulsed dye laser. *J Am Acad Dermatol* 1996; 35: 64–68.
108. Erceg A, Bovenschen HJ, van de Kerkhof PC, et al. Efficacy of the pulsed dye laser in the treatment of localized recalcitrant plaque psoriasis: a comparative study. *Br J Dermatol* 2006; 155: 110–114.
109. Hern S, Allen MH, Sousa AR, et al. Immunohistochemical evaluation of psoriatic plaques following selective photothermolysis of the superficial capillaries. *Br J Dermatol* 2001; 145: 45–53.
110. Housman TS, Rohrback JM, Fleischer AB, Jr, et al. Phototherapy utilization for psoriasis is declining in the United States. *J Am Acad Dermatol* 2002; 46: 557–559.
111. Fleischer AB, Jr, Clark AR, Rapp SR, et al. Commercial tanning bed treatment is an effective psoriasis treatment: results from an uncontrolled clinical trial. *J Invest Dermatol* 1997; 109: 170–174.

Chapter 5

Systemic and Topical PUVA Therapy

Warwick L. Morison and Elisabeth G. Richard

SYSTEMIC PUVA THERAPY

In this section, psoralen and ultraviolet A (PUVA) therapy will refer to oral methoxsalen photochemotherapy in which a patient ingests methoxsalen and is subsequently exposed to an indoor artificial source of ultraviolet A (UVA) (320–400 nm) radiation [1–3]. This therapy has been used for treating moderate to severe psoriasis for nearly four decades. During this time, it has undergone intense scrutiny, and its benefits and risks have been clearly defined. Successful use of PUVA therapy requires a well-informed physician, trained staff, and an educated, motivated patient. Although this can bc said of all psoriasis treatment, it is particularly true for PUVA therapy because of the complexity of the regimen.

Patient Selection

A careful evaluation of the patient is necessary because PUVA therapy is often a long-term treatment. Good documentation is likewise essential, and an evaluation form ensures that no essential points are missed (Table 5.1). The absolute and relative contraindications to PUVA therapy need to be kept in mind throughout the evaluation (Table 5.2) [4]. Laboratory investigations are not required except as suggested on the basis of the history and examination. Photosensitizing medications are not a contraindication to treatment, but their use should be noted.

The most common indication for PUVA therapy is disabling psoriasis unresponsive to topical therapy. Because the definition of disability can vary among individuals, it is best determined on a case-by-case basis as a consensus between physician and patient. It is unwise to treat minimal disease with PUVA therapy for two reasons. First, such treatment has a poor risk/benefit ratio. Second, PUVA therapy rarely achieves complete clearance. A person with 1% body involvement cleared of 95% of the disease may still be an unhappy patient. In contrast, a person with 50% body involvement who achieves 95% clearance will be delighted. PUVA therapy is indicated as the initial treatment for a few patients because of explosive onset of widespread psoriasis. Finally, PUVA therapy is indicated for some patients as they cycle off methotrexate or other systemic therapy.

When considering the use of PUVA therapy, the alternative treatment considered for most patients is ultraviolet B (UVB) phototherapy—either broadband (BB) or narrowband (NB). In this decision, three important differences must be kept in mind:

- PUVA therapy is more effective than UVB phototherapy in clearing psoriasis in most patients, although NB-UVB may be comparable in moderate psoriasis [5].

TABLE 5.1 Evaluation of the Patient

Patient
Past medical and family history
Pregnancy, lactation, birth control
Other disease, medications, photosensitivity
Social and geographic
Motivation and intelligence
Psoriasis
Nature, extent, severity
Previous treatment and response
Arthritis
Effect of exposure to sunlight
Full skin examination
Laboratory investigations, if suggested by history
anti-nuclear antibody, anti-Ro, anti-La
Hepatic function
Ophthalmologic examination: Repeat yearly

TABLE 5.2 Contraindications to PUVA Therapy

Absolute
Xeroderma pigmentosum
Lupus erythematosus
Lactation
Relative
History or family history of melanoma
History of nonmelanoma skin cancer, extensive solar damage
Previous treatment with ionizing radiation or arsenic
Previous treatment with cyclosporine
Pemphigus and pemphigoid
Uremia and hepatic failure
Severe myocardial disease or other infirmity likely to make standing for a prolonged period difficult or hazardous
Immunosuppression
Pregnancy
Young age
Inability to comprehend details of the treatment

- PUVA therapy is a much more convenient and effective maintenance treatment.
- UVA radiation is more penetrating than UVB radiation; that is, UVA penetrates through a greater depth of tissue

Factors that suggest use of UVB phototherapy include the following:

1. The disease
    - Psoriasis of recent initial onset. It is possible that long-term maintenance treatment will be unnecessary. The extreme example of this is acute guttate psoriasis, which should always be initially treated with UVB phototherapy.

- Thin, macular psoriasis.
- A history of rapid and easy clearance on exposure to sunlight.
- Psoriasis with a demonstrated photosensitivity to UVA but not UVB radiation.

2. The patient
    - Pregnancy, lactation, or intention to become pregnant.
    - Young age: A child with psoriasis may have a lifetime of disease ahead, and it is best to use the safest treatments first and leave the more potent treatments for later.
3. Skin type I that always burns, never tans; or a past history of X-ray or arsenic treatment. These patients are prone to PUVA-induced skin cancer.
4. Illiteracy or low intelligence.
5. Patient preference for avoiding oral medications.

Factors that suggest use of PUVA therapy include the following:

1. The disease
    - A long history of psoriasis. This suggests that maintenance therapy will be an almost certain requirement.
    - Thick plaques.
    - Involvement of the palms and soles. NB-UVB therapy may improve psoriasis at these sites but seldom clears the disease [6].
    - Nail disease.
    - Psoriasis with a demonstrated photosensitivity to UVB but not UVA radiation.
    - Failure to respond to UVB phototherapy.
    - Active, aggressive disease with a marked inflammatory component.
    - Erythrodermic and pustular psoriasis are the extreme examples of this situation.
2. The patient
    - Skin types III and higher. Pigmentation appears to be less of an obstacle to successful clearance with PUVA therapy than with UVB phototherapy.
    - Geographic, social, or occupational factors that necessitate keeping treatments to a minimum.
    - In addition to these considerations, there are two factors that are not easily quantified: physician and patient preference. Some physicians feel more comfortable with one or another treatment. A common reason for a patient's treatment choice is that a relative's or friend's disease responded to that particular therapy.

Education of Patients

Before the start of PUVA therapy, it is essential to inform patients fully about the procedure. This will help to ensure that the treatment is performed correctly and that the patient takes the necessary precautions to avoid adverse effects. It will also prepare the patient for the possibility of adverse side effects. The initial discussion about PUVA therapy usually takes 20–30 minutes and can be reinforced by providing a handout explaining the treatment and its potential problems. A follow-up discussion between the patient and the nurse or technician prior to the first treatment completes the initial introduction. During the course of therapy, the nurse should also regularly question patients about the number and timing of the psoralen capsules they have taken, their use of eye protection, and their avoidance of exposure to sunlight on the days of treatment.

Pharmacology and Photobiology

PUVA therapy involves a phototoxic interaction between a psoralen (the photosensitizer) and a waveband of UVA radiation. The exact cellular mechanism of the phototoxic reaction is unknown but is thought to involve penetration of psoralen into the cell; then, UVA radiation causes linkage of the psoralen to pyrimidine bases, forming C_4 cycloadducts. These adducts inhibit DNA synthesis and epidermal proliferation and may cause cell apoptosis through activation of the p53 pathway. Cytokines and chemokines are reduced by PUVA, in addition to the immunosuppressive and antiproliferative effects. Present evidence indicates that psoriasis is an autoimmune disease involving activated T lymphocytes in the skin, and these T lymphocytes are presumably a target for PUVA therapy either directly or through an effect on keratinocytes [7].

Pharmacology Psoralens occur naturally in a large number of plants and are responsible for inducing phytophotodermatitis, which is simply a phototoxic reaction in the skin. Several psoralens are used in PUVA therapy, but only methoxsalen (8-methoxypsoralen) is approved for use in treating psoriasis in the United States. Bergapten (5-methoxypsoralen) is available for treatment in Europe.

Several features of the pharmacology of psoralens are important in therapy. Psoralens are poorly soluble in water; this limits their absorption from the gastrointestinal tract. Liquid formulations partially overcome this problem and are more completely absorbed than crystalline forms. There is a significant first-pass removal by the liver, however, because this is saturable—as the dose is raised, the proportion of active compound reaching the skin rises. Finally, there are large interindividual and smaller intraindividual variations in absorption, and this is reflected in the height and timing of the peak level in skin and blood.

Photobiology Psoralens must absorb photons in order to photosensitize; they must, therefore, be exposed to a source of radiation that emits a waveband that includes their absorption spectrum. Early studies suggested that the peak of the action spectrum for psoralen photosensitization was between 340 and 380 nm, which led to the use of fluorescent bulbs with a peak emission of approximately 355–365 nm. A more recent work [8] indicates that the peak of the spectrum is between 320 and 340 nm. Because the same fluorescent bulbs have good emission at these shorter wavelengths, they continue to be the most commonly used PUVA lamps. These fluorescent bulbs are usually placed in a cylindrical chamber for whole-body exposure or in a specialized apparatus for hand and foot treatment. Banks of metal halide lamps are also used for whole-body treatment, and single lamps can be used for treating localized disease. Other sources of UVA radiation should not be used for PUVA therapy at this time because the cutaneous responses to them in combination with psoralens have not been determined or clinically evaluated. The sun is not a safe source of UVA radiation in combination with methoxsalen because severe phototoxic reactions are common, even when sophisticated radiometry is used [9].

Units of Measurement

The units used in therapy are as follows:

- *Radiant energy* is the amount of radiation and is expressed in joules (J): 1 J = 10^3 mJ.
- *Radiant power* is the rate of delivery of energy and is expressed in watts (W): W = J/second, 1 W = 10^3 mW.
- *Irradiance* is the radiant power/unit area (1 cm^2) at a given surface and is expressed in W/cm^2, which is measured by a radiometer.
- *Exposure dose* is the radiant energy delivered/unit area of a given surface in a given exposure time and is expressed in J/cm^2; exposure dose = irradiance × exposure time.

Cutaneous Responses

PUVA therapy produces erythema and pigmentation of normal and psoriatic skin. These responses are markedly influenced by several factors: Dose, individual susceptibility (e.g., the patient's skin type), prior exposure to UV radiation, and body site (e.g., the limbs can tolerate approximately twice the dose tolerated by the trunk and face).

Erythema from PUVA therapy appears later and lasts longer than sunlight-induced erythema. It usually appears 24–48 hours after treatment but may be delayed as long as 72–96 hours (Figure 5.1). The more intense the erythema, the later it appears and the later it reaches a maximum. PUVA-induced erythema also has a steeper dose–response curve than UVB or sunlight-induced erythema (Figure 5.2). Thus, the dose required to produce 4+ erythema with blistering is only a few multiples of the dose that produces 1+ erythema. These features are important in therapy because small alterations in the frequency and timing of treatment or the dose of UVA radiation can result in painful erythema. Erythema is usually associated with a deep, burning pruritus, which may last for weeks.

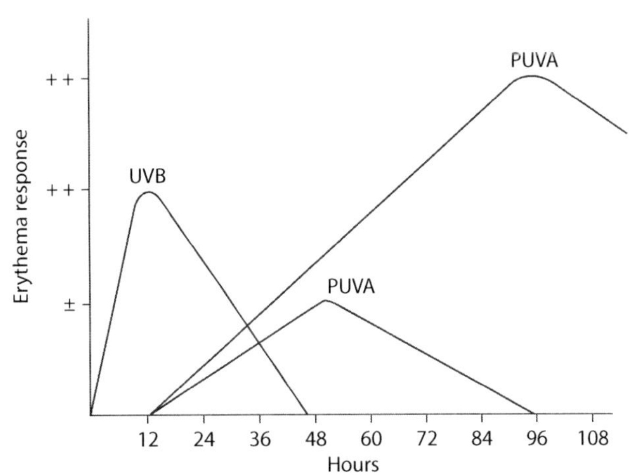

FIGURE 5.1 Time course for PUVA- and UVB-induced erythema. Note that more intense erythema peaks later.

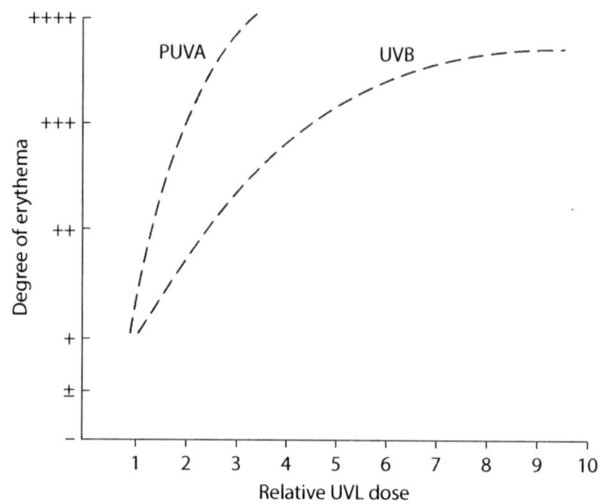

FIGURE 5.2 Dose–response curve for erythema following exposure to PUVA and UVB radiation.

Erythema is followed by pigmentation in all patients who possess functioning melanocytes. This pigmentation is darker and lasts longer than the pigmentation following a comparable sunlight-induced erythema.

Dosage and Administration

A liquid formulation of methoxsalen is available in the United States as 10 mg gelatin capsules (Oxsoralen Ultra, Valeant Pharmaceuticals). This formulation is taken at a dosage of 0.4 mg/kg body weight (Table 5.3) one hour prior to the exposure to UVA radiation. It is best to avoid food for an hour before and after ingestion because food slows and diminishes absorption of the drug. Higher dosages of the medication are frequently associated with nausea.

The starting dosages of UVA radiation, the increments of each treatment, and the suggested maximum final clearing doses are usually determined by the skin type of the individual (Table 5.4). Some centers use a determination of the minimum phototoxic dose (MPD) to decide upon a starting dose of UVA radiation [10]. Treatments in the clearance phase of therapy are usually given two or three times each week, with 48 hours or more between treatments to allow assessment of any erythemal reaction from the last exposure [11]. If no erythema occurs following treatment, the UVA dosage should be increased at the next therapy session. If erythema occurs but clears between sessions, the previous exposure dosage should be maintained at the next treatment. If the erythema has not cleared, the treatment should be cancelled unless the erythema is very localized and the area can be shielded with clothing or zinc oxide ointment.

An alternative schedule (more frequently used in Europe) consists of four treatments each week on Monday, Tuesday, Thursday, and Friday with a rest day on Wednesday to assess any cumulative erythema. The starting dosages of UVA radiation for this schedule are lower (Table 5.5), and the dosage is increased every third treatment. This schedule is more effective in clearing psoriasis but is associated with more phototoxicity. It is most useful in patients with thick plaques who have skin type III or higher or in any patients who have skin type V or VI.

TABLE 5.3 Dose Schedule for Methoxsalen (Oxsoralen Ultra) by Patient Weight

In lb	In kg	Drug Dose (mg)
≤66	≤30	10
66–143	30–65	20
144–200	66–91	30
≥200	≥91	40

TABLE 5.4 Dosages of Ultraviolet A Radiation for Bi- and Triweekly Schedules

	Ultraviolet A Radiation Dosage (J/cm²)		
Skin Type	**Initial**	**Increments**	**Final**
I	1.5	0.5	5
II	2.5	0.5	8
III	3.5	0.5–1.0	12
IV	4.5	1.0	14
V	5.5	1.0	16
VI	6.5	1.0–1.5	20

TABLE 5.5 Dosages of Ultraviolet A Radiation for Monday, Tuesday, Thursday, and Friday Schedule

	Ultraviolet A Radiation Dosage (J/cm²)	
Skin Type	**Initial**	**Increments**
I	0.5	0.5
II	1.5	0.5
III	2.5	0.5
IV	3.5	1.0
V	4.5	1.0
VI	5.5	1.5

An additional exposure to the limbs is given if there is significant involvement of this area because disease on the limbs (particularly the lower legs) is slower to clear than on the trunk. Disease on the palms and soles is also an indication for additional treatment. The starting dosage for these additional treatments is half the whole-body exposure, but the increments are the same.

When the disease is adequately controlled, the frequency of treatment is reduced to once a week for four weeks, then to every other week for two months, and finally to monthly treatment to provide maintenance therapy and to prevent recurrence of psoriasis. During this progressive reduction in frequency of treatment, any significant flare up of disease is best managed by a return to the previous level of therapy or even to the initial (clearance treatment) level. It is important for the patient to understand that weekly and less frequent treatment seldom produces any clearance of disease and is strictly maintenance therapy.

When the frequency of treatment has been reduced to one exposure each month, the decision as to whether to continue maintenance therapy depends on many factors, including the duration and severity of disease, the skin type of the individual, and the personal wishes of the patient. Most patients choose to cease treatment after a few months. Typically, a course of PUVA therapy lasts less than six months. However, in the few patients with chronic, active disease, PUVA therapy may be continued for years. There is no formalized upper limit to the amount of treatment that can be given. An individual decision must be made for each patient based upon disability from the disease, adverse effects, and therapeutic alternatives.

Precautions

There are three points during treatment at which protection must be considered:

1. During radiation, the eyes require protection by UV-opaque goggles, the male genitalia should be covered by underpants or an athletic supporter unless there is significant disease there, and the face usually should be shielded because it is seldom affected by psoriasis and it receives high ambient exposure to UV radiation.
2. Following ingestion of psoralen, the eyes should be shielded by UV-opaque sunglasses when exposed to sunlight for at least the remainder of that day. Particular attention to eye protection is essential in patients with aphakia. The skin should also be protected by clothing or a broad-spectrum sunscreen. Exposure to sunlight should be minimized.
3. On nontreatment days, the patients should be encouraged to minimize exposure to sunlight because sunlight-induced tanning complicates treatment and increases photoaging. Outdoor use of UV-opaque sunglasses throughout PUVA therapy should be encouraged.

Combination Therapy

PUVA therapy is often combined with another treatment to achieve more rapid clearance at a lower dose of UVA radiation. When the disease is clear, the second therapy is usually stopped and control of psoriasis is maintained by PUVA therapy alone. The main indications for combination therapy are listed in Table 5.6.

PUVA and Broadband–Ultraviolet B Phototherapy The patient is exposed to UVA and UVB radiation simultaneously. Fortunately, erythemal reactions from the two treatments are not cumulative. (In fact, the cause of an erythema can be determined from the

TABLE 5.6 Indications for Combination Therapy

Previous failed or partial response to PUVA therapy
Erythrodermic or generalized pustular psoriasis
Asbestos and coral–plaque psoriasis
Photosensitive psoriasis
Skin types V and VI
Social or geographic limitations on therapy

time course because a UVB-induced erythema appears on the day of treatment while a PUVA-induced erythema is delayed for at least 24 hours.) This combination is useful in two situations. First, as initial therapy on a three times a week schedule using a high-dosage UVB protocol (starting dosage of 70% of minimal erythema dose with increments of 17% each subsequent treatment) and a regular three times a week PUVA schedule [12]. Second, UVB therapy may be added to the schedule of a PUVA patient who is showing a slow response to treatment and/or is near the desired upper limit of the dose of UVA radiation. In this situation, the dosage of UVA radiation is usually held constant, while the starting dosage of UVB is 30–150 mJ/cm^2 for skin types I–VI with increments of 20% each subsequent treatment.

PUVA plus Acitretin This combination is widely used in Europe although there has been some disagreement as to its efficacy [13,14]. An analysis of the various studies indicates it is useful provided two criteria are met: acitretin is given in a dosage of at least 1 mg/kg body weight, and it is commenced at least 10–14 days before PUVA therapy. The usual limitations on use of acitretin apply (e.g., women of childbearing potential should be strictly excluded), and close monitoring is required. Isotretinoin plus PUVA therapy has been reported to be an alternative combination treatment [15], but the data to support this are not strong.

PUVA plus Methotrexate Methotrexate is begun three weeks before PUVA therapy in a dosage of 2.5–5.0 mg at 12-hour intervals for three doses each week. This is continued through the clearance phase of PUVA therapy [16]. The usual precautions of methotrexate therapy apply (see Chapter 9 on methotrexate), and blood tests to monitor the treatment are required before and during therapy. Unexpected and unexplained phototoxic episodes marked the original evaluation of this protocol, but greater experience with the treatment has found that these events are very infrequent.

PUVA plus Biologic Agents There are a limited number of published studies evaluating the combination of the biologic agents with phototherapy; however, in reality, these combinations are being used in real-world practice. The main concern is whether these combinations will be associated with an increased rate of skin cancer. From the rheumatology literature, across all biologic therapies, treatment with biologics was associated with an increased risk of nonmelanoma skin cancer (NMSC) but not solid tumors or lymphoproliferative malignancies. Further work is needed to elucidate the long-term safety of PUVA in combination with the biologics. The importance of routine skin cancer screening in these patients is emphasized given the recognized increase rate of skin cancers in patients receiving biologic therapies [17–21].

Efficacy

Most studies of the efficacy of PUVA therapy have been patient series, and few have been adequately controlled. A systematic review of systemic treatments of psoriasis found that PUVA therapy cleared (100%) approximately 70% of patients and gave a good response (75%–100% clearance) in 83% of patients [22].

Improvement in disease (flattening of plaques and decreased scaling) usually occurs after 6–10 treatments, followed by clearance of most lesions after 20–30 treatments. If the disease does not respond in this way, the reason for failure must be determined. The most common cause is missed treatments: The patient has been receiving one exposure or less each week, maximizing pigmentation and minimizing clearance. The next most common cause of treatment failure is a low methoxsalen concentration in the skin, which is suggested by a lack of pigmentation of normal skin. Possible reasons for this include a failure to take the medication, low absorption of methoxsalen, and concomitant use of medications such as carbamazepine or phenytoin sodium, which activate microsomal enzymes in the liver. In addition, certain medications such as lithium, antimalarials, and systemic corticosteroids make psoriasis unstable and often result in a failure to respond. Finally, there remains a group of patients whose disease fails to respond to therapy for unknown reasons. For these patients, some other approach to treatment must be found.

Disease of the nails responds in approximately 70% of affected patients but usually requires three to four months of treatment. Involvement of the scalp and intertriginous areas requires supplemental topical or excimer laser therapy.

Side Effects

It is crucially important for patients to know that almost everyone undergoing PUVA therapy experiences some adverse effects from the treatment. It is equally important for them to know what those effects might be. Because most of the problems are short term, minor, and easily corrected, a full discussion will prepare the patient and will help avoid misunderstanding or worse.

Short-Term Side Effects The short-term side effects of PUVA therapy are listed in Table 5.7. Nausea from methoxsalen results when a central mechanism is triggered by high serum levels of the drug. The sequential measures to overcome this problem are to ingest the drug with food, to schedule treatments late in the day, and to reduce the dosage by 10 mg. Rarely, use of an antiemetic may be required. Symptoms related to the central nervous system (CNS) occur in most patients, but few voluntarily complain of them. Headache, dizziness, insomnia, depression, and hyperkinesis are common side effects that seldom interfere with treatment.

The major short-term problem is phototoxicity. At least 10% of patients will have a phototoxic event of sufficient magnitude to warrant interruption of treatment. Patients should be warned of this in advance so they will check for erythema or other changes in their skin. The main causes of phototoxic events are variable absorption of methoxsalen, treatment on a day when erythema has not sufficiently cleared or on consecutive days, and passing the patient's cumulative threshold for erythema. There is no specific treatment for PUVA-induced phototoxicity, and supportive measures such as cool baths, moisturizers, and antipruritics provide only partial relief.

Long-Term Side Effects The most common long-term problem related to PUVA therapy is photoaging of the skin. Its occurrence depends on the amount of therapy and on the skin type of the patient. Dryness and wrinkling of the skin are early changes and largely reversible. Freckling, telangiectasia, and keratoses occur later and are probably irreversible.

TABLE 5.7 Short-Term Side Effects

Due to methoxsalen
Gastrointestinal disturbance
Central nervous system symptoms
Bronchoconstriction
Toxic hepatitis
Drug fever
Exanthema
Phototoxicity
Erythema
Pruritus
Subacute phototoxicity
Photo-onycholysis
Friction blisters
Phytophotodermatitis
Koebner phenomenon
New rash
Polymorphous light eruption
Lupus erythematosus
Seborrheic dermatitis of the face
Herpes simplex
Nonphototoxic reactions
Cardiovascular stress
Hypertrichosis

NMSC occurs more frequently in long-term PUVA patients. The increase in NMSC is noted in patients with more than 150 treatments, and risk increases with the greater number of lifetime treatments. These NMSCs were predominantly squamous cell carcinomas (SCCs) as opposed to basal cell carcinomas (BCCs), and the risk of SCC was greatly increased compared to population incidence data [23–26]. Patients with skin types I and II account for much of this increase; prior exposure to X-ray, arsenic, or high dosages of sunlight and UVB radiation appears to increase the risk. Prior to development of skin cancer, affected patients almost always have extensive photoaging changes, and such patients should be closely monitored. The lesions are mainly on the trunk and lower limbs; the male genitalia also have a significant incidence [27]. Treatment with cyclosporine subsequent to exposure to PUVA therapy appears to greatly increase the risk of skin cancer [28]. This agent, and perhaps other immunosuppressants, is relatively contraindicated in patients who have been treated with PUVA therapy.

An increased incidence of melanoma starting approximately 15 years after treatment with PUVA therapy has been reported in one study [29]. The risk is greater in patients exposed to high dosages of PUVA therapy and appears to be increasing with time. Greater frequency of melanoma has not been reported in other cohorts.

The occurrence of cataracts has been a concern since the introduction of PUVA therapy for psoriasis because these were observed in mice and other rodents. However, possibly because eye protection has been used by most patients, cataracts in PUVA patients have not occurred with increased frequency [30,31]. Other potential long-term adverse effects that have been sought but not observed include immune suppression, autoimmune phenomena, systemic neoplasia, and hepatic damage.

TOPICAL PUVA THERAPY

Direct application of psoralen to the skin, combined with subsequent exposure to UVA radiation, has been used for the treatment of psoriasis for almost as long as oral PUVA therapy. The first approach used a dilute solution of trimethylpsoralen (TMP) in a bath [32,33], and subsequent studies have used methoxsalen and 5-methoxypsoralen in bath solutions as well as creams and lotions. Topical PUVA therapy is used most widely used in Europe and it appears. And it appears to be much less popular elsewhere. In addition, because methoxsalen is the only psoralen available for use in the United States, this section will only discuss treatment with this agent. The suggested advantages of topical PUVA therapy are

- Marked reduction of systemic exposure to methoxsalen so that gastrointestinal side effects and risk of cataracts are virtually eliminated.
- Possible improved efficacy.
- Possible reduced risk of skin cancer.

The efficacy of any topical PUVA protocol will be determined by how aggressive the dosimetry is with respect to drug and radiation—an aggressive topical PUVA protocol will be more effective than a conservative oral PUVA protocol and vice versa. There is no information on the potential carcinogenicity of topical PUVA therapy using methoxsalen in humans. The lower dosage of UVA radiation required for topical PUVA therapy is often mentioned as an advantage for this treatment, but this is likely to be irrelevant because it is probably the number of adducts formed in DNA that determines therapeutic effect and long-term side effects.

Patient Selection

The indications and contraindications are the same as for oral PUVA therapy. Erythrodermic psoriasis is best treated with combination treatment due to the difficulty in differentiating between exacerbations of psoriasis and PUVA-induced erythema. Generalized pustular psoriasis is likewise an indication for combination treatment due to the risk of exacerbation by erythema.

Pharmacology and Photobiology

Presumably the mechanism of action of topical PUVA therapy is the same as oral PUVA therapy, but there is no direct evidence for this. Intraepidermal T lymphocytes appear to be a major target [34].

Pharmacology The kinetics of psoralen absorption and photosensitivity after topical application depend on several variables. When normal skin is immersed in a dilute solution of methoxsalen (such as in bath or soak PUVA therapy), photosensitivity is maximal in the first

10 minutes after the immersion and is greatly decreased 40–60 minutes later; after four hours, no photosensitivity is evident [35,36]. In contrast, maximum photosensitivity is reached 40–60 minutes after application of methoxsalen in an alcohol/glycerol lotion [37] and can persist for a week or more [38]. Psoriatic skin allows faster absorption, while palmoplantar skin has peak photosensitivity 40 minutes after bathing in a dilute solution, and this persists for an hour or more [39]. Repeated exposures to bath PUVA produces increased photosensitivity with the MPD reduced by as much as 60% after five exposures [40]. Finally, bathing time is important because increasing this time from 5 to 10 minutes also reduces the MPD by 60% [41]. It is assumed that antipsoriatic activity correlates with photosensitivity, but this is not definitely established. Plasma levels of methoxsalen are very low or undetectable in most patients treated with topical PUVA therapy. In one study [42], it was found that the severity of disease correlated with plasma levels after bath PUVA with detectable levels in the half of the patients with the most severe disease. Limited application of a 0.1% solution yielded undetectable levels in all patients [43].

Photobiology The action spectrum for topical methoxsalen photosensitivity is maximal at 330 nm, but there is photoreactivity from 313 to 350 nm [44]. This broad action spectrum probably explains why narrowband (311 nm) radiation and broadband UVA lamps have similar efficacy in psoriasis in combination with methoxsalen bath treatment [45]. The time course of erythema is probably similar for topical and oral PUVA therapy.

Dosage and Administration

There are no established protocols for topical PUVA therapy; instead, there are various published procedures, some of which have been studied in detail. There are two sources of methoxsalen: Oxsoralen lotion 1% (70% alcohol, propylene glycol, acetone, and water) and Oxsoralen Ultra 10 mg capsules (alcohol solution in a soft gelatin capsule).

Bath PUVA Various concentrations of methoxsalen have been used. A 0.5% final concentration in bath water is a conservative dose but appears to be effective [46]. This can be achieved by heating five capsules in three cups of water or using 10 mL of the 1% Oxsoralen lotion and adding it to 100 L of bath water at body temperature. The patient bathes for 15 minutes, wetting all areas up to the neck, pats dry, and then is immediately exposed to UVA radiation. Higher concentrations of methoxsalen have been used. In one study, 30 mL Oxsoralen lotion was added to 80 L bath water to give a final concentration of 3.75 mg/L [47]. There is a good correlation between the MPD in a group of individuals and the methoxsalen concentration in bath water [48].

The starting dosage of UVA radiation should be determined by measuring the MPD before initiating whole body treatment. At a bath water methoxsalen concentration of 0.5 mg/L, a suitable range of dosages for testing is 1.0, 2.0, 4.0, 6.0, 8.0, 10.0, 12.0, and 14.0 J/cm^2 with erythema responses read at 72 hours; the median MPD will be around 6 J/cm^2 [48]. The initial dosage of UVA radiation is one square below the MPD. Treatments are given two or three times weekly, and the dosage should not be increased until five treatments are given—after which a 1 J/cm^2 increase per treatment is usually tolerated. Selecting an initial dosage based on the skin type of the individual can be hazardous because there is a poor correlation between skin type and MPD, particularly for skin types II and III [49].

Soak PUVA This is a topical therapy for treatment of diseases on the palms and soles, and the protocols used have been similar to those for bath PUVA. A volume of approximately 5 L tap water in a basin and concentrations of 0.5 mg/L methoxsalen [50] to as high as 20 mg/L [51] have been used.

Cream PUVA Methoxsalen has been used topically in a cream base for treatment of widespread and local disease [52]. The kinetics of photosensitivity are similar to bath PUVA—irradiation is performed immediately after removal of the cream, and photosensitivity is lost within two hours.

Lotion PUVA Direct application of Oxsoralen lotion to plaques of psoriasis is not an acceptable treatment. This form of PUVA produces prolonged photosensitivity and a high frequency of bullous erythema and intense pigmentation that can persist for a year or more.

Precautions

The precautions required with topical PUVA therapy are essentially the same as those for oral PUVA, with minor variations. Following bath PUVA therapy, four hours' avoidance of sun exposure appears to be adequate. Eye protection should be used because detectable serum levels are found in some patients.

Side Effects

Short-Term Side Effects Phototoxicity is the main adverse effect, and its frequency depends on the aggressiveness of the treatment protocol. Erythema, pruritus, and pain are similar in appearance and duration to that seen with oral PUVA. Gastrointestinal disturbances and CNS symptoms are not seen with topical PUVA therapy.

Long-Term Side Effects There is no information in humans on the long-term safety of topical methoxsalen PUVA therapy. A lower risk of skin cancer has been reported with TMP bath therapy than with oral PUVA therapy using methoxsalen [53–55]; this may be based on a lower carcinogenic potential of TMP [56]. However, based on this mouse study, there is no reason to expect bath and oral methoxsalen PUVA to have different risks for skin cancer. Because of the very low serum levels seen with topical PUVA therapy, the potential risk of cataracts should be nonexistent.

Patient Monitoring

The nurse or technician must determine the response to the last treatment prior to each exposure. The patient is asked about the occurrence of any erythema and, if the response is in doubt, the patient should be examined. Inquiry should also be made about the occurrence of, or alteration in, any pruritus. An evaluation by the physician is required after every 6–10 treatments (more frequently if problems develop or decision points are reached).

A chart is kept for each patient to record the number of treatments, the dosages given, and what areas were treated (Figure 5.3). Remarks about progress and/or problems should be noted

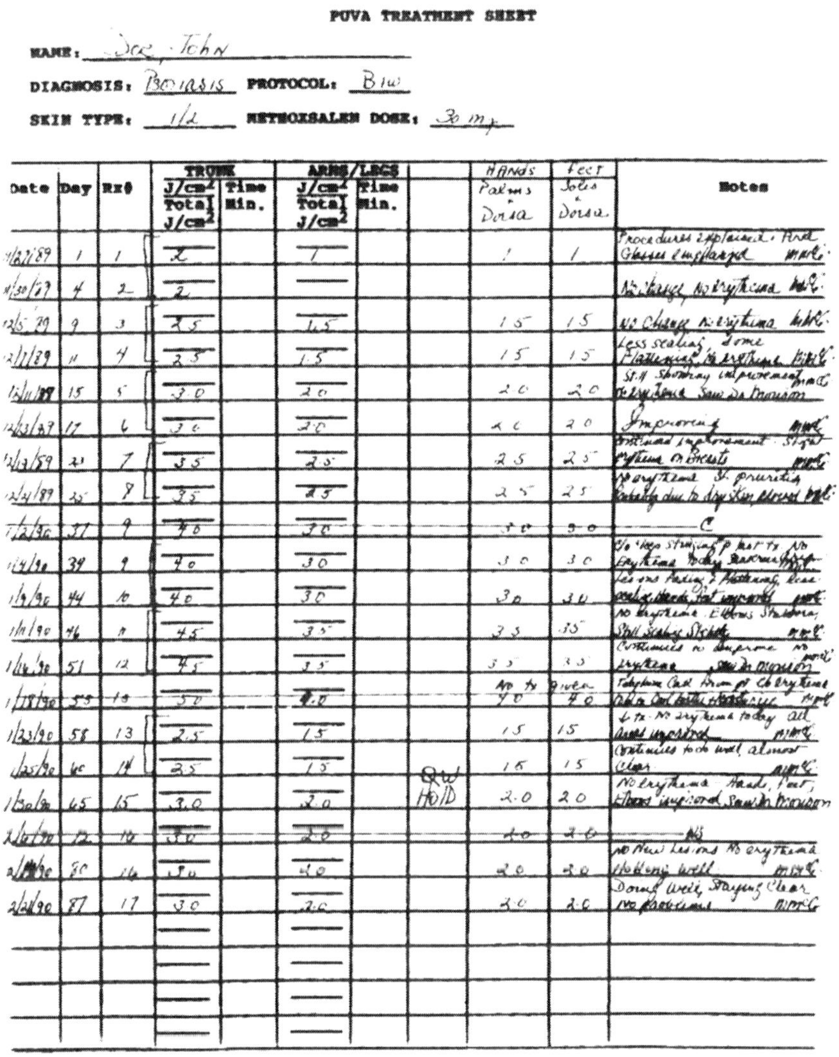

PUVA TREATMENT SHEET

NAME: Doe, John

DIAGNOSIS: Psoriasis PROTOCOL: Biw

SKIN TYPE: 1/2 METHOXSALEN DOSE: 30 mg

Date	Day	Rx#	TRUNK J/cm² Total J/cm²	TRUNK Time Min.	ARMS/LEGS J/cm² Total J/cm²	ARMS/LEGS Time Min.		Hands Palms & Dorsa	Feet Soles & Dorsa	Notes
11/27/89	1	1	2		1			1	1	Procedures explained. And Glasses [illegible]
11/30/89	4	2	2							No change, No erythema
12/5/89	9	3	2.5		1.5			1.5	1.5	No change no erythema
12/7/89	11	4	2.5		1.5			1.5	1.5	Less scaling, some flattening, no erythema
12/11/89	15	5	3.0		2.0			2.0	2.0	Still showing improvement no erythema [illegible]
12/13/89	17	6	3.0		2.0			2.0	2.0	Improving
12/19/89	23	7	3.5		2.5			2.5	2.5	Continued improvement. Slight erythema on Breasts
12/21/89	25	8	3.5		2.5			2.5	2.5	No erythema. Sl. pruritis probably due to dry skin [illegible]
1/2/90	37	9	4.0		3.0			3.0	3.0	C
1/4/90	39	9	4.0		3.0			3.0	3.0	[illegible] No erythema today [illegible]
1/9/90	44	10	4.0		3.0			3.0	3.0	Lesions fading & flattening, [illegible] hands, feet improved
1/11/90	46	11	4.5		3.5			3.5	3.5	No erythema. Elbows [illegible] Still scaling slightly
1/16/90	51	12	4.5		3.5			3.5	3.5	Continues to improve. No erythema [illegible]
1/18/90	53	13	5.0		4.0			4.0 No tx given	4.0	Telephone call from pt c/o erythema [illegible]
1/23/90	58	13	2.5		1.5			1.5	1.5	[illegible] tx. No erythema today. All areas improved
1/25/90	60	14	2.5		1.5			1.5	1.5	Continues to do well, almost clear
1/30/90	65	15	3.0		2.0		QW HOLD	2.0	2.0	No erythema. Hands, feet, elbows improved [illegible]
2/6/90	72	16	3.0		2.0			2.0	2.0	NS
2/[illegible]/90	80	16	3.0		2.0			2.0	2.0	No new lesions. No erythema. Holding well
2/21/90	87	17	3.0		2.0			2.0	2.0	Doing well, staying clear. No problems

FIGURE 5.3 Sample patient chart for PUVA therapy.

for each treatment. Cancelled treatments and no-shows should be prominently recorded. An accurate chart often provides the key to the origin of treatment problems.

Finally, patients need to be sensitized to the need to examine their skin for the development of any new lesions. This educational task is a joint responsibility of the nurse and the physician. During the initial evaluation, at follow-up evaluations, and through written patient instructions, patients should be encouraged to call the caregiver's attention to freckles, moles, or any other lesions that are new or changed to ensure early detection of long-term problems.

Equipment

Safe and effective treatment requires accurate delivery of a measured dose of radiation. The output of bulbs and lamps declines with age and, therefore, must be monitored. Some radiators are equipped with an internal radiometer that constantly measures the output of the lamps. The dose of radiation is punched into the keyboard, and the machine stops when the correct dose is delivered. An alarm that shuts off the machine if it malfunctions is a very useful safety feature with such a system. Other radiators require external monitoring with a handheld radiometer. The dose is then read off a chart of doses and irradiances. Both systems require periodic checks with another instrument to ensure their accuracy. A log should be kept that records dates of relamping and all readings of the output of the system.

REFERENCES

1. Parrish JA, Fitzpatrick TB, Tanenbaum L, et al. Photochemotherapy of psoriasis with oral methoxsalen and longwave ultraviolet. *N Engl J Med* 1974; 291: 1207–1211.
2. Morison WL. *Phototherapy and Photochemotherapy of Skin Disease*, 3rd ed. New York: Taylor & Francis; 2005.
3. Abel EA. *Photochemotherapy in Dermatology*. New York: Igaku-Shoin; 1992.
4. American Academy of Dermatology. Guidelines of care for the management of psoriasis and psoriatic arthritis. Section 5: guidelines of care for the treatment of psoriasis with phototherapy and photochemotherapy. *J Am Acad Dermatol* 2010; 62: 114–135.
5. Tanew A, Radakovic-Fijan S, Schemper M, et al. Narrowband UV-B phototherapy vs photochemotherapy in the treatment of chronic plaque-type psoriasis. *Arch Dermatol* 1999; 135: 519–524.
6. Nordal EJ, Christensen OB. Treatment of chronic hand dermatoses with UVB-TL01. *Acta Derm Venereol* 2004; 84: 302–304.
7. Stern RS. Psoralen and ultraviolet A light therapy for psoriasis. *N Engl J Med* 2007; 357: 682–690.
8. Farr PM, Diffey BL, Higgins EM, et al. The action spectrum between 320 and 400 nm for clearance of psoriasis by psoralen photochemotherapy. *Br J Dermatol* 1991; 124: 443–448.
9. Parrish JA, White AD, Kingsbury T, et al. Photochemotherapy of psoriasis using methoxsalen and sunlight. *Arch Dermatol* 1977; 133: 1529–1532.
10. Wolff K, Gschnait F, Honigsmann H, et al. Phototesting and dosimetry for photochemotherapy. *Br J Dermatol* 1977; 96: 1–10.
11. Melski JW, Tanenbaum L, Parrish JA, et al. Oral methoxsalen photochemotherapy for the treatment of psoriasis: a cooperative clinical trial. *J Invest Dermatol* 1977; 68: 328–335.
12. Momtaz-TK, Parrish JA. Combination of psoralens and ultraviolet A and ultraviolet B in the treatment of psoriasis vulgaris: a bilateral comparison study. *J Am Acad Dermatol* 1984; 10: 481–486.
13. Fritch PO, Honigsmann H, Jaschke E, et al. Augmentation of oral methoxsalen–photochemotherapy with an oral retinoic acid derivative. *J Invest Dermatol* 1978; 70: 178–182.
14. Parker S, Coburn P, Lawrence C, et al. A randomized double-blind comparison of PUVA-etretinate and PUVA-placebo in the treatment of chronic plaque psoriasis. *Br J Dermatol* 1984; 110: 215–220.
15. Honigsmann H, Wolff K. Isotretinoin-PUVA for psoriasis. *Lancet* 1983; 1: 236.
16. Morison WL, Momtaz K, Parrish JA, et al. Combined methotrexate PUVA therapy in the treatment of psoriasis. *J Am Acad Dermatol* 1982; 6: 46–51.
17. Heffernan MP. Combining traditional systemic and biologic therapies for psoriasis. *Semin Cutan Med Surg* 2010; 29: 67–69.
18. Wolfe F, Michaud K. Biologic treatment of rheumatoid arthritis and the risk of malignancy: analyses from a large US observational study. *Arthritis Rheum* 2007; 56(9): 2886–2895.
19. Kircik L, Bagel J, Korman N, et al. Utilization of narrow-band ultraviolet light B therapy and etanercept for the treatment of psoriasis (UNITE): efficacy, safety, and patient-reported outcomes. *J Drugs Dermatol* 2008; 7(3): 245–253.
20. Gambichler T, Tigges C, Scola N, et al. Etanercept plus narrowband ultraviolet B phototherapy of psoriasis is more effective than etanercept monotherapy at 6 weeks. *Br J Dermatol* 2011; 164(6): 1383–1386.
21. Inzinger M, Heschl B, Weger W, et al. Efficacy of psoralen plus ultraviolet A therapy vs. biologics in moderate to severe chronic plaque psoriasis: retrospective data analysis of a patient registry. *Br J Dermatol* 2011; 165(3): 640–645.

22. Spuls PI, Witkamp L, Bossuyt PMM, et al. A systematic review of five systemic treatments for severe psoriasis. *Br J Dermatol* 1997; 137: 943–949.
23. Stern RS, Thibodeau LA, Kleinerman RA, et al. Risk of cutaneous carcinoma in patients treated with oral methoxsalen photochemotherapy for psoriasis. *N Eng J Med* 1979; 300: 809–813.
24. Stern RS, Lange R. Non-melanoma skin cancer occurring in patients treated with PUVA five to ten years after first treatment. *J Invest Dermatol* 1988; 91: 120–124.
25. Henseler T, Christophers E, Honigsmann H, et al. Skin tumors in the European PUVA study. *J Am Acad Dermatol* 1987; 16: 108–116.
26. Stern RS, PUVA Follow-Up Study. The risk of squamous cell and basal cell cancer associated with psoralen and ultraviolet A therapy: a 30-year prospective study. *J Am Acad Dermatol* 2012; 66: 553–562.
27. Stern RS. Genital tumors among men with psoriasis exposed to psoralens and ultraviolet A radiation (PUVA) and ultraviolet B radiation. The Photochemotherapy Follow-up Study. *N Engl J Med* 1990; 322: 1093–1097.
28. Marcil I, Stern RS. Squamous-cell cancer of the skin in patients given PUVA and cyclosporin: nested cohort crossover study. *Lancet* 2001; 358: 1042–1045.
29. Stern RS. The risk of melanoma in association with long-term exposure to PUVA. *J Am Acad Dermatol* 2001; 44: 755–761.
30. Stern RS, Parrish JA, Fitzpatrick TB. Ocular findings in patients treated with PUVA. *J Invest Dermatol* 1985; 85: 269–273.
31. Malanos, D, Stern RS. Psoralen plus ultraviolet A does not increase the risk of cataracts: a 25-year prospective study. *J Am Acad Dermatol* 2007; 57: 231–237.
32. Fischer T, Alsins J. Treatment of psoriasis with trioxsalen baths and dysprosium lamps. *Acta Dermatovener (Stockh)* 1976; 56: 383–390.
33. Hannuksela M, Karvonen J. Trioxsalen bath plus UVA effective and safe in the treatment of psoriasis. *Br J Dermatol* 1978; 99: 703–707.
34. Coven T, Murphy F, Gilleaudeau P, et al. Trimethylpsoralen bath PUVA is a remittive treatment for psoriasis vulgaris. *Arch Dermatol* 1998; 134: 1263–1268.
35. Neumann NJ, Kerscher M, Ruzicka T, et al. Evaluation of PUVA bath phototoxicity. *Acta Derm Venereol (Stockholm)* 1997; 77: 385–387.
36. Gruss C, Behrens S, Reuther T, et al. Kinetics of photosensitivity in bath-PUVA photochemotherapy. *J Am Acad Dermatol* 1998; 39: 443–446.
37. Meffert H, Andersen K, Sonnichsen N. Phototoxicity and antipsoriatic effect of a topical methoxypsoralen solution in relation to the application time. *Photodermatology* 1984; 1: 191–194.
38. Gange RW, Levins P, Murray J, et al. Prolonged skin photosensitization induced by methoxsalen and subphototoxic UVA irradiation. *J Invest Dermatol* 1984; 82: 219–222.
39. Diffey B. Time course of activity of topical 8-methoxypsoralen. *Br J Dermatol* 1992; 127: 654–659.
40. Koulu L, Jansen C. Skin phototoxicity variations during repeated bath PUVA exposures to 8-methoxpsoralen and trimethylpsoralen. *Clin Exp Dermatol* 1984; 9: 64–69.
41. Dolezal E, Seeber A, Honigsmann H, et al. Correlation between bathing time and photosensitivity in 8-methoxypsoralen (8-MOP) bath PUVA. *Photodermatol Photoimmunol Photomed* 2000; 16: 183–185.
42. Gomez M, Azana J, Arranz I, et al. Plasma levels of 8-methoxypsoralen after bath- PUVA for psoriasis: relationship to disease severity. *Br J Dermatol* 1995; 133: 37–40.
43. Hallman C, Koo J, Omohundro C, et al. Plasma levels of 8-methoxypsoralen after topical paint PUVA on nonpalmoplantar psoriatic skin. *J Am Acad Dermatol* 1994; 31: 273–275.
44. Cripps D, Lowe N, Lerner A. Action spectra of topical psoralens: a re-evaluation. *Br J Dermatol* 1982; 107: 77–82.
45. Ortel B, Perl S, Kinaciyan T, et al. Comparison of narrow-band (311 nm) UVB and broad-band UVA after oral or bath-water 8-methoxypsoralen in the treatment of psoriasis. *J Am Acad Dermatol* 1993; 29: 736–740.
46. Vallat V, Battat L, Heftler N, et al. PUVA bath therapy with 8-methoxypsoralen. In: Weinstein GD, Gottlieb AB, eds. *Therapy of Moderate-to-Severe Psoriasis*. Portland, OR: National Psoriasis Foundation; 1994, pp. 39–55.
47. Lowe N, Weingarten D, Bourget T, et al. PUVA therapy for psoriasis: comparison of oral and bath-water delivery of 8-methoxypsoralen. *J Am Acad Dermatol* 1986; 14: 754–760.
48. Tanew A, Kipfelsperger T, Seeber A, et al. Correlation between 8-methoxypsoralen bath-water concentration and photosensitivity in bath-PUVA treatment. *J Am Acad Dermatol* 2001; 44: 638–642.

49. Schiener R, Behrens-Williams S, Pillekamp H, et al. Does the minimal phototoxic dose after 8-methoxypsoralen baths correlate with the individual's skin phototype? *Photodermatol Photoimmunol Photomed* 2001; 17: 156–158.
50. Grundmann-Kellmann M, Behrens S, Peter R, et al. Treatment of severe recalcitrant dermatoses of the palms and soles with PUVA-bath versus PUVA-cream therapy. *Photodermatol Photoimmunol Photomed* 1999; 15: 87–89.
51. Taylor C, Baron E. Hand and foot PUVA soaks: an audit of the Massachusetts General Hospital's experience from 1994 to 1998. *Photodermatol Photoimmunol Photomed* 1999; 15: 188–192.
52. Grundmann-Kollmann M, Tegeder I, Ochsendorf F, et al. Kinetics and dose–response of photosensitivity in cream psoralen plus ultraviolet A photochemotherapy: comparative *in vivo* studies after topical application of three standard preparations. *Br J Dermatol* 2001; 144: 991–995.
53. Berne B, Fischer T, Michaelsson G, et al. Long-term safety of trioxsalen bath PUVA treatment: an 8-year follow-up of 149 psoriasis patients. *Photodermatol* 1984; 1: 18–22.
54. Lindelof B, Sigurgeirsson B, Tegner E, et al. Comparison of the carcinogenic potential of trioxsalen bath PUVA and oral methoxsalen PUVA. *Arch Dermatol* 1992; 128: 1341–1344.
55. Hannuksela A, Pukkala E, Hannuksela M, et al. Cancer incidence among Finnish patients with psoriasis treated with trioxsalen bath PUVA. *J Am Acad Dermatol* 1996; 35: 685–689.
56. Hannuksela M, Stenback F, Lahti A. The carcinogenic properties of topical PUVA. A lifelong study in mice. *Arch Dermatol Res* 1986; 278: 347–351.

Chapter 6

Goeckerman Therapy

Rishu Gupta and John Y. M. Koo

INTRODUCTION

Goeckerman therapy for the treatment of psoriasis was first described in 1925 by Dr. William Goeckerman at the Mayo Clinic [1]. The treatment involves ultraviolet B (UVB) phototherapy and crude coal tar (CCT) [1]. Topical corticosteroids are often used as needed for the most erythematous or stubborn areas of inflammation. Dr. Goeckerman discovered that these agents act synergistically when used together [1]. Goeckerman therapy has long been considered the "gold standard" for psoriasis and is highly effective with a long duration of therapeutic effect [2,3]. Furthermore, this regimen does not have internal side effects. Goeckerman therapy was initially formulated for the treatment of psoriasis, but a modified version has been successfully used for the treatment of other skin conditions such as eczema [4]. The regimen can also be tailored for generalized pruritus, prurigo nodularis, pityriasis lichenoides chronica, erythroderma, and other related skin disorders.

EFFICACY

Goeckerman therapy is one of the oldest treatment modalities available for moderate to severe psoriasis. Even with the development of biologics, the authors consider it one of the most effective treatments for psoriasis. A published study in a peer-reviewed journal revealed that 100% of patients with moderate to severe psoriasis (n=25) treated at the University of California, San Francisco achieved 75% improvement from baseline on the Psoriasis Assessment and Severity Index (PASI 75) after three months [5]. The therapy is also known to have a fairly rapid onset of action because 24/25 of the patients only needed two months to achieve PASI 75. In another study, Menter et al. administered the regimen to 300 patients with psoriasis. One hundred percent of the patients achieved 90% or more clearing of their baseline psoriasis lesions. The average time needed to achieve this primary endpoint of 90% efficacy was only 18 days [2]. In comparison, biologics have reported (in clinical trials) that only 35%–67% of patients achieved PASI 75 at three months [6]. Though the comparison is not derived from a direct head-to-head study, it does reaffirm the notion that Goeckerman therapy is a highly effective option even in the era of biologics. Goeckerman therapy can also be used in treatment refractory cases and has been reported to induce remission for patients who have failed multiple biologics or other systemic treatments [7].

Goeckerman therapy has one of the longest reported average lengths of remission out of all the psoriasis treatments [8]. Psoriasis is a chronic disease that typically returns even after successful induction of remission. Longer duration of remission from a treatment modality can reduce cost of therapy and improve the quality of life for patients. The average length of remission has been reported to range from 9.5 months to more than a year [2,3,8]. If the psoriasis does flare up, the Goeckerman regimen can be repeated. Unlike biologics or some other psoriasis therapies, patients do not develop physiological resistance (tachyphylaxis) to Goeckerman. Furthermore, in the authors' experience, repeated admissions often require fewer treatment days to achieve clearance.

The main topical agent used in Goeckerman therapy is crude coal tar (CCT). Topical tar has been used medicinally for psoriasis and other dermatological disorders since ancient times [9]. There are thousands of compounds within topical tar. Even though tar has been used effectively for many years, the specific therapeutic ingredient(s) in tar and the molecular mechanisms of the therapy are unknown [9]. Regardless, the use of tar in Goeckerman therapy plays a critical role in enhancing efficacy. In addition, the combination of topical tar with UVB phototherapy has a synergistic efficacy.

SAFETY

Goeckerman therapy has an excellent side effect profile especially in comparison to other systemic therapies for psoriasis. The side effects of Goeckerman are minor and usually tolerable. These include folliculitis and phototoxic reaction. Biologics are associated with potentially serious adverse conditions such as cancer, serious infections, and cardiovascular events. Oral therapies, such as cyclosporine and methotrexate, can also put the patient at risk for serious end organ toxicity affecting the liver and kidney. Goeckerman therapy does not have the same side effects as oral or biologic medications. Furthermore, because the safety profile is excellent, Goeckerman therapy can be used for many types of patients including the elderly, children, those with a history of cancer, immunosuppressed patients, pregnant females, and patients with other comorbidities.

Historically, there have been concerns about the carcinogenic effects of tar. However, clinical and epidemiological studies following patients for an extended period of time have not observed an increased risk of cutaneous or internal malignancy with the topical use of tar [10–12]. The U.S. Food and Drug Administration also reviewed multiple studies and ultimately declared that coal tar was safe and effective for the use in patients with psoriasis and other skin conditions [13]. Finally, Goeckerman therapy should not be used to treat patients with pustular psoriasis because it has been the author's experience that tar tends to exacerbate pustulation.

ADMINISTRATION OF GOECKERMAN THERAPY

Goeckerman therapy was initially performed as an inpatient treatment for days to weeks until the psoriasis cleared. However, changes in reimbursement and managed care have led to the transition of the therapy from inpatient facilities to outpatient daycare centers. In the outpatient daycare centers, patients are typically treated for a minimum of four to eight hours/day, five days/week until the psoriasis clears.

Typically, patients start off the morning with an assessment of their skin. If the patient is found to be erythrodermic or exhibits intense, bright-red inflammation, a "cool down" procedure (mentioned in the section on "Cool Down Procedure") is performed prior to starting UVB phototherapy or topical tar. Once the inflammation has decreased and there is less concern that it will be aggravated by UVB phototherapy or topical tar, the Goeckerman regimen is started. The patients are given UVB phototherapy in the morning after which topical tar and steroids are applied to the skin. The topical therapy is subsequently occluded by plastic wrap to keep the medication on the skin and to improve efficacy by allowing for better penetration of the active ingredients. After four hours, the patient can remove the occlusive dressing and wash off any remaining topical medication. If the topical therapies are left on for less than four hours, the efficacy of the treatment may be compromised. Before leaving for the day, a second iteration of topical therapy is applied (usually topical steroids or 20% liquid carbonis detergens [LCD]) or the patient is given instructions to apply it before bed.

The daily administration of phototherapy and topical tar is repeated until the psoriasis clears. Each morning, the dosimetry of UVB is increased upwards. If the patient experiences erythema or burning, the phototherapy is held until the symptoms resolve—at which point the dosimetry is usually reduced. The strength of tar can also be titrated as tolerated. Initially, 2% CCT is applied to the skin. However, if the patient does not experience any reaction to the tar after several days, then 5% and then 10% CCT can be applied. For thicker plaques, special tar formulations containing 2%, 5%, or 10% salicylic acid can also be applied to the lesions with a similar upward titration as the strength of CCT.

The typical duration of the treatment is 30 days. However, for severely recalcitrant cases, the treatment may be continued for as long as it takes the psoriasis to clear. In the experience of the authors, complete clearance is more often associated with a longer duration of remission.

To most effectively maintain remission, patients are encouraged to receive outpatient UVB phototherapy three times a week for at least the first three months, along with daily application of topical medications. After three months, the frequency of phototherapy can be decreased to twice/week followed by once/week if the patient maintains clearance.

COOL DOWN PROCEDURE

When patients present with erythrodermic or near erythrodermic skin, the patient must undergo a "cool down" procedure. These patients have intense cutaneous inflammation that can actually be worsened by UVB phototherapy or topical tar. Therefore, before starting Goeckerman therapy, medium strength to superpotent topical steroids are applied to the whole body under occlusion. This is done on a daily basis until the erythema is reduced, and the patient is able to receive phototherapy and topical tar.

CONCLUSION

Goeckerman therapy is one of the oldest and most effective treatments available for psoriasis. It is not associated with malignancy, serious infection, or major organ toxicity, which may occur from other treatment modalities for moderate to severe psoriasis. Given the excellent safety profile, Goeckerman therapy is a valuable treatment option for moderate to severe psoriasis in patients who cannot tolerate systemic or biologic therapy. This includes patients who have a history of cancer, chronic infection, or multiple comorbidities, or those who are elderly or pregnant. Goeckerman therapy should be considered in patients with moderate to severe psoriasis who are determined to commit the time and effort to improving their psoriasis.

There were no funding sources for this paper.

Dr. John Koo is a speaker for AbbVie, Leo, and Stiefel-GSK. Dr. Koo conducts research for Amgen, Janssen, Novartis, Photomedex, Galderma, Merck, and Pfizer. Dr. Koo has no stocks, employment, or board memberships with any pharmaceutical company. None of the grants were directly related to this study.

REFERENCES

1. Goeckerman WH. The treatment of psoriasis. *Northwest Med* 1925; 24: 229–230.
2. Menter A, Cram DL. The Goeckerman regimen in two psoriasis day care centers. *J Am Acad Dermatol* 1983; 9(1): 59–65.
3. de Miguel R, el-Azhary R. Efficacy, safety, and cost of Goeckerman therapy compared with biologics in the treatment of moderate to severe psoriasis. *Int J Dermatol* 2009; 48(6): 653–658.
4. Dennis M, Bhutani T, Koo J, et al. Goeckerman therapy for the treatment of eczema: a practical guide and review of efficacy. *J Dermatolog Treat* 2013; 24: 2–6.
5. Lee E, Koo J. Modern modified 'ultra' Goeckerman therapy: a PASI assessment of a very effective therapy for psoriasis resistant to both prebiologic and biologic therapies. *J Dermatolog Treat* 2005; 16(2): 102–107.
6. Kim IH, West CE, Kwatra SG, et al. Comparative efficacy of biologics in psoriasis: a review. *Am J Clin Dermatol* 2012; 13(6): 365–374.
7. Serrao R, Davis MD. Goeckerman treatment for remission of psoriasis refractory to biologic therapy. *J Am Acad Dermatol* 2009; 60(2): 348–349.
8. Koo J, Lebwohl M. Duration of remission of psoriasis therapies. *J Am Acad Dermatol* 1999; 41(1): 51–59.
9. Paghdal KV, Schwartz RA. Topical tar: back to the future. *J Am Acad Dermatol* 2009; 61(2): 294–302.
10. Maughan WZ, Muller SA, Perry HO, et al. Incidence of skin cancers in patients with atopic dermatitis treated with ocal tar. A 25-year follow-up study. *J Am Acad Dermatol* 1980; 3(6): 612–615.
11. Pittelkow MR, Perry HO, Muller SA, et al. Skin cancer in patients with psoriasis treated with coal tar. A 25-year follow-up study. *Arch Dermatol* 1981; 117(8): 465–468.
12. Roelofzen JH, Aben KK, Oldenhof UT, et al. No increased risk of cancer after coal tar treatment in patients with psoriasis or eczema. *J Invest Dermatol* 2010; 130(4): 953–961.
13. Food and Drug Administration, HHS. Dandruff, seborrheic dermatitis, and psoriasis drug products containing coal tar and menthol for over-the-counter human use; amendment to the monograph. Final rule. *Fed Regist* 2007; 72(43): 9849–9852.

Chapter 7

Combination, Rotational, and Sequential Therapies

Jason Emer and Mark G. Lebwohl

INTRODUCTION

In patients with moderate to severe psoriasis, remission can be difficult to achieve and sustain; thus, short- and long-term maintenance agents are needed. Combination, rotational, and sequential therapies rely on the use of lower-dose therapeutic agents to minimize toxicity. In the case of combination therapy, additive or synergistic effects may result in enhanced efficacy; however, the dangers of additive toxicity or of immunosuppression must be considered. Apparent synergistic enhancement is seen with most paired combinations of the four major conventional therapies for severe psoriasis: acitretin, phototherapy, cyclosporine, and methotrexate (MTX). Over the past few years, our greater understanding of the immune system's involvement in the etiology of psoriasis has led to a number of treatments that target specific steps in the immunopathogenesis of the disease. Thus, combination therapies using the systemic agent mycophenolate mofetil and the newer biologic agents (i.e., infliximab, etanercept, and adalimumab) have recently been reported. Using two or more therapies is often necessary for most patients with moderate to severe psoriasis, but picking a combination that serves to balance safety and efficacy needs careful consideration. Topical, systemic, and ultraviolet therapies may be used in combination, rotational, or sequential therapy in patients with moderate to severe psoriasis. This chapter will not only emphasize the use of multiple therapeutic agents in combination therapy but will also review rotational and sequential therapeutic options.

ROTATIONAL THERAPY

The concept of rotational therapy was first introduced by Weinstein and White [1]. At that time, ultraviolet B (UVB) plus tar, psoralen plus ultraviolet A (PUVA), MTX, and etretinate were the treatments available for severe psoriasis. Weinstein and White advocated using each form of therapy for one to two years and then switching to the next form. By rotating these treatments, the cumulative toxicity of each individual form of therapy could be minimized, thus reducing the carcinogenesis of PUVA, the hepatic fibrosis and need for liver biopsies with MTX, and the musculoskeletal toxicity of retinoids. It was suggested that as new therapies were developed (i.e., cyclosporine, mycophenolate mofetil, and biologic agents), they could be added to the rotation allowing for even further reduction in cumulative toxicity.

The selection of a treatment is based on the clinical presentation of psoriasis and the type of contraindications that exist. In some cases, monotherapy adequately controls disease and has the advantage of lower cost and greater adherence by the patient. However, for a number or reasons—including inability to clear current lesions, loss of efficacy, adverse effects, or cumulative or acute toxicity—a single modality may not be adequate. Some treatments are appropriate for continuous use (i.e., acitretin, calcipotriol, and biologics) because they maintain efficacy and have very low cumulative toxicity potential. In contrast, some medications are not indicated for chronic use (i.e., topical steroids, PUVA, cyclosporine, and MTX) because cutaneous atrophy or tachyphylaxis to topical steroids, photocarcinogenicity of PUVA, kidney damage and hypertension secondary to cyclosporine, and liver fibrosis caused by MTX are concerns in the long term [2,3].

With most of the new biologic agents, nephrotoxicity and hepatotoxicity are not major side effects and these agents could theoretically be added in rotation to minimize cumulative doses of cyclosporine or MTX. It is easy to imagine the scenario of rotating a patient off MTX after two to three years of therapy to avoid a liver biopsy, or after one year of cyclosporine therapy onto a biologic agent, with the potential for longer remission [4]. Because chronic use of biologic agents is not associated with major organ toxicity, there is less need to rotate to other therapies if the biologic agent is effective.

COMBINATION THERAPY

Combination therapy has been used for a long time, but the concept of using low-dosage combinations of different treatments to minimize toxicity and enhance efficacy was formally introduced at a consensus conference chaired by Dr. Alan Menter and funded by the National Psoriasis Foundation in 1994 [5]. The concept was to minimize toxicity and enhance efficacy by combining lower dosages of different systemic therapies. Since then, many useful combinations have been studied with only a handful of combinations to be completely avoided (i.e., cyclosporine–PUVA, cyclosporine–UVB, coal tar–PUVA, and acitretin–MTX) or closely monitored (i.e., UVB–MTX, UVB–PUVA, PUVA–MTX, and cyclosporine–MTX).

With the advent of newer biologic medications for the treatment of psoriasis, the principles of combination therapy have become even more important. For recalcitrant psoriatic disease, periods of combination therapy with traditional systemic medications overlapping with the newer biologic therapies will be commonplace. Biologic agents have alternative mechanisms of action compared to traditional therapies and, theoretically, these combinations will have an added benefit. It has been hypothesized that combinations with multiple biologic agents will be used to treat multiple diseases concurrently, although increased immunosuppression and financial burden may limit use. It is prudent only to combine agents with differing adverse effect profiles in order to obtain synergistic enhancement and few adverse effects.

SEQUENTIAL THERAPY

Formally introduced by Dr. John Koo, the concept of sequential therapy makes use of a "rabbit to turtle" approach where the therapeutic strategy involves a deliberate sequence starting with a more efficacious but riskier agent (i.e., "rabbit"). For long-term maintenance, a less efficacious but safer agent (i.e., "turtle") is used. As originally stated, sequential therapy involves three phases: a clearing phase, which uses a rapidly acting therapy often with greater side effects; a transitional phase, defined as adding a second therapy while gradually tapering the first therapy; and a maintenance phase, consisting of long-term treatment with the second agent alone. As an example, cyclosporine at maximal dosage was used for the clearing phase followed by the addition of acitretin during the transitional phase. Once maximal dosages of acitretin were tolerated, cyclosporine was gradually tapered and acitretin was continued for long-term maintenance. Phototherapy with UVB or PUVA was added if additional improvement was needed for maintenance [6]. This algorithm has since evolved to include topical agents as well as other systemic therapies (i.e., biologic agents).

TOPICAL THERAPY IN COMBINATION, ROTATIONAL, AND SEQUENTIAL THERAPIES WITH OTHER TOPICAL AGENTS

Topical agents are probably the most common medications used in combination therapy. When combining topical agents with phototherapy or with other topical medications, caution must be used because treatments can inactivate one another or, alternatively, can enhance the efficacy and toxicity of particular agents. For example, the addition of tars to anthralin regimens was advocated in the early 1980s because it was noted that tar reduced the cutaneous effects caused by anthralin [7–10]. However, it was subsequently noted that tar inactivates anthralin, and this effect is therefore responsible for the reduced irritation [10]. Calcipotriene is likewise a relatively unstable molecule that is easily inactivated by acidic compounds. For example, salicylic acid completely inactivates calcipotriene on contact. Other agents, such as topical hydrocortisone valerate and ammonium lactate, also inactivate calcipotriene over time. Halobetasol propionate cream and ointment, however, were found to be entirely compatible with calcipotriene ointment for up to two weeks [11].

Before it was known that calcipotriene and halobetasol ointments were compatible, the agents were used separately in the morning or evening or on different days in combination and sequential regimens. In one study, it was shown that once-daily calcipotriene and once-daily halobetasol ointments were superior to either of the individual agents used twice daily for two weeks [12]. A sequential regimen was then developed in which the first two weeks of calcipotriene and halobetasol ointments were followed by a regimen in which halobetasol ointment was used twice daily on weekends and calcipotriene ointment was used twice daily on weekdays for six months [13]. The latter regimen was found to be superior to a traditional weekend pulse therapy regimen of superpotent steroids alone. Tazarotene has likewise been shown to be compatible with numerous topical corticosteroids [14]. Regimens combining tazarotene with topical corticosteroids have demonstrated increased efficacy and reduced irritation [15,16].

TOPICAL THERAPY COMBINED WITH PHOTOTHERAPY

The use of topical therapy with phototherapy offers unique advantages and disadvantages. For example, some treatments, such as salicylic acid and tar, block UVB [17]. Other medications can be affected by ultraviolet light if applied prior to phototherapy. For example, UVA inactivates calcipotriene [18], and both UVA and UVB inactivate calcitriol [19]. Other medications pose unique problems. Tars, which were part of the original Goeckerman regimen, caused a photosensitive reaction known as tar smarts when applied prior to UVA irradiation [20]. Two weeks of treatment with tazarotene increases the erythemogenicity of UVB, suggesting that phototherapy doses should be reduced by approximately one-third in patients being treated with tazarotene [21]. UVA doses should likewise be reduced by 1–2 J/cm^2 in patients treated with tazarotene and PUVA, or the tazarotene may make the patients more prone to burning.

The combination of tazarotene and UVB has been shown to result in greater improvement than with UVB and vehicle or UVB alone [22]. Tazarotene has also been shown to improve the response to narrowband UVB, as has calcipotriene [23]. Another study failed to show a beneficial effect with the addition of calcipotriene to narrowband UVB [24].

The effect of calcipotriene on a broadband UVB phototherapy regimen has also been questioned. In a bilateral comparison controlled trial, UVB plus calcipotriene was slightly more effective than UVB with vehicle [25]. At least two other publications support the increased efficacy of UVB when calcipotriene is added [26,27]. A third study showed that UVB added to a calcipotriene regimen was no more effective than the calcipotriene alone [28]. It has been shown that calcipotriene used in combination with twice weekly UVB phototherapy is as effective as three times weekly UVB phototherapy [29].

In a bilateral comparison study in which PUVA on one side of the body was compared to PUVA and calcipotriene ointment on the other side, the side treated with both therapies cleared more quickly with lower UVA dosages than the side treated with PUVA alone, supporting a role for calcipotriene in reducing cumulative doses and in photocarcinogenesis of PUVA [30]. Tazarotene has likewise been used in combination with PUVA [31] but, as noted earlier, UVA doses should be lowered by 1–2 J/cm^2 when tazarotene is added to a PUVA regimen [21].

A leading controversy in the combination of topical agents with phototherapy relates to the concomitant use of topical corticosteroids with UVB and PUVA. One study examined patients treated with UVB phototherapy three times a week. Approximately half the patients applied potent topical corticosteroids twice daily until clear, and the other half applied control medication. Although there was a trend toward slightly more rapid clearing in the patients treated with topical corticosteroids, the differences were not significant, nor did those patients require fewer treatments or lower dosages of UVB to achieve clearing. Nonetheless, those patients had a longer average duration of remission [32]. In contrast, a study by Horwitz et al. showed that patients treated with a modified Goeckerman regimen and hydrocortisone valerate cream relapsed after 5.9 weeks compared to 17.9 weeks for patients treated with the modified Goeckerman regimen alone, suggesting that topical corticosteroids shorten the duration of remission [33]. Other studies have confirmed the absence of beneficial effects when topical corticosteroids are added to UVB phototherapy regimens [34,35]. In contrast, topical corticosteroids may have a beneficial role when used with PUVA. Psoriatic disease appears to clear with fewer treatments and lower UVA dosage when corticosteroids are added to a PUVA regimen [36–38].

PHOTOTHERAPY AND SYSTEMIC AGENTS

The addition of systemic therapy to a phototherapy regimen has numerous benefits. Most important is that the number of phototherapy visits can be reduced by the addition of systemic therapy, thus minimizing the dose-related photodamage and carcinogenicity of treatment, such as PUVA [39]. A number of publications have suggested that broadband UVB phototherapy is not carcinogenic [40,41]. The addition of systemic therapy to UVB phototherapy allows for more rapid and more effective clearing than monotherapy with UVB, as well as faster clearing with lower UVB doses and less photodamage. Also, the total dosages and toxicities of systemic agents can be minimized by combining phototherapy with those agents in either a combination, rotational, or sequential regimen.

Combination therapy involves the use of lower dosages of phototherapy with lower dosages of systemic agents, to minimize the overall toxicities of either treatment as monotherapy. In rotational therapy, patients are given a rest period from any given monotherapeutic treatment, thus minimizing the total cumulative dosage of either treatment alone. In sequential therapy, clearing is initiated with a powerful systemic agent such as cyclosporine, MTX, or a fast-acting biologic therapy, which can overlap with phototherapy until improvement is noted. Then, the fast-acting systemic agent is gradually tapered because phototherapy would be left as long-term therapy.

Retinoids and Phototherapy

Both etretinate and its active metabolite acitretin have been studied in conjunction with phototherapy. In high dosages, retinoids are associated with numerous mucocutaneous side effects including hair loss, cheilitis, thinning of nail plates, development of pyogenic granulomas, and dry or sticky skin. Systemic toxicities include hyperlipidema and bony changes, such as osteophyte formation, osteoporosis, and diffuse idiopathic skeletal hyperostosis (DISH), which is associated with long-term usage [6].

When combining retinoids with UVB phototherapy, lower dosages (such as 10–25 mg/day) can be used to minimize mucocutaneous side effects and to reduce long-term cumulative dosages. Several studies have examined the combination of acitretin or etretinate with broadband UVB [42,43]. All studies have shown that the addition of low-dose retinoids allows for a marked reduction in UVB exposure and much more effective clearing. In current practice, acitretin in dosages of 10–25 mg/day is started one to two weeks before initiating UVB phototherapy (Table 7.1). Therapeutic dosages of UVB should be reduced by one-third to one-half to avoid burning, especially if retinoids are added in the middle of a course of phototherapy. Retinoids work by thinning the stratum corneum allowing for more penetration by UVB and thus increasing the erythemogenicity. Thinning of the stratum corneum occurs

TABLE 7.1 Combination Therapy: Acitretin and UVB or PUVA

Start acitretin 10–25 mg/day.
After 1–2 weeks, add UVB 10–50 mJ/cm^2 or methoxalen + UVA 0.5–3 J/cm^2 according to skin type.
Daily acitretin should be continued and phototherapy administered three times/week with incremental increase in light dosage (10–30 mJ/cm^2 UVB or 0.25–2 J/cm^2 UVA).

over a one-week period, so the increased susceptibility to burning may not be apparent until several days after oral retinoids are initiated.

As with broadband UVB, retinoids increase the efficacy of narrowband UVB [44]. Retinoids likewise increase the efficacy of PUVA, and the combination of retinoids and PUVA is among the most powerful psoriasis treatments available. Published studies have demonstrated faster clearing with lower dosages of UVA when combined with retinoids [45]. When used with PUVA, retinoids have the added advantage of suppressing the development of skin cancers during the treatment period.

Although the use of retinoids is generally avoided in women of childbearing potential, isotretinoin combined with ultraviolet phototherapy is often effective in this population [46]. Further, the risk period of teratogenicity from isotretinoin is shorter (one month) than with acitretin or etretinate (two years or more).

Methotrexate and Phototherapy

The combination of MTX and broadband UVB phototherapy has been used for many years in the treatment of psoriasis [47]. In one study, three weekly doses of MTX 15 mg were given before starting UVB phototherapy. Standard dosages of UVB were used and MTX was continued for several weeks until complete clearing, at which point the MTX was discontinued and the patient was maintained with UVB. The total dosage of MTX used in this regimen is usually under 200 mg for an entire course. MTX can be used with narrowband UVB in regimens similar to those with broadband UVB.

One major side effect of concern is radiation recall, which has been reported for a number of chemotherapy agents used in patients after radiation or ultraviolet-induced burns. These patients develop erythema and burning at previously burned sites even though they are no longer exposed to ultraviolet light or radiation.

The combination of MTX and PUVA is somewhat controversial; however, both treatments have been used successfully at lower dosages of MTX and UVA, producing faster and more effective clearing [48]. There is some evidence that patients treated with MTX and PUVA have a higher risk of squamous cell carcinoma [49].

Cyclosporine and Phototherapy

The development of squamous cell carcinoma in patients treated with cyclosporine for the prevention of organ transplant rejection is well known [50] and has led to great concern about the combination of phototherapy with cyclosporine, particularly with PUVA [39,51]. There is less concern about combining UVB with cyclosporine [40,41]. Nevertheless, most clinicians avoid using phototherapy with cyclosporine, and some have advocated using cyclosporine during severe flaring psoriasis and then tapering the cyclosporine dosage once PUVA is initiated [52].

Combinations of Biologic Agents with Phototherapy

Although experience with biologic agents in combination with phototherapy for psoriasis is limited, these agents appear to be safer than cyclosporine with respect to development of malignancies. In some studies, etanercept has not been reported to increase the risk of skin carcinoma when used by patients with rheumatoid arthritis or psoriasis [53,54], although one paper documents the development of squamous cell carcinomas in seven patients after treatment with etanercept [55]. A large observational study reported a 1.2-fold increase in nonmelanoma skin cancer in etanercept-treated patients with rheumatoid arthritis and a 1.7-fold increase with infliximab. There were also 2.4- and 2.6-fold increases in the risk of melanoma with etanercept and infliximab, respectively [56].

Realistically, combination therapy with UVB and PUVA will be performed with the biologic agents, and caution should be exercised especially with patients in whom skin cancer subsequently developed after PUVA therapy. UVB therapy combined with biologic agents is well tolerated, without evidence of significant laboratory abnormalities and with a trend toward greater and more rapid efficacy [57–61].

The most recent addition to our armamentarium of biologics, ustekinumab, has been used successfully in combination with narrowband UVB. In a bilateral comparison trial, 10 patients were treated with ustekinumab at weeks 0 and 4. Narrowband UVB treatments were started after the first injection of ustekinumab and were administered three times/week. At week 6, Psoriasis Area and Severity Index 75 was achieved in 78% of patients on the narrowband-treated side but only 11% on the contralateral side [62].

SYSTEMIC THERAPY

For patients responsive to conventional psoriasis therapy, the combination of systemic agents offers a way to reduce dosages and toxicities of those agents while maintaining improvement in psoriasis. For patients with the most refractory disease, the combination of systemic agents offers the most effective way of clearing their skin but must be used cautiously because some combinations can be dangerous. The toxicity of each of the components of a combination regimen must be considered. Nonetheless, there are multiple combinations of systemic agents that can be used safely.

Systemic, rotational, and sequential therapy can be applied to systemic agents with the goal of a quick resolution by gradually reducing the most dangerous drug in the combination while maintaining therapeutic response with the safest medication. In some instances, remission allows for drug holidays during which therapy is not required. Systemic therapies that have overlapping toxicities may result in severe side effects, and some of these combinations must be avoided. For example, the combinations of MTX and hydroxyurea or mycophenolate mofetil can result in bone marrow toxicity, MTX and acitretin can cause severe hepatotoxicity, and PUVA and cyclosporine can cause cutaneous skin carcinogenesis. On the other hand, certain combinations may be better tolerated or more beneficial. Some of the more common combinations include MTX and cyclosporine, acitretin and cyclosporine, and acitretin and phototherapy. As new biologic agents are introduced, they may be of benefit in combination or sequential therapy. Fortunately, most of the biologic agents are neither nephrotoxic nor hepatotoxic, although they are immunosuppressive and should be used with caution when combined with any other immunosuppressive agent.

TABLE 7.2 Dividing Drugs by Major Acute Toxicities to Select Combinations That Avoid Overlap

Bone Marrow Suppression	Immunosuppression	Other
Methotrexate	Cyclosporine	Acitretin
Hydroxyurea	Mycophenolate mofetil	Sulfasalazine
6-Thioguanine	Biologics	

For purposes of safety, systemic drugs can be classified according to their major toxicities (Table 7.2). To minimize toxicity while maximizing efficacy, attempts should be made to avoid combinations of drugs with toxicities that might be additive or synergistic. Bone marrow toxicity may be one of the most serious complications of combined therapy. As stated, MTX and hydroxyurea both affect the bone marrow. Although these two agents have been used together [63], additive bone marrow toxicity is the main obstacle to their concomitant use. In general, physicians should avoid combining agents that individually cause bone marrow toxicity. On the occasions when those combinations must be overlapped, both the dosages and duration of overlap should be minimized.

Table 7.2 includes acute, life-threatening toxicities such as bone marrow suppression or immunosuppression. Numerous drugs (i.e., nonsteroidal anti-inflammatory drugs [NSAIDs], antifungal medications, statins, calcium channel blockers, angiotensin-converting enzyme [ACE] inhibitors, etc.) are known to increase MTX levels, which can lead to increased bone marrow toxicity [64,65]. Drugs such as sulfasalazine that do not have any of these toxicities can be safely added to most of the therapies listed. For example, the combination of sulfasalazine and MTX has been used safely [66,67].

Of the newer biologic agents, infliximab and etanercept have been routinely prescribed with MTX for rheumatoid arthritis [68–77]. The combination of MTX and infliximab has also been used for patients with recalcitrant erythrodermic psoriasis and psoriatic arthritis who were unresponsive to MTX, cyclosporine, and acitretin monotherapy [78]. There is also evidence that MTX used with infliximab prevents the development of antichimeric antibodies [71]. Etanercept has been used in patients with severe psoriasis in combinational [79] and rotational therapy [80] with MTX. Adalimumab has also been studied in combination with MTX for patients with active rheumatoid arthritis showing significant, rapid, and sustained improvement of disease activity over 24 weeks compared to MTX plus placebo [81]. Additional studies with adalimumab have documented similar results, advocating that adalimumab is well tolerated and provides significant improvement when combined with a concomitant standard antirheumatic therapy such as MTX [82–84]. Ustekinumab has been anecdotally used in combination with methotrexate and with cyclosporine for psoriasis and psoriatic arthritis [85,86]. Nonetheless, further larger-scale clinical trials should be done before routine use of biologic agents with other systemic therapies.

Side effects other than those listed in Table 7.2, such as hepatotoxicity, can occur and warrant additional monitoring. For example, etretinate has been used safely and effectively in combination with MTX for the treatment of erythrodermic and pustular psoriasis [85–88].

However, because of the potential for additive hepatotoxicity, liver function tests should be checked one week after initiation and at least monthly thereafter. There is no evidence that hepatotoxicity from acitretin is a cumulative phenomenon as compared to the hepatotoxic effects of MTX and the nephrotoxic effects of cyclosporine. The combination of biologics with MTX requires no additional monitoring above and beyond what is performed for each of the agents as monotherapy [69,88,89].

Retinoids are among the safest agents we have for the treatment of psoriasis and have been combined not only with medications that affect the bone marrow, but also with medications that may be immunosuppressive. In fact, retinoids such as acitretin may suppress the development of squamous cell carcinomas that occur as a result of immunosuppressive therapies such as cyclosporine [90,91]. Because etretinate may raise plasma concentrations of MTX [92], a complete blood count and platelet count should be obtained one week after combining the two treatments and should be repeated at least monthly (Table 7.3). The limited effect of retinoids on the immune system makes them suitable for human immunodeficiency virus (HIV)-positive patients with severe psoriasis.

The major side effect seen with acitretin is teratogenicity, and the risk can be prolonged with concomitant ingestion of ethanol [93]. When treating a woman of childbearing age, both her reproductive status and the agent's pregnancy category should be considered.

TABLE 7.3 Blood Monitoring Recommendations When Combining Systemic Therapies[a]

Combination Therapy	Monitoring Modifications
MTX + acitretin	Liver function tests: Baseline, 1 week, at least monthly for 3 months, then every 3 months, if normal
	CBC + platelets: Baseline, 1 week, and at least monthly
	Lipids: Baseline, 1–2 weeks, monthly for 3 months, every 3 months, if stable
Acitretin + cyclosporine	Lipids: Baseline, 2-week intervals first month, monthly until stable for several months. Then every 3 months
	Chem screen including: BUN, creatinine, Mg^{++}, LFTs, uric acid: Baseline, 2 weeks, 4 weeks, and monthly thereafter
MTX + cyclosporine	CBC platelets: Baseline, repeat every 1–2 weeks first month, then monthly
	Chem screen including LFTs, lipids, BUN, creatinine, Mg^{++}, uric acid: Baseline, repeat every 1–2 weeks first month, then monthly
Biologics + MTX	In addition to MTX monitoring obtain baseline PPD and chest X-ray if PPD is positive
Cyclosporine + mycophenolate mofetil	CBC + differential + platelets: Baseline, every 1–2 weeks first month, at least monthly thereafter
	Chem screen including LFTs, lipids, BUN, creatinine, Mg^{++}, uric acid: Every 2 weeks first month and monthly thereafter

Note: MTX, methotrexate; BUN, blood urea nitrogen; Mg^{++}; Magnesium; LFTs, liver function tests; PPD, purified protein derivative.

[a] Liver biopsy monitoring + pregnancy monitoring recommendations are not changed.

Biologic therapy is pregnancy category B; however, the safety data are limited to animal studies [94].

Monotherapy with retinoids is not as effective as monotherapy with cyclosporine or with MTX and, as a consequence, attempts to taper patients off cyclosporine onto acitretin are not always successful [95]. The effectiveness of acitretin is increased when combined with either phototherapy or systemic therapies [96]. Acitretin results in a gradual clearing of psoriatic lesions, requiring a longer duration of treatment to achieve peak effect as compared to rapidly acting agents like cyclosporine or MTX. Only a handful of studies combining acitretin with biologic agents exist in the literature, and these patients tolerated therapy without any significant adverse effects. These publications have reported combining acitretin with etanercept, adalimumab, and infliximab. All the study results confirm that the combination of acitretin and a biologic agent is a promising method for the treatment of refractory psoriasis [97–99]. Nonetheless, more data are needed to determine the long-term safety, efficacy, and remission rates of this combination.

The combination of retinoids with cyclosporine has been used safely, although this combination is not always effective [100]. It should be recognized, however, that published cases of retinoids used in conjunction with cyclosporine usually document patients whose psoriasis is severe and refractory to conventional therapy. Thus, this combination may be useful in selected patients. Because retinoids and cyclosporine can cause hyperlipidemia, serum lipids should be monitored at baseline every two weeks after using the combination for the first month and at least monthly thereafter.

The combination of agents that are immunosuppressive with agents that affect the bone marrow is particularly effective. It should be recognized that agents affecting the bone marrow are also immunosuppressive, so physicians must be particularly vigilant about the possibility that opportunistic infections might arise. Theoretically, because biologic agents target specific steps in the pathogenesis of psoriasis, they should be less immunosuppressive than agents such as cyclosporine that have more broad effects on T cells. The one systemic treatment used for psoriasis that is not immunosuppressive is acitretin, and in all likelihood, this agent could safely be combined with any of the biologic agents entering the market [101]. When considering a combination of any of the biologic agents with any traditional systemic therapy, the potential for additive immunosuppression should be considered. In the majority of cases that report an increase in serious infections of patients on biologic medications, it should be pointed out that those patients were either on other immunosuppressive agents (i.e., MTX, cyclosporine, corticosteroids, mercaptopurine, and mycophenolate mofetil) or were debilitated because of underlying systemic illness [102–114]. Although caution should be exercised with this proposed combination, the frequency of infection with these agents appears to be small. The most noteworthy has been the development of tuberculosis; thus, purified protein derivate tests and, if indicated, chest radiographs to rule out the possibility of latent tuberculosis [115] should be obtained at baseline and yearly thereafter [115]. Etanercept has been successfully used as combination therapy in an uncontrolled study of six patients with recalcitrant severe psoriasis [116].

TABLE 7.4 Principles to Consider in Transitioning Patients to Biologics

Drug	Time to Onset (Week)	Time to Onset of Major Therapeutic Effects (Week)
Adalimumab	Within 2	~4
Etanercept	Within 2	4–8
Infliximab	Within 2	2–4
Ustekinumab	Within 2	~4

TABLE 7.5 Transitioning from Traditional Systemic Medications to Biologics

Drug	How and When to Taper	Additional Information
MTX	Begin taper at 4 weeks	Adjust according to clinical response
	Begin at 8–12 weeks for alefacept	No increase in bone marrow or liver toxicity observed
Cyclosporine	Begin taper at 4 weeks	Adjust according to clinical response
	Begin at 8–12 weeks for alefacept	No increase in nephrotoxicity or hypertension
	Taper daily dose by 50 mg each week	No acute drug interactions
Acitretin	Begin taper at 4 weeks	Adjust according to clinical response
	Begin at 8–12 weeks for alefacept	
	25 mg qod × 4 weeks; can be maintained for long term if needed	

In addition, both etanercept and infliximab are routinely used with MTX for rheumatoid arthritis, although they are not usually used this way for psoriasis [70,71,100,117].

Thus, because biologic agents are not significantly hepatotoxic, nephrotoxic, or myelotoxic, they will most likely be used with MTX, cyclosporine, acitretin, or mycophenolate mofetil (Tables 7.4 and 7.5). Concern over additive immunosuppression should temper the use of these combinations until more data are available. Acitretin is not immunosuppressive and is considered the safest agent to combine with biologic therapies. Hence, more clinical trials are needed to assess the safety of combining biologic agents with the currently approved systemic therapies for severe psoriasis.

The grouping of MTX and cyclosporine was the first combination to be used that included an immunosuppressive agent with one that primarily affects the bone marrow [118,119]. Recently, cyclosporine with mycophenolate mofetil [120–122] and with hydroxyurea [123] has been used as combinational therapies. Because MTX is hepatotoxic and cyclosporine is metabolized in the liver, and because cyclosporine is nephrotoxic and MTX is excreted through the kidneys, this combination was initially thought to be unsafe [124]. Rheumatologists subsequently showed that combination therapy with cyclosporine and MTX was more effective in the treatment of rheumatoid arthritis than MTX monotherapy [125]. Later, cyclosporine and MTX were also effectively combined to treat severe psoriatic arthritis [126]. In one study, combination therapy in 19 patients helps improve symptoms of psoriasis and psoriatic arthritis. With long-term therapy, six patients showed elevations of serum creatinine that improved with reduction in the dosage of cyclosporine, while in three patients, impaired renal function did not normalize [118].

When used as a monotherapy, cyclosporine can induce rapid clearance of plaques in a large majority of patients with attainment of 60%–80% reduction at 8–12 weeks, respectively [127]. When combining MTX and cyclosporine, maximal dosages are seldom necessary [118].

As detailed earlier, cyclosporine therapy has been extensively confirmed with sequential acitretin use [4,128] and more recently implicated as effective in combination with etanercept [116,129,130]. Further, two cases of patients with rheumatoid arthritis and hepatitis C were treated with simultaneous cyclosporine and tumor necrosis factor-α (TNF-α)-blockers etanercept and adalimumab. No side effects were noted, thus the authors concluded that combination therapy with cyclosporine and TNF-α-blockers should be considered safe and well tolerated in the treatment of hepatitis C virus (HCV)-positive rheumatoid arthritis (RA) patients [131].

In addition, in a recent study, seven of nine patients whose psoriasis had failed to clear with cyclosporine alone, or who were unable to tolerate higher dosages of cyclosporine, experienced improvement when mycophenolate mofetil was added to their regimen. The maximum dosage of mycophenolate mofetil was 3 g/day, and the mean dosage of cyclosporine was 2.5 mg/kg/day [120]. The addition of mycophenolate mofetil to a cyclosporine regimen does not necessitate any modification in cyclosporine dosage, although patients may be able to reduce their cyclosporine dosages gradually. Attempts to switch patients from cyclosporine to mycophenolate mofetil in cases of severe psoriasis are only occasionally successful. Mycophenolate mofetil monotherapy is not nearly as effective as cyclosporine. In one study, eight patients treated with long-term cyclosporine were changed to mycophenolate mofetil. Five of the patients experienced significant exacerbations of their psoriasis, while three patients had only mild recurrences of psoriasis. All six patients who had impaired renal function as a result of the cyclosporine therapy experienced improvement in renal function following the switch to mycophenolate mofetil [121].

Again, the use of phototherapy such as UVB and PUVA is not recommended in combination with cyclosporine because of the increased risk of potential skin malignancies [50]; however, phototherapy may be added at lower doses as a patient is about to finish a tapering course of cyclosporine to aid in relapse prevention.

In addition to the potential for added immunosuppression, close attention must be paid to liver function tests, blood urea nitrogen, creatinine, complete blood cell count, and platelet counts when combining cyclosporine and other systemic therapies such as MTX, mycophenolate mofetil, hydroxyurea, and biologic agents.

SUMMARY

Severe cases of psoriasis often require a combination of therapies. By using this strategy in the right context, we should be able to improve patient outcomes. However, combining various systemic agents requires careful monitoring. More clinical data are required to determine an accurate evidence-based protocol. Ultimately, the improved therapeutic efficacy resulting from combination, rotational, and sequential therapeutic strategies can have a profound impact on the patient's quality of life and thus is a powerful tool for dermatologists in treating psoriatic disease.

REFERENCES

1. Weinstein GD, White GM. An approach to the treatment of moderate to severe psoriasis with rotational therapy. *J Am Acad Dermatol* 1993; 28(3): 454–459.
2. Van de kerkhof PC. Therapeutic strategies: rotational therapy and combinations. *Clin Exp Dermatol* 2001; 26(4): 356–361.
3. Lebwohl M, Menter A, Koo J, et al. Combination therapy to treat moderate to severe psoriasis. *J Am Acad Dermatol* 2004; 50(3): 416–430.
4. Lebwohl M. Combining the new biologic agents with our current psoriasis armamentarium. *J Am Acad Dermatol* 2003; 49(2): S118–S124.
5. Menter MA, See JA, Amend WJ, et al. Proceedings of the Psoriasis Combination and Rotation Therapy Conference. Deer Valley, Utah, Oct. 7–9, 1994. *J Am Acad Dermatol* 1996; 34(2 Pt 1): 315–321.
6. Koo J. Systemic sequential therapy of psoriasis: a new paradigm for improved therapeutic results. *J Am Acad Dermatol* 1999; 41(3 Pt 2): S25–S28.
7. Schulze HJ, Steigleder GK. Experiences in half-side treatment with tar additive to cignolin-salicylic-acid-white-vaseline therapy of psoriasis vulgaris [in German]. *Z Hautkr* 1984; 59(10): 654–656.
8. Schulze HJ, Steigleder GK, Pullmann H, et al. The effect of a tar admixture to dithranolsalicylic-acid-white-petrolatum therapy on the cytokinetics of psoriasis [in German]. *Z Hautkr* 1984; 59(5): 288–290, 295–297.
9. Steigleder GK, Schulze HJ. A new Cologne therapy scheme—addition of tar to cignoline-salicylic acid-white vaseline therapy in psoriasis vulgaris [in German]. *Z Hautkr* 1984; 59(3): 188, 191–192.
10. Muller R, Naumann E, Detmar M, et al. Stability of cignolin (dithranol) in ointments containing tar with and without the addition of salicylic acid. Oxidation to danthron and dithranol dimer [in German]. *Hautarzt* 1987; 38(2): 107–111.
11. Patel B, Siskin S, Krazmien R, et al. Compatibility of calcipotriene with other topical medications. *J Am Acad Dermatol* 1998; 38(6 Pt 1): 1010–1011.
12. Lebwohl M, Siskin SB, Epinette W, et al. A multicenter trial of calcipotriene ointment and halobetasol ointment compared with either agent alone for the treatment of psoriasis. *J Am Acad Dermatol* 1996; 35(2 Pt 1): 268–269.
13. Lebwohl M, Yoles A, Lombardi K, et al. Calcipotriene ointment and halobetasol ointment in the long-term treatment of psoriasis: effects on the duration of improvement. *J Am Acad Dermatol* 1998; 39(3): 447–450.
14. Hecker D, Worsley J, Yueh G, et al. *In vitro* compatibility of tazarotene with other topical treatments of psoriasis. *J Am Acad Dermatol* 2000; 42(6): 1008–1011.
15. Lebwohl M, Lombardi K, Tan MH. Duration of improvement in psoriasis after treatment with tazarotene 0.1% gel plus clobetasol propionate 0.05% ointment: comparison of maintenance treatments. *Int J Dermatol* 2001; 40(1): 64–66.
16. Lebwohl MG, Breneman DL, Goffe BS, et al. Tazarotene 0.1% gel plus corticosteroid cream in the treatment of plaque psoriasis. *J Am Acad Dermatol* 1998; 39(4 Pt 1): 590–596.
17. Lebwohl M, Martinez J, Weber P, et al. Effects of topical preparations on the erythemogenicity of UVB: implications for psoriasis phototherapy. *J Am Acad Dermatol* 1995; 32(3): 469–471.
18. Lebwohl M, Hecker D, Martinez J, et al. Interactions between calcipotriene and ultraviolet light. *J Am Acad Dermatol* 1997; 37(1): 93–95.
19. Lebwohl M, Quijije J, Gilliard J, et al. Topical calcitriol is degraded by ultraviolet light. *J Invest Dermatol* 2003; 121(3): 594–595.
20. Diette KM, Gange RW, Stern RS, et al. Coal tar phototoxicity: characteristics of the smarting reaction. *J Invest Dermatol* 1985; 84(4): 268–271.
21. Hecker D, Worsley J, Yueh G, et al. Interactions between tazarotene and ultraviolet light. *J Am Acad Dermatol* 1999; 41(6): 927–930.
22. Koo JY, Lowe NJ, Lew-Kaya DA, et al. Tazarotene plus UVB phototherapy in the treatment of psoriasis. *J Am Acad Dermatol* 2000; 43(5 Pt 1): 821–828.
23. Schiener R, Behrens-Williams SC, Pillekamp H, et al. Calcipotriol vs. tazarotene as combination therapy with narrowband ultraviolet B(311 nm): efficacy in patients with severe psoriasis. *Br J Dermatol* 2000; 143(6): 1275–1278.
24. Brands S, Brakman M, Bos JD, et al. No additional effect of calcipotriol ointment on low-dose narrow-band UVB phototherapy in psoriasis. *J Am Acad Dermatol* 1999; 41(6): 991–995.

25. Hecker D, Lebwohl M. Topical calcipotriene in combination with UVB phototherapy for psoriasis. *Int J Dermatol* 1997; 36(4): 302–303.
26. Molin L. Topical calcipotriol combined with phototherapy for psoriasis. The results of two randomized trials and a review of the literature. Calcipotriol-UVB Study Group. *Dermatology* 1999; 198(4): 375–381.
27. Kokelj F, Lavaroni G, Guadagnini A. UVB versus UVB plus calcipotriol (MC 903) therapy for psoriasis vulgaris. *Acta Derm Venereol* 1995; 75(5): 386–387.
28. Kragballe K. Combination of topical calcipotriol (MC 903) and UVB radiation for psoriasis vulgaris. *Dermatologica* 1990; 181(3): 211–214.
29. Ramsay CA, Schwartz BE, Lowson D, et al. Calcipotriol cream combined with twice weekly broadband UVB phototherapy: a safe, effective and UVB-sparing antipsoriatic combination treatment. The Canadian Calcipotriol and UVB Study Group. *Dermatology* 2000; 200(1): 17–24.
30. Speight EL, Farr PM. Calcipotriol improves the response of psoriasis to PUVA. *Br J Dermatol* 1994; 130(1): 79–82.
31. Behrens S, Grundmann-Kollmann M, Peter RU, et al. Combination treatment of psoriasis with photochemotherapy and tazarotene gel, a receptor-selective topical retinoid. *Br J Dermatol* 1999; 141(1): 177.
32. Dover JS, McEvoy MT, Rosen CF, et al. Are topical corticosteroids useful in phototherapy for psoriasis? *J Am Acad Dermatol* 1989; 20(5 Pt 1): 748–754.
33. Horwitz SN, Johnson RA, Sefton J, et al. Addition of a topically applied corticosteroid to a modified Goeckerman regimen for treatment of psoriasis: effect on duration of remission. *J Am Acad Dermatol* 1985; 13(5 Pt 1): 784–791.
34. Petrozzi JW. Topical steroids and UV radiation in psoriasis. *Arch Dermatol* 1983; 119(3): 207–210.
35. LeVine MJ, Parrish JA. The effect of topical fluocinonide ointment on phototherapy of psoriasis. *J Invest Dermatol* 1982; 78(2): 157–159.
36. Hanke CW, Steck WD, Roenigk HH, Jr. Combination therapy for psoriasis. Psoralens plus longwave ultraviolet radiation with betamethasone valerate. *Arch Dermatol* 1979; 115(9): 1074–1077.
37. Schmoll M, Henseler T, Christophers E. Evaluation of PUVA, topical corticosteroids and the combination of both in the treatment of psoriasis. *Br J Dermatol* 1978; 99(6): 693–702.
38. Gould PW, Wilson L. Psoriasis treated with clobetasol propionate and photochemotherapy. *Br J Dermatol* 1978; 98(2): 133–136.
39. Stern RS, Laird N, Melski J, et al. Cutaneous squamous-cell carcinoma in patients treated with PUVA. *N Engl J Med* 1984; 310(18): 1156–1161.
40. Larko O, Swanbeck G. Is UVB treatment of psoriasis safe? A study of extensively UVB-treated psoriasis patients compared with a matched control group. *Acta Derm Venereol* 1982; 62(6): 507–512.
41. Pittelkow MR, Perry HO, Muller SA, et al. Skin cancer in patients with psoriasis treated with coal tar. A 25-year follow-up study. *Arch Dermatol* 1981; 117(8): 465–468.
42. Ruzicka T, Sommerburg C, Braun-Falco O, et al. Efficiency of acitretin in combination with UV-B in the treatment of severe psoriasis. *Arch Dermatol* 1990; 126(4): 482–486.
43. Orfanos CE, Steigleder GK, Pullmann H, et al. Oral retinoid and UVB radiation: a new, alternative treatment for psoriasis on an out-patient basis. *Acta Derm Venereol* 1979; 59(3): 241–244.
44. Halasz CL. Narrowband UVB phototherapy for psoriasis: results with fixed increments by skin type (as opposed to percentage increments). *Photodermatol Photoimmunol Photomed* 1999; 15(2): 81–84.
45. Tanew A, Guggenbichler A, Honigsmann H, et al. Photochemotherapy for severe psoriasis without or in combination with acitretin: a randomized, double-blind comparison study. *J Am Acad Dermatol* 1991; 25(4): 682–684.
46. Anstey A, Hawk JL. Isotretinoin-PUVA in women with psoriasis. *Br J Dermatol* 1997; 136(5): 798–799.
47. Paul BS, Momtaz K, Stern RS, et al. Combined methotrexate–ultraviolet B therapy in the treatment of psoriasis. *J Am Acad Dermatol* 1982; 7(6): 758–762.
48. Morison WL, Momtaz K, Parrish JA, et al. Combined methotrexate-PUVA therapy in the treatment of psoriasis. *J Am Acad Dermatol* 1982; 6(1): 46–51.
49. Stern RS, Laird N. The carcinogenic risk of treatments for severe psoriasis. Photochemotherapy follow-up study. *Cancer* 1994; 73(11): 2759–2764.
50. Frezza EE, Fung JJ, van Thiel DH. Non-lymphoid cancer after liver transplantation. *Hepatogastroenterology* 1997; 44(16): 1172–1181.

51. Marcil I, Stern RS. Squamous-cell cancer of the skin in patients given PUVA and ciclosporin: nested cohort crossover study. *Lancet* 2001; 358(9287): 1042–1045.
52. Korstanje MJ, Hulsmans RF. Combination therapy cyclosporin A—PUVA in psoriasis. *Acta Derm Venereol* 1990; 70(1): 89–90.
53. Klareskog L, Moreland L, Cohen S, et al. Global safety and efficacy of up to five years of etanercept (Enbrel) therapy. *Arthritis Rheum* 2001; 44: S77.
54. Gottlieb AB, Leonardi CL, Goffe BS, et al. Etanercept monotherapy in patients with psoriasis: a summary of safety, based on an integrated multistudy database. *J Am Acad Dermatol* 2006; 54(3 Suppl 2): S92–S100.
55. Smith KJ, Skelton HG. Rapid onset of cutaneous squamous cell carcinoma in patients with rheumatoid arthritis after starting tumor necrosis factor alpha receptor IgG1-Fc fusion complex therapy. *J Am Acad Dermatol* 2001; 45(6): 953–956.
56. Wolfe F, Michaud K. Biologic treatment of rheumatoid arthritis and the risk of malignancy: analyses from a large US observational study. *Arthritis Rheum* 2007; 56: 2886–2895.
57. Kircik L, Bagel J, Korman N, et al. Utilization of narrow-band ultraviolet light B therapy and etanercept for the treatment of psoriasis (UNITE): efficacy, safety, and patient-reported outcomes. *J Drugs Dermatol* 2008; 7(3): 245–253.
58. Ortonne JP, Khemis A, Koo JY, et al. An open-label study of alefacept plus ultraviolet B light as combination therapy for chronic plaque psoriasis. *J Eur Acad Dermatol Venereol* 2005; 19(5): 556–563.
59. Scheinfeld N. Alefacept: its safety profile, off-label uses, and potential as part of combination therapies for psoriasis. *J Dermatolog Treat* 2007; 18(4): 197–208.
60. Koo JY, Bagel J, Sweetser MT, et al. Alefacept in combination with ultraviolet B phototherapy for the treatment of chronic plaque psoriasis: results from an open-label, multicenter study. *J Drugs Dermatol* 2006; 5(7): 623–628.
61. Legat FJ, Hofer A, Wackernagel A, et al. Narrowband UV-B phototherapy, alefacept, and clearance of psoriasis. *Arch Dermatol* 2007; 143(8): 1016–1022.
62. Wolf P, Weger W, Legat FJ, et al. Treatment with 311-nm ultraviolet B enhanced response of psoriatic lesions in ustekinumab-treated patients: a randomized intraindividual trial. *Br J Dermatol* 2012; 166(1): 147–153.
63. Sauer GC. Combined methotrexate and hydroxyurea therapy for psoriasis. *Arch Dermatol* 1973; 107(3): 369–370.
64. Tracy TS, Krohn K, Jones DR, et al. The effects of a salicylate, ibuprofen, and naproxen on the disposition of methotrexate in patients with rheumatoid arthritis. *Eur J Clin Pharmacol* 1992; 42(2): 121 125.
65. Wallace CA, Smith AL, Sherry DD. Pilot investigation of naproxen/methotrexate interaction in patients with juvenile rheumatoid arthritis. *J Rheumatol* 1993; 20(10): 1764–1768.
66. Islam MN, Alam MN, Haq SA, et al. Efficacy of sulphasalazine plus methotrexate in rheumatoid arthritis. *Bangladesh Med Res Counc Bull* 2000; 26(1): 1–7.
67. O'Dell JR, Leff R, Paulsen G, et al. Treatment of rheumatoid arthritis with methotrexate and hydroxychloroquine, methotrexate and sulfasalazine, or a combination of the three medications: results of a two-year, randomized, double-blind, placebo-controlled trial. *Arthritis Rheum* 2002; 46(5): 1164–1170.
68. Lipsky PE, van der Heijde DM, St Clair EW, et al. Infliximab and methotrexate in the treatment of rheumatoid arthritis. Anti-Tumor Necrosis Factor Trial in Rheumatoid Arthritis with Concomitant Therapy Study Group. *N Engl J Med* 2000; 343(22): 1594–1602.
69. Weinblatt ME, Kremer JM, Bankhurst AD, et al. A trial of etanercept, a recombinant tumor necrosis factor receptor: Fc fusion protein, in patients with rheumatoid arthritis receiving methotrexate. *N Engl J Med* 1999; 340(4): 253–259.
70. Schmeling H, Mathony K, John V, et al. A combination of etanercept and methotrexate for the treatment of refractory juvenile idiopathic arthritis: a pilot study. *Ann Rheum Dis* 2001; 60(4): 410–412.
71. Maini RN, Breedveld FC, Kalden JR, et al. Therapeutic efficacy of multiple intravenous infusions of anti-tumor necrosis factor alpha monoclonal antibody combined with low- dose weekly methotrexate in rheumatoid arthritis. *Arthritis Rheum* 1998; 41(9): 1552–1563.
72. Kristenesn LE, Saxne T, Nilsson JA, et al. Impact of concomitant DMARD therapy on adherence to treatment with etanercept and infliximab in rheumatoid arthritis. Results from a six-year observational study in southern Sweden. *Arthritis Res Ther* 2006; 8(6): R174.

73. Emery P, Breedveld FC, Hall S, et al. Comparison of methotrexate monotherapy with a combination of methotrexate and etanercept in active, early, moderate to severe rheumatoid arthritis (COMET): a randomised, double-blind, parallel treatment trial. *Lancet* 2008; 372(9636): 375–382.
74. Lee YH, Woo JH, Rho YH, et al. Meta-analysis of the combination of TNF inhibitors plus MTX compared to MTX monotherapy, and the adjusted indirect comparison of TNF inhibitors in patients suffering from active rheumatoid arthritis. *Rheumatol Int* 2008; 28(6): 553–559.
75. Hyrich KL, Symmons DP, Watson KD, et al. Comparison of the response to infliximab or etanercept monotherapy with the response to cotherapy with methotrexate or another disease-modifying antirheumatic drug in patients with rheumatoid arthritis: results from the British Society for Rheumatology Biologics Register. *Arthritis Rheum* 2006; 54(6): 1786–1794.
76. Gibofsky A, Palmer WR, Goldman JA, et al. Real-world utilization of DMARDs and biologics in rheumatoid arthritis: the RADIUS (Rheumatoid Arthritis Disease- Modifying Anti-Rheumatic Drug Intervention and Utilization Study) study. *Curr Med Res Opin* 2006; 22(1): 169–183.
77. van der Heijde D, Klareskog L, Rodriguez-Valverde V, et al. Comparison of etanercept and methotrexate, alone and combined, in the treatment of rheumatoid arthritis: two-year clinical and radiographic results from the TEMPO study, a double-blind, randomized trial. *Arthritis Rheum* 2006; 54(4): 1063–1074.
78. Heikkila H, Ranki A, Cajanus S, et al. Infliximab combined with methotrexate as long-term treatment for erythrodermic psoriasis. *Arch Dermatol* 2005; 141(12): 1607–1610.
79. Driessen RJ, van de Kerkhof PC, de Jong EM. Etanercept combined with methotrexate for high-need psoriasis. *Br J Dermatol* 2008; 159(2): 460–463.
80. Yamauchi PS, Lowe NJ. Etanercept therapy allows the tapering of methotrexate and sustained clinical responses in patients with moderate to severe psoriasis. *Int J Dermatol* 2008; 47(2): 202–204.
81. Weinblatt ME, Keystone EC, Furst DE, et al. Adalimumab, a fully human anti-tumor necrosis factor alpha monoclonal antibody, for the treatment of rheumatoid arthritis in patients taking concomitant methotrexate: the ARMADA trial. *Arthritis Rheum* 2003; 48(1): 35–45.
82. Lovell DJ, Ruperto N, Goodman S, et al. Adalimumab with or without methotrexate in juvenile rheumatoid arthritis. *N Engl J Med* 2008; 359(8): 810–820.
83. Furst DE, Schiff MH, Fleischmann RM, et al. Adalimumab, a fully human anti-tumor necrosis factor-alpha monoclonal antibody, and concomitant standard antirheumatic therapy for the treatment of rheumatoid arthritis: results of STAR (Safety Trial of Adalimumab in Rheumatoid Arthritis). *J Rheumatol* 2003; 30(12): 2563–2571.
84. Weisman MH, Moreland LW, Furst DE, et al. Efficacy, pharmacokinetic, and safety assessment of adalimumab, a fully human anti-tumor necrosis factor-alpha monoclonal antibody, in adults with rheumatoid arthritis receiving concomitant methotrexate: a pilot study. *Clin Ther* 2003; 25(6): 1700–1721.
85. Allegue Rodriguez F, Sendagorta Gomendio E, Freire Murgueytio P, et al. Treatment of erythrodermic and pustulous psoriasis with a combination of methotrexate and etretinate [in Spanish]. *Med Cutan Ibero Lat Am* 1988; 16(1): 43–49.
86. Rosenbaum MM, Roenigk HH, Jr. Treatment of generalized pustular psoriasis with etretinate (Ro 10–9359) and methotrexate. *J Am Acad Dermatol* 1984; 10(2 Pt 2): 357–361.
87. Tuyp E, MacKie RM. Combination therapy for psoriasis with methotrexate and etretinate. *J Am Acad Dermatol* 1986; 14(1): 70–73.
88. Cutolo M. Etanercept improves rheumatoid arthritis partially responsive to methotrexate. *Clin Exp Rheumatol* 2001; 19(6): 626–627.
89. Bankhurst AD. Etanercept and methotrexate combination therapy. *Clin Exp Rheumatol* 1999; 17(6 Suppl 18): S69–S72.
90. van de Kerkhof PC, de Rooij MJ. Multiple squamous cell carcinomas in a psoriatic patient following high-dose photochemotherapy and cyclosporin treatment: response to long-term acitretin maintenance. *Br J Dermatol* 1997; 136(2): 275–278.
91. Bavinick JN, Tieben LM, Van der Woude FJ, et al. Prevention of skin cancer and reduction of keratotic skin lesions during acitretin therapy in renal transplant recipients: a double-blind, placebo-controlled study. *J Clin Oncol* 1995; 13(8): 1933–1938.
92. Larsen FG, Nielsen-Kudsk F, Jakobsen P, et al. Interaction of etretinate with methotrexate pharmacokinetics in psoriatic patients. *J Clin Pharmacol* 1990; 30(9): 802–807.

93. Larsen FG, Jakobsen P, Knudsen J, et al. Conversion of acitretin to etretinate in psoriatic patients is influenced by ethanol. *J Invest Dermatol* 1993; 100(5): 623–627.
94. Remicade [product information]. *Physicians' Desk Reference*. Montvale, NJ: Medical Economics Company; 2002, p. 1181.
95. Salomon D, Mesheit J, Masgrau-Peya E, et al. Acitretin does not prevent psoriasis relapse related to cyclosporin A tapering. *Br J Dermatol* 1994; 130(2): 257–258.
96. Lebwohl M. Acitretin in combination with UVB or PUVA. *J Am Acad Dermatol* 1999; 41(3 Pt 2): S22–S24.
97. Smith EC, Riddle C, Menter MA, et al. Combining systemic retinoids with biologic agents for moderate to severe psoriasis. *Int J Dermatol* 2008; 47(5): 514–518.
98. Tobin AM, Kirby B. Successful treatment of recalcitrant acrodermatitis continua of Hallopeau with adalimumab and acitretin. *Br J Dermatol* 2005; 153(2): 445–446.
99. Gisondi P, Del Giglio M, Cotena C, et al. Combining etanercept and acitretin in the therapy of chronic plaque psoriasis: a 24-week, randomized, controlled, investigator-blinded pilot trial. *Br J Dermatol* 2008; 158(6): 1345–1349.
100. Kuijpers AL, van Dooren-Greebe JV, van de Kerkhof PC. Failure of combination therapy with acitretin and cyclosporin A in 3 patients with erythrodermic psoriasis. *Dermatology* 1997; 194(1): 88–90.
101. Cather J, Menter A. Combining traditional agents and biologics for the treatment of psoriasis. *Semin Cutan Med Surg* 2005; 24(1): 37–45.
102. Stack WA, Richardson PD, Logan RP, et al. Nocardia asteroids lung abscess in acute ulcerative colitis treated with cyclosporine. *Am J Gastroenterol* 2001; 96(7): 2255–2256.
103. Cainelli F, Concia E, Vento S. Cryptococcal meningitis during cyclosporin treatment in a patient with psoriasis. *Br J Dermatol* 2000; 143(6): 1327–1328.
104. Rolland Y, Cantagrel A, Laroche M, et al. *Pneumocystic carinii* pneumopathy in rheumatoid polyarthritis treated by methotrexate in a patient with pulmonary asbestosis [in French]. *Rev Med Interne* 1998; 19(8): 581–583.
105. Bresnihan B, Cunnane G. Infection complications associated with the use of biologic agents. *Rheum Dis Clin North Am* 2003; 29(1): 185–202.
106. Cursiefen C, Grunke M, Dechant C, et al. Multiple bilateral eyelid molluscum contagiosum lesions associated with TNF alpha-antibody and methotrexate therapy. *Am J Ophthalmol* 2002; 134(2): 270–271.
107. True DG, Penmetcha M, Peckham SJ. Disseminated cryptococcal infection in rheumatoid arthritis treated with methotrexate and infliximab. *J Rheumatol* 2002; 29(7): 1561–1563.
108. Warris A, Bjomeklett A, Gaustad P. Invasive pulmonary aspergillosis associated with infliximab therapy. *N Engl J Med* 2001; 344(14): 1099–1100.
109. Slifman NR, Gershon SK, Lee JH, et al. Listeria monocytogenes infection as a complication of treatment with tumor necrosis factor alpha-neutralizing agents. *Arthritis Rheum* 2003; 48(2): 319–324.
110. Matzkies FG, Manger B, Schmitt-Haendle M, et al. Severe septicaemia in a patient with polychondritis and Sweet's syndrome after initiation of treatment with infliximab. *Ann Rheum Dis* 2003; 62(1): 81–82.
111. Helbling D, Breitbach TH, Krause M. Disseminated cytomegalovirus infection in Crohn's disease following anti-tumour necrosis factor therapy. *Eur J Gastroenterol Hepatol* 2002; 14(12): 1393–1395.
112. Tai TL, O'Rourke KP, McWeeney M, et al. Pneumocystis carinii pneumonia following a second infusion of infliximab. *Rheumatology (Oxford)* 2002; 41(8): 951–952.
113. Lee JH, Slifman NR, Gershon SK, et al. Life-threatening histoplasmosis complicating immunotherapy with tumor necrosis factor alpha antagonists infliximab and etanercept. *Arthritis Rheum* 2002; 46(10): 2565–2570.
114. Bongartz T, Sutton AJ, Sweeting MJ, et al. Anti-TNF antibody therapy in rheumatoid arthritis and the risk of serious infections and malignancies. Systematic review and meta-analysis of rare harmful effects in randomized controlled trials. *JAMA* 2006; 295(19): 2275–2285.
115. Keane J, Gershon S, Wise RP, et al. Tuberculosis associated with infliximab, a tumor necrosis factor alpha-neutralizing agent. *N Engl J Med* 2001; 345(15): 1098–1104.
116. Iyer S, Yamauchi P, Lowe NJ. Etanercept for severe psoriasis and psoriatic arthritis: observations on combination therapy. *Br J Dermatol* 2002; 146(1): 118–121.

117. Kirby B, Marsland AM, Carmichael AJ, et al. Successful treatment of severe recalcitrant psoriasis with combination infliximab and methotrexate. *Clin Exp Dermatol* 2001; 26(1): 27–29.
118. Clark CM, Kirby B, Morris AD, et al. Combination treatment with methotrexate and cyclosporin for severe recalcitrant psoriasis. *Br J Dermatol* 1999; 141(2): 279–282.
119. Aydin F, Canturk T, Senturk N, et al. Methotrexate and ciclosporin combination for the treatment of severe psoriasis. *Clin Exp Dermatol* 2006; 31(4): 520–524.
120. Ameen M, Smith HR, Barker JN. Combined mycophenolate mofetil and cyclosporin therapy for severe recalcitrant psoriasis. *Clin Exp Dermatol* 2001; 26(6): 480–483.
121. Davison SC, Morris-Jones R, Powles AV, et al. Change of treatment from cyclosporin to mycophenolate mofetil in severe psoriasis. *Br J Dermatol* 2000; 143(2): 405–407.
122. Pedraz J, Dauden E, Delgado-Jiminez Y, et al. Sequential study on the treatment of moderate-to-severe chronic plaque psoriasis with mycophenolate mofetil and cyclosporin. *J Eur Acad Dermatol Venereol* 2006; 20(6): 702–706.
123. Kirby B, Harrison PV. Combination low-dose cyclosporin (Neoral) and hydroxyurea for severe recalcitrant psoriasis. *Br J Dermatol* 1999; 140(1): 186–187.
124. Korstanje MJ, van Breda Vriesman CJ, van de Staak WJ. Cyclosporine and methotrexate: a dangerous combination. *J Am Acad Dermatol* 1990; 23(2 Pt 1): 320–321.
125. Tugwell P, Pincus T, Yocum D, et al. Combination therapy with cyclosporine and methotrexate in severe rheumatoid arthritis. The Methotrexate–Cyclosporine Combination Study Group. *N Engl J Med* 1995; 333(3): 137–141.
126. Mazzanti G, Coloni L, De Sabbata G, et al. Methotrexate and cyclosporin combined therapy in severe psoriatic arthritis. A pilot study. *Acta Derm Venereol Suppl (Stockh)* 1994; 186: 116–117.
127. Lebwohl M, Ellis C, Gottlieb A, et al. Cyclosporine consensus conference: with emphasis on the treatment of psoriasis. *J Am Acad Dermatol* 1998; 39(3): 464–475.
128. Short MW, Vaughan TK. Sequential therapy using cyclosporine and acitretin for treatment of total body psoriasis. *Cutis* 2004; 74(3): 185–188.
129. Yamauchi PS, Lowe NJ. Cessation of cyclosporine therapy by treatment with etanercept in patients with severe psoriasis. *J Am Acad Dermatol* 2006; 54(3 Suppl 2): S135–S138.
130. Kamarashev J, Lor P, Forster A, et al. Generalised pustular psoriasis induced by cyclosporin a withdrawal responding to the tumour necrosis factor alpha inhibitor etanercept. *Dermatology* 2002; 205(2): 213–216.
131. Bellisai F, Giannitti C, Donvito A, et al. Combination therapy with cyclosporine A and anti-TNF-alpha agents in the treatment of rheumatoid arthritis and concomitant hepatitis C virus infection. *Clin Rheumatol* 2007; 26(7): 1127–1129.

Chapter 8

Systemic Retinoids

Daniel C. Butler, Tina Bhutani, Ethan C. Levin, Eva Wang, and John Y. M. Koo

INTRODUCTION

The systemic retinoids have been used for a multitude of purposes including the treatment of psoriasis (acitretin), nodulocystic or recalcitrant acne (isotretinoin), and cutaneous T-cell lymphoma (bexarotene). This chapter will focus on general recommendations for the treatment of psoriasis [1] in combination with other systemic agents, [2] for use in children, and [3] in special populations (e.g., immunocompromised and hepatitis B or C positive patients). Acitretin will also be evaluated as a chemopreventive agent.

CHEMISTRY AND PHARMACOLOGY

Figure 8.1 shows the chemical structures of acitretin and etretinate. Etretinate is a lipophilic ethyl-ester prodrug that is metabolized to its active metabolite, acitretin. It has a much longer half-life than acitretin (120 days vs. 50 hours) [1]. Etretinate is approximately 50 times more lipophilic than acitretin and can be detected in serum for up to two years after cessation of treatment. For this reason, etretinate was removed from the U.S. market and replaced by acitretin in 1997. Concurrent ethanol consumption during acitretin therapy can result in transesterification to etretinate [1,2]. The amount of ethanol required has not been quantified. Acitretin is pregnancy category X and is contraindicated in women of childbearing age who may wish to become pregnant during treatment and up to three years after discontinuing this medication. Patients should be advised to take acitretin with food to increase absorption and bioavailability [1,3].

MECHANISM OF ACTION

Retinoids act on retinoic acid receptors (RAR α, β, γ) and retinoid X receptors (RXR α, β, γ) [4–6]. Acitretin is a second-generation systemic retinoid that binds poorly but activates all three RAR subtypes. Unlike other systemic antipsoriatic medications that function predominantly via immunosuppressive mechanisms, acitretin's antipsoriatic effects are thought to be secondary to interaction with nuclear receptors, resulting in enhancement of skin cell differentiation and maturation and leading to antiproliferative effects.

MONOTHERAPY

Plaque-Type Psoriasis

There are several studies documenting the efficacy of acitretin for plaque psoriasis [7–10]. One study compared the efficacy of acitretin (n = 127) with etretinate (n = 41). Patients

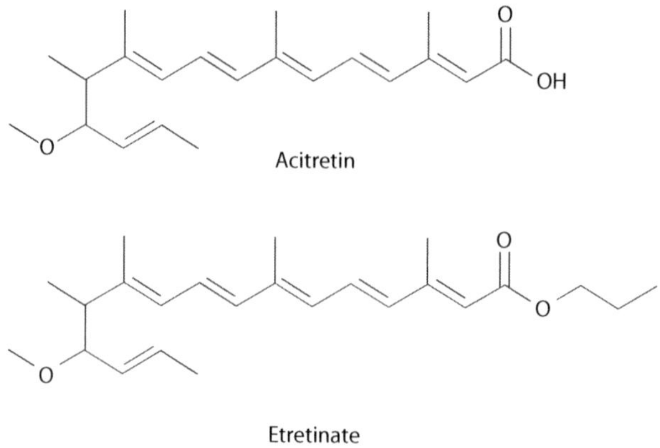

FIGURE 8.1 The chemical structures of acitretin and etretinate.

received an initial dose of 40 mg/day with dose adjustments as needed. The average dose was 0.54 mg/kg/day and 0.65 mg/kg/day for acitretin and etretinate, respectively. The percentage of patients achieving a 75% or greater improvement in their Psoriasis Area and Severity Index score (PASI 75) after 12 weeks was 52% for acitretin and 45% for etretinate [8]. Another open-label multicenter Canadian study ($n = 63$) treated patients with an initial dose of 50 mg/day of acitretin for four weeks followed by individual dose adjustments as needed. The percent of patients with at least PASI 75 improvement after 12 weeks was 34% [9].

Acitretin may be dosed starting with 25 mg or less/day, increasing 10–25 mg every two to four weeks [10]. Optimal dosing ranges from 10 to 50 mg/day. Patients should expect to see improvement after three to six months of therapy. Faster responses may be obtained with higher dosing (50–75 mg/day), but dose-associated side effects may be poorly tolerated. Once the patient has cleared, acitretin can be tapered to the lowest effective dose required for long-term maintenance. To avoid intolerable side effects such as hair loss, xerosis, cracked lips, and so on, the authors recommend starting with a lower dose of 10–25 mg/day rather than the higher dose used in the aforementioned older studies.

Pustular Psoriasis

Acitretin can be very effective as monotherapy for long-term control of pustular psoriasis. One uncontrolled, multicenter study in Japan ($n = 385$) reported improvement in 84% of patients treated with etretinate, compared with methotrexate (76%), cyclosporine (71%), and oral psoralen plus ultraviolet A (PUVA) phototherapy (46%) [11].

Patients can be started on an initial dose of 25 mg/day. Those with severe, generalized disease may require higher starting doses (50–75 mg/day). Patients may see resolution of pustules in as little as 10 days after starting therapy. Once pustulation is resolved, acitretin may be decreased to the lowest effective dose (e.g., 10 mg/day or 25 mg every other day).

The safety and efficacy of acitretin has not been established in pediatric patients because no clinical trials have been conducted in this population [1]. One case report described an eight-year-old male with generalized pustular psoriasis successfully treated with induction therapy consisting of two weeks of cyclosporine (1 mg/kg/day, tapered to 0.5 mg/kg/day) followed by weekly narrowband ultraviolet B (NB-UVB) phototherapy and acitretin (0.3 mg/kg/day) [12].

Isotretinoin (half-life 10–20 hours) may be preferable for females of childbearing potential. Only experienced practitioners who are involved with government-mandated registry programs should use this medication [13].

Erythrodermic Psoriasis

Acitretin may be started at an initial dose of 25 mg/day and increased as tolerated by 10–25 mg every two to four weeks. Sequential therapy is often helpful for patients presenting with exfoliative erythrodermic psoriasis [14]. The physician may start induction therapy with cyclosporine (5 mg/kg/day divided twice daily) for three to four weeks for rapid clearing. Acitretin (25 mg/day) may then be started and increased as tolerated while cyclosporine is tapered to discontinuation. Acitretin can be used for long-term maintenance. Patients with refractory disease may benefit from adding NBUVB, broadband ultraviolet B (BBUVB), or PUVA.

COMBINATION THERAPY

Acitretin and PUVA

Therapy combining a systemic retinoid such as acitretin with PUVA (Re-PUVA) generally results in increased efficacy, decreased number and duration of treatments, and decreased cumulative UVA exposure compared to placebo [15–17]. In fact, Re-PUVA is the only treatment modality other than Goeckerman therapy for which there is at least one clinical study showing all patients achieving PASI 75 after 12 weeks [16,18,19]. One randomized, placebo-controlled study reported clearing or near clearing in 96% of patients receiving Re-PUVA (n = 23) compared to 80% of patients receiving PUVA plus placebo (n – 25) [15]. The median cumulative UVA dose was 42% lower in Re-PUVA-treated patients. Another study compared acitretin (n = 17) versus etretinate (n = 17) (40 mg/day for two weeks then 20 mg/day) in combination with bath PUVA three times weekly. After 10 weeks, all patients achieved at least a 90% improvement in PASI score from baseline [16].

Concomitant use of acitretin may reduce the rate of cutaneous carcinogenesis that is associated with PUVA [20–23]. One case report described a patient who developed three squamous cell cancers (SCCs) after more than 14 years of PUVA treatment [22]. He developed an additional 21 SCCs after switching to cyclosporine. Acitretin therapy (60 mg/day) was initiated. The authors noted a decreased rate of development of new tumors within the first two years of treatment and no new tumors four years thereafter. Another nested cohort study (n = 135) compared each patient's incidence of SCC and basal cell carcinoma (BCC) with or without retinoids [23]. Patients were followed from 1985 to 2000 and were required to have used acitretin or etretinate for at least 26 weeks/year. There was a 30% reduction in SCC incidence associated with retinoid use. The SCC incidence quickly approached preretinoid use if the retinoid was discontinued.

Bath or soak PUVA is an alternative for patients who cannot tolerate oral PUVA. It has several advantages including no gastrointestinal toxicity, faster recovery from phototoxicity, and lower carcinogenic potential. Soak Re-PUVA can be used to treat patients with pustular, erythrodermic, and plaque psoriasis, especially those with a poor response to PUVA monotherapy. One open-label study (n = 4) treated patients with acitretin (0.5 mg/kg/day) plus bath PUVA three to five times weekly. All patients achieved at least a PASI 90 response after four weeks, with no relapse after three months [24].

Acitretin therapy (25 mg/day) may be started two weeks prior to or at initiation of phototherapy. UVA dosimetry should be advanced more slowly to reduce the risk of ultraviolet radiation–induced erythema; a side effect thought to be secondary to retinoid-induced thinning of stratum corneum, resulting in increased epidermal transmission of UV radiation [25]. If acitretin is added to a patient's regimen, his or her UVA dose should be reduced by 50% to avoid burning ("delayed retinoid burn") [26]. If no phototoxicity occurs, light may be increased back to the patient's baseline dosimetry. Once clearing is obtained, the patient should be transitioned to maintenance therapy with low-dose acitretin, Re-PUVA, or PUVA monotherapy.

Acitretin and Broadband Ultraviolet B Phototherapy

Acitretin can also be used to enhance the effects of broadband ultraviolet B (BB-UVB) phototherapy, resulting in lower cumulative doses of BB-UVB and fewer treatments [27–29]. One such study showed higher improvement in patients treated with acitretin (50 mg/day) plus BB-UVB (74%) versus BB-UVB monotherapy (35%) [28]. Another placebo-controlled study reported the percentage of patients who achieved a PASI 75 response was 79% in patients treated with acitretin (35 mg/day) for four weeks followed by acitretin (25 mg/day) plus BB-UVB. In comparison, the percentage of patients with PASI 75 response who received placebo and BB-UVB was 35% [29].

Practitioners may find it helpful to "prime" patients by starting acitretin (25 mg/day) two weeks prior to initiating phototherapy. Patients with an inadequate response to phototherapy may also benefit from adding acitretin (25 mg/day). As with PUVA, dosimetry should be reduced by 50% one week after starting acitretin (delayed retinoid burn) [26]. If there is no phototoxicity, patients may be advanced back to their baseline dose.

Acitretin and NB-UVB

NB-UVB has a spectrum of activity specific for psoriasis (311–313 nm) and is therefore preferred over other forms of phototherapy for the treatment of psoriasis. A retrospective study (n = 40) reported a PASI 75 or greater in 72.5% of patients receiving acitretin (25 mg/day) and NB-UVB three times weekly [30].

Combination Therapy with Other Systemic Agents

Acitretin may be used in combination with other systemic agents to enhance their effects. Sequential therapy with cyclosporine and acitretin is one such regimen [14]. Lipid profiles should be monitored when using these two agents because they both can cause a reversible elevation in cholesterol and triglycerides.

Acitretin is not approved by the U.S. Food and Drug Administration (FDA) for concomitant use with methotrexate due to a theoretical risk of hepatitis from combined use of etretinate and methotrexate, even though there are very few such cases reported in the world's medical literature to date [31]. However, a chart review (n = 18) of patients treated with both acitretin and methotrexate failed to find any cases of hepatotoxicity [32]. Two patients with mildly elevated liver function tests (LFTs) admitted to ethanol consumption and chose to discontinue therapy instead of abstaining from ethanol. Contrary to the FDA warning, the authors concluded that adding methotrexate to acitretin therapy is not an absolute contraindication.

Studies evaluating combination acitretin with biologics prove to be safe and effective. In a study of 60 patients, one 25 mg injection of etanercept weekly combined with 0.4 mg/kg of acitretin proved more effective than twice-weekly injections of etanercept or acitretin alone [33]. Another case series (n = 8) described five patients treated with both etanercept (25–50 mg once to twice weekly) and acitretin (25–50 mg every other day to daily) [34]. One of the patients changed from etanercept to adalimumab 40 mg weekly but continued acitretin. The combination has also proven effective for resistant cases of acral psoriasis [35]. The most serious adverse effect, development of non-Hodgkin lymphoma, was observed in one patient who used the combination for three years. Three other patients developed cutaneous squamous cell carcinoma (SCC), but all three had histories positive for SCC [36]. Other reported effects were transient and included mild elevations in cholesterol and liver enzymes.

Chemoprevention

Oral retinoids induce maturation and differentiation on a cellular level, which is thought to be protective against certain cancers. The most compelling literature details retinoids and the prevention of nonmelanoma skin cancers, which has translated to the clinical use specifically for this protective effect. Acitretin is widely used in the transplant population to suppress the risk of skin cancer related to immunosuppression. In psoriasis, acitretin is useful for skin cancer suppression especially for those patients on combination therapy with cyclosporine and PUVA phototherapy. In addition, the use of oral retinoids is beneficial in the prevention of cutaneous T cell lymphoma, acute promyelocytic leukemia, head and neck cancers, liver cancer, breast cancer, and neuroblastoma. However, these beneficial effects do not apply to all cancers; there is concern regarding the harmful effects for smokers and the development of lung cancer [37]. Considering the elevated risk of malignancies within the psoriasis population, the chemopreventative properties offer an additional, compelling reason for their use.

TOXICITY AND ADVERSE REACTIONS

Acitretin has a side effect profile similar to other systemic retinoids. However, most data reporting on adverse effects is based on high-dose (≥25 mg/day) therapy. Adverse effects are much less common with low-dose (≤5 mg/day) acitretin therapy. Postanalysis of clinical trials reported lower incidences of adverse effects in patients taking lower doses [38]. The incidence of specific adverse effects will be discussed in this section.

Teratogenicity

Acitretin, like other systemic retinoids, is teratogenic and carries a category X pregnancy rating. Exposure during the first three to six weeks of gestation causes toxic effects on neural crest development. Types of major anomalies include central nervous system (CNS) (meningomyelocele, meningoencephalocele, and multiple synostosis), craniofacial (high palate and anophthalmia), and musculoskeletal (syndactyly, absence of terminal phalanges, and hip malformations) [1].

As stated earlier, ethanol consumption can induce conversion of acitretin to etretinate. Based on current recommendations, female patients should refrain from ethanol consumption during treatment as well as for an additional two months after discontinuation of therapy. Females of childbearing potential should be advised to use two forms of contraception during treatment and for at least three years after treatment discontinuation. Practitioners must obtain two negative pregnancy tests prior to starting acitretin therapy. Patients need be informed of the risk of fetal birth defects if exposed to acitretin, and informed consent needs to be obtained as part of a government-mandated safety program [1].

There is scant data regarding transmission of acitretin through seminal fluid. Currently, the FDA has not mandated avoiding semen exposure to women of childbearing potential from male patients receiving acitretin.

Mucocutaneous Toxicity

The most common side effects with acitretin therapy include cheilitis and xerosis. The incidence of cheilitis is greater than or equal to 75% with high-dose acitretin and 70% with low-dose acitretin [34]. Skin peeling occurs in 50%–75% of patients using high-dose acitretin compared to 30% in patients on low-dose acitretin. The incidence of xerosis is about 25%–50% with high-dose acitretin, versus 4% with low-dose acitretin. These effects are dose dependent and may be relieved with routine skin care (bland emollients, lip balms, and eye drops) or by decreasing the dose of acitretin.

Some patients report a "sticky sensation" with their skin after initiating acitretin therapy. This may be due to increased mucus deposition [39]. Retinoid dermatitis is a rare adverse effect characterized by erythema, pruritus, and scaling that can be mistaken for a psoriatic flare. This reaction can develop fairly quickly after initiating acitretin [38]. Practitioners should reassure patients that this is a transient reaction that does not require cessation of therapy. Symptomatic treatment with bland emollients and low-strength topical corticosteroids is often helpful. Should these measures fail to provide relief, dose reduction may be necessary.

Nonscarring alopecia is a dose-related side effect that may occur several weeks into treatment. The incidence of alopecia is approximately 50%–75% with high-dose acitretin and 13% with low-dose acitretin [38]. Alopecia will often resolve six to eight weeks after therapy is discontinued. A few cases of permanent alopecia have been reported; however, causation by acitretin has not been established.

Nail abnormalities such as onychorrhexis, onychoschizia, and periungual pyogenic granulomas may also occur, especially with prolonged therapy. The incidence of such nail disorders is about 25%–50% with high-dose acitretin versus 0% with low-dose acitretin [1,38]. Treatment consists of reducing the dose or discontinuing acitretin.

Musculoskeletal

The most common musculoskeletal side effects are myalgias and arthralgias. Myalgias can occur in the presence or absence of elevated creatinine phosphokinase. Arthralgias may occur in a small percentage of patients. This will often resolve with discontinuation of therapy.

Diffuse idiopathic skeletal hyperostosis (DISH) syndrome is most commonly associated with isotretinoin therapy. One study conducted a radiographic survey with age- and sex-matched patients receiving etretinate therapy to evaluate the association of etretinate with DISH-like bony abnormalities [40]. There was radiographic evidence of calcification in 84% of patients ($n = 38$) receiving high-dose etretinate (mean dose 0.8 mg/kg/day) after an average of five years. The study's author noted that bone toxicity typically occurs with high-dose, long-term, chronic use. He further speculated that the rate of bone toxicity might be similar between acitretin and etretinate because acitretin is the active metabolite of etretinate. He also cautioned that there might be a period of time that passes before acitretin toxicity is observed because this medication had only been available for a few years at the time of this publication.

These results have not been confirmed in other studies. In the three largest prospective studies including a total of more than 600 patients, *de novo* hyperostosis was not strongly associated with the use of systemic retinoids and was seen in less than 1% of cases followed [41–43]. Further, this may have been due to normal aging processes rather than acitretin therapy. In another study, a chart review conducted at the University of California, San Francisco Psoriasis Center ($n = 49$), investigators failed to find any confirmed cases of DISH syndrome in patients treated with at least one year (average duration two years) of etretinate or acitretin over the last 20 years [44]. Based on these study results, there appears to be no convincing evidence that hyperostosis occurs in patients treated with low-dose acitretin.

Premature epiphyseal closure is of particular concern in pediatric patients receiving systemic retinoids. Premature epiphyseal closure and bony hyperostosis have been reported in patients treated with isotretinoin and rarely etretinate but not acitretin [40–42,45,46]. One case series ($n = 8$) did not find bony changes in patients treated with etretinate [40]. Another report discussed two patients previously treated with etretinate for five years who later presented with severe bony changes consisting of bilateral ossification of the interosseous ligament and resulting in bridging of the radius and ulna, preventing forearm rotation [46].

Neurological

Cases of pseudotumor cerebri (idiopathic intracranial hypertension) have been associated with systemic retinoid therapy, but the incidence is unclear. A review of the literature [47] did not find any evidence-based data supporting a relationship between acitretin monotherapy and pseudotumor cerebri. One clinical trial evaluating acitretin for the treatment of psoriasis reported cases of pseudotumor cerebri in association with other oral retinoids when used concomitantly with tetracycline-class antibiotics [48]. Tetracycline antibiotics, especially minocycline, are thought to decrease cerebral spinal fluid absorption by interacting with cyclic adenosine monophosphate on arachnoid villi [48,49]. Pseudotumor cerebri has also been reported with isotretinoin when used as monotherapy or in combination with tetracycline-class antibiotics [50–53].

One study (n = 525) reported a rate of pseudotumor cerebri of less than 1% in patients receiving acitretin monotherapy [1]. Another study (n = 331) reviewing case reports of ocular side effects in association with systemic retinoids found 21 cases of intracranial hypertension associated with retinoids, three of which were linked specifically to acitretin [54]. The authors concluded that the three cases were sufficient to infer a "probable" causal relationship by World Health Organization (WHO) criteria of intracranial hypertension secondary to acitretin therapy. Despite these findings, there is a lack of evidence-based data to support a definite causal relationship between acitretin and pseudotumor cerebri. Further investigation is recommended to determine whether these associations can be supported by scientific data, or if they are due to class labeling.

Nevertheless, practitioners should counsel patients on signs and symptoms of pseudotumor cerebri (severe headaches, nausea, and visual changes). Oral retinoids should not be prescribed in combination with oral tetracycline-class antibiotics. Ophthalmological examination to rule out papilledema is necessary if pseudotumor cerebri is suspected.

Psychiatric

A suicide-depression warning is included in the prescribing information as per the FDA; however, there are no convincing case reports in the literature associating acitretin with depression or suicide. John Koo feels that this may be a "class label" by the FDA, reflecting the controversy in regard to depression and suicide involving isotretinoin.

Gastrointestinal

Hypertriglyceridemia and hypercholesterolemia occur in approximately 66% and 33% of patients, respectively [55]. However, these data are based on high-dose therapy. Most cases of hypertriglyceridemia and hypercholesterolemia are mild and can be managed medically without discontinuing acitretin therapy. Fulminant hepatitis secondary to severely elevated serum triglycerides has been reported in rare cases [1]. Patients should be counseled about lifestyle changes such as decreasing dietary fat intake and increasing regular exercise. If hypercholesterolemia does not respond to lifestyle changes, a lipid-lowering agent may be necessary [55].

Patients with hypertriglyceridemia who do not respond to lifestyle changes may require the addition of gemfibrozil (600 mg twice daily). If triglycerides are more than 499 mg/dL despite gemfibrozil therapy, the retinoid dose should be decreased by 50%. If triglycerides are more than 800 mg/dL, the retinoid should be discontinued at once to eliminate risk of pancreatitis.

Once hypertriglyceridemia is well controlled, systemic retinoid therapy may be restarted. If triglycerides remain elevated despite statin therapy, prescription strength omega-3-acid ethyl esters (P-OM3) may be useful [56].

The patient may also be referred back to their primary care physician for management of this problem. Combination therapy of a statin with gemfibrozil is contraindicated secondary to an increased risk of rhabdomyolysis.

Abnormal LFTs may occur in up to 25%–30% of patients on high-dose therapy [55]. However, liver abnormalities are rare in patients receiving low-dose therapy [38]. Elevation in LFTs is typically seen after two to eight weeks of acitretin and is transient; severe or persistent elevations are rare. Patients with transaminase levels greater than two times the upper limit of normal should have their acitretin dose decreased by 50% and their LFTs rechecked in two weeks. Acitretin may also be discontinued until LFTs normalize and then restarted at a lower dose with close laboratory monitoring. Patients should also be counseled to abstain from alcohol or acetaminophen consumption to reduce their risk of hepatotoxicity. If LFTs remain persistently elevated at greater than two times the upper limit of normal, hepatology consultation should be considered.

A history of hepatitis B or C is not an absolute contraindication for acitretin therapy. A case report described a patient with hepatitis C and psoriasis that worsened while receiving interferon-α therapy [57]. Baseline laboratories showed normal serum transaminase levels, and the patient was started on acitretin (1 mg/kg/day). The patient's skin was almost clear after 6 months and clear after 10 months of acitretin therapy. He remained clear during his one-year follow-up. The authors suggested that patients with viral hepatitis might be candidates for acitretin therapy if they have normal baseline serum transaminase levels. Overall, acitretin is not absolutely contraindicated in patients with pre-existing liver disease but should be used with caution [55].

Immunosuppression

Acitretin is the only systemic agent that does not function by predominantly immunosuppressive mechanisms. For this reason, acitretin is therefore safe for use in immunocompromised individuals, such as patients with human immunodeficiency virus (HIV). A single-center pilot study (n = 11) evaluated the safety and efficacy of acitretin monotherapy in patients treated with acitretin for 20 weeks [58]. They reported good-to-excellent responses in PASI score in 54% of patients, and the remaining patients (34%) demonstrated complete clearing. Immunosuppression was not increased with acitretin.

FOLLOW-UP

Baseline labs (complete blood count, LFTs, and fasting lipid profile) should be obtained with monthly follow-up while dose adjustments are being made. In a typical low-dose use of 25 mg/day or less, frequency of monitoring may be decreased to every two to three months once dosing has stabilized and prior lab work is not concerning for hepatotoxicity or hyperlipidemia.

Routine liver biopsy is not required in patients receiving long-term acitretin. A prospective study (n = 128) monitoring patients taking acitretin (25–50 mg/day) over a two-year period did not find any progressive hepatotoxicity. Pre- and post-acitretin liver biopsies showed either no changes (59%), improvement (24%), or worsening (14%) in patients. The biopsy results showing hepatotoxicity could not be correlated with acitretin therapy or with the degree of LFT abnormalities [59].

Females of childbearing potential must have two negative pregnancy tests prior to initiating acitretin and monthly pregnancy testing during treatment [1]. Acitretin is not recommended in females of childbearing potential; isotretinoin has a shorter half-life and may be a more appropriate choice even though this medication is off-label when used in psoriasis.

REFERENCES

1. Stiefel Laboratories. Soriatane (acitretin) prescribing information. Coral Gables, FL: Stiefel Laboratories, 2007.
2. Larsen FG, Jakobsen P, Knudsen J, et al. Conversion of acitretin to etritinate in psoriatic patients is influenced by ethanol. *J Invest Dermatol* 1998; 100: 623–627.
3. McNamara PJ, Jewell RC, Jensen BK, et al. Food increases the bioavailability of acitretin. *J Clin Pharmacol* 1988; 28: 1051–1055.
4. Chandraratna RA. Rational design of receptor-selective retinoids. *J Am Acad Dermatol* 1998; 39: S124–S128.
5. Kang S, Li SY, Voorhees JJ. Pharmacology and molecular action of retinoids and vitamin D in skin. *J Invest Dermatol Symposium Proc* 1996; 1: 15–21.
6. Rowe A. Retinoids X receptors. *Int J Biochem Cell Biol* 1997; 29: 276–278.
7. Leon A, Nguyen A, Letsinger J, et al. An attempt to formulate an evidence-based strategy in the management of moderate-to-severe psoriasis: A review of the efficacy and safety of biologics and prebiologic options. *Exp Opin Pharmacother* 2007; 8(5): 617–632.
8. Kragballe K, Jansen CT, Geiger JM, et al. A double-blind comparison of acitretin and etretinate in the treatment of severe psoriasis. *Acta Derm Venereol* 1989; 69: 35–40.
9. Murray HE, Anhalt AW, Lessard R, et al. A 12-month treatment of severe psoriasis with acitretin: Results of a Canadian open multicenter trial. *J Am Acad Dermatol* 1991; 24: 598–602.
10. Ling MR. Acitretin: Optimal dosing strategies. *J Am Acad Dermatol* 1999; 41(3): S2–S6.
11. Ozawa A, Ohkido M, Haruki Y, et al. Treatment of generalized pustular psoriasis: A multicenter study in Japan. *J Dermatol* 1999; 26: 141–149.
12. Kim HS, Kim GM, Kim SY. Two-stage therapy for childhood generalized pustular psoriasis: Low-dose cyclosporin for induction and maintenance with acitretin/narrowband ultraviolet B phototherapy. *Pediatr Dermatol* 2006; 23(3): 306–308.
13. iPLEDGE.(2013). Retrieved June 1, 2013, Available from: https://www.ipledgeprogram.com
14. Koo J. Systemic sequential therapy of psoriasis: A new paradigm for improved therapeutic results. *J Am Acad Dermatol* 1999; 41: S25–S28.
15. Tanew A, Guggenbichler A, Honigsmann H, et al. Photochemotherapy for severe psoriasis without or in combination with acitretin: A randomized, double-blind comparison study. *J Am Acad Dermatol* 1991; 26: 682–684.
16. Lauharanta J, Geiger JM. A double-blind comparison of acitretin and etretinate in combination with bath PUVA in the treatment of extensive psoriasis. *Br J Dermatol* 1989; 121: 107–112.
17. Saurat JH, Geiger JM, Amblard P, et al. Randomized double-blind multicenter study comparing acitretin-PUVA, etretinate-PUVA, and placebo-PUVA in the treatment of severe psoriasis. *Dermatologica* 1988; 177: 218–224.
18. Green C, Lakshmipathi T, Johnson BE, Ferguson J. A comparison of the efficacy and relapse rates of narrowband UVB (TL-01) monotherapy vs. etretinate (re-TL-01) vs. etretinate-PUVA (re-PUVA) in the treatment of psoriasis patients. *Br J Dermatol* 1992; 127(1): 5–9.
19. Lee E, Koo J. Modern modified "ultra" Goeckerman therapy: A PASI assessment of a very effective therapy for psoriasis resistant to both prebiologic and biologic therapies. *J Dermatol Treat* 2005; 16(2): 102–107.

20. Stern RS, Liebman EJ, Väkevä L. PUVA Follow-up study: Oral psoralen and ultraviolet light (PUVA) treatment of psoriasis and persistent risk of nonmelanoma skin cancer. *J Natl Cancer Inst* 1998; 90(17): 1278–1284.
21. Lindelof B, Sigurgeirsson B, Tegner E, et al. PUVA and cancer: A large-scale epidemiologic study. *Lancet* 1991; 338: 91–93.
22. van De Kerkohof PC, De Rooij MJ. Multiple squamous cell carcinomas in a psoriatic patient following high-dose photochemotherapy and cyclosporine treatment: Response to long-term acitretin maintenance. *Br J Dermatol* 1997; 136: 275–278.
23. Nijsten TE, Stern RS. Oral retinoid use reduces cutaneous squamous cell carcinoma risk in patients with psoriasis treated with psoralen-UVA: A nested cohort study. *J Am Acad Dermatol* 2003; 49(4): 644–650.
24. Muchenberger S, Schof E, Simon JC. The combination of oral acitretin and bath PUVA for the treatment of severe psoriasis. *Br J Dermatol* 1997; 137: 587–589.
25. Yamauchi PS, Rizk D, Kormili T, et al. Systemic retinoids. In: Weinstein GD, Gottlieb AB, eds. *Therapy of Moderate-to-Severe Psoriasis*. New York: Marcel Dekker Inc, 2003: 137–150.
26. Busse K, Koo J. Introducing the delayed retinoid burn: A case report and discussion of this potential risk of retinoid-phototherapy combination management. *J Am Acad Dermatol* 2011; 64(5): 1011–1012.
27. Iest J, Boer J. Combined treatment of psoriasis with acitretin and UVB phototherapy compared with acitretin alone and UVB alone. *Br J Dermatol* 1989; 120: 665–670.
28. Lowe N, Prystowsky JH, Bourget T, et al. Acitretin plus UVB therapy for psoriasis: Comparisons with placebo plus UVB and acitretin alone. *J Am Acad Dermatol* 1991; 24: 591–594.
29. Ruzicka T, Sommerburg C, Braun-Falco O, et al. Efficiency of acitretin in combination with UV-B in the treatment of severe psoriasis. *Arch Dermatol* 1990; 126: 482–486.
30. Spuls PI, Rozenblit M, Lebwohl M. Retrospective study of the efficacy of narrowband UVB and acitretin. *J Dermatol Treat* 2003; 14(suppl 2): 17–20.
31. Zachariae H. Methotrexate and etretinate as concurrent therapies in the treatment of psoriasis. *Arch Dermatol* 1984; 120(2): 155.
32. Lowenthal KE, Horn PJ, Kalb RE. Concurrent use of methotrexate and acitretin revisited. *J Dermatol Treat* 2008; 19: 22–26.
33. Gisondi P, Del Giglio M, Cotena C, Girolomoni G. Combining etanercept and acitretin in the therapy of chronic plaque psoriasis: A 24-week, randomized, controlled, investigator-blinded pilot trial. *Br J Dermatol* 2008; 158: 1345–1349.
34. Conley J, Nanton J, Dhawan S, et al. Novel combination regimens: Biologics and acitretin for the treatment of psoriasis—A case series. *J Dermatol Treat* 2006; 17: 86–89.
35. Ingram JR, Anstey AV, Piguet V. Combination treatment with a tumour necrosis factor antagonist and an oral retinoid: Efficacy in severe acral psoriasis? *Br J Dermatol* 2012; 167: 937–963.
36. Smith E, Riddle C, Menter A, et al. Combining systemic retinoids with biologic agents for moderate to severe psoriasis. *Int J Dermatol* 2008; 47: 514–518.
37. Bhutani T, Koo J. A review of the chemopreventative effects of oral retinoids for internal neoplasms. *J Am Acad Dermatol* 2011; 10(11): 1292–1298.
38. Stiefel [package insert]. *Triangle Park*, NC: Stiefel Laboratories; 2013.
39. Hartevelt MM, Bavinck JN, Kootte AMM, et al. Incidence of skin cancer after renal transplantation in the Netherlands. *Transplantation* 1990; 49: 506–509.
40. Gilbert M, Ellis CN, Voorhees JJ. Lack of skeletal radiographic changes during short-term etretinate therapy for psoriasis. *Dermatologica* 1986; 172: 160–163.
41. Katz HI, Waalen J, Leach EE. Acitretin in psoriasis: An overview of adverse effects. *J Am Acad Dermatol* 1999; 41(3 Pt 2): S7–S12.
42. Van Dooren-Greebe RJ, Lemmens JA, De Boo T, et al. Prolonged treatment with oral retinoids in adults: No influence on the frequency and severity of spinal abnormalities. *Br J Dermatol* 1996; 134(1): 71–76.
43. Orfanos CE. Retinoids: The new status. Maintenance therapy, disorders of resorption in "non-responders", interactions and interferences with drugs, treatment of children and bone toxicity, acitetin and 13-cis-acitretin. *Hautarzt* 1989; 40(3): 123–129.
44. Lee E, Koo J. Single-center retrospective study of long-term use of low-dose acitretin (Soriatane®) for psoriasis. *J Dermatol Treat* 2004; 15: 8–13.
45. Prendiville J, Bingham EA, Burrows D. Premature epiphyseal closure—A complication of etretinate therapy in children. *J Am Acad Dermatol* 1986; 15(6): 1259–1262.

46. Guit GL, Obermann WR, van der Schroeff JG, et al. Cortical hyperostosis and enthesopathy due to long-term etretinate administration. *Diagn Imaging Clin Med* 1986; 55: 214–218.
47. Starling J, Koo J. Evidence based or theoretical concern? Pseudotumor cerebri and depression as acitretin side effects. *J Drugs Dermatol* 2005; 4: 690–696.
48. Stuart BH, Litt IF. Tetracycline-associated intracranial hypertension in an adolescent: A complication of systemic acne therapy. *J Pediatr* 1978; 92: 679–680.
49. Walters BN, Gubbay SS. Tetracycline and benign intracranial hypertension: Report of 5 cases. *Br Med J (Clin Res Ed)* 1981; 282: 19–20.
50. Bigby M, Stern RS. Adverse reactions to isotretinoin. A report from the Adverse Drug Reaction Reporting System. *J Am Acad Dermatol* 1988; 18(3): 543–552.
51. Lee AG. Pseudotumor cerebri after treatment with tetracycline and isotretinoin for acne. *Cutis* 1995; 55(3): 165–168.
52. Roytman M, Frumkin A, Bohn TG. Pseudotumor cerebri caused by isotretinoin. *Cutis* 1988; 42(5): 399–400.
53. Fraunfelder FW, Fraunfelder FT, Corbett JJ. Isotretinoin-induced intracranial hypertension. *Ophthalmology* 2004; 111(6): 1248–1250.
54. Fraunfelder FW, Fraunfelder FT. Evidence for a probable causal relationship between tretinoin, acitretin, and etretinate and intracranial hypertension. *J Neuro-Ophthalmol* 2004; 24(3): 214–216.
55. Otley CC, Stasko T, Tope WD, et al. Chemoprevention of nonmelanoma skin cancer with systemic retinoids: Practical dosing and management of adverse effects. *Dermatol Surg* 2006; 32: 562–568.
56. Davidson MH, Stein EA, Bays HE, et al. COMBination of prescription Omega-3 with Simvastatin (COMBOS) Investigators: Efficacy and tolerability of adding prescription omega-3 fatty acids 4 g/d to simvastatin 40 mg/d in hypertriglyceridemic patients: An 8-week, randomized, double-blind, placebo-controlled study. *Clin Ther* 2007; 29(7): 1354–1367.
57. Erkek E, Karaduman A, Akcan Y, et al. Psoriasis associated with HCV and exacerbated by interferon alpha: Complete clearance with acitretin during interferon alpha treatment for chronic active hepatitis. *Dermatology* 2000; 201: 179–180.
58. Buccheri L, Katchen BR, Karter AJ, et al. Acitretin therapy is effective for psoriasis associated with human immunodeficiency virus infection. *Arch Dermatol* 1997; 133(6): 711–715.
59. Roenigk HH, Jr, Callen JP, Guzzo CA, et al. Effects of acitretin on the liver. *J Am Acad Dermatol* 1999; 41: 584–588.

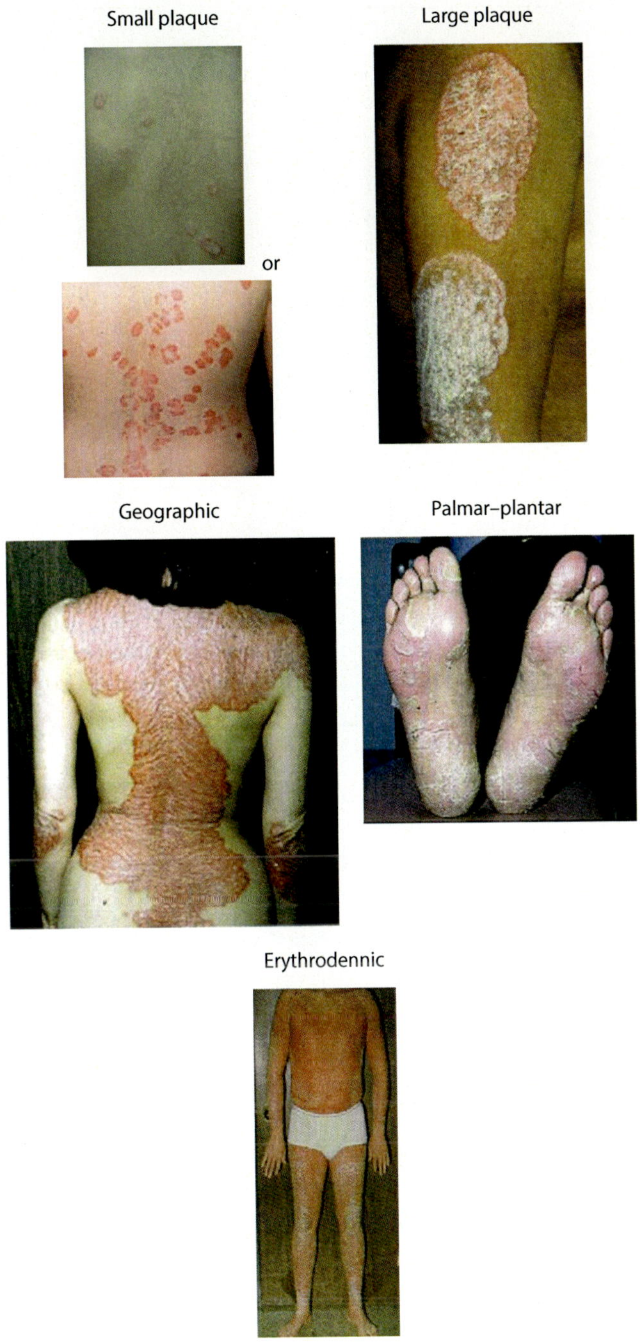

FIGURE 1.1 Morphological variants of psoriasis: Is this one disease?

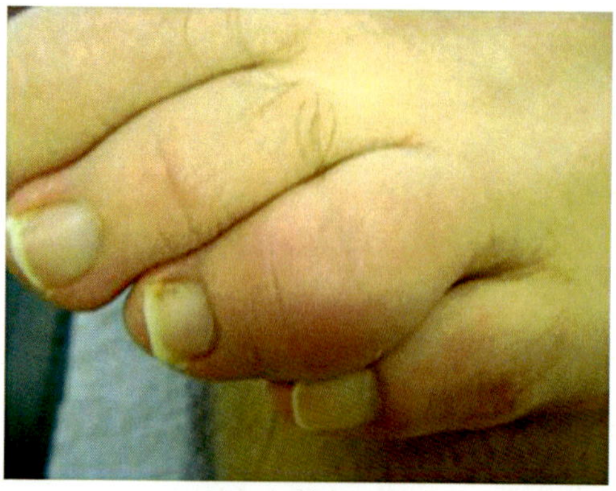

(a)

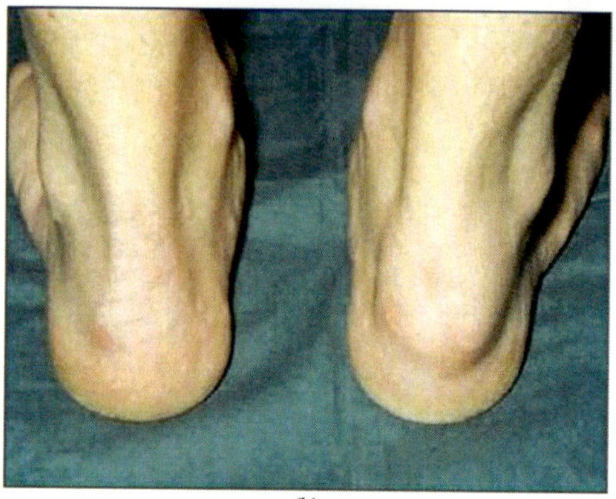

(b)

FIGURE 1.2 (a) Dactylitis, left fourth toe, and (b) enthesitis of achilles tendon.

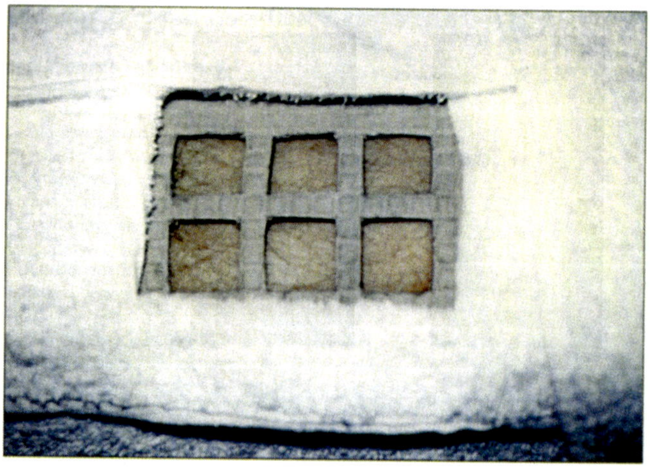

FIGURE 4.1 When conducting formal MED testing, a different amount of UVB radiation is applied sequentially to each opening in the template, which is made of an opaque material such as a thick piece of cardboard. The increment of UVB exposure is usually 15 or 30 seconds when a UVB box with fluorescent lights is used.

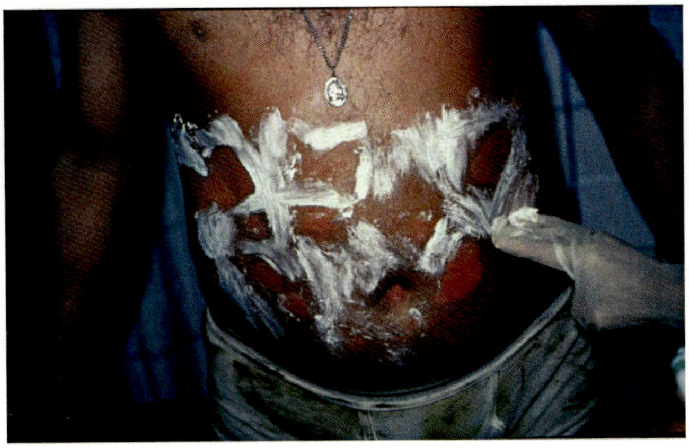

FIGURE 4.4 Because noninvolved skin burns much more easily than psoriatic plaques, zinc oxide paste is used to protect the noninvolved skin in between the psoriatic plaques before the patient is treated with a high-intensity UVB source such as a hot quartz lamp.

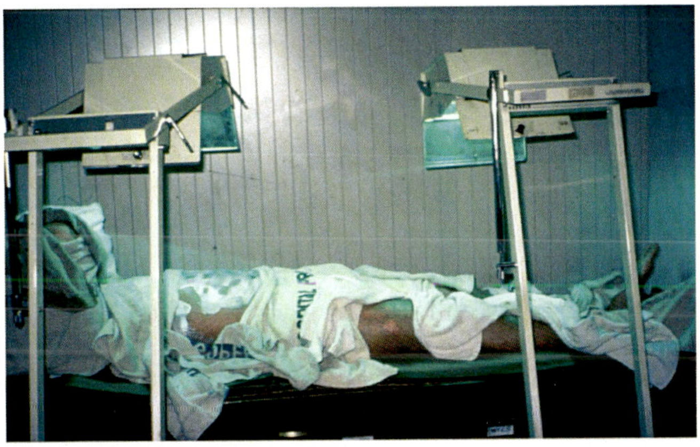

FIGURE 4.5 Because patients are treated lying down, one advantage of a hot quartz lamp is that it is relatively easy to cover the noninvolved areas with towels to avoid unnecessary exposure to UVB.

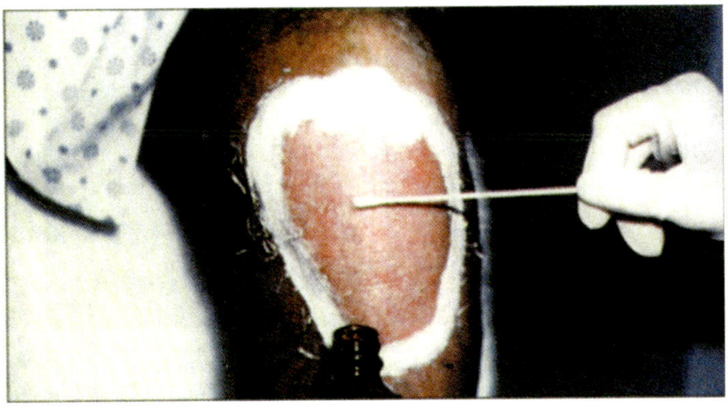

FIGURE 4.6 The application of topical "paint" PUVA therapy to selected, resistant psoriatic plaque. Zinc oxide paste is sometimes used to prevent inadvertent application of 0.1% Oxsoralen solution to the noninvolved skin.

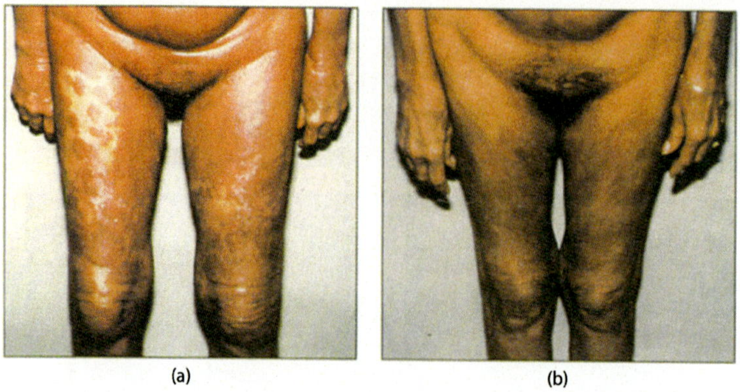

FIGURE 4.7 Erythrodermic patient with psoriasis and intense leg edema (a) before and (b) after short-term cyclosporine followed by long-term UVB phototherapy. This therapeutic regimen makes use of the powerful anti-inflammatory property of cyclosporine while minimizing the risk of systemic effects, which may be associated with long-term use of cyclosporine.

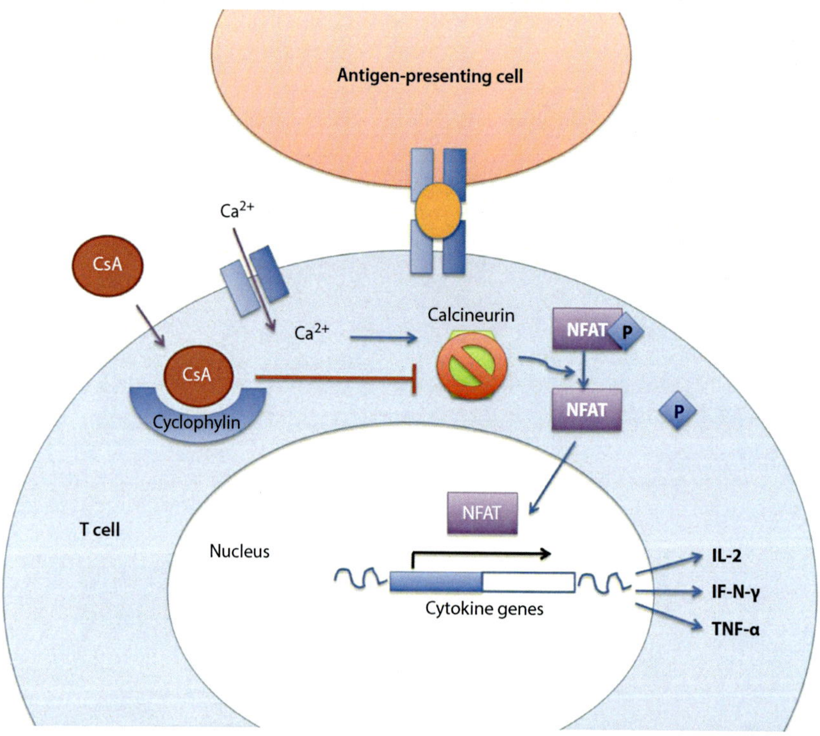

FIGURE 10.1 Cyclosporine mechanism of action: T cells are activated through interactions with the major histocompatibility complex and costimulatory molecules of an antigen-presenting cell. This initiates a complex signaling pathway, which results in an influx of calcium ions from the endoplasmic reticulum and extracellular environment into the T cell. Ultimately, this leads to the activation of the enzyme calcineurin, which in turn activates nuclear factor of activated T cells (NFAT). NFAT is a transcription factor that needs to be dephosphorylated (activated) by calcineurin in order to localize to the nucleus of the cell and to increase cytokine gene expression. By inhibiting calcineurin, cyclosporine prevents transcription of NFAT-dependent genes critical to the pathogenesis of psoriasis, such as IL-2, INF-γ, and TNF-α. (Reprinted with permission from Bryn Mawr Communications: Practical Dermatology, Bhutani T et al., *Prac Dermatol*, 28–32, 2010.)

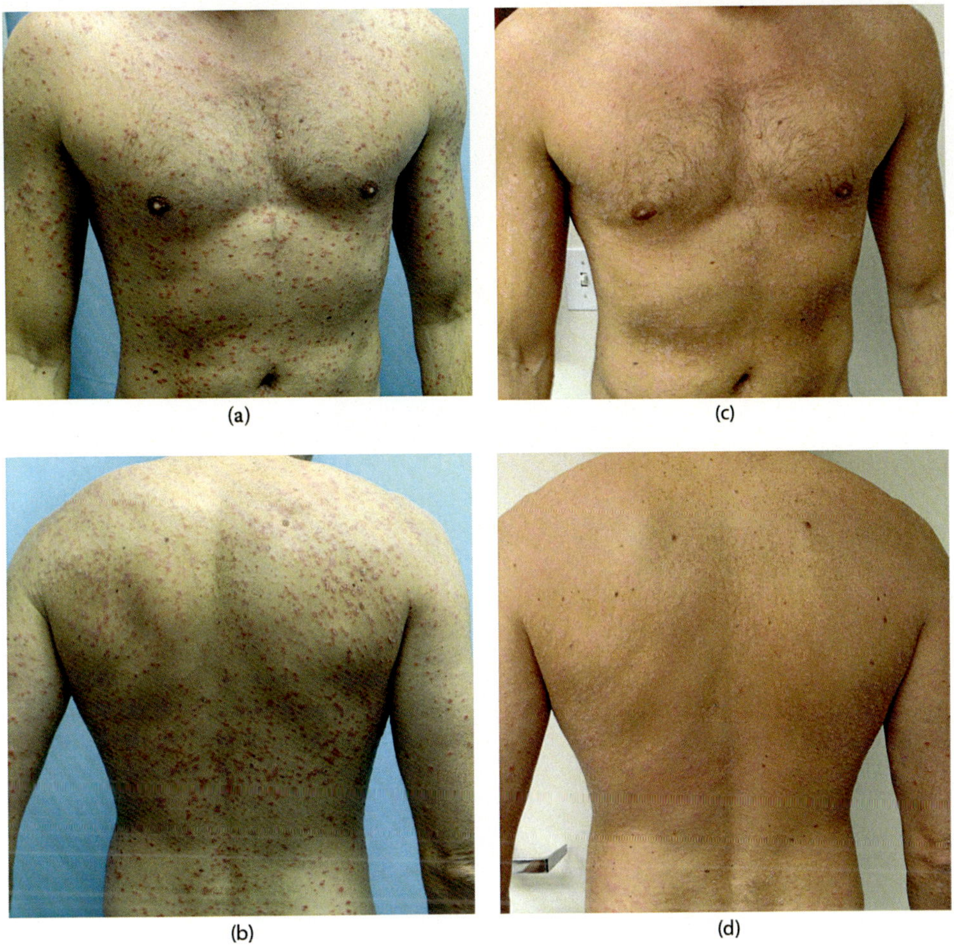

FIGURE 10.2 Representative patient with severe flare of guttate psoriasis at baseline (a, b) and two weeks after starting cyclosporine 5 mg/kg/day (c, d).

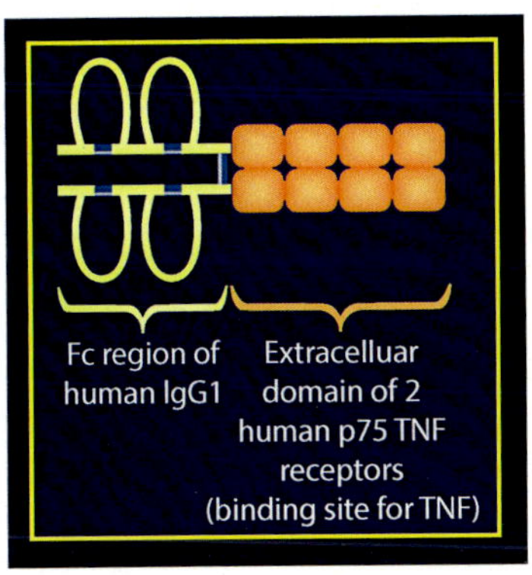

FIGURE 11.1 Structure of etanercept.

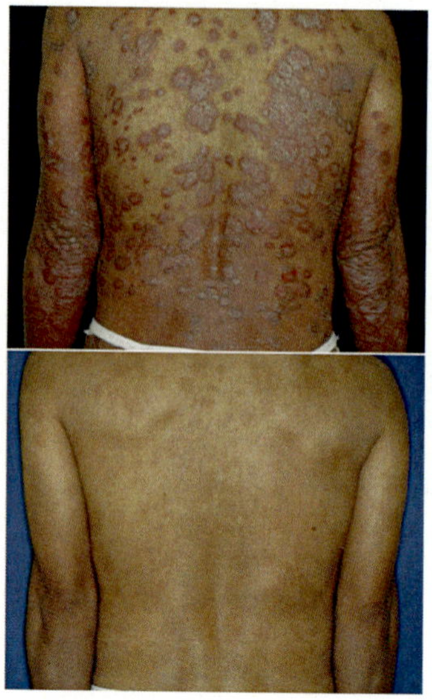

FIGURE 13.3 Representative patient with severe psoriasis at baseline (top) and following 52 weeks of treatment with ustekinumab (bottom).

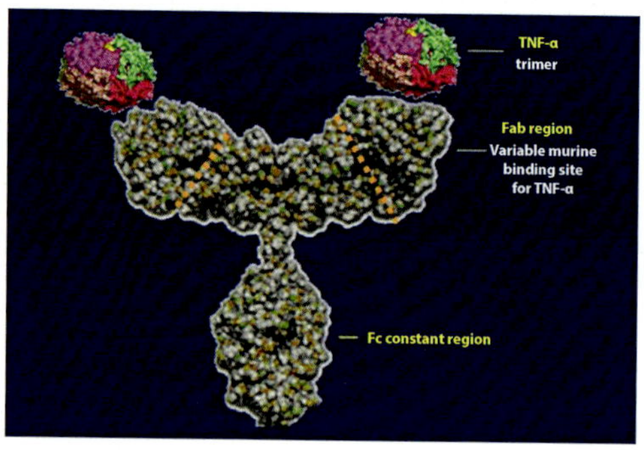

FIGURE 14.1 Infliximab molecule. (Adapted from Knight DM et al., *Mol Immunol* 30, 1443–1453, 1993; Infliximab.)

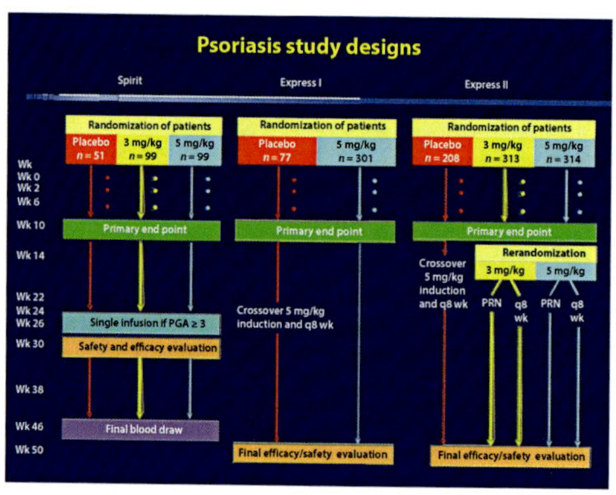

FIGURE 14.2 Infliximab psoriasis clinical trial study designs. (Adapted from Menter A et al., *J Am Acad Dermatol* 56, 31.e1–15, 2007; Gottlieb AB et al., *J Am Acad Dermatol* 51, 534–542, 2004; and Reich K et al., *Lancet* 366, 1367–1374, 2005.)

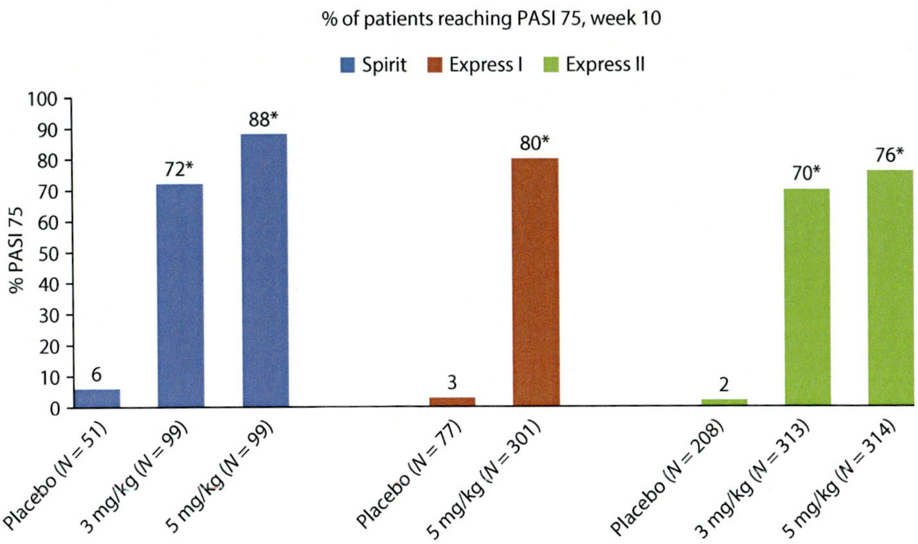

FIGURE 14.3 PASI 75 responses at week 10 in infliximab psoriasis clinical trials. $^*p < 0.001$ for comparison with placebo. (Adapted from Menter A et al., *J Am Acad Dermatol* 56, 31.e1–15, 2007; Gottlieb AB et al., *J Am Acad Dermatol* 51, 534–542, 2004; and Reich K et al., *Lancet* 366, 1367–1374, 2005.)

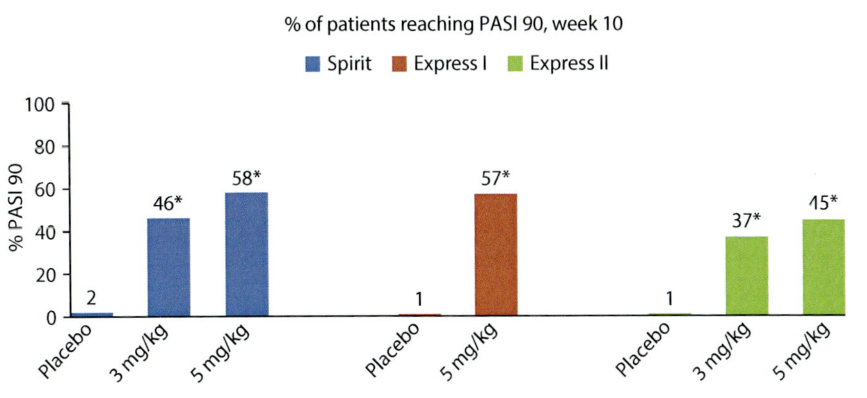

FIGURE 14.4 PASI 90 responses at week 10 in infliximab psoriasis clinical trials. $^*p < 0.001$ for comparison with placebo. (Adapted from Menter A et al., *J Am Acad Dermatol* 56, 31.e1–15, 2007; Gottlieb AB et al., *J Am Acad Dermatol* 51, 534–542, 2004; and Reich K et al., *Lancet* 366, 1367–1374, 2005.)

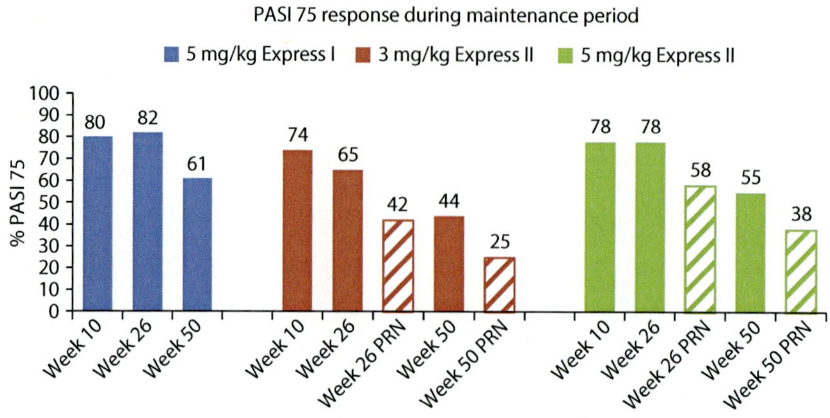

FIGURE 14.5 Maintenance of clinical response: Percent of PASI 75 responders at weeks 10, 26, and 50 from EXPRESS I and II Study. *Note:* Week 10 reflects only those patients who were randomized to continue in the maintenance phase of the studies. "PRN" dosing: patients treated with infliximab if they have less than PASI 75 improvement from baseline (week 0) during monthly assessments. (Adapted from Menter A et al., *J Am Acad Dermatol* 56, 31.e1–15, 2007; Reich K et al., *Lancet* 366, 1367–1374, 2005.)

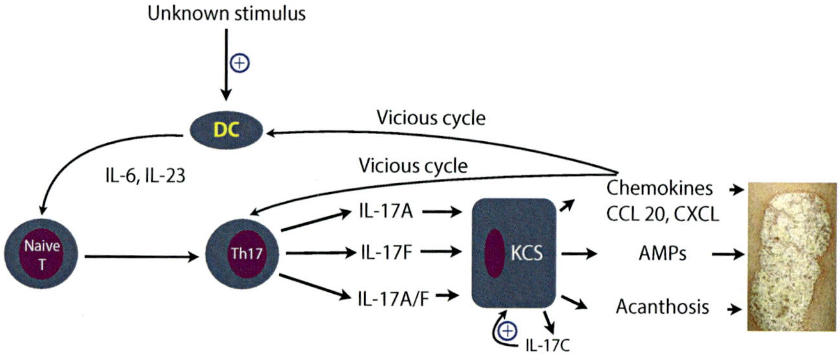

FIGURE 16.1 IL-17 in psoriasis pathogenesis. An unknown stimulus leads to activation of dendritic cells (DCs). These cells produce IL-6 and IL-23, which drive differentiation of naïve T cells into Th17 cells [11,12]. Th17 cells produce IL-17A, IL-17F, and IL-17A/F, which stimulate keratinocytes (KCS) to proliferate and to produce proinflammatory antimicrobial peptides (AMPs) and chemokines (e.g., CCL20). Chemokines such as CCL20 recruit inflammatory dendritic cells and Th17 cells into the active psoriasis lesion. Other chemokines play a role in neutrophil recruitment (CXCL) and angiogenesis. Keratinocytes also produce IL-17C, which acts via an autocrine mechanism to amplify the response IL-17A. IL-17C also acts on endothelial cells to augment expression of TNF-α, which further amplifies the inflammatory pathway [13].

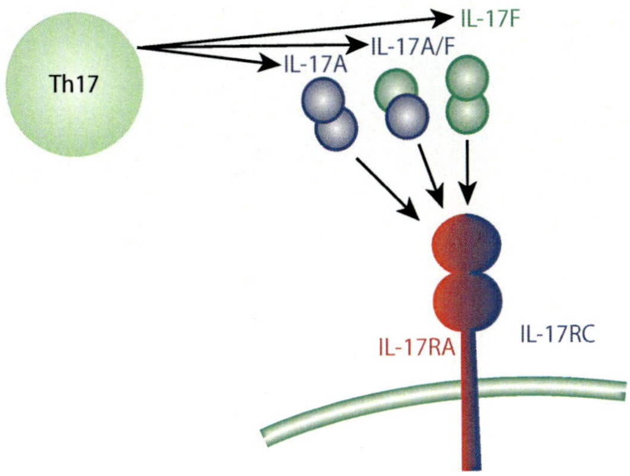

FIGURE 16.2 Th17 cells secrete IL-17A, IL-17F, and IL-17A/F. These three cytokines share the same heterodimer receptor complex, two subunits of which are IL-17RA and IL-17RC.

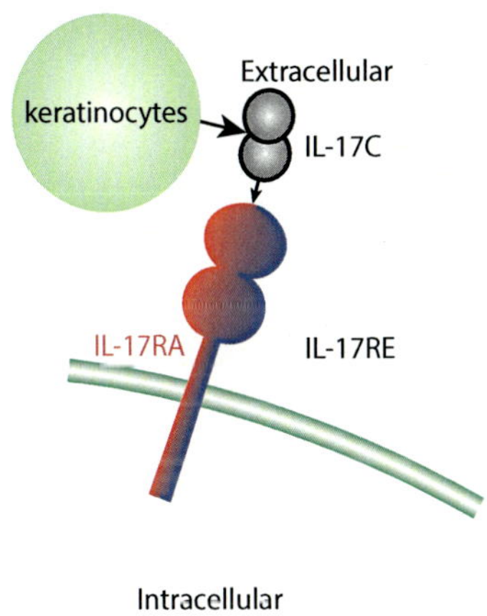

FIGURE 16.3 Keratinocytes secrete IL-17C. The receptor is a heterodimer composed of IL-17RE and IL-17RA. This receptor is expressed predominantly on epithelial cells.

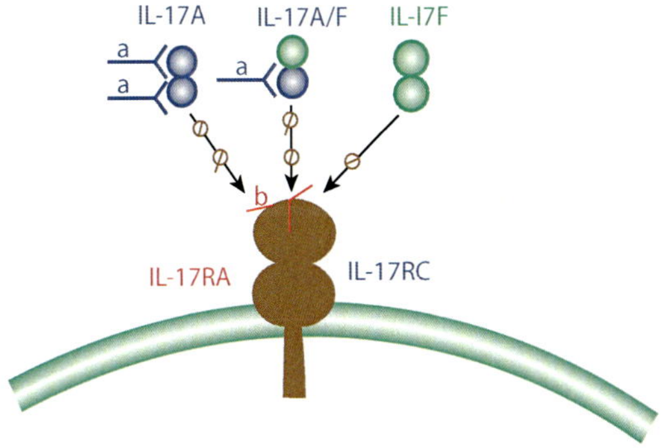

FIGURE 16.4 Antibody (a) (e.g., secukinumab, ixekizumab) selectively binds IL-17A. This prevents IL-17A and IL-17A/F from interacting with its receptor. Blocking antibody (b) (e.g., brodalumab) antagonizes the receptor, keeping it in an inactive state even in the presence of IL-17A, IL-17A/F, or IL-17F.

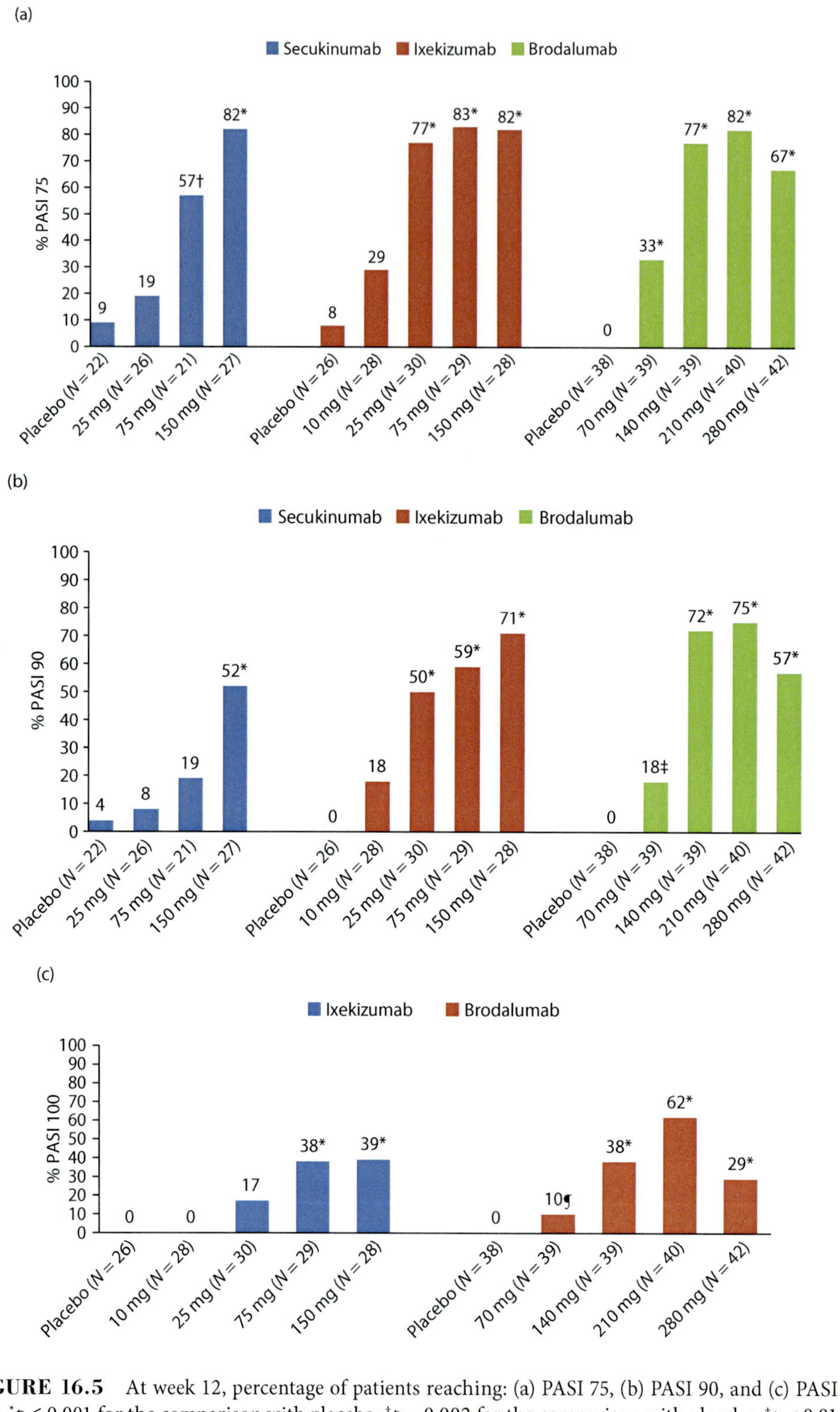

FIGURE 16.5 At week 12, percentage of patients reaching: (a) PASI 75, (b) PASI 90, and (c) PASI 100. *$p \leq 0.001$ for the comparison with placebo; †$p = 0.002$ for the comparison with placebo; ‡$p < 0.01$ for the comparison with placebo; ¶$p < 0.05$ for the comparison with placebo.

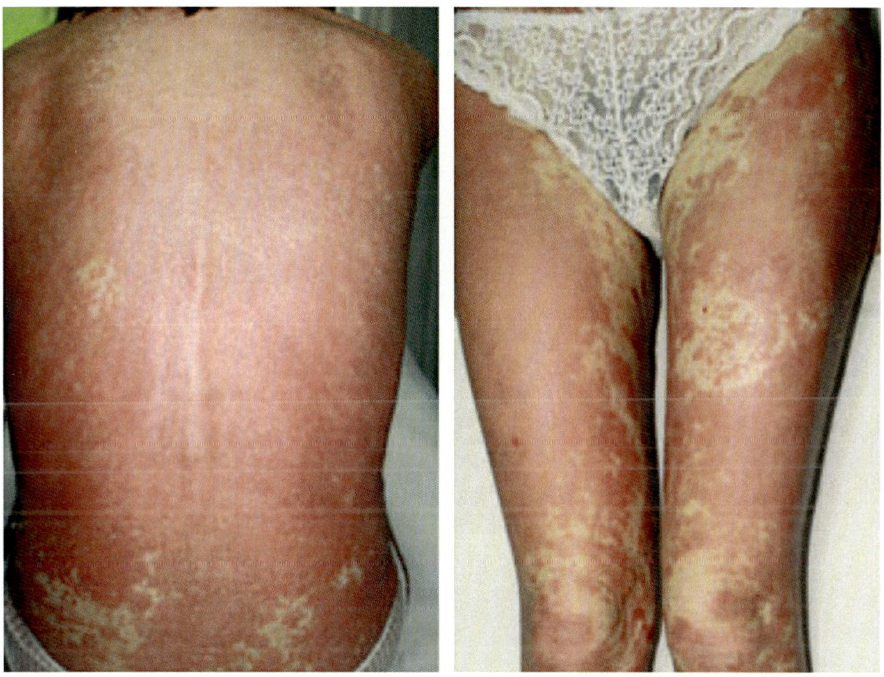

(a) (b)

FIGURE 17.1 Erythrodermic psoriasis. (a) Erythematous, diffuse, confluent plaque covering most of the back with few islands of sparing. (b) Large, coalescing erythematous patches with islands of sparing involving the bilateral lower extremities. (Reprinted from Santos-Juanes J et al.: Ustekinumab induces rapid clearing of erythrodermic psoriasis after failure of antitumor necrosis factor therapies. *Br J Dermatol*. 2010. 162, 1144–6. Copyright Wiley-VCH Verlag GmbH & Co. KGaA. Reproduced with permission.)

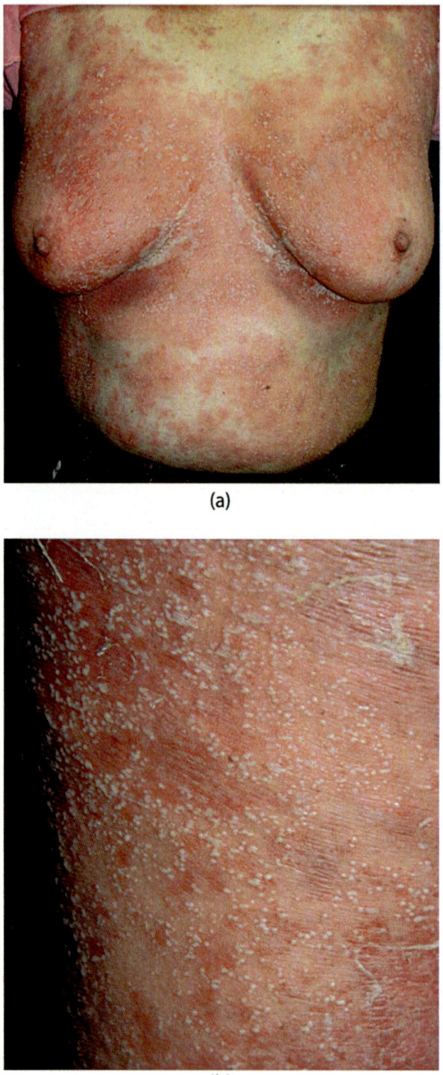

(a)

(b)

FIGURE 17.2 Generalized pustular psoriasis. (a) Extensive erythematous plaques with multiple pustules distributed over the upper trunk, breasts and abdomen. There is adherent scale along the underside of the breasts. (b) Numerous sterile pustules on a deeply erythematous plaque. (Wu MC, Lee JY: Generalized flare of pustular psoriasis induced by PEGylated interferon-alpha2b therapy for chronic hepatitis C. *Aust J Dermatol*. 2012. 53, e69–72. Copyright Wiley-VCH Verlag GmbH & Co. KGaA. Reproduced with permission.)

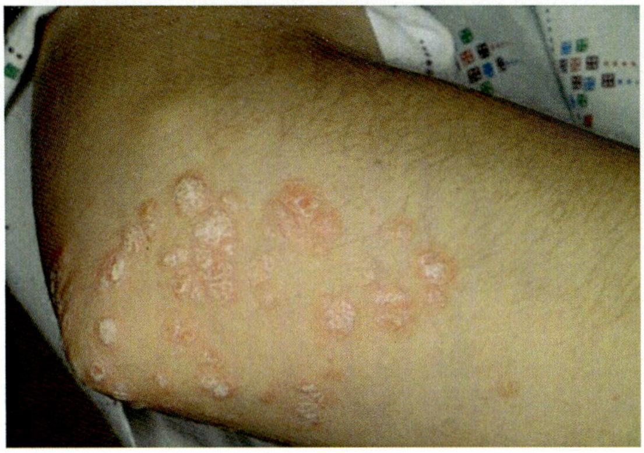

FIGURE 18.1 Extensor surfaces of knees and elbows are the most commonly involved areas in children. This older child has involvement of the right elbow with round to oval erythematous plaques with overlying silver scale.

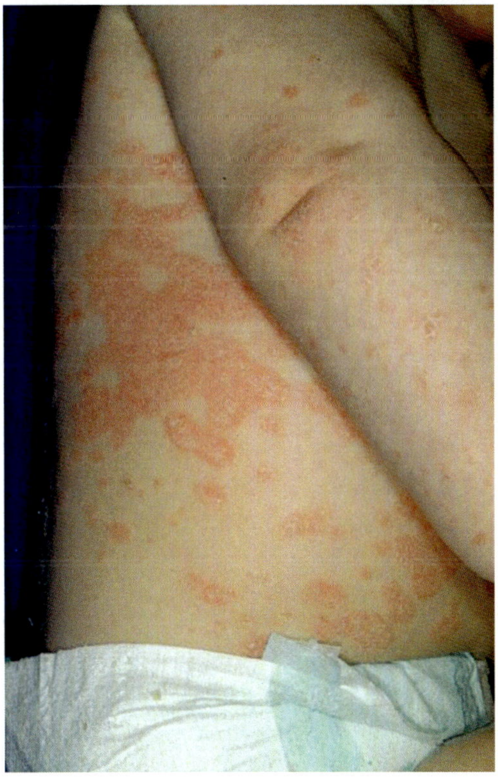

FIGURE 18.2 Small coalescing plaques on the right side of the trunk of an infant. In comparison with the psoriatic plaques in the older child in Figure 18.1, the scale on these plaques is thinner and finer.

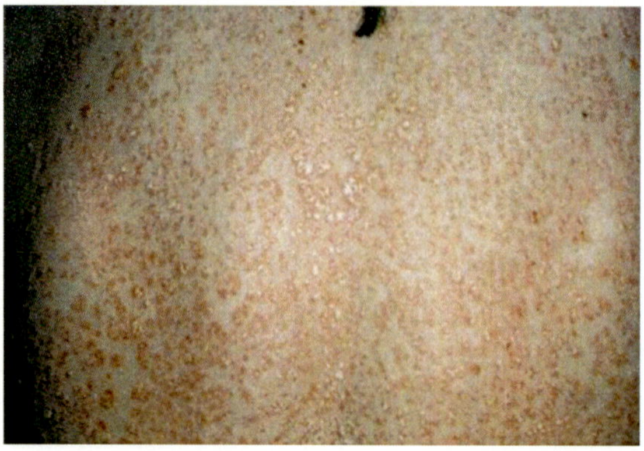

FIGURE 18.3 The small guttate plaques of psoriasis, most common on the trunk, are frequently the presenting feature of pediatric psoriasis, especially following streptococcal infection. Note that the patient shows peripheral residual postinflammatory hypopigmentation at sites of resolution.

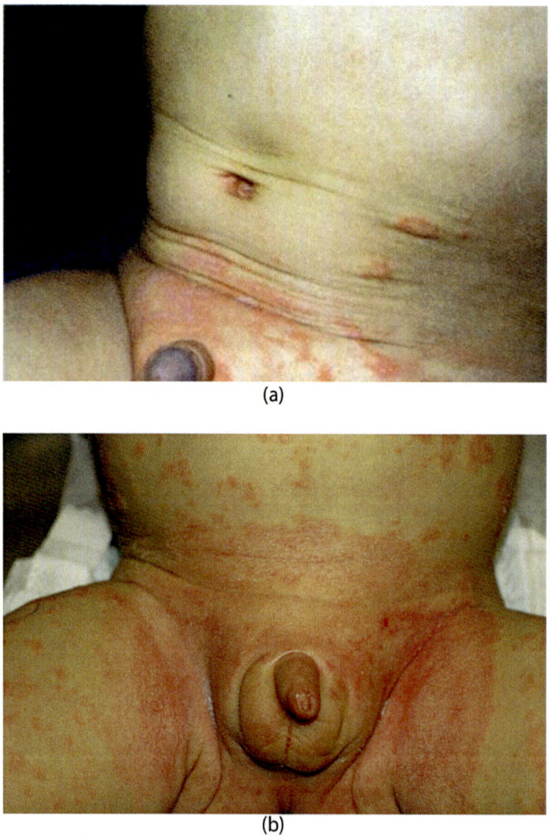

FIGURE 18.4 Diaper area psoriasis shows brightly erythematous, well-demarcated plaques. (a) Well demarcated plaques on the lateral diaper area. (b) Frontal view of diaper area shows brightly erythematous, well demarcated plaques.

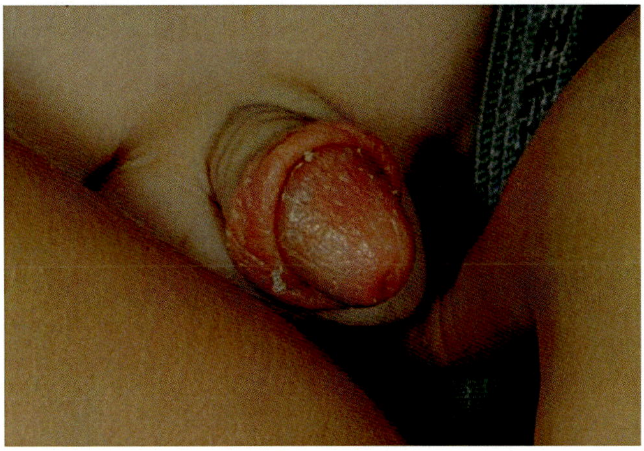

FIGURE 18.5 Penile psoriasis with erythema and scaling.

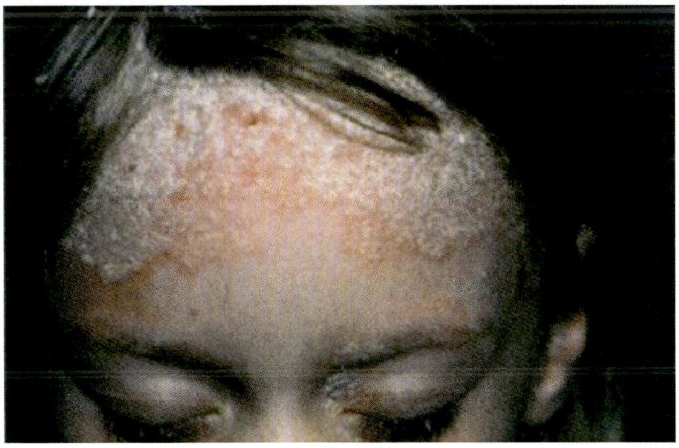

FIGURE 18.6 Facial psoriasis is more common in children than in adults.

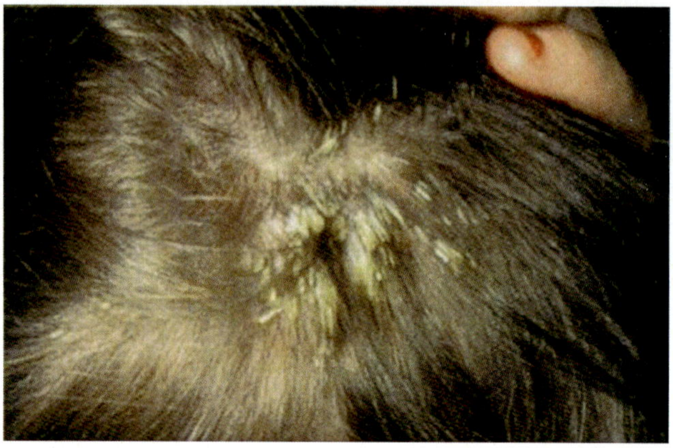

FIGURE 18.7 Pityriasis amiantacea is characterized by plaques of mild to moderate erythema and scalp scaling with distinct scale that encases and is adherent to the hair shaft.

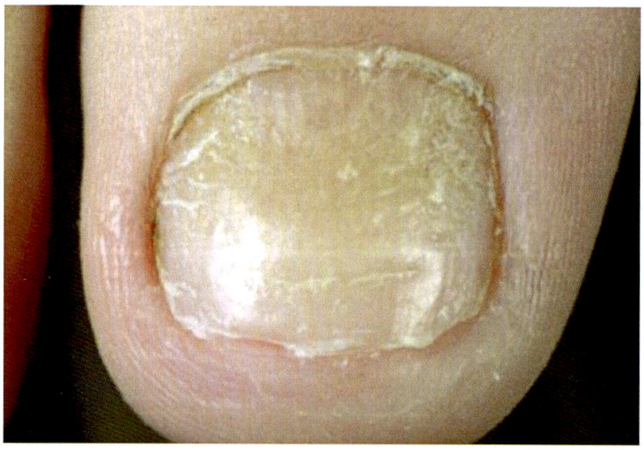

FIGURE 18.8 Nail psoriasis is more common in adolescents than in young children and is characterized by nail pitting, discoloration, onycholysis, and/or subungual hyperkeratosis.

Chapter 9

Methotrexate

Gerald D. Weinstein and Edward W. B. Jeffes III

A half-century has passed since Gubner made the serendipitous observation that aminopterin, a folic acid, improved the lesions of psoriasis during a trial to assess its anti-inflammatory effects in patients with psoriatic arthritis [1]. These observations were transferred into clinical trials using a daily dosage of aminopterin [2]. In the late 1950s, methotrexate (MTX) replaced aminopterin. During the next two decades, alternate dosage schedules were developed based on cell cycle information and cancer chemotherapy concepts. Until the development of psoralen plus ultraviolet A (PUVA) in 1975, ultraviolet B (UVB), tar phototherapy, and MTX were the only effective treatments for moderate to severe psoriasis. MTX was approved for psoriasis by the U.S. Food and Drug Administration (FDA) without the usual, at least by current standards, large double-blinded clinical trials. MTX usage for psoriasis appeared to be "grandfathered in," in part related to guidelines for MTX therapy of psoriasis discussed later in this chapter. Thus, there are no large double-blinded, placebo-controlled clinical trials to quantitate efficacy and safety of the drug for psoriasis. Reliance for its usefulness is based on many years of clinical experience and on numerous clinical retrospective studies with more emphasis on side effects than efficacy [3–6]. In past years, it has been estimated that approximately 25,000–30,000 patients were receiving MTX therapy in the United States, although current data are not available.

Because MTX was approved for the treatment of rheumatoid arthritis (RA) in 1988, it has become one of the main choices of therapy for RA. With a majority of these patients being treated with MTX in doses similar to psoriasis, much more data has become available on the relative safety of this drug. Guidelines developed by rheumatology and dermatology organizations are similar but differ in their requirements for liver biopsy prior to MTX therapy. The decision not to perform liver biopsies in RA patients reflects a lack of significant liver toxicity found in comparison to that discussed in detail in the dermatology literature [7].

PATIENT SELECTION

Patients with psoriasis involving more than 15%–20% body surface area (BSA) are considered to have moderate to severe disease. Further thinking and experience have suggested that many patients may have less severe disease but have lesions in more visible areas of the body, such as the face, hands, or other areas of occupational or social importance. Examples of patients requiring MTX with only mild to moderate disease or less than 15% BSA might include those with careers in which appearance is of importance. It is estimated that this population comprises approximately 20%–30% of psoriatic patients in the United States [8].

TABLE 9.1 Indications for the Use of Methotrexate in Psoriasis

Plaque psoriasis
Erythrodermic psoriasis
Pustular psoriasis (acute and localized)
Psoriatic arthritis
Extensive psoriasis unresponsive to other available therapies
Psoriasis that significantly impacts a patient's economic or psychological well-being
Lack of response to phototherapy, PUVA, or retinoids

Thus, in recent years, the criteria for using therapies such as MTX have changed from a more rigid percent body involvement to that of the location of the disease and its impact on quality of life concerns [9]. This extent/location of disease warrants more aggressive forms of therapy when topical therapy is not effective. The options for treatment include phototherapy, PUVA, retinoids, MTX, cyclosporine, and, more recently, biologics, based in part on quality of life concerns. The information in this chapter is based in part on the concepts that evolved in a series of guidelines that were developed from 1972 to 2008 on MTX use for psoriasis [7,10–13].

INDICATIONS FOR THE USE OF MTX FOR PSORIASIS

MTX is indicated for the treatment of patients with moderate to severe psoriasis that is unresponsive to topical therapy and for patients with joint involvement. We have learned from many years of experience that administration of MTX for psoriasis must be an individualized decision. It is used in patients with moderate-to-extensive plaque lesions as well as other variants of psoriasis including erythrodermic psoriasis, acute pustular psoriasis (of von Zumbusch), psoriatic arthritis, and localized pustular psoriasis (Table 9.1). Its use is justified in less severe patients when the condition of the psoriasis jeopardizes the patients' economic, psychosocial, or physical well-being.

MTX is an extremely effective drug for psoriasis. In the authors' opinion, MTX and phototherapy (narrowband ultraviolet B [NB-UVB]) modalities should generally be the initial forms of therapy for most moderate to severe psoriasis patients. If phototherapy becomes ineffective and/or has been used so extensively that the risks of side effects are increasing, then switching to MTX would be the next line of therapy [14]. In many patients, however, MTX may well be the initial choice of therapy if phototherapy is not an option. For patients being cared for by a nondermatologist considering the use of MTX, dermatologic consultation is recommended.

CONTRAINDICATIONS FOR THE USE OF MTX

Until the advent of biologics, MTX was the most frequently used treatment for moderate to severe psoriasis since the 1960s. In general, relative contraindications to therapy with MTX are disease processes that may enhance the toxicity of MTX, particularly liver, kidney, and hematopoietic diseases (Table 9.2). Absolute contraindications exist for female patients, who are pregnant or nursing and for females or males attempting to conceive. Significant anemia, leukopenia, and thrombocytopenia are also absolute contraindications.

TABLE 9.2 Contraindications to Methotrexate Therapy

Relative
Liver disease
Significantly abnormal LFTs
Cirrhosis or severe degrees of histologically proven fibrosis
Recent or active hepatitis
Excessive alcohol consumption
Kidney disease
Significantly decreased renal function (elevated Cr and BUN; decreased Cr clearance). Decreased renal function is frequently seen in elderly individuals and compensation can be made using lower than standard doses of MTX
Hematopoietic abnormalities
Mild to moderate leukopenia, anemia, or thrombocytopenia
Active severe infectious diseases
HIV, tuberculosis, etc.
Immunocompromised state
Obesity
Diabetes mellitus
Recent vaccination (live vaccines are of particular concern)
Active peptic ulcer
Unreliable patient
Absolute
Females that are pregnant or nursing
Male or female patients attempting to conceive a child
Concurrent use of trimethoprim-sulfamethoxazole
Severe leukopenia, anemia, or thrombocytopenia

Over the past 50 years, experience with MTX for chemotherapy of neoplastic diseases, psoriasis, and arthritis has produced extensive guidelines about how to use MTX safely. An appropriate history and physical examination should allow the physician to detect any contraindications to therapy with MTX. When treating malignant diseases, significantly larger doses are used that result in much more toxicity than would be acceptable in treating patients with psoriasis. In selected patients, circumstances may arise in which relative contraindications may be waived when it is considered that benefits of therapy may outweigh potential risks.

MECHANISM OF ACTION

Although MTX has been used for more than 50 years, its mechanism of action in psoriasis is not fully delineated. The current knowledge is that MTX may be effective in psoriasis by acting as both an antimetabolite [15] and an immunomodulatory agent [16]. MTX acts as an antimetabolite by blocking the synthesis of deoxyribonucleic acid (DNA) via inhibition of dihydrofolic acid reductase, thus preventing the donation of methyl groups during synthesis of purine and pyrimidine nucleotides (particularly, thymidylate) [17]. Thymidylate, one of the four DNA precursors, is necessary for DNA synthesis and cell division.

MTX's antimetabolite activity led to theories that it may exert a therapeutic effect in psoriasis by directly interfering with epidermal cell proliferation. Psoriatic skin contains twice as many proliferating cells and eight times as many cells in the synthesis (*S*) phase of cell division as normal skin. In addition, the proliferating cells have a cell cycle of 36 hours, which is eight times faster than normal [18]. Previous studies of MTX's mechanism of action indicate that after systemic or intralesional administration, MTX inhibits DNA synthesis in psoriatic epidermal cells, followed within several hours by the cessation of mitoses [15]. These data for many years suggested a direct effect of MTX on decreasing the rapidly proliferating psoriatic keratinocyte population.

In more recent years, several studies have explored MTX's role in disrupting keratinocyte hyperproliferation. The results of these data are conflicting. Schwartz et al. [19] suggested that MTX did not reduce the viability of keratinocytes but did inhibit cell growth and induce cell maturation and terminal differentiation. A few years later, Jeffes et al. [20] showed that MTX does not inhibit keratinocytes cell growth. It was the lymphocytes in psoriatic lesions that were vulnerable to MTX's cytotoxic effects rather than keratinocytes. In 1998, Heenen et al. [21] concluded that low-dose MTX can induce apoptosis in keratinocytes. Data suggest that MTX's therapeutic benefit in psoriasis patients probably does not result from inhibition of keratinocyte proliferation [22], inhibition of keratinocytes mitoses, keratinocyte cell damage, and keratinocytes cell death [15].

In addition to psoriasis, MTX has been found to be effective in the treatment of a number of inflammatory autoimmune diseases including RA and inflammatory bowel disease [23]. Based on this—along with the discovery that cyclosporine, an immunologically active drug, was effective for psoriasis (another serendipitous observation in psoriasis therapy)—much evidence has accumulated for an immunologic basis for psoriasis and has redirected research efforts toward MTX's possible role in immunomodulation. *In vitro* studies have revealed that keratinocytes are relatively resistant to MTX in culture at clinical concentrations reached in low dose MTX therapy [24]. In comparison, activated lymphocytes are sensitive to MTX at concentrations of approximately 100-fold lower than those needed to affect keratinocytes. Based on the long experience with the use of MTX, in low doses, it may have a major immunosuppressant effect on psoriatic disease but does not appear to produce a clinically immunosuppressive effect in patients. Several studies in recent years have shown that MTX has multiple effects on T cells, which are key players in the immunopathogenesis of psoriasis. Evidence now suggests that MTX has cytotoxic effects on T cells [19], reduces cutaneous lymphocyte-associated antigen (CLA) expression [25,26], reduces peripheral T cells [25], and induces T-cell apoptosis [27].

PRETHERAPEUTIC EVALUATION/CONTRAINDICATIONS

The pretherapy evaluation starts with an appropriate history and physical examination that concentrates mainly on the patient's renal and liver function (Tables 9.3 and 9.4). MTX is excreted mainly by the kidneys; therefore, any underlying renal disease must be detected. This is especially important in older individuals, who are more likely to have decreased renal excretory function, which could cause both higher and extended MTX blood levels resulting in increased toxicity at otherwise standard doses. A routine urinalysis, serum creatinine (Cr), blood urea nitrogen (BUN), and glomerular filtration rate (GFR) are the standard tests for renal function. A more sensitive test of kidney excretion is the Cr clearance over 24 hours.

TABLE 9.3 Risk Factors with Methotrexate Therapy

- History of current excessive alcohol consumption (MTX toxicity is associated with a history of total lifetime alcohol intake before MTX therapy. The exact amount of alcohol that confers risk is unknown and differs among persons.)
- Persistent abnormal liver chemistry studies
- History of liver disease including chronic hepatitis B or C
- Family history of inheritable liver disease
- History of diabetes mellitus and/or obesity (probably of secondary importance)
- History of significant exposure to hepatotoxic drugs or chemicals

TABLE 9.4 Pretherapy Evaluation

- History (including risk factors for liver and kidney disease) and physical examination
- Liver function tests (aspartate aminotransferase, alanine aminotransferase, alkaline phosphatase)
- Renal function tests (serum Cr, BUN, GFR, 24-hour urine, or Cr clearance)
- CBC with platelet count
- Chest X-ray (optional per history)
- Liver biopsy (before or shortly after initiation of therapy in patients with risk factors for liver disease)
- HIV antibody determinations for patients at risk for AIDS
- Some suggest TB testing

Cr clearance of less than 50 mL/min is indicative of at least moderate renal failure and may be a relative contraindication to therapy. In patients with slightly decreased 24-hour urine Cr clearance rates (if MTX is going to be used), lower doses of MTX should be employed. In these patients, more vigilant monitoring for MTX toxicity will be necessary.

CURRENT STATUS OF PRETREATMENT OR EARLY LIVER BIOPSY (AS OF 2008)

In the history of MTX use for psoriasis, the issue of liver toxicity risk has received the most discussion and concern. The 2009 guidelines for MTX and psoriasis [13] discuss this issue in detail and are summarized here. Although thorough histories, physical examinations, and liver function tests (LFTs) may identify some patients with preexisting risk factors for liver disease, the liver biopsy still remains the most reliable test for liver damage. In most studies in which patients had no significant risk factors, liver biopsies have found very few patients with fibrosis or cirrhosis.

DOSAGE/ADMINISTRATION

Dosage regimens for MTX in psoriasis have gone through several stages of evolution. Initially, an empirically derived schedule was based on daily small doses of aminopterin and later, MTX [28]. This daily schedule was subsequently found to produce greater liver toxicity. Using experience from oncologic therapy schedules with MTX, weekly doses of intramuscular (IM) MTX were found to be effective in psoriasis [29]. This regimen was then adapted for use as a single weekly oral dose [10]. The triple-dose schedule (MTX at 12-hour intervals for three doses each week) was proposed in 1971 to provide a therapeutic level of MTX for approximately 36 hours, the duration of the psoriatic cell cycle [30].

TABLE 9.5 Dermatologists' Preferences for Methotrexate Dosing Schedules: Results of a 1984 Survey

Dosing Schedule	Percentage
Weekly divided oral doses	74
Weekly single oral dose	16[a]
Weekly IM dose	3
Other dosing schedule	7

Source: Data from Peckham PE et al., *Arch Dermatol* 123, 1303–1307, 1987.

[a] May now be more frequently used.

MTX is administered for psoriasis therapy principally by two schedules: the triple-dose weekly regimen or a single weekly dose, either orally or intramuscularly. In 1984, a majority of dermatologists used the triple-dose schedule (Table 9.5) [8]. The triple-dose regimen is initiated with a test dose of 5 mg (2.5 mg every 24 hours for two doses) for the first one to two weeks. The concept of a small test dose was initiated to avoid possible serious side effects if a patient had an undiagnosed medical condition or an allergic sensitivity to MTX. Early use of MTX was given with much larger doses than are currently used and, as a result, severe side effects occurred. After the test dose, if laboratory results are normal and there is no unusual sensitivity to the test dose, the first triple dose is started at a dose of one 2.5 mg tablet every 12 hours for three doses (1/1/1), totaling 7.5 mg for the week. One to two weeks later, if there are no adverse effects, the dose is increased to four tablets (2/1/1), for a total of 10 mg. Over the following weeks the dose is increased by one 2.5 mg tablet/week every two to four weeks, depending on the effectiveness of the drug and the patient's ability to tolerate a given dosage regimen. In the typical 70-kg patient, the dose is usually plateaued at 2/2/2 (15 mg/week), although larger patients or those with resistant psoriasis may require a higher dosage. This schedule is continued until the patient's psoriasis is under adequate control. Most patients begin to see improvement in six to eight weeks.

The dose schedule using single, weekly, oral doses is initiated with a 5.0–7.5 mg test dose and is subsequently increased by 2.5 mg every two to four weeks. The total weekly maintenance dose is usually between 7.5 and 25 mg. Typical maintenance MTX doses in the range of 12.5–15 mg/week are common. Dosages as high as 37.5 mg/week may be required for effectiveness, particularly in patients with a larger habitus or those with severe disease. For unreliable patients, MTX may be administered in weekly intramuscular (IM) doses. The IM route may also be used when the effectiveness of oral MTX has diminished or if gastrointestinal (GI) side effects are limiting treatment.

Alternative methods of administration are used by rheumatologists including self-administered subcutaneous injections and oral solutions of MTX [31]. If oral administration of MTX solution is needed, withdraw 0.1 mL (or more) of the 50 mg/2 mL aqueous solution (typically for parenteral administration), which is equal to a 2.5 mg tablet, and mix with a small amount of water. Oral administration by tablet or the equivalent solution has equal effectiveness. Regardless of the dosage schedule or route of administration, the same principles previously described for adjusting doses for individual patients to minimize the cumulative MTX dose should be followed (Table 9.6).

To minimize side effects (in particular, severe liver toxicity), MTX doses should be kept as low as possible to achieve and maintain "adequate control" of the disease. Total clearing of lesions is *not* the intended goal of therapy because that may require continuing increases in weekly dosages approaching toxicity. At the point of optimal response, the dose is titrated down every month by one tablet until the lowest effective maintenance dose is achieved. When possible, attempts should be made to discontinue therapy for several months at a time. The summer months are often a good time for a drug holiday because the natural course of psoriasis tends to improve with increased sun exposure. This limits the cumulative dose, extends the time interval between liver biopsies, and permits longer duration of MTX therapy. New MTX patients are seen weekly for two to three weeks, then biweekly, and finally monthly as they develop a response pattern (Table 9.7). Clinical responses are titrated by one tablet up or down at monthly visits.

The maximum duration that a patient should be maintained on MTX is not defined. Therefore, as clearance is achieved, the dose of MTX should be tapered with a goal of

TABLE 9.6 Instructions to Patients Taking Methotrexate for Psoriasis

- Great care is needed when taking MTX.
- MTX is taken only three times/week or as a single weekly dose orally or by injection (not daily).
- Take only the prescribed, correct dose of MTX at the *same time and day(s) each week*.
- Do *not begin or change* the dosage of *any medication* (including nonprescription medications) unless your physician has approved it.
- Avoid alcoholic beverages.
- If you have side effects or any symptoms of dehydration, notify your physician before the next dose.
- If you develop cough, fever, shortness of breath, or any have any problems with sore throat; infections, including skin infections; or skin or mouth ulcers, *stop MTX and contact your physician.*
- See your physician regularly, usually every four weeks (more frequently at the beginning of therapy).
- Do not miss doctor's appointments or blood tests.
- Notify your physician at once if an accidental overdose has occurred.

TABLE 9.7 Drug Dose Schedules

(1) Divided oral dose schedule

2.5–5.0 mg at 12-hour intervals for 3 doses each week.

Gradually increase by 2.5 mg/week, every 2–4 weeks, with appropriate monitoring of laboratory tests.

Total dose generally not to exceed 6–9 tablets/week (15–22.5 mg).

(2) Weekly single oral dosage ranges from 7.5–37.5 mg/week

If single weekly doses are administered by IM or IV, the doses can go as high as 50 mg/week.

Intravenous drips of MTX should not be used due to persistent blood absorption, which may produce significant toxicity.

TABLE 9.8 Duration of Methotrexate Treatments to Achieve a Cumulative Dose of 1.5 g

Weekly Dosage (mg)	Months to 1.5 g
7.5	50
15.0	25
22.5	17

achieving the lowest possible maintenance schedule. If a patient can be maintained with as little as two to three tablets/week, the calculated cumulative dose would be 260–400 mg/year. Using a 1.0–1.5 g cumulative dose as the dose range within which liver changes may develop (Table 9.8) [12], a patient could receive low dose MTX continuously for more than three years. If a patient is able to tolerate rest periods off MTX each year, then even longer durations of MTX could be used before reaching this cumulative dose range. However, if a patient were to require higher maintenance doses, for example, 15 mg/week (2/2/2), then a cumulative dose warranting concern about liver toxicity could be reached in 1.5–2.0 years. At that time, stopping MTX and "rotating" to another form of therapy is recommended [14]. At a future point, the patient could restart therapy with MTX, hopefully with some reversal of any cumulative liver toxicity [14,32,33]. If MTX must be continued, a liver biopsy would have to be considered.

MONITORING THERAPY

Patients on MTX are monitored for the drug's effect on hematopoietic, kidney, and liver function as they are reflected in laboratory tests (Table 9.9).

The 2009 guidelines [13] suggest that: A complete blood cell count (CBC) should be obtained one week after the initial dose of MTX, then every two to four weeks over the next few months. Once a patient is consistently stable, the laboratories should be followed at least every three months. The need for closer monitoring will depend on the laboratory results and the risk factors of the patient. A CBC should be obtained at least seven days after the last dose because MTX causes a depression in the leukocyte and platelet counts that is most evident approximately 7–14 days after drug administration. Dosage reduction or a brief interruption of therapy is warranted when leukocyte and/or platelet counts drop below low normal levels. The appearance of oral mucosal ulcerations, previously used to clinically monitor MTX toxicity, is now infrequently observed due to the use of lower dosage regimens and careful monitoring of hematopoietic function.

Kidney function tests, BUN, and serum Cr should be evaluated every two to three months. A GFR should be calculated for patients at high risk for decreased kidney function even if they exhibit normal BUN and Cr.

LFTs, aspartate aminotransferase (AST), alanine aminotransferase (ALT), alkaline phosphatase, and serum albumin, should be evaluated every one to three months during therapy. Because MTX can cause a transient and clinically insignificant elevation in liver enzymes one to three days after drug administration, these tests should also be obtained at least five to seven days after the last dose. If liver enzymes are significantly elevated at that time,

TABLE 9.9 Monitoring Ongoing Therapy

CBC and platelet count

Monitor every 2–4 weeks after initiating treatment with MTX. Once the patient is consistently stable, can extend up to 3 months in between monitoring laboratory tests.

Serum chemistries

Liver function (aspartate aminotransferase, alanine aminotransferase, alkaline phosphatase, albumin) should be monitored every 1–3 months. Renal function (BUN, Cr) should be monitored every 2–3 months and a GFR should be calculated in at risk patients, particularly elderly patients.

Chest X-ray

Monitor annually if there are pulmonary symptoms. A chest X-ray should be performed in the event of acute pulmonary changes that might suggest a "MTX pneumonitis," seen rarely in psoriatics but more frequently in RA patients taking MTX.

Liver biopsy

- In patients without risk factors: First biopsy between 1–4 g cumulative MTX.
- In patients with risk factors: First biopsy after 2–4 months of therapy. Subsequent biopsies after each 1.0 g cumulative dose.

MTX therapy should be interrupted for one to two weeks and the tests repeated before restarting therapy. In most cases, the LFTs will return to normal within two weeks. However, if significant elevations persist, a liver biopsy should be considered before continuing MTX therapy. The use of liver biopsies to monitor evidence of liver toxicity has greatly diminished to the point that they are now rarely being done. This change has been led by reluctance of the gastroenterologists (due to the risk of procedure) and by rheumatologists (due to the low incidence of side effects seen in RA patients). Dermatologists are influenced by this and the fact that lower doses are used in psoriasis.

LIVER BIOPSY RECOMMENDATIONS

Controversy still exists on the need for a pretreatment/early liver biopsy. The most recent recommendations from the 2009 National Psoriasis Foundation Consensus Conference [13] suggest that patients should be stratified based on their risk factors as discussed here.

Risk Factors for Hepatic Toxicity from MTX

The risk factors include: history or current alcohol consumption, persistent abnormal liver chemistry studies (including chronic hepatitis B or C), family history of heritable liver disease, diabetes, obesity, significant exposure to hepatotoxic drugs or chemicals, lack of folate supplementation, and hyperlipidemia.

Patients with No Risk Factors

If there is no evidence of significant risk factors, it is rare for life-threatening liver disease to occur within the first 1.0–1.5 g of cumulative MTX. On this basis, the "guidelines" have been revised to not obtain a liver biopsy until a patient has received this cumulative dose of MTX [12]. More recent data suggest that the first liver biopsy is not required until a cumulative MTX dose of 3.5–4.0 g is reached [34,35], if five of nine serum AST levels are elevated over a 12-month period, or if serum albumin drops under the normal [13,36].

Patients with Risk Factors

If risk factors are found prior to initiating MTX, and MTX is still indicated, it is advisable that a liver biopsy be performed early on. Because it is possible that some patients will not continue taking MTX after the first few months due to adverse effects, lack of effectiveness, or other reasons, it is reasonable to postpone the biopsy until after this initial period. If the drug is effective and its use will continue for long-term therapy, there is more incentive for a patient to accept the decision for a liver biopsy. There is no information available that short-term use of MTX will cause clinically significant liver disease. A repeat liver biopsy should occur once a cumulative dose of 1.0–1.5 g is reached or if the patient is found to have persistently elevated, clinically significant liver chemistry values. It is suggested that the liver biopsy be performed at least two weeks after the last dose of MTX to minimize any acute histologic liver changes. Despite the risk factors, clinical experience has suggested that a liver biopsy may not be warranted in certain patient populations (listed here). In the decision process, LFTs should be obtained frequently at approximately two-month intervals.

- Elderly patient population
- Patients with acute illness and/or severe exacerbation of psoriasis
- Patients with medical contraindications for a biopsy (e.g., cardiac instability, bleeding)
- Patients with limited life expectancy

The risk of liver biopsy versus the risk of continued MTX therapy must be carefully assessed in these patients. Occasionally, there are also reluctant patients who refuse a liver biopsy. In the absence of evidence of liver changes, it then becomes the option of the physician to continue using MTX or consider the availability of other therapies, using risk/benefit considerations. It is recommended that the patient's chart reflect the discussions. We would suggest that the patient sign such a notation in the chart.

SIDE EFFECTS

Short-term side effects of MTX such as nausea, anorexia, and fatigue are dose-related and rapidly reversible with a decrease in dosage or with a brief interruption in therapy. Alternatively, rotating between triple-dose and weekly oral or IM dosage may alleviate severe symptoms that may otherwise cause a patient to discontinue MTX therapy. However, utilizing the IM route does not necessarily reduce GI side effects. In patients on higher doses of MTX, nausea may be psychologically triggered in anticipation of the next dose. Food and occasional anti-emetic drugs may be necessary to permit drug administration. Table 9.10 lists the side effects that are associated with MTX.

FOLIC AND FOLINIC ACID SUPPLEMENTS

Folate supplementation decreases the incidence of GI, hematologic, and hepatotoxic abnormalities without affecting the action of MTX [37]. Some experts recommend all patients receive folate supplementation while others believe supplementation is only necessary when patients exhibit side effects.

In several reports, it has been suggested that concomitant administration of oral folic acid (1–5 mg/day) can reduce side effects such as nausea and megaloblastic anemia.

TABLE 9.10 Reported Side Effects with Methotrexate

Nausea/Vomiting
Anorexia
Fatigue
Anemia
Thrombocytopenia
Leukopenia
Hepatotoxicity/cirrhosis
Mucositis
Photosensitivity
Alopecia
Acral erythema
Skin necrosis
Pneumonitis
Pulmonary fibrosis
Infections
Nail hyperpigmentation
Erythroderma

Folinic acid (the direct antidote for MTX), if given on days when MTX is not administered, will also reduce these side effects [38,39]. Folinic acid can be administered orally in three consecutive 5 mg doses every 12 hours, once weekly. The first dose of folinic acid should be taken 12 hours after the last dose of MTX. Immediate oral or intravenous administration of folinic acid (20 mg) should be considered in cases of severe leukopenia or thrombocytopenia [13].

LIVER TOXICITY

The major limitation in the use of MTX is the potential for severe drug-induced liver fibrosis and cirrhosis. Even with lower dosage regimens, long-term use of MTX can cause life-threatening cirrhosis [40]. Data from several studies suggest that MTX's effects on the liver are mainly related to the cumulative dose. The incidence of cirrhosis is 3% in the range of 1.5–2.0 g cumulative dose and as high as 20%–26% with a cumulative dose of 4.0 g. The incidence of MTX-induced cirrhosis in the United States appears to be lower than in the Scandinavian populations, although the reasons for this are unclear [41,42]. A history of heavy alcohol consumption, intravenous drug use, or the presence of diabetes mellitus, obesity, suboptimal renal function, or preexisting liver pathology is a risk factor for the development of severe liver toxicity [11]. These risk factors are specifically of concern in psoriatic patients because, compared to the general population, they tend to have a higher incidence of obesity, diabetes, and alcoholism [43]. We recommend that any patient with moderate to severe psoriasis avoid or at least minimize alcohol consumption in order to maintain the option for future MTX use.

Fortunately, fibrosis or cirrhosis due to MTX can be detected and may improve once therapy with MTX is discontinued, as demonstrated by repeat liver biopsies [33]. Some researchers believe that MTX-related cirrhosis is "not aggressive," as evidenced by little

TABLE 9.11 Classification of Liver Biopsy Findings

Grade I	Normal; mild fatty infiltration/portal inflammation
Grade II	Moderate to severe fatty infiltration/portal tract inflammation
Grade III	A. Mild fibrosis
	B. Moderate to severe fibrosis
Grade IV	Cirrhosis
Clinical interpretation of liver biopsy results	
Grade I or II	Continue MTX therapy
Grade III A	May continue MTX therapy. Repeat biopsy after 6 months of continuous MTX therapy
Grade III B	Discontinue MTX therapy
Grade IV	Discontinue MTX therapy

or no progression of liver histopathology in patients with documented cirrhosis who continued on MTX [32]. However, most would agree that if the liver biopsy shows Grade III B or Grade IV (moderate to severe fibrosis or cirrhosis), MTX should be discontinued (Table 9.11). Severe liver diseases, as well as a few deaths, have occurred in patients receiving long-term MTX. To the authors' knowledge, most of the problems have occurred in situations where there have been significant deviations from appropriate patient/doctor safeguards [40].

Liver toxicity can often be detected by monitoring liver enzymes, as described earlier. Unfortunately, these tests are not always reliable. In fact, severe liver disease, including cirrhosis, can be present in the absence of elevated liver enzymes [44]. As a result, other tests of liver function have been investigated as indicators of liver disease that might obviate the need for liver biopsies. Ultrasound and radiographic imaging have been found to be unreliable [45–48], although one investigator argues that—given the risks of liver biopsy—ultrasound, if performed by an experienced specialist, is a justified screening method and urges reevaluation of the guidelines for routine liver biopsy [49]. Levels of serum aminoterminal propeptide of type III procollagen (PIIINP) have been correlated with liver histology [50] and are a measurement commonly used in the United Kingdom to detect liver disease. In psoriatic patients without arthritis, high levels of PIIINP appear to be an indicator of liver fibrosis. Patients with coexistent arthritis often have high levels of PIIINP in the absence of liver fibrosis. On a more practical note, this test is not FDA approved and thus not commercially available in the United States.

To date, liver biopsy remains the gold standard for evaluating MTX-induced liver toxicity in patients. Unfortunately, this procedure is not without risk and carries a general complication rate of 2.2% and a mortality rate of 9/100,000 [51]. The risks associated with liver biopsy tend to be lower in patients with psoriasis than with other diseases. Most adverse events occur in patients with GI problems related to other diseases. Although uncommon, the risk of severe and life-threatening liver damage due to MTX outweighs the risk of liver biopsy. It is obvious that a qualified gastroenterologist who performs frequent liver biopsies should be consulted on appropriate patients. In addition, the pathologist should be familiar with the liver pathology classifications in MTX-treated patients as described in the 1998 guidelines to provide the best clinicopathologic correlations [12].

HEMATOLOGIC COMPLICATIONS

Myelosuppression is one of the most concerning complications associated with MTX therapy, although it should be easily avoidable with proper evaluation and monitoring. Lack of folate supplementation, renal impairment, advanced age, and concomitant drug use increase the risk for myelosuppression. A "test dose" of MTX ranging from 5 to 15 mg may be given followed by laboratory tests to evaluate hematologic values over the following one to two weeks. Patients with decreased renal function need to be evaluated with a test dose prior to initiating treatment. These patients also need more frequent laboratory monitoring and slower titration to the therapeutic effect.

Regular laboratory monitoring is necessary because pancytopenia can occur at any time during treatment. Pancytopenia occurs most frequently after an increase in dosage, thus more frequent laboratory monitoring may be needed during these periods. Patients should be reminded of the many drug interactions and the importance of keeping all physicians up to date on any medication changes.

MTX OVERDOSAGE

Causes for MTX overdosage are patient/physician/nurse/pharmacist errors, impaired renal function, or concomitant administration of drugs such as trimethoprin or trimethoprim-sulfamethoxazole (Bactrim, Septra, and generics). Leucovorin calcium, the antidote for MTX toxicity, should be initiated if an overdose is suspected (Table 9.12). Early treatment with leucovorin is crucial because its effectiveness decreases as the time interval from the last dose of MTX increases. In overdoses of MTX used for cancer chemotherapy, the success of antidote administration greatly decreases if the last dose of MTX was received more than 24–48 hours prior to rescue [52].

When MTX toxicity develops secondary to decreased renal function, leucovorin administration should be prolonged because MTX blood levels will be elevated for a longer time. If serum Cr concentration has increased to more than or equal to 50% of baseline, leucovorin should be given intravenously at 100 mg/m^2 every three hours until MTX concentration is less than 0.01 μmol/L. Alkalinization of the urine by means of sodium bicarbonate and fluid administration may be necessary to prevent precipitation of MTX in the renal tubules. All cases of suspected overdosage require vigilant monitoring for development of hematologic or other toxic effects.

TABLE 9.12 Leucovorin Rescue after Methotrexate Overdose

Serum MTX Level (μmol/L)	Leucovorin Dose (mg)
5×10^{-7}	20[a]
1×10^{-6}	100
2×10^{-6}	200
$\geq 2 \times 10^{-6}$	Proportionately increased

[a] The initial 20 mg dose of leucovorin is given parenterally, with subsequent doses given every 6 hours, either orally or parenterally.

TABLE 9.13 Medications That Interact with Methotrexate (Abbreviated List)

• Trimethoprim–sulfamethoxazole: most common offender
• NSAIDs: salicylates, naproxen, ibuprofen, indomethacin
• Other antibiotics: penicillins, sulfonamides, ciprofloxacin, tetracyclines
• Other sulfonamides: furosemide, probenacid, sulfasalazine, thiazides
• Misc: barbiturates, colchicine, dipyramidole, phenytoin, dapsone

Note: NSAIDs = nonsteroidal anti-inflammatory agents.

DRUG INTERACTIONS

Reports of interactions between MTX and other drugs have been observed (Table 9.13) but, fortunately, are not common. Mechanisms of some drug interactions include interference with protein binding, renal tubular secretion, or intracellular transport of MTX [53]. Other drugs may affect the efficacy or increase the toxicity of MTX. Barbiturates, phenylbutazone, phenytoin, probenecid, salicylates, and sulfonamides can displace MTX from serum albumin, causing elevated levels of free MTX and enhancing potential toxicity. Nonsteroidal anti-inflammatory agents, phenylbutazone, probenecid, salicylates, and sulfonamides can compete with MTX for active renal tubular secretion, thus increasing the half-life of MTX. Dipyridamole can interfere with intracellular transport of MTX and also prolong its effects. The combination of MTX and trimethoprim can cause severe suppression of bone marrow function and is best avoided [54].

MTX can be ineffective if given concomitantly with folic acid or vitamin preparations that contain folic acid. Folic acid, or more specifically folinic acid, may bypass MTX inhibition of the dihydrofolic acid pathway. In a patient not responding to MTX, concurrent medications should be reviewed for any vitamin preparations that may contain folic acid.

MTX in combination with other systemic therapies for psoriasis should be used with caution. Historically, many of the early cases of severe side effects and deaths occurred with the concomitant use of systemic corticosteroids and MTX. MTX-induced leukopenia together with steroid suppression of immune function led to overwhelming infections. It is thus well appreciated that the combination of MTX and systemic corticosteroids should be avoided as much as possible. In one report, 2 out of 10 patients on combined therapy with MTX and etretinate developed life-threatening, drug-induced hepatitis [32]. Cyclosporine and MTX, through their respective toxicities (renal and liver, respectively) and metabolic pathways (liver and renal, respectively), can cause elevated levels of both drugs, thereby increasing the risk of severe side effects from both drugs [55].

FERTILITY

MTX is a known abortifacient and teratogen (category X drug in pregnancy) even at the low doses commonly used in psoriasis. A report of 10 pregnancies occurring in eight women receiving MTX for rheumatic disease included five normal infants delivered at full term, three spontaneous abortions, and two elective abortions [56]. Fetal skeletal, cardiac, and central nervous system abnormalities have been associated with MTX use in pregnancy [57], although there are reports of normal offspring born to women who had previously received higher doses of MTX for choriocarcinoma [58,59]. Nonetheless, female patients should take all precautions to avoid pregnancy while taking MTX and for at least one month or, more conservatively, three to four months after discontinuing MTX.

Oligospermia [60] and sperm abnormalities have been reported in men receiving MTX, yet we are aware of five male patients on MTX who fathered normal offspring. Nonetheless, it is recommended that male patients taking MTX avoid fathering offspring during therapy and for three to four months after discontinuing therapy.

PULMONARY COMPLICATIONS

Pneumonitis due to MTX has been reported in at least 20 patients with RA [61]. One patient, a 39-year-old female, also had psoriasis and had been treated with MTX 15 mg/week on a triple-dose regimen for five months prior to developing symptoms of nonproductive cough and progressive dyspnea [62]. The occurrence of MTX-pneumonitis in psoriatics appears rarely in contrast to RA patients on MTX. However, unexplained pulmonary symptoms in an MTX-treated patient should be evaluated for MTX-pneumonitis and the drug discontinued, at least temporarily.

INFECTIOUS COMPLICATIONS

A review of case reports of infectious complications of low-dose MTX therapy includes varicella zoster, *Pneumocystis carinii* pneumonia, nocardiosis, and cryptococcosis [63]. The patients described were all receiving low-dose MTX for arthritic conditions. Three cases of disseminated histoplasmosis in patients receiving low-dose MTX for psoriasis were also reported. Two had received a total of 7 and 8 g of MTX, respectively, and the third had received only 160 mg. Opportunistic infections should be considered in patients on MTX therapy who have unexplained prolonged fever.

COST OF MTX THERAPY

In deciding appropriate therapy, one must consider the cost/benefit ratio as well as the risk/benefit ratios of different treatments. The limitations of health care resources have restricted access to some forms of therapy narrowing treatment options. For patients with moderate to severe psoriasis, the treatments available include phototherapy, PUVA, MTX, retinoids, and cyclosporine. Several biologics that are available are significantly more expensive than the treatments listed here. In 1997, the average annual cost for UVB was approximately US$1850 and MTX costs ranged from US$1500 to US$2150. For comparison, PUVA and etretinate were approximately US$3000 and cyclosporine was US$4000. These estimates did not include physicians' fees [64].

CONCLUSION

In the authors' opinion, we have been fortunate to have had access to MTX for the past half-century. It is amazing that no other folic acid antagonists (after aminopterin) have become available to improve on the effectiveness and safety of MTX for the treatment of psoriasis as well as for cancer chemotherapy. Most psoriasis patients do not develop resistance to intermittent or continued therapy in contrast to what happens in some forms of leukemia.

Adverse events from short-term or continued use of MTX have been relatively limited with the exception of the concern for hepatic toxicity. In the early years of MTX use, more problems were found when there was inadequate information on how to use the drug safely. In recent years, in the authors' opinion, the prior problems of liver damage have been minimized because we have: (i) selected patients more carefully for this drug, (ii) tested patients more frequently for liver disease, and (iii) perhaps most importantly, treated psoriasis by rotating the additional new therapies so that MTX is not used as frequently or for prolonged periods. In our experience, the number of episodes of severe liver disease in recent years has been rare. This does not mean that MTX cannot cause problems but from the knowledge acquired from the other physicians and malpractice litigation, these difficulties appear to come in situations where there is abuse by patients [40] or inappropriate use. Given this long and fortuitous experience, it remains an important drug for the therapy of moderate to severe psoriasis.

REFERENCES

1. Gubner R. Effect of aminopterin on epithelial tissues. *AMA Arch Derm Syphilol* 1951; 64(6): 688–699.
2. Rees RB, Bennett JH, Bostick WL. Aminopterin for psoriasis. *AMA Arch Derm* 1955; 72(2): 133–143.
3. Kuijpers AL, van de Kerkhof PC. Risk-benefit assessment of methotrexate in the treatment of severe psoriasis. *Am J Clin Dermatol* 2000; 1(1): 27–39.
4. Wollina U, Stander K, Barta U. Toxicity of methotrexate treatment in psoriasis and psoriatic arthritis—Short and long-term toxicity in 104 patients. *Clin Rheumatol* 2001; 20(6): 406–410.
5. Kumar B, Saraswat A, Kaur I. Short-term methotrexate therapy in psoriasis: A study of 197 patients. *Int J Dermatol* 2002; 41(7): 444–448.
6. Van Dooren-Greebe RJ, Kuijpers AL, Mulder J, et al. Methotrexate revisited: Effects of long-term treatment in psoriasis. *Br J Dermatol* 1994; 130(2): 204–210.
7. Roenigk HH, Jr, Maibach HI, Weinstein GD. Use of methotrexate in psoriasis. *Arch Dermatol* 1972; 105(3): 363–365.
8. Peckham PE, Weinstein GD, McCullough JL. The treatment of severe psoriasis. A national survey. *Arch Dermatol* 1987; 123: 1303–1307.
9. Krueger GG, Feldman SR, Camisa C, et al. Two considerations for patients with psoriasis and their clinicians: What defines mild, moderate, and severe psoriasis? What constitutes a clinically significant improvement when treating psoriasis? *J Am Acad Dermatol* 2000; 43(2 Pt 1): 281–285.
10. Roenigk HH, Jr, Auerbach R, Maibach HI, et al. Methotrexate guideline—Revised. *J Am Acad Dermatol* 1982; 6(2): 145–155.
11. Roenigk HH, Jr, Auerbach R, Maibach HI, et al. Methotrexate in psoriasis: Revised guidelines. *J Am Acad Dermatol* 1988; 19(1 Pt 1): 145–156.
12. Roenigk HH, Jr, Auerbach R, Maibach HI, et al. Methotrexate in psoriasis: Consensus conference. *J Am Acad Dermatol* 1998; 38(3): 478–485.
13. Kalb RE, Strober B, Weinstein GD, et al. Methotrexate and psoriasis: 2009 National Psoriasis Foundation Consensus Conference. *J Am Acad Dermatol* 2009; 60(5): 824–837.
14. Weinstein GD, White GM. An approach to the treatment of moderate to severe psoriasis with rotational therapy. *J Am Acad Dermatol* 1993; 28(3): 454–459.
15. Weinstein GD, Goldfaden G, Frost P. Methotrexate. Mechanism of action on DNA synthesis in psoriasis. *Arch Dermatol* 1971; 104: 236–243.
16. Law JH, Koo B, Koo JYM. Methotrexate update: Mechanism of action in psoriasis therapy. *Psoriasis Forum* 2008; 14(1): 17–28.
17. Olsen EA. The pharmacology of methotrexate. *J Am Acad Dermatol* 1991; 25: 306–318.
18. Weinstein GD, McCullough JL, Ross PA. Cell kinetic basis for pathophysiology of psoriasis. *J Invest Dermatol* 1985; 85: 579–583.

19. Schwartz PM, Barnett SK, Atillasoy ES, et al. Methotrexate induces differentiation of human keratinocytes. *Proc Natl Acad Sci U S A* 1992; 89(2): 594–598.
20. Jeffes EW, III, McCullough JL, Pittelkow MR, et al. Methotrexate therapy of psoriasis: Differential sensitivity of proliferating lymphoid and epithelial cells to the cytotoxic and growth-inhibitory effects of methotrexate. *J Invest Dermatol* 1995; 104(2): 183–188.
21. Heenen M, Laporte M, Noel JC, et al. Methotrexate induces apoptotic cell death in human keratinocytes. *Arch Dermatol Res* 1998; 290(5): 240–245.
22. Pol A, Bergers M, Schalkwijk J. Comparison of antiproliferative effects of experimental and established antipsoriatic drugs on human keratinocytes, using a simple 96-well-plate assay. *In Vitro Cell Dev Biol Anim* 2003; 39(1–2): 36–42.
23. Weinblatt ME, Coblyn JS, Fox DA, et al. Efficacy of low-dose methotrexate in rheumatoid arthritis. *N Engl J Med* 1985; 312(13): 818–822.
24. Jeffes EW, III, Lee GC, Said S, et al. Elevated numbers of proliferating mononuclear cells in the peripheral blood of psoriatic patients correlate with disease severity. *J Invest Dermatol* 1995; 105: 733–738.
25. Sigmundsdottir H, Johnston A, Gudjonsson JE, et al. Methotrexate markedly reduces the expression of vascular E-selectin, cutaneous lymphocyte-associated antigen and the numbers of mononuclear leucocytes in psoriatic skin. *Exp Dermatol* 2004; 13(7): 426–434.
26. Johnston A, Gudjonsson JE, Sigmundsdottir H, et al. The anti-inflammatory action of methotrexate is not mediated by lymphocyte apoptosis, but by the suppression of activation and adhesion molecules. *Clin Immunol* 2005; 114(2): 154–163.
27. Herman S, Zurgil N, Deutsch M. Low dose methotrexate induces apoptosis with reactive oxygen species involvement in T lymphocytic cell lines to a greater extent than in monocytic lines. *Inflamm Res* 2005; 54(7): 273–280.
28. Rees RB, Bennett JH, Maibach HI, et al. Methotrexate for psoriasis. *Arch Dermatol* 1967; 95: 2–11.
29. Vanscott EJ, Auerbach R, Weinstein GD. Parenteral methotrexate in psoriasis. *Arch Dermatol* 1964; 89: 550–556.
30. Weinstein GD, Frost P. Methotrexate for psoriasis. A new therapeutic schedule. *Arch Dermatol* 1971; 103(1): 33–38.
31. Zackheim HS. Subcutaneous administration of methotrexate. *J Am Acad Dermatol* 1992; 26: 1008.
32. Zachariae H. Methotrexate side-effects. *Br J Dermatol* 1990; 122 (Suppl 36): 127–133.
33. Newman M, Auerbach R, Feiner H, et al. The role of liver biopsies in psoriatic patients receiving long-term methotrexate treatment. Improvement in liver abnormalities after cessation of treatment. *Arch Dermatol* 1989; 125: 1218–1224.
34. Aithal GP, Haugk B, Das S, et al. Monitoring methotrexate-induced hepatic fibrosis in patients with psoriasis: Are serial liver biopsies justified? *Aliment Pharmacol Ther* 2004; 19: 391–399.
35. Thomas JA, Aithal GP. Monitoring liver function during methotrexate therapy for psoriasis: Are routine biopsies really necessary? *Am J Clin Dermatol* 2005; 6: 357–363.
36. Erickson AR, Reddy V, Vogelgesang SA, et al. Usefulness of the American College of Rheumatology recommendations for liver biopsy in methotrexate-treated rheumatoid arthritis patients. *Arthritis Rheum* 1995; 38: 1115–1119.
37. Strober BE, Menon K. Folate supplementation during methotrexate therapy for patients with psoriasis. *J Am Acad Dermatol* 2005; 53: 652–659.
38. Ortiz Z, Shea B, Suarez-Almazor ME, et al. The efficacy of folic acid and folinic acid in reducing methotrexate gastrointestinal toxicity in rheumatoid arthritis. A metaanalysis of randomized controlled trials. *J Rhematol* 1998; 25: 36–43.
39. Duhra P. Treatment of gastrointestinal symptoms associated with methotrexate therapy for psoriasis. *J Am Acad Dermatol* 1993; 28: 466–469.
40. Gilbert SC, Klintmalm G, Menter A, et al. Methotrexate-induced cirrhosis requiring liver transplantation in three patients with psoriasis. A word of caution in light of the expanding use of the "steroid-sparing" agent. *Arch Intern Med* 1990; 150: 889–891.
41. Zachariae H, Kragballe K, Sogaard H. Methotrexate-induced liver cirrhosis. Studies including serial liver biopsies during continued treatment. *Br J Dermatol* 1980; 102: 407–412.
42. Nyfors A. Liver biopsies from psoriatics related to Methotrexate therapy. 2. Findings before and after methotrexate therapy in 88 patients. A blind study. *Acta Pathol Microbiol Scand* 1976; 84: 262–270.

43. Herron MD, Hinckley M, Hoffman MS, et al. Impact of obesity and smoking on psoriasis presentation and management. *Arch Dermatol* 2005; 141: 1527–1534.
44. Weinstein GD, Roenigk H, Maibach HI, et al. Psoriasis-liver-methotrexate interactions. *Arch Dermatol* 1973; 108(1): 36–42.
45. Rademaker M, Webb JA, Lowe DG, et al. Magnetic resonance imaging as a screening procedure for methotrexate induced liver damage. *Br J Dermatol* 1987; 117: 311–316.
46. Geronemus RG, Auerbach R, Tobias H. Liver biopsies versus upsilon liver scans in methotrexate-treated patients with psoriasis. *Arch Dermatol* 1982; 118: 649–651.
47. Mitchell D, Johnson RJ, Testa HJ, et al. Ultrasound and radionuclide scans-poor indicators of liver damage in patients treated with methotrexate. *Clin Exp Dermatol* 1987; 12: 243–245.
48. Coulson IH, McKenzie J, Neild VS, et al. A comparison of liver ultrasound with liver biopsy histology in psoriatics receiving long-term methotrexate therapy. *Br J Dermatol* 1987; 116: 491–495.
49. Verschuur AC, van Everdingen JJ, Cohen EB, et al. Liver biopsy versus ultrasound in methotrexate-treated psoriasis: A decision analysis. *Int J Dermatol* 1992; 31(6): 404–409.
50. Zachariae H, Aslam HM, Bjerring P, et al. Serum aminoterminal propeptide of type III procollagen in psoriasis and psoriatic arthritis: Relation to liver fibrosis and arthritis. *J Am Acad Dermatol* 1991; 25(1 Pt 1): 50–53.
51. Piccinino F, Sagnelli E, Pasquale G, et al. Complications following percutaneous liver biopsy. A multicentre retrospective study on 68276 biopsies. *J Hepatol* 1986; 2: 165–173.
52. Bertino JR. "Rescue" techniques in cancer chemotherapy: Use of leucovorin and other rescue agents after methotrexate treatment. *Semin Oncol* 1977; 4(2): 203–216.
53. Evans WE, Christensen ML. Drug interactions with methotrexate. *J Rheumatol* 1985; 12 (Suppl 12): 15–20.
54. Groenendal H, Rampen FH. Methotrexate and trimethoprim/sulfamethoxazole-A potentially hazardous combination. *Clin Exp Dermatol* 1990; 15: 358–360.
55. Korstanje MJ, van Breda Vriesman CJ, van de Staak WJ. Cyclosporine and methotrexate: A dangerous combination. *J Am Acad Dermatol* 1990; 23(2 Pt 1): 320–321.
56. Kozlowski RD, Steinbrunner JV, MacKenzie AH, et al. Outcome of first-trimester exposure to low-dose methotrexate in eight patients with rheumatic disease. *Am J Med* 1990; 88: 589–592.
57. Lloyd ME, Carr M, McElhatton P, et al. The effects of methotrexate on pregnancy, fertility, and lactation. *QJM* 1999; 92: 551–563.
58. Ayhan A, Ergeneli MH, Yuce K, et al. Pregnancy after chemotherapy for gestational trophoblastic disease. *J Reprod Med* 1990; 35: 522–524.
59. Nabers J, Splinter TA, Wallenburg HCS, et al. Choriocarcinoma with lung metastases during pregnancy with successful delivery and outcome after chemotherapy. *Thorax* 1990; 45(5): 416–418.
60. Sussman A, Leonard JM. Psoriasis, methotrexate and oligospermia. *Arch Dermatol* 1980; 116: 215–217.
61. Ridley MG, Wolfe CS, Mathews JA. Life threatening acute pneumonitis during low dose methotrexate treatment for rheumatoid arthritis: A case report and review of the literature. *Ann Rheum Dis* 1988; 47: 784–788.
62. Schwartz GF, Anderson ST. Methotrexate induced pneumonitis in a young woman with psoriasis and rheumatoid arthritis. *J Rheumatol* 1990; 17: 980.
63. Witty LA, Steiner F, Curfman M, et al. Disseminated histoplasmosis in patients receiving low-dose methotrexate therapy for psoriasis. *Arch Dermatol* 1992; 128: 91–93.
64. Lee GC, Weinstein GD. Comparative cost-effectiveness of different treatments for psoriasis. In: Rajagopalan R, Scherertz EF, Anderson RT, eds. *Care and Management of Skin Diseases*. New York: Marcel Dekker, 1998; 269–298.

Chapter 10

Cyclosporine

Ethan C. Levin and Charles N. Ellis

INTRODUCTION

The evidence of psoriasis as an immune-mediated disease can be traced back to 1979, when cyclosporine was first used in kidney transplant patients to prevent graft rejection [1]. Some of these patients also had psoriasis, which improved after starting cyclosporine. Prior to this serendipitous observation, psoriasis was thought to be a disease of keratinocyte hyperproliferation. However, after this discovery, there was a dramatic shift in the focus of psoriasis research from keratinocyte biology to immunology. Besides being extremely effective in the treatment of psoriasis [2–26], cyclosporine has helped redefine the disease, inspiring the development of other medications that have similar immunologic targets.

PHARMACOLOGY

Mechanism of Action

Cyclosporine is a cyclic polypeptide composed of 11 amino acids whose therapeutic action is derived through the inhibition of calcineurin. To understand the mechanism of action of cyclosporine, it is important to first review the process of T-cell activation. T cells are activated through interactions with the major histocompatibility complex and costimulatory molecules of an antigen-presenting cell. This initiates a complex signaling pathway, which results in an influx of calcium ions from the endoplasmic reticulum and extracellular environment into the T cell. Ultimately, this leads to the activation of the enzyme calcineurin, which in turn activates nuclear factor of activated T cells (NFAT). NFAT is a transcription factor that needs to be dephosphorylated (activated) by calcineurin in order to localize to the nucleus of the cell and increase cytokine gene expression. Therefore, by inhibiting calcineurin, cyclosporine prevents transcription of NFAT-dependent genes (Figure 10.1). This includes genes critical to the pathogenesis of psoriasis, such as interleukin-2 (IL-2), interferon-γ (INF-γ), and tumor necrosis factor-α (TNF-α). Because IL-2 is needed for T-cell proliferation and differentiation, blocking IL-2 expression with cyclosporine was thought to be the principal mechanism for disease improvement in psoriasis. However, with advances in immunology and molecular biology, the understanding of how cyclosporine works has become more complex. For example, Th17 and Th22 cells have been identified as subsets of helper T cells that are critical drivers in psoriasis and other inflammatory conditions [27–29]. In addition, NFAT, which was originally named after T cells, is now recognized as a ubiquitous transcription factor found in a wide variety of immune cells including the lymphoid and myeloid lineages [30]. Therefore, one might hypothesize that cyclosporine has a broader immunosuppressive effect that can target any immune cell regulated by calcineurin/NFAT signaling (Table 10.1). This hypothesis was supported by a study that showed decreased expression of genes characteristic of both the Th1 (IFNγ, Stat1) and Th17 (p19, IL-17, IL-22, chemokine ligand 20 [CCL20]) pathways

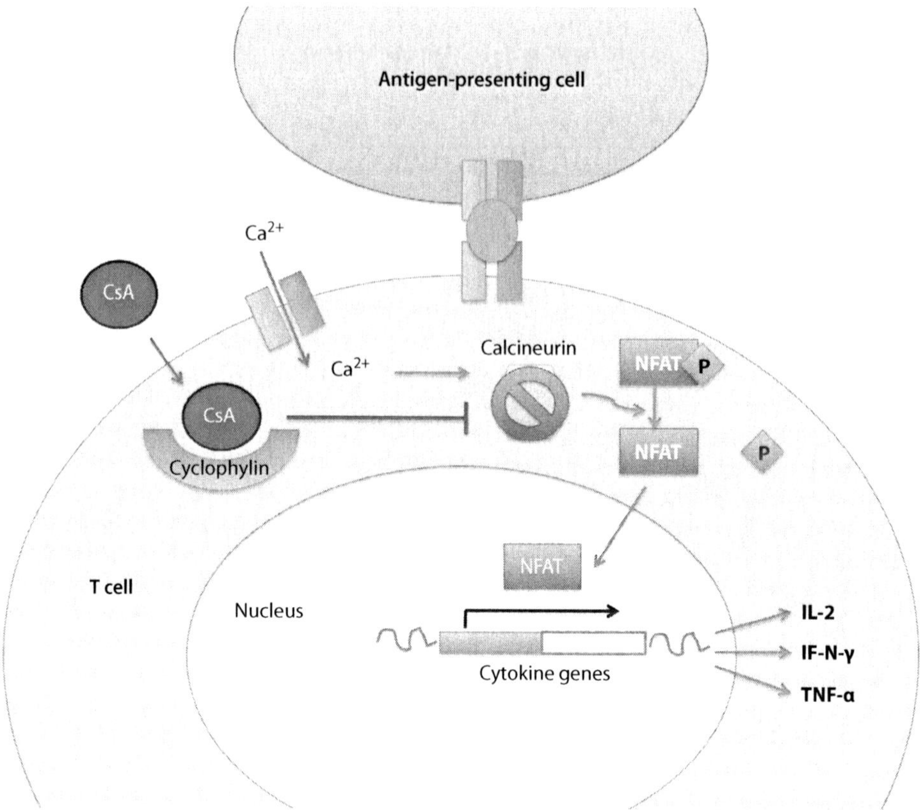

FIGURE 10.1 (See color insert.) Cyclosporine mechanism of action: T cells are activated through interactions with the major histocompatibility complex and costimulatory molecules of an antigen-presenting cell. This initiates a complex signaling pathway, which results in an influx of calcium ions from the endoplasmic reticulum and extracellular environment into the T cell. Ultimately, this leads to the activation of the enzyme calcineurin, which in turn activates nuclear factor of activated T cells (NFAT). NFAT is a transcription factor that needs to be dephosphorylated (activated) by calcineurin in order to localize to the nucleus of the cell and to increase cytokine gene expression. By inhibiting calcineurin, cyclosporine prevents transcription of NFAT-dependent genes critical to the pathogenesis of psoriasis, such as IL-2, INF-γ, and TNF-α. (Reprinted with permission from Bryn Mawr Communications: Practical Dermatology, Bhutani T et al., *Prac Dermatol*, 28–32, 2010.)

TABLE 10.1 Anti-Inflammatory Effects of Cyclosporine in Psoriasis

Cell Type	Gene Product
Naïve T cell	IL-2
Th1	IFNγ, Stat1
Th17	IL-17, IL-22, p19, CCL20
Tip-dendritic cell	IL-23, TNF, iNOS

in psoriatic skin after treatment with cyclosporine [31]. Furthermore, there was decreased expression of genes produced by a subset of monocyte-derived dendritic cells (DCs), known as "Tip-DCs" (TNF–and inducible nitric oxide synthase [iNOS]–producing inflammatory DCs). These cells are a newly recognized population of DCs in psoriasis that produce inflammatory cytokines and activate epidermal keratinocytes [32–34]. In psoriasis, cyclosporine decreased expression of three Tip-DC gene products—IL-23, TNF, and iNOS [31]. In fact, these genes had the strongest correlation with disease remission when measured over the entire treatment period. Cyclosporine may also decrease inflammatory cell trafficking in the skin through alterations in adhesion molecule production [35] and inhibit monocyte production of IL-12 [36].

Metabolism

Cyclosporine is primarily eliminated by the liver, and the parent compound has a terminal half-life of approximately 20 hours [38]. Many of the metabolites of cyclosporine circulate in the blood, and some of them have immunosuppressive activity.

CLINICAL USE IN PSORIASIS

Efficacy

Cyclosporine has a rapid onset of action and is one of the most efficacious systemic treatments for psoriasis. In a double-blind study that compared the efficacy of the two different formulations of cyclosporine (Neoral® and Sandimmune®) for the treatment of severe psoriasis, about 80% of patients in both groups achieved Psoriasis Area and Severity Index (PASI) 75 by week 12 [39]. Many of the other pivotal clinical trials using cyclosporine were conducted before PASI 75 became a common endpoint of psoriasis treatment. Nonetheless, when adequate treatment doses were used (2.5–5 mg/kg/day), the vast majority of patients who completed 12–16 weeks of therapy had significant improvement in their psoriasis [19,26,40–42].

Patient Selection

Typical Patient Cyclosporine therapy should be limited to the treatment of patients with moderate to severe psoriasis, including those with substantial total body surface area involvement (at least 10%, but likely in practice greater than 20%) and those who are disabled by psoriasis (e.g., palmoplantar involvement). Current data suggest that cyclosporine is effective for all types of psoriasis [43–49]. In patients with severe pustular or erythrodermic psoriasis, cyclosporine is recommended by the National Psoriasis Foundation as one of the first-line therapies [43,50]. The drug has also been shown to improve the condition of patients with psoriatic arthritis [51]. Although cyclosporine would be useful in the treatment of milder forms of psoriasis and for psoriasis of the scalp or nails, its side effect profile (discussed later in this chapter) generally discourages this.

Because cyclosporine is recommended for short-term use (see "Duration of Usage"), it is appropriate for patients who are not able to continue their previous therapy, either temporarily or permanently. It may be used as a part of rotational or sequential therapy for psoriasis (for details, see Chapter 7) as a way of reducing toxicities from systemic agents. Cyclosporine may be useful for patients with severe, sudden flares of psoriasis because

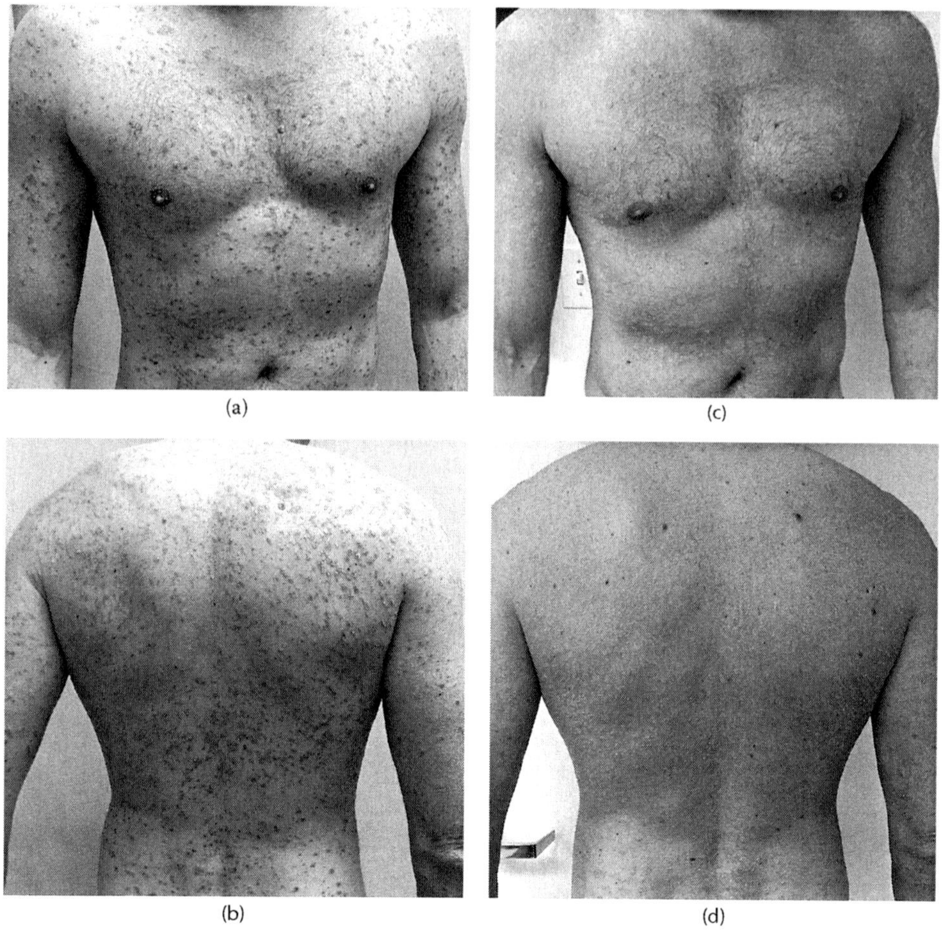

FIGURE 10.2 (See color insert.) Representative patient with severe flare of guttate psoriasis at baseline (a, b) and two weeks after starting cyclosporine 5 mg/kg/day (c, d).

dosages in the top range of 5 mg/kg/day usually have a rapid onset of action (see Figure 10.2). Cyclosporine may also be useful for major life events such as weddings because it can provide substantial clearing of disease. Not only is cyclosporine more affordable than the newer biologic therapies, it usually does not require preauthorization from insurance companies, which may be considerations when speed of onset and cost are concerns. However, in using cyclosporine, a careful explanation is required to ensure that the patient does not later demand long-term cyclosporine therapy. Most dermatologists are familiar with this quandary, which also occurs with the use of systemic corticosteroids for the treatment of various dermatoses. Patients who are unlikely to accept the eventual discontinuation of the drug may represent poor candidates for therapy.

Contraindications

General Advice Because cyclosporine can produce nephrotoxicity, patients who take it should have adequate renal function and should not be taking other drugs concurrently that reduce kidney activity, such as nonsteroidal anti-inflammatory agents.

TABLE 10.2 Contraindications to Cyclosporine Therapy for Psoriasis

Strong Contraindications	Relative Contraindications
Uncontrolled hypertension	Patients who are unlikely to agree to the intermittent use of the drug
Renal disease	Patients with treated hypertension
Sensitivity to components of the medication	Gout
Pregnancy, nursing	Patients taking nephrotoxic drugs (Table 10.3)
Cancer (or history of cancer especially lymphoma)[a]	Elderly patients
Migraines, strokes, other major vascular-related problems (especially in the central nervous system or critical organs, e.g., cardiac angina)	Drug interactions (Table 10.3)
Patients requiring live vaccinations during therapy	Significant hepatic disease
Patients unavailable for regular follow-up	Gingivitis or excessive dental plaque
Active infection	Immunodeficiency of any cause, including due to other psoriasis therapy

[a] Treated basal cell carcinomas usually do not represent contraindications.

Cyclosporine may increase serum uric acid levels, resulting in difficulty for patients with gout. Since cyclosporine is an immunosuppressant, patients should not take the medication if they have active infections including human immunodeficiency virus (HIV), known cancer (especially a history of lymphoma or related nonsolid malignancy), or if they would be harmed by being immunosuppressed for any other reason.

Patients with high blood pressure, migraines, or other vascular-related medical problems (e.g., strokes) have relative contraindications to cyclosporine use. Because cyclosporine causes vasoconstriction, these problems may be exacerbated. Hypertension, whether preexisting or induced by cyclosporine therapy, should be controlled; patients with hypertension may be at increased risk for nephrotoxicity from cyclosporine.

Elderly patients require special consideration because renal function declines with age and elderly patients are more likely to have some of the problems listed earlier. Other medications may represent contraindications (see later in this chapter).

Cyclosporine is contraindicated in patients with a hypersensitivity to any of the components of the medication, although this is extremely rare.

If a patient has a preexisting condition that could be made worse by the known side effects of cyclosporine, such relative contraindications must be considered. (These are discussed in more detail in the sections on "Side Effects of Cyclosporine.")

Patients who are given cyclosporine should be available for follow-up. Table 10.2 summarizes contraindications to cyclosporine therapy for psoriasis.

Pregnancy and Pediatric Use

As with other medications, cyclosporine should not be given to pregnant women unless clearly necessary. However, it is reassuring that in more than 100 pregnancies in women receiving cyclosporine (most of whom took the drug throughout the entire pregnancy because they were transplant recipients), the only consistent findings were premature birth at 28–36 weeks and low birth weight for gestational age [38]. The U.S. Food and Drug Administration (FDA) labels cyclosporine pregnancy category C—there are no adequate studies in pregnant women. The drug is not known to be mutagenic or teratogenic when it is administered at the appropriate dosage; it was only shown to be teratogenic in rodents at five times the normally administered dosage [38].

The immune function of infants exposed to cyclosporine while in utero does not appear to be affected [52]. One study included five infants whose mothers took cyclosporine for an average of more than 200 days during pregnancy. There were not any differences in the measure of immune function in these infants compared to unexposed controls. Some of the parameters measured included immunoglobulin levels, *in vitro* secretion of IL-2 and IFN-γ by peripheral blood mononuclear cells, and antibody response to hepatitis B vaccination [52].

Patients taking cyclosporine should not nurse because the drug is excreted in breast milk. However, even in cases of breastfeeding, the risk may be minimal. In a lactation study of a breastfeeding mother with psoriasis on cyclosporine 3.2 mg/kg/day, the dose received by the infant through the breast milk was less than 2% of the therapeutic dose for an infant [53]. Infant exposure to anything less than 10% of the therapeutic dose is not considered clinically significant [54]. In addition, cyclosporine has been used in infants and children for nondermatological indications and for skin conditions including psoriasis without any unexpected side effects [38,55].

Drug and Food Interactions

Medication, food, and supplement interactions need to be considered to evaluate for possible contraindications in the administration of cyclosporine.

Cyclosporine is metabolized in the gut and liver by CYP3A4 (formerly called cytochrome P-450IIIA4) enzymes, which also metabolize numerous other drugs [56]. (See Table 10.3 for specific examples that use this system.) Any drug or substance that also uses CYP3A4 enzymes may change the bioavailability of cyclosporine. Therefore, patients should be instructed to report all medications taken over the course of cyclosporine therapy so that physicians can address any potential interactions. Grapefruit and grapefruit juice inhibit CYP3A4 and may increase cyclosporine blood levels to an unpredictable degree.

Patients using cyclosporine therapy should avoid drugs that cause renal damage. Because immunosuppression beyond that caused by cyclosporine is undesirable, patients should not be receiving other immunosuppressive agents unless the combination is specifically designed to reduce the side effects of both agents without causing excessive immunosuppression.

Dosage

Dosage Forms Novartis Pharmaceuticals Corp. produces two forms of cyclosporine: Sandimmune® (cyclosporine) and Neoral® (cyclosporine modified), both of which are

TABLE 10.3 Selected Interactions of Other Medications with Cyclosporine

Medications or dietary agents that inhibit hepatic CYP3A4 activity and may increase the blood concentration of cyclosporine	**Medications or dietary agents that increase the risk of hyperkalemia**
Erythromycin, clarithromycin, azithromycin, cephalosporins, doxycycline	Nonsteroidal anti-inflammatory agents, especially indomethacin
Quinupristin/dalfopristin	Certain antihypertensives
Ketoconazole, fluconazole, itraconazole, voriconazole	Angiotensin-converting inhibitors
Oral contraceptives	β-Adrenergic blockers
Cimetidine	Digitalis
Diltiazem, nicardipine, verapamil	Heparin
Danazol	Potassium-containing products
Androgenic steroids	Salt substitutes
Methylprednisolone	Potassium in penicillins
Allopurinol	Potassium iodides
Bromocriptine	Certain foods and food supplements
Metoclopromide	**Drugs that increase or decrease immunosuppression**
Cochicine	Various
Amiodarone	**Other drug interactions with cyclosporine**
Disulfiram or acute alcohol use	Digitalis levels elevated (risk: digitalis toxicity)
Norfloxacin, ciprofloxacin	Lovastatin levels elevated (risk: rhabdomyolysis)
Valproic acid	Vaccines (if substantial immunosuppression exists, could reduce efficacy of vaccine or the patient receiving or exposed to persons receiving live vaccines could be infected)
Grapefruit and grapefruit juice	**Medications or dietary agents that induce hepatic CYP3A4 activity and may decrease the blood concentration of cyclosporinea**
HIV protease inhibitors (e.g., indinavir, nelfinavir, ritonavir, saquinavir)	Griseofulvin
Medications that cause potential synergistic nephrotoxicity	Nafcillin
Nonsteroidal anti-inflammatory drugs: azapropazon, diclofenac, naproxen, sulindac, and others	Carbamazepine
Colchicine	Chronic alcohol use
Diuretics	Octreotide
Gentamycin, tobramycin, vancomycin	Orlistat
Cimetidine, ranitidine	Phenobarbital
Aminoglycosides	Phenytoin
Melphalan	Pioglitazone, rosiglitazone
Amphotericin B	Rifampin
Ketoconazole	St. John's wort
Trimethoprim–sulfamethoxazole	Ticlopidine
Tacrolimus	

[a] These agents are of less medical concern in the treatment of psoriasis than the others in this table because the risk of cyclosporine toxicity is reduced; however, the psoriasis may not respond as well.

available either in 25 or 100 mg capsules or in 50 mL bottles of an oral solution containing 100 mg cyclosporine/mL. The solution requires the patient to follow specific instructions for mixing with a beverage [38].

Oral cyclosporine should be divided into two doses daily, which is thought to reduce the side effect profile. The medication can also be taken three or four times a day, although it is unclear whether this provides any additional benefit. Sandimmune is known for inconsistent absorption, even within the same patient. On the other hand, Neoral is much more consistent. Furthermore, Neoral has a 10%–54% greater bioavailability than Sandimmune [39,41,57–59]. Only Neoral has been approved by the FDA for marketing as a treatment for psoriasis.

Generic versions of cyclosporine USP (25 or 100 mg capsules) and cyclosporine USP modified (25, 50, and 100 mg capsules, as well as 100 mg/mL solution) are available. Although generics meet FDA tests for bioavailability equivalent to the reference drugs Sandimmune and Neoral, some uncertainty exists as to whether the formulations are interchangeable in practice. Although variations in bioavailability are more critical in the treatment of transplant rejection, patients with psoriasis should be instructed to notify their physicians if they receive different capsules than usual from their pharmacists. In such cases, changes in clinical or laboratory results could be related to drug absorption.

It is recommended that patients take cyclosporine at a standard time of the day, in particular with respect to meals. In separate studies, preprandial administration has been shown to increase peak drug levels and efficacy in treating psoriasis when compared to same-dose postprandial administration [60,61].

In general, patients' responses to cyclosporine represent a combination of the dosage and time on therapy. For example, in our study of Sandimmune, about two-thirds of the patients receiving 5 mg/kg/day were clear or nearly clear of psoriasis after two months of therapy [19]. However, only about one-third of the patients receiving 3 mg/kg/day had achieved that response in the same period. Longer periods of treatment tend to achieve continued clearing in many patients.

No consistently effective formulation of topical cyclosporine has been developed; the drug does not penetrate well through skin. Intralesional injection of Sandimmune into psoriatic plaques has been attempted; however, the discomfort is prohibitive and impractical for most patients [62–64].

Dosage Regimens According to the package insert, the initial dose of cyclosporine USP modified should be 2.5 mg/kg/day, divided into two equal doses for a duration of four weeks [65,66]. To achieve the desired clinical effect, the dose can then be increased 0.5 mg/kg/day every two weeks to a maximum of 4 mg/kg/day. However, many authorities including the National Psoriasis Foundation recommend higher maximum doses of up to 5 or 6 mg/kg/day, if needed [67]. The recommended dosing for cyclosporine is based on ideal body weight. This dose may be subtherapeutic for obese patients, who may benefit from dosing based on actual body weight.

The low starting-dose approach (i.e., starting at 2.5 mg/kg/day) described on the package insert is appropriate in patients with stable moderate to severe psoriasis. However, in patients with severe psoriasis that is recalcitrant to other treatments or when rapid control of a flare is needed, a high starting-dose approach (i.e., 5.0 mg/kg/day) is justified (e.g., Figure 10.2). The high starting-dose approach is especially useful in cases of erythrodermic or generalized pustular psoriasis, where a quick response can reduce the likelihood of developing potentially life-threatening complications (see Chapter 17).

One study compared these two dosing strategies over three months, in which study investigators either increased the dose in the low starting-dose group (2.5 mg/kg/day) or decreased the dose in the high starting-dose group (5.0 mg/kg/day), based on disease response [68]. After 12 weeks, more patients in the high starting-dose group achieved PASI 75 than patients in the low starting dose-group and did so in a shorter average time. In addition, there were no significant differences in total adverse events or adverse events requiring intervention between the two groups.

Doses of cyclosporine higher than 5 mg/kg/day may result in faster clearing, but the risk of side effects increases. Although psoriasis is not mentioned in the labeling for Sandimmune in the United States, the recommended maximum dosage is 5 mg/kg/day. Maximum dosages of the two forms of cyclosporine as discussed herein should not be exceeded unless there is documented poor absorption of the drug [69].

If the patient shows no improvement after receiving 5 mg/kg/day (or the patient's own highest tolerated dosage if lower) for three to four months, cyclosporine should be stopped with a gradual taper over the next month. Such a period of maximal dosing should be sufficient to determine that the patient will not be successfully treated with cyclosporine and there is little point in continuing.

In our experience, most patients require 3–4 mg/kg/day of Neoral to achieve and maintain a desired clearing. Once near-clearing is achieved, the daily dosage may be reduced by 0.5 mg/kg/day every month until recurrence becomes apparent. For most patients, 2.5–3.0 mg/kg/day is an effective dosage in the maintenance period [70–72]. Similar to methotrexate usage, it is reasonable to adjust the dosage so that the patient maintains a small amount of psoriasis; if the psoriasis were completely cleared, the patient might be receiving more cyclosporine than necessary. However, this is not easily accomplished with cyclosporine. Cyclosporine often acts as a switch for psoriasis. When an adequate dose of cyclosporine is administered, the disease is turned off. Breakthrough of psoriasis while the patient is receiving an adequate dosage of cyclosporine rarely occurs. When cyclosporine is stopped or tapered, the disease will recur; the drug does not permanently alter the natural course of the disease [73].

In the case of persistent and intolerable side effects, the dosage should be decreased by 1 mg/kg. If the side effects persist, further dosage reduction is required. It should be noted that in cases where higher doses cannot be tolerated due to side effects, "ultra-low" dose cyclosporine (1–2 mg/kg/day) may be considered. In a recent Japanese study using an average dose of 1.5 mg/kg/day, about half of the patients achieved PASI 75 by week 12 [74].

Throughout maintenance administration, side effects should be judged reasonable and therapeutic response should be adequate, or cyclosporine should be discontinued.

Duration of Usage

Cyclosporine is recommended as an intermittent therapy for psoriasis; the U.S. labeling recommends that treatment courses not exceed one year, although international standards suggest that two years of treatment are acceptable. Most studies suggest that effective results can be achieved with a short-term course of cyclosporine that lasts from six months to one year [39,42,70,75]. If a patient has been on therapy for one year, it is time to taper off cyclosporine and begin a different treatment if at all possible. For some patients, cyclosporine may be the only option for severe, treatment-resistant psoriasis. In these patients, it may be appropriate to extend the use of cyclosporine for up to two years, which is consistent with the international guidelines. The exact length of time one needs to take a break from cyclosporine before it can be restarted has never been officially defined, but in worldwide practice, it is generally understood to be at least three months. In addition, the patient's serum creatinine level should be near its original baseline before restarting cyclosporine. Continuous, uninterrupted use over many years should be avoided due to the long-term side effects. In a few select cases, patients have been able to extend therapy for more than five years, but this requires vigilant monitoring because of the increasing risk of side effects [76–80].

Transitioning Off of Cyclosporine

There is no single correct method for transitioning patients from cyclosporine to another agent. The optimal strategy depends on a number of factors including patient preference, natural history of the psoriasis, and the availability of various other therapies. However, in most cases, the authors recommend starting the next medication at least one month *before* tapering the cyclosporine. Overlapping therapy is off-label and requires consent from the patient. Given that cyclosporine is one of the most efficacious systemic agents approved to treat psoriasis, no matter what agent the patient is transitioned to, there is likely to be an "efficacy gap." To bridge this gap, we recommend choosing the next-most efficacious agent available, such as adalimumab or ustekinumab. The chosen agent can be started according to the normal dosing schedule in combination with cyclosporine. After one month of overlap, the cyclosporine should be tapered over the next two to three months until the patient is transitioned to a single agent. This method may give the patient the best chance at maintaining remission *off* of cyclosporine and, when explained as such to the patient, is usually well received. Another advantage of this method is the increased dosing frequency or dosing amount when starting a biologic medication, which further helps to bridge the gap in efficacy with cyclosporine. There are numerous case reports describing successful transition of cyclosporine to biologic agents [81–86].

When biologic therapy is not medically appropriate or not available to the patient, acitretin may be considered. Short-term overlapping therapy with acitretin is usually possible without significant side effects [87]. Although there is some concern about transitioning from cyclosporine directly to ultraviolet (UV) phototherapy, acitretin can provide a buffer period before beginning UV phototherapy and theoretically may inhibit skin malignancies that might occur from any residual immunosuppression.

Cyclosporine may also be transitioned to another systemic immunosuppressant, such as methotrexate, as long as the overlap period is short. This is reasonable because cyclosporine and methotrexate have different organ toxicities.

It should be noted that there are some rare patients with psoriasis who go into remission while on cyclosporine [42]. This may become apparent during maintenance dosing of the medication, when successively lower doses are tolerated without any return of psoriasis. In these patients, it may be most appropriate to attempt to gradually taper the cyclosporine without transitioning to another agent.

Recurrence of Psoriasis after Cyclosporine Treatment

Predictions may be made about the recurrence of psoriasis after cyclosporine is stopped. In our experience, recurrence reflects the severity and intensity of the patient's psoriasis when untreated. Thus, patients with stable, chronic plaque psoriasis are likely to have a gradual recurrence, while patients with brittle, highly inflammatory, and active psoriasis should expect a quicker recurrence. Recurrence of psoriasis to an extent beyond that of the patient's pretherapy condition is unusual.

Psoriasis therapies may be categorized into those that are remittive and those that are not; usually this is a function of whether the therapy depletes the pathogenic T cells or merely suppresses them. Cyclosporine is not remittive. Thus, the relapse rate after stopping cyclosporine is probably not significantly different from that when other major nonremittive therapies are discontinued in patients with moderate to severe psoriasis [73].

Side Effects of Cyclosporine

Miscellaneous Side Effects The side effects associated with cyclosporine are usually dose dependent (Table 10.4) [19]. The two most clinically significant side effects are hypertension and nephrotoxicity (discussed in the following section). When using cyclosporine at 3–5 mg/kg/day, it is reasonable to expect an increase in mean arterial blood pressure of 5 mmHg [88]. Although the exact mechanism of cyclosporine-associated hypertension is unknown, vasoconstriction and increased sodium uptake by the renal tubules are likely important factors [89–91]. Cyclosporine use may also be associated with hyperlipidemia. Both hyperlipidemia and hypertension require intervention, which should begin with dietary changes and an increase in physical activity. If these measures are unsuccessful, pharmacological intervention or cyclosporine dose reduction may be necessary.

Cyclosporine is remarkably well tolerated when used in low dosages for the treatment of dermatological disease. Many of the frequently reported side effects may spontaneously resolve after several weeks of therapy. This includes headaches, temperature hypersensitivity, paresthesias, nausea, and malaise. Hypertrichosis is of minimal concern to most patients; however, women may find it more troublesome than men. Gingival hyperplasia

TABLE 10.4 Side Effects of Relatively Common Frequency When Cyclosporine Is Used in Dermatologic Dosages

Clinical Symptoms		
	Early onset, tend to resolve during therapy	
		Malaise, fatigue
		Nausea
		Headaches
		Achiness in muscles and joints
		Hand tremor
		Paresthesias
		Distal sensitivity to hot or cold
	Onset at any time, persist during therapy	
		Hypertrichosis
		Gingival hyperplasia[a]
Clinical signs		
	Onset at any time	
	Hypertension[b]	
Laboratory changes		
	Increased	
		Creatinine[c]
		Urea nitrogen
		Lipids[b]
		Bilirubin[d]
		Uric acid
		Potassium[b]
	Decreased	
		Magnesium[e]
		Glomerular filtration rate[c]

Note: Side effects in bold represent the most important ones (including nephrotoxicity).
[a] May improve with increased dental hygiene.
[b] May require cyclosporine dosage adjustment or addition of specific therapy.
[c] May require cyclosporine dosage adjustment.
[d] Usually asymptomatic and does not require intervention.
[e] May require replacement therapy.

may be minimized by careful dental hygiene. Hyperbilirubinemia is typically asymptomatic and does not require dosage reduction. Hyperuricemia and gout are not usually problems in nontransplant patients.

Cyclosporine is known for causing hyperkalemia and hypomagnesemia in some patients. Hyperkalemia may respond to a low-potassium diet or a thiazide diuretic. Hypomagnesemia may require replacement therapy, although serum magnesium levels may be misleading in the setting of short-term cyclosporine use. Magnesium is primarily an intracellular cation and less than 1% of the total body store is found in the serum. Studies have shown that short-term cyclosporine use is associated with an intracellular shift of magnesium [92–94], and thus serum magnesium levels in these patients may be poor indicators of total body magnesium. However, long-term use of cyclosporine is associated with renal magnesium wasting as a result of the nephrotoxic effects of the medication [95,96]. Given that magnesium replacement therapy is highly unlikely to harm the patient, the authors recommend magnesium supplementation as needed.

Renal Toxicities Cyclosporine-induced renal toxicity is a major concern [97–105]. Serum creatinine levels may increase within a few weeks of beginning cyclosporine as a result of its early, reversible, vasoconstrictive effect [19]. As a general rule, renal effects can be minimized by low-dosage cyclosporine, and by adjusting the dosage if the serum creatinine rises 25%–30% above baseline on two occasions (separated by two weeks) [106]. In this situation, it is reasonable to decrease the dose of cyclosporine by 0.5–1.0 mg/kg/day every two weeks until the creatinine is no more than 10% higher than the baseline level. Fish oil supplements [107] or amlodipine [108,109] may be able to minimize renal toxicity. Measurements of glomerular filtration rate may be useful in following renal function in patients who have abnormal creatinine levels.

Nevertheless, there remains concern that cyclosporine could induce progressive renal failure in some patients. Histological changes in the kidney including tubular atrophy and interstitial fibrosis do occur after one year or more of treatment [87,106,110]. However, cyclosporine nephrotoxicity is thought to be at least partially reversible. Even patients with impaired renal function after five years of continuous cyclosporine showed gradual improvement after stopping the medication [76]. In our experience and in the literature [111], no patients treated as described for less than one year have developed any renal dysfunction that has affected their normal daily lives. Although most of the patients received therapy for six months or less, some were treated for as long as three years. Renal biopsies are unlikely to be needed in patients treated with intermittent dosing.

If we assume that a patient has normal kidney function prior to beginning cyclosporine therapy, one concern is to what degree his or her normal renal reserve is expended following cyclosporine treatment and to what extent this is a practical issue. It is known that everyone has reduced kidney function with aging; in addition, some people receive additional drugs or other agents that exacerbate or cause kidney damage. How all these factors interact requires further study.

There is a late point in renal damage that is irreversible and leads to a very slow but progressive decline of renal function. In the intermittent treatment of psoriasis with cyclosporine, it is expected that this point would not be reached. However, a patient's kidney function must be monitored so that therapy may be stopped if laboratory test results exceed those recommended. This should prevent progressive declines in renal function.

Cancer and Infection Risk The risk of lymphoma or other cancer as a direct result of cyclosporine therapy for psoriasis is low [69,112]. One retrospective study included 272 patients treated with cyclosporine for at least one month with more than 10 years of median follow-up time. The overall risk of cancer, including lymphoma and skin cancer, was not different compared to the general population [113]. Because cyclosporine is used at low, intermittent dosages in patients with psoriasis, and additional immunosuppression (such as with systemic corticosteroids) is not used simultaneously as it is in transplant patients, the risk of tumors is much lower than in graft recipients [69]. There may be a slight increase in nonmelanoma skin cancers in patients treated with cyclosporine for psoriasis [114,115]. If patients have received psoralen and ultraviolet A (PUVA) prior to cyclosporine therapy, there is an increased risk of squamous cell carcinoma of the skin equivalent to that associated with 200 PUVA treatments [114,116].

In one case, cyclosporine therapy was associated with the onset of cutaneous T-cell lymphoma (CTCL) that disappeared when the cyclosporine was stopped [117]. Some patients who appear to develop CTCL during cyclosporine therapy are found in retrospect likely to have had the condition prior to beginning cyclosporine [118]. Patients with atypical psoriasis or psoriasis that has been thought to be spongiotic dermatitis or eczema clinically or histologically in the past may actually have CTCL. Because cyclosporine may exacerbate CTCL, such patients, if identified, should avoid cyclosporine.

Benign lymphocytic infiltrates have been reported during cyclosporine treatment of psoriasis [119]. Increased risk of common infections (including warts, impetigo, and tineas) is not encountered in our experience [19]. Despite occasional reports of unusual infections in patients receiving cyclosporine, the incidence is extremely rare.

Although cyclosporine has been used safely in patients with hepatitis C infection, even possibly having an antiviral effect [120,121], it is still not recommended as first- or second-line therapy. There may be a rebound effect associated with discontinuing the cyclosporine, leading to the recurrence and progression of hepatitis C [122].

Monitoring

Table 10.5 offers monitoring guidelines. The most important laboratory test is measurement of the serum creatinine [69]. Before initiating therapy, it is imperative to establish a baseline creatinine level for each patient (see Table 10.5 for a suggested protocol). If creatinine levels ever exceed the baseline reading by 25%–30%, the patient's cyclosporine dosage must be reduced. Similarly, increases in blood pressure beyond normal should trigger decreases in dose or addition of antihypertensive medication.

Blood levels of cyclosporine are rarely useful, except to demonstrate poor absorption or noncompliance [123–125]. In the rare person who fails to respond adequately to cyclosporine, a blood level may provide information that the patient is a nonresponder as opposed to not absorbing or taking the drug. At the dosage used in the treatment of psoriasis, it is extremely unlikely that a patient would achieve such a high blood level of cyclosporine that the dosage would be reduced on this account alone. Expected blood levels are lower than those desired in transplant patients, and therefore may be lower than the "normal" values given by the laboratory [123]. In most patients, the dosing is titrated by clinical response or side effects, and blood levels usually provide little helpful information.

TABLE 10.5 Suggested Monitoring of Patients Taking Cyclosporine and Responses to Findings

Obtain at least two pretherapy measurements of serum creatinine to determine a baseline; the values should be within 20% or additional measures should be obtained.
Baseline screening for HIV and hepatitis B and C may be indicated in high-risk patients.
At baseline, after 2 and 4 weeks, and then monthly, obtain measurements of
Blood pressure
Serum
Creatinine (for baseline, see earlier)
Urea nitrogen
Lipids (once stable, may be assessed less often)
Bilirubin, liver function tests
Uric acid
Magnesium
Electrolytes
A review of any new medications.
For hypertension, reduce cyclosporine dosage if possible or treat the high blood pressure.
If serum creatinine exceeds baseline by 25%–30%, reduce cyclosporine dosage. If serum magnesium below normal range, give replacement therapy.
Although bilirubin usually increases, therapy is rarely warranted and dosage reduction usually not needed.
Other laboratory abnormalities should be addressed if significantly abnormal.
Outpatient creatinine clearance tests tend to be unreliable; creatinine clearance can be calculated from formulas based on the serum creatinine but this often adds little additional information. Glomerular filtration rates (GFRs) may be measured by qualified physicians, usually nephrologists; a rate significantly below expected for a patient would serve as a contraindication for cyclosporine therapy. However, there is no consensus that routine measurements of GFR are necessary when cyclosporine is used at dermatological dosages.

Combination Therapy

Using topical drugs, such as anthralin, topical corticosteroids, or vitamin D analogs (such as calcipotriene), concurrently with cyclosporine improves clearance rates, often at lower cyclosporine dosages [12,126–128]. In one study, patients were treated with cyclosporine 2 mg/kg/day combined with either calcipotriol/betamethasone dipropionate ointment or emollient. At eight weeks, more than twice as many patients treated with calcipotriol/betamethasone dipropionate ointment reached PASI 75 than those treated with emollient (87% vs. 37%, $P = 0.0001$) [129]. This is consistent with another study in which improvement rate was four times higher when patients used cyclosporine and calcipotriene ointment versus cyclosporine and placebo [130].

Because most systemic therapies for psoriasis would provide additive immunosuppression (e.g., methotrexate, phototherapy, or biologic therapies), it would be ideal to avoid their use with cyclosporine. In most patients, cyclosporine is so effective that other therapies are not required unless they can be clearly shown to reduce side effects of both agents. However, in a few cases, coadministration of mycophenolate mofetil with cyclosporine has helped clear psoriasis in patients unresponsive to cyclosporine alone [131]. Combining methotrexate and cyclosporine allowed for lower dosages of each in the treatment of 19 patients with severe psoriasis [132]; in patients with rheumatoid arthritis who are not fully responding to methotrexate, the U.S. label for cyclosporine indicates the additive benefit of cyclosporine.

There have been anecdotal reports using the combination of cyclosporine with a TNF-α inhibitor. One prospective case series included seven patients with refractory psoriasis that were treated with a combination of cyclosporine 200 mg/day and etanercept 50 mg/week. Six of seven patients achieved PASI 90 by week seven. Further, these patients were able to maintain their response with lower doses of cyclosporine and etanercept for up to one year of follow-up without any serious adverse events or serious infections reported [133]. However, another report described a patient who developed lymphoma while on cyclosporine and infliximab for psoriasis [134]. Five months after discontinuing cyclosporine, a full remission occurred.

Phototherapy engenders the risk of inducing skin cancers during the modest immunosuppression of cyclosporine, and there is an admonition for using both together in the U.S. label for cyclosporine modified. Furthermore, cyclosporine with PUVA was of less benefit than an oral retinoid with PUVA in one study [135].

The combination of an oral retinoid with cyclosporine may not provide additional benefit in psoriasis [136]. The combination is more frequently used in transplant recipients, in which the addition of acitretin may reduce the development of skin cancers. Both retinoids and cyclosporine may cause lipid elevations [137,138]; however, if hyperlipidemia is induced, it generally can be treated with antilipid agents. Rather than being used simultaneously with cyclosporine in psoriasis, acitretin is a useful therapy to follow cyclosporine.

Other Calcineurin Inhibitors

Topical pimecrolimus and tacrolimus are used in some forms of psoriasis and in body areas where penetration into the skin occurs more readily.

Because the clinical utility of cyclosporine is mitigated by its side effect profile, there is an interest in the use of other systemically administered calcineurin inhibitors that may be safer for patients. Several have been studied, including pimecrolimus, tacrolimus, and voclosporin, formerly ISA247 [139–143]. Studies involving these medications in psoriasis have generally compared them to placebo, rather than to cyclosporine, and have been of relatively short duration (less than a year), limiting the ability to compare their efficacy or side effects head-to-head with cyclosporine. Development of oral pimecrolimus has been stopped. At this writing, there is no current development of oral tacrolimus as a psoriasis therapy, although the drug is available for off-label use in the United States; in limited earlier studies, the drug appeared to have efficacy and side effect profiles similar to oral cyclosporine [142,143]. At the time of this writing, voclosporin development is focused on indications other than psoriasis.

REFERENCES

1. Mueller W, Herrmann B. Cyclosporin A for psoriasis [letter]. *N Engl J Med* 1979; 301: 555.
2. Ellis CN, Gorsulowsky DC, Hamilton TA, et al. Cyclosporine improves psoriasis in a double-blind study. *JAMA* 1986; 256: 3110–3116.
3. Muller W, Graf U. Die behandlung der psoriasis-arthritis mit cyclosporin A, einem neuen immunosuppressivum. *Schweiz Med Wochenschr* 1981; 111: 408–413.

4. Harper JI, Keat ASC, Staughton RCD. Cyclosporine for psoriasis. *Lancet* 1984; 2: 981–982.
5. van Hooff JP, Leunissen KML, Staak WVD. Cyclosporin and psoriasis. *Lancet* 1985; 1: 335.
6. Marks J. Psoriasis. *Br Med J* 1986; 293: 509.
7. Griffiths CEM, Powles AV, Leonard JN, et al. Clearance of psoriasis with low dose cyclosporin. *Br Med J* 1986; 293: 731–732.
8. Brookes DB. Clearance of psoriasis with low dose cyclosporin. *Br Med J* 1986; 293: 1098–1099.
9. van Joost T, Heule F, Stolz E, et al. Short-term use of cyclosporin A in severe psoriasis. *Br J Dermatol* 1986; 114: 615–620.
10. Wentzell JM. Baughman RD, O'Connor GT, et al. Cyclosporine in the treatment of psoriasis. *Arch Dermatol* 1987; 123: 163–165.
11. Picascia DD, Garden JM, Freinkel RK, et al. Treatment of resistant severe psoriasis with systemic cyclosporine. *J Am Acad Dermatol* 1987; 17: 408–414.
12. Griffiths CEM, Powles AV, Baker BS, et al. Combination of cyclosporine A and topical corticosteroid in the treatment of psoriasis. *Transplant Proc* 1988; 20 (Suppl 4): 50–52.
13. van Joost T, Bos JD, Heule F, et al. Low-dose cyclosporin A in severe psoriasis: a double-blind study. *Br J Dermatol* 1988; 118: 183–190.
14. Meinardi MMHM, Bos JD. Cyclosporine maintenance therapy in psoriasis. *Transplant Proc* 1988; 20 (Suppl 4): 42–49.
15. Finzi AF, Mozzanica N, Cattaneo A, et al. Effectiveness of cyclosporine treatment in severe psoriasis: a clinical and immunologic study. *J Am Acad Dermatol* 1989; 21: 91–97.
16. Heule F, Bousema MT, Laeijendecker R, et al. Three long-term regimens with cyclosporin for psoriasis vulgaris. *Acta Derm Venereol Suppl (Stockh)* 1989; 146: 171–175.
17. Meinardi MMHM, de Rie MA, Bos JD. Oral cyclosporin A in the treatment of psoriasis: an overview of studies performed in the Netherlands. *Br J Dermatol* 1990; 122 (Suppl 36): 27–31.
18. Timonen P, Friend D, Abeywickrama K, et al. Efficacy of low-dose cyclosporin A in psoriasis: results of dose-finding studies. *Br J Dermatol* 1990; 122 (Suppl 36): 33–39.
19. Ellis CN, Fradin MS, Messana JM, et al. Cyclosporine for plaque-type psoriasis. Results of a multidose, double-blind trial. *N Engl J Med* 1991; 324: 277–284.
20. Powles AV, Baker BS, Valdimarsson H, et al. Four years of experience with cyclosporine A for psoriasis. *Br J Dermatol* 1990; 122 (Suppl 36): 13–19.
21. Tegelberg-Stassen MJAM, Lammers A, Van Floten WA, et al. Responsiveness of moderate psoriatic skin lesions to 1, 2, or 3 mg/kg/day cyclosporin A: a multicenter study. *Eur J Dermatol* 1992; 2: 147–150.
22. Dubertret L, Grossman R, Perrussel M, et al. Low-dose cyclosporin A in psoriasis. In: Wolff K, ed. *Cyclosporin A and The Skin, International Congress and Symposium Series No. 192*. London: Royal Society of Medicine Services; 1992, p. 13 [abstract].
23. Christophers E, Mrowietz U, Henneicke HH, et al. Cyclosporin A in psoriasis: interim results of a multicentre dose-finding study in severe chronic plaque-type psoriasis. In: Wolff K, ed. *Cyclosporin A and The Skin, International Congress and Symposium Series No. 192*. London: Royal Society of Medicine Services, 1992, pp. 21–26.
24. Mahrle G, Schulze HJ, Farber L. Cyclosporin A vs. etretinate in the treatment of psoriasis: preliminary results. In: Wolff K, ed. *Cyclosporin A and The Skin, International Congress and Symposium Series No. 192*. London: Royal Society of Medicine Services, 1992, pp. 27–28.
25. Flytstrom I, Stenberg B, Svensson A, et al. Methotrexate vs. cyclosporin in psoriasis: effectiveness, qualify of life and safety. A randomized controlled trial. *Br J Dermatol* 2008; 158(1): 116–121.
26. Heydendael VM, Spuls PI, Opmeer BC, et al. Methotrexate versus cyclosporine in moderate-to-severe chronic plaque psoriasis. *N Engl J Med* 2003; 349(7): 658–665.
27. Eyerich S, Eyerich K, Pennino D, et al. Th22 cells represent a distinct human T cell subset involved in epidermal immunity and remodeling. *J Clin Invest* 2009; 119(12): 3573–3585.
28. Chen W, Jin W, Hardegen N, et al. Conversion of peripheral CD4+CD25- naive T cells to CD4+CD25+ regulatory T cells by TGF-beta induction of transcription factor Foxp3. *J Exp Med* 2003; 198(12): 1875–1886.
29. Veldhoen M, Hocking RJ, Atkins CJ, et al. TGFbeta in the context of an inflammatory cytokine milieu supports de novo differentiation of IL-17-producing T cells. *Immunity* 2006; 24(2): 179–189.
30. Macian F. NFAT proteins: key regulators of T-cell development and function. *Nat Rev Immunol* 2005; 5(6): 472–484.

31. Haider AS, Lowes MA, Suarez-Farinas M, et al. Identification of cellular pathways of "type 1," Th17 T cells, and TNF- and inducible nitric oxide synthase-producing dendritic cells in autoimmune inflammation through pharmacogenomic study of cyclosporine A in psoriasis. *J Immunol* 2008; 180(3): 1913–1920.
32. Satpathy AT, Wu X, Albring JC, et al. Re(de)fining the dendritic cell lineage. *Nat Immunol* 2012; 13(12): 1145–1154.
33. Lowes MA, Chamian F, Abello MV, et al. Increase in TNF-alpha and inducible nitric oxide synthase-expressing dendritic cells in psoriasis and reduction with efalizumab (anti-CD11a). *Proc Natl Acad Sci U S A* 2005; 102(52): 19057–19062.
34. Nestle FO, Kaplan DH, Barker J. Psoriasis. *N Engl J Med* 2009; 361(5): 496–509.
35. Wong RL, Winslow CM, Cooper KD. The mechanisms of action of cyclosporin A in the treatment of psoriasis. *Immunol Today* 1993; 14: 69–74.
36. Tada Y, Asahina A, Takekoshi T, et al. Interleukin 12 production by monocytes from patients with psoriasis and its inhibition by cyclosporin A. *Br J Dermatol* 2006; 154: 1180–1183.
37. Bhutani T, Busse K, Koo J. Revisiting cyclosporine in the age of biologics: update on efficacy and mechanism of action. *Prac Dermatol* 2010: 28–32.
38. Novartis Pharmaceuticals Corporation. Neoral; Sandimmune. Physician's Desk Reference, 2007.
39. Koo J. A randomized, double-blind study comparing the efficacy, safety and optimal dose of two formulations of cyclosporine, Neoral and Sandimmune, in patients with severe psoriasis. OLP302 Study Group. *Br J Dermatol* 1998; 139: 88–95.
40. Ho VC, Griffiths CE, Albrecht G, et al. Intermittent short courses of cyclosporine (Neoral(R)) for psoriasis unresponsive to topical therapy: a 1-year multicentre, randomized study. The PISCES Study Group. *Br J Dermatol* 1999; 141(2): 283–291.
41. Berth-Jones J, Henderson CA, Munro CS, et al. Treatment of psoriasis with intermittent short course cyclosporine (Neoral). *Br J Dermatol* 1997; 136: 527–530.
42. Ho VC, Griffiths CE, Berth-Jones J, et al. Intermittent short courses of cyclosporine microemulsion for the long-term management of psoriasis: a 2-year cohort study. *J Am Acad Dermatol* 2001; 44: 643–651.
43. Robinson A, Van Voorhees AS, Hsu S, et al. Treatment of pustular psoriasis: from the Medical Board of the National Psoriasis Foundation. *J Am Acad Dermatol* 2012; 67(2): 279–288.
44. Nogita T, Mitsuishi T, Terajima S, et al. Efficacy of cyclosporin in two cases of erythrodermic psoriasis [letter]. *J Dermatol* 1991; 18: 302–304.
45. Reitamo S, Mustakallio KK. Cyclosporine in erythrodermic psoriasis. *Acta Derm Venereol Suppl (Stockh)* 1989; (Suppl 146): 140–141.
46. Korstanje MJ, Bessems PJMJ, van de Staak WJBM. Combination therapy cyclosporine etretinate effective in erythrodermic psoriasis [letter]. *Dermatologica* 1989; 179: 94.
47. Sutthipisal N, Sriwatsantsak J, Sirimachan S, et al. The use of low dose cyclosporine A in a case of recalcitrant erythrodermic psoriasis. *J Int Med Res* 1988; 16: 485–488.
48. Korstanje MJ, Bessems PJMJ, Hulsmans RFHJ. Pustular psoriasis and acrodermatitis continua (Hallopeau) need high doses of systemic cyclosporine A [letter]. *Dermatologica* 1989; 179: 90–91.
49. Feliciani C, Zampetti A, Forleo P, et al. Nail psoriasis: combined therapy with systemic cyclosporine and topical calcipotriol. *J Cutan Med Surg* 2004; 8(2): 122–125.
50. Rosenbach M, Hsu S, Korman NJ, et al. Treatment of erythrodermic psoriasis: from the medical board of the National Psoriasis Foundation. *J Am Acad Dermatol* 2010; 62(4): 655–662.
51. Gupta AK, Matteson EL, Ellis CN, et al. Cyclosporine in the treatment of psoriatic arthritis. *Arch Dermatol* 1989; 125: 507–510.
52. Biggioggero M, Borghi MO, Gerosa M, et al. Immune function in children born to mothers with autoimmune diseases and exposed in utero to immunosuppressants. *Lupus* 2007; 16(8): 651–656.
53. Mazzuoccolo LD, Andrada R, Pellerano G, et al. Levels of cyclosporine in breast milk and passage into the circulation of the infant of a mother with psoriasis. *Int J Dermatol* 2013. [Epub ahead of print]
54. Armenti VT, Radomski JS, Moritz MJ, et al. Report from the National Transplantation Pregnancy Registry (NTPR): outcomes of pregnancy after transplantation. *Clin Transpl* 2004: 103–114.
55. Pereira TM, Vieira AP, Fernandes JC, et al. Cyclosporine A treatment in severe childhood psoriasis. *J Eur Acad Dermatol Venereol* 2006; 20(6): 651–656.

56. Watkins PB. The role of cytochromes P-450 in cyclosporine metabolism. *J Am Acad Dermatol* 1990; 23: 1301–1311.
57. Somerville MF, Scott DG. Neoral—new cyclosporine for old? *Br J Rheumatol* 1997; 36: 1113–1115.
58. Gulliver WP, Murphy GF, Hannaford VA, et al. Increased bioavailability and improved efficacy, in severe psoriasis, of a new microemulsion formulation of cyclosporine. *Br J Dermatol* 1996; 135 (Suppl 48): 35–39.
59. Elder CA, Moore M, Chang CT, et al. Efficacy and pharmacokinetics of two formulations of cyclosporine A in patients with psoriasis. *J Clin Pharmacol* 1995; 35: 865–875.
60. Umezawa Y, Mabuchi T, Ozawa A. Preprandial vs. postprandial pharmacokinetics of cyclosporine in patients with psoriasis. *Int J Dermatol* 2007; 46(8): 880–882.
61. Hashizume H, Ito T, Yagi H, et al. Efficacy and safety of preprandial versus postprandial administration of low-dose cyclosporine microemulsion (Neoral) in patients with psoriasis vulgaris. *J Dermatol* 2007; 34(7): 430–434.
62. Ho VC, Griffiths CEM, Ellis CN, et al. Intralesional cyclosporine in the treatment of psoriasis. A clinical, immunologic, and pharmacokinetic study. *J Am Acad Dermatol* 1990; 22: 94–100.
63. Burns MK, Ellis CN, Eisen D, et al. Intralesional cyclosporine for psoriasis: relationship of dose, tissue levels, and efficacy. *Arch Dermatol* 1992; 128: 786–790.
64. Powles AV, Baker BS, McFadden J, et al. Intralesional injection of cyclosporine in psoriasis. *Lancet* 1988; 1: 537.
65. Neoral [package insert].
66. Griffiths CE, Dubertret L, Ellis CN, et al. Cyclosporine in psoriasis clinical practice: an international consensus statement. *Br J Dermatol* 2004; 150 (Suppl 67): 11–23.
67. Rosmarin DM, Lebwohl M, Elewski BE, et al. Cyclosporine and psoriasis: 2008 National Psoriasis Foundation Consensus Conference. *J Am Acad Dermatol* 2010; 62(5): 838–853.
68. Yoon HS, Youn JI. A comparison of two cyclosporine dosage regimens for the treatment of severe psoriasis. *J Dermatol Treat* 2007; 18(5): 286–290.
69. Fradin MS, Ellis CN, Voorhees JJ. Management of patients and side effects during cyclosporine therapy for cutaneous disorders. *J Am Acad Dermatol* 1990; 23: 1265–1275.
70. Shupack J, Abel E, Bauer E, et al. Cyclosporine as maintenance therapy in patients with severe psoriasis. *J Am Acad Dermatol* 1997; 36: 423–432.
71. Ellis CN, Fradin MS, Hamilton TA, et al. Duration of remission during maintenance cyclosporine therapy for psoriasis. Relationship to maintenance dose and degree of improvement during initial therapy. *Arch Dermatol* 1995; 131: 791–795.
72. Mahrle G, Schulze HJ, Farber L, et al. Low-dose short-term cyclosporine versus etretinate in psoriasis: improvement of skin, nail, and joint involvement. *J Am Acad Dermatol* 1995; 32: 78–88.
73. Higgins E, Munro C, Marks J, et al. Relapse rates in moderately severe chronic psoriasis treated with cyclosporine A. *Br J Dermatol* 1989; 121(1): 71–74.
74. Shintani Y, Kaneko N, Furuhashi T, et al. Safety and efficacy of a fixed dose cyclosporine microemulsion (100 mg) for the treatment of psoriasis. *J Dermatol* 2011; 38(10): 966–972.
75. Finzi AF. Individualized short-course cyclosporine therapy in psoriasis. *Br J Dermatol* 1996; 135 (Suppl 48): 31–34.
76. Powles AV, Hardman CM, Porter WM, et al. Renal function after 10 years' treatment with cyclosporine for psoriasis. *Br J Dermatol* 1998; 138: 443–449.
77. Lowe NJ, Wieder JM, Rosenbach A, et al. Long-term low-dose cyclosporine therapy for severe psoriasis: effects on renal function and structure. *J Am Acad Dermatol* 1996; 35(5 Pt 1): 710–719.
78. Grossman RM, Chevret S, Abi-Rached J, et al. Long-term safety of cyclosporine in the treatment of psoriasis. *Arch Dermatol* 1996; 132: 623–629.
79. Mrowietz U, Farber L, Henneicke-von Zepelin HH, et al. Long-term maintenance therapy with cyclosporine and post-treatment survey in severe psoriasis: results of a multicenter study. German Multicenter Study. *J Am Acad Dermatol* 1995; 33: 470–475.
80. Peluso AM, Bardazzi F, Tosti A, et al. Intermittent cyclosporine A treatment of severe plaque psoriasis. Long-term follow-up of 26 patients. *Acta Derm -Venereol Suppl* 1994; 186: 90–91.
81. Iyer S, Yamauchi P, Lowe NJ. Etanercept for severe psoriasis and psoriatic arthritis: observations on combination therapy. *Br J Dermatol* 2002; 146(1): 118–121.
82. Yamauchi P, Lowe N. Cessation of cyclosporine therapy by treatment with etanercept in patients with severe psoriasis. *J Am Acad Dermatol* 2006; 54(3): S135–S138.

83. Ricotti C, Kerdel FA. Subacute annular generalized pustular psoriasis treated with etanercept and cyclosporine combination. *J Drugs Dermatol* 2007; 6(7): 738–740.
84. Kress D. Etanercept therapy improves symptoms and allows tapering of other medications in children and adolescents with moderate to severe psoriasis. *J Am Acad Dermatol* 2006; 54(3): S126–S128.
85. Cather JC, Menter A. Combining traditional agents and biologics for the treatment of psoriasis. *Semin Cutan Med Surg* 2005; 24(1): 37–45.
86. Strober BE, Clarke S. Etanercept for the treatment of psoriasis: combination therapy with other modalities. *J Drugs Dermatol* 2004; 3(3): 270–272.
87. Young EW, Ellis CN, Messana JM, et al. A prospective study of renal structure and function in psoriasis patients treated with cyclosporine. *Kidney Int* 1994; 46: 1216–1222.
88. Robert N, Wong GW, Wright JM. Effect of cyclosporine on blood pressure. *Cochrane Database Syst Rev* 2010; (1): CD007893.
89. Hoorn EJ, Walsh SB, McCormick JA, et al. Pathogenesis of calcineurin inhibitor-induced hypertension. *Am J Nephrol* 2012; 25(3): 269–275.
90. Curtis JJ, Luke RG, Jones P, et al. Hypertension in cyclosporine-treated renal transplant recipients is sodium dependent. *Am J Med* 1988; 85(2): 134–138.
91. Porter GA, Bennett WM, Sheps SG. Cyclosporine-associated hypertension. National High Blood Pressure Education Program. *Arch Intern Med* 1990; 150(2): 280–283.
92. Barton CH, Vaziri ND, Mina-Araghi S, et al. Effects of cyclosporine on magnesium metabolism in rats. *J Lab Clin Med* 1989; 114(3): 232–236.
93. Nozue T, Kodama T, Kobayashi A. Improved method for the determination of the magnesium concentration of mononuclear blood cells. *Clin Chim Acta* 1991; 203(2–3): 411–412.
94. Palestine AG, Austin HA, 3rd, Nussenblatt RB. Renal tubular function in cyclosporine-treated patients. *Am J Med* 1986; 81(3): 419–424.
95. Barton CH, Vaziri ND, Martin DC, et al. Hypomagnesemia and renal magnesium wasting in renal transplant recipients receiving cyclosporine. *Am J Med* 1987; 83(4): 693–699.
96. June CH, Thompson CB, Kennedy MS, et al. Profound hypomagnesemia and renal magnesium wasting associated with the use of cyclosporine for marrow transplantation. *Transplantation* 1985; 39(6): 620–624.
97. Feutren G, Mihatsch MJ. Risk factors for cyclosporine-induced nephropathy in patients with autoimmune diseases. *N Engl J Med* 1992; 326: 1654–1660.
98. Powles AV, Carmichael D, Hulme B, et al. Renal function after long-term low-dose cyclosporine for psoriasis. *Br J Dermatol* 1990; 122: 665–669.
99. Gilbert SC, Emmett M, Menter A, et al. Cyclosporine therapy for psoriasis: serum creatinine measurements are an unreliable predictor of decreased renal function. *J Am Acad Dermatol* 1989; 21: 470–474.
100. Messana JM, Rocher LL, Ellis CN, et al. Effects of cyclosporine on renal function in psoriasis patients. *J Am Acad Dermatol* 1990; 23: 1288–1293.
101. Feutren G, Laburte C, Krupp P. Safety and tolerability of cyclosporine A in psoriasis. In: Wolff K, ed. *Cyclosporine A and The Skin, International Congress and Symposium Series No. 192*. London: Royal Society of Medicine Services; 1992, pp. 3–12.
102. Feutren G, Abeywickrama K, Friend D, et al. Renal function and blood pressure in psoriatic patients treated with cyclosporine A. *Br J Dermatol* 1990; 122 (Suppl 36): 57–69.
103. Mason J. Renal side effects of cyclosporine A. *Br J Dermatol* 1990; 122 (Suppl 36): 71–77.
104. Mason J, Moore LC. Indirect assessment of renal dysfunction in patients taking cyclosporine A for autoimmune diseases. *Br J Dermatol* 1990; 122 (Suppl 36): 79–84.
105. Mihatsch MJ, Thiel G, Ryffel B. Renal side-effects of cyclosporine A with special reference to autoimmune diseases. *Br J Dermatol* 1990; 122 (Suppl 36): 101–115.
106. Mihatsch MJ, Wolff K. Consensus conference on cyclosporine A for psoriasis, February 1992. *Br J Dermatol* 1992; 126: 621–623.
107. Stool TJ, Korstanje MJ, Bilo HJ, et al. Does fish oil protect renal function in cyclosporine-treated psoriasis patients? *J Intern Med* 1989; 226(6): 437–441.
108. Raman G, Feehally J, Coates R, et al. Renal effects of amlodipine in normotensive renal transplant recipients. *Nephrol Dial Transplant* 1999; 14: 384–388.
109. Raman GV, Campbell SK, Farrer A, et al. Modifying effects of amlodipine on cyclosporine A-induced changes in renal function in patients with psoriasis. *J Hypertens Suppl* 1998; 16: S39–S41.

110. Zachariae H, Hansen HE, Kragballe K, et al. Morphologic renal changes during cyclosporine treatment of psoriasis. *J Am Acad Dermatol* 1992; 26: 415–419.
111. Koo JYM, Lee CS, Maloney JE. Cyclosporine and related drugs. In: Wolverton SE, ed. *Comprehensive Dermatologic Drug Therapy*. Philadelphia, PA: WB Saunders; 2001, pp. 205–229.
112. Behnam SM, Behnam SE, Koo JY. Review of cyclosporine immunosuppressive safety data in dermatology patients after two decades of use. *J Drugs Dermatol* 2005; 4(2): 189–194.
113. Vakeva L, Reitamo S, Pukkala E, et al. Long-term follow-up of cancer risk in patients treated with short-term cyclosporine. *Acta Derm Venereol Suppl* 2008; 88(2): 117–120.
114. Paul CF, Ho VC, McGeown C, et al. Risk of malignancies in psoriasis patients treated with cyclosporine: a 5 yr cohort study. *J Invest Dermatol* 2003; 120(2): 211–216.
115. Lain EL, Markus RF. Early and explosive development of nodular basal cell carcinoma and multiple keratoacanthomas in psoriasis patients treated with cyclosporine (case reports). *J Drugs Dermatol* 2004; 3: 680–682.
116. Marcil I, Stern RS. Squamous-cell cancer of the skin in patients given PUVA and cyclosporine: nested cohort crossover study. *Lancet* 2001; 358: 1042–1045.
117. Kirby B, Owen CM, Blewitt RW, et al. Cutaneous T-cell lymphoma developing in a patient on cyclosporine therapy. *J Am Acad Dermatol* 2002; 47: S165–S167.
118. Zackheim HS, Koo J, LeBoit PE, et al. Psoriasiform mycosis fungoides with fatal outcome after treatment with cyclosporine. *J Am Acad Dermatol* 2002; 47: 155–157.
119. Gupta AK, Cooper KD, Ellis CN, et al. Lymphocytic infiltrates of the skin in association with cyclosporine therapy. *J Am Acad Dermatol* 1990; 23: 1137–1141.
120. Bellisai F, Giannitti C, Donvito A, et al. Combination therapy with cyclosporine A and anti-TNF-alpha agents in the treatment of rheumatoid arthritis and concomitant hepatitis C virus infection. *Clin Rheumatol* 2007; 26(7): 1127–1129.
121. Imafuku S, Tashiro A, Furue M. Cyclosporine treatment of psoriasis in a patient with chronic hepatitis C. *Br J Dermatol* 2007; 156(6): 1367–1369.
122. Creemers P, Pascoe MD, Pontin AR, et al. Rebound effect of the allogenic T-cell response to donor and third-party lymphocytes after cyclosporine withdrawal in renal transplant recipients. *Transpl Immunol* 1998; 6(4): 261–264.
123. Mockli G, Kabra PM, Kurtz TW. Laboratory monitoring of cyclosporine levels: guidelines for the dermatologist. *J Am Acad Dermatol* 1990; 23: 1275–1279.
124. Feutren G, Friend D, Timonen P, et al. Predictive value of cyclosporine A level for efficacy or renal dysfunction in psoriasis. *Br J Dermatol* 1990; 122 (Suppl 36): 85–93.
125. Ieiri I, Nakayama J, Murakami H, et al. Evaluation of the therapeutic range of whole blood cyclosporine concentration in the treatment of psoriasis. *Int J Clin Pharmacol Ther* 1996; 34: 106–111.
126. Kokelj F, Torsello P, Plozzer C. Calcipotriol improves the efficacy of cyclosporine in the treatment of psoriasis vulgaris. *J Eur Acad Dermatol Venereol* 1998; 10: 143–146.
127. Gottlieb SL, Heftler NS, Gilleaudeau P, et al. Short-contact anthralin treatment augments therapeutic efficacy of cyclosporine in psoriasis: a clinical and pathologic study. *J Am Acad Dermatol* 1995; 33: 637–645.
128. Bagot M, Grossman R, Pamphile R, et al. Additive effects of calcipotriol and cyclosporine A: from *in vitro* experiments to *in vivo* applications in the treatment of severe psoriasis. *C R Acad Sci III* 1994; 317: 282–286.
129. Vena GA, Galluccio A, Pezza M, et al. Combined treatment with low-dose cyclosporine and calcipotriol/betamethasone dipropionate ointment for moderate-to-severe plaque psoriasis: a randomized controlled open-label study. *J Dermatol Treat* 2012; 23(4): 255–260.
130. Grossman RM, Thivolet J, Claudy A, et al. A novel therapeutic approach to psoriasis with combination calcipotriol ointment and very low-dose cyclosporine: results of a multicenter placebo-controlled study. *J Am Acad Dermatol* 1994; 31: 68–74.
131. Ameen M, Smith HR, Barker JN. Combined mycophenolate mofetil and cyclosporine therapy for severe recalcitrant psoriasis. *Clin Exp Dermatol* 2001; 26: 480–483.
132. Clark CM, Kirby B, Morris AD, et al. Combination treatment with methotrexate and cyclosporine for severe recalcitrant psoriasis. *Br J Dermatol* 1999; 141: 279–282.
133. Lee EJ, Shin MK, Kim NI. A clinical trial of combination therapy with etanercept and low dose cyclosporine for the treatment of refractory psoriasis. *Ann Dermatol* 2010; 22(2): 138–142.
134. Mahe E, Descamps V, Grossin M, et al. CD30+ T-cell lymphoma in a patient with psoriasis treated with cyclosporine and infliximab. *Br J Dermatol* 2003; 149(1): 170–173.

135. Petzelbauer P, Honigsmann H, Langer K, et al. Cyclosporine A in combination with photochemotherapy (PUVA) in the treatment of psoriasis. *Br J Dermatol* 1990; 123: 641–647.
136. Korstanje MJ, van de Staak WJ. Combination-therapy cyclosporine-A—etretinate for psoriasis. *Clin Exp Dermatol* 1990; 15: 172–173.
137. Ellis CN, Voorhees JJ. Etretinate therapy. *J Am Acad Dermatol* 1987; 16: 267–291.
138. Halioua B, Saurat JH. Risk: benefit ratio in the treatment of psoriasis with systemic retinoids. *Br J Dermatol* 1990; 122 (Suppl 36): 135–150.
139. Gottlieb AB, Griffiths CE, Ho VC, et al. Oral pimecrolimus in the treatment of moderate to severe chronic plaque-type psoriasis: a double-blind, multicentre, randomized, dose-finding trial. *Br J Dermatol* 2005; 152(6): 1219–1227.
140. Papp K, Bissonnette R, Rosoph L, et al. Efficacy of ISA247 in plaque psoriasis: a randomised, multicentre, double-blind, placebo-controlled phase III study. *Lancet* 2008; 371(9621): 1337–1342.
141. Bissonette R, Papp K, Poulin Y, et al. A randomized, multicenter, double-blind, placebo-controlled phase 2 trial of ISA247 in patients with chronic plaque psoriasis. *J Am Acad Dermatol* 2006; 54(3): 472–478.
142. Jegasothy BV, Ackerman CD, Todo S, et al. Tacrolimus (FK 506)—a new therapeutic agent for severe recalcitrant psoriasis. *Arch Dermatol* 1992; 128: 781–785.
143. The European FK 506 Multicentre Psoriasis Study Group. Systemic tacrolimus (FK 506) is effective for the treatment of psoriasis in a double-blind, placebo-controlled study. *Arch Dermatol* 1996; 132: 419–423.

Chapter 11

Etanercept

Shannon Famenini, Eric Y. Sako,
Daniel C. Butler, and Jashin J. Wu

INTRODUCTION

The use of tumor necrosis factor (TNF) antagonists has significantly enhanced the treatment of moderate to severe psoriasis. Among these, etanercept (Enbrel®) was the first to receive approval from U.S. Food and Drug Administration (FDA) for the treatment of plaque psoriasis in 2004. Etanercept is a combination of two human TNF receptors bound to the Fc portion of an IgG1, the region that interacts with cell surface receptors to activate the complement system. This medication is administered subcutaneously and has shown good clinical outcomes for psoriasis and psoriatic arthritis (PsA). In this chapter, we will review the structure, pharmacokinetics, side effects, efficacy, and the recommended treatment regimens of etanercept.

MECHANISM OF ACTION

TNF-α (TNF-α) binds two different receptors, TNFR-1 and TNFR-2, which initiates a cascade of cellular signaling resulting in the production and release of cytokines that serve to recruit other inflammatory cells. Binding of TNF on vascular endothelial cells increases leukocyte adhesion and trans-endothelial migration [1,2]. An upregulation of TNFR-1 and TNFR-2 is found in dermal blood vessels of psoriatic lesions [3]. Serum of psoriatic patients also showed increased levels of TNF-α.

Etanercept is a fully humanized, soluble, recombinant fusion protein that exerts its effect by competitively binding to TNF, thereby preventing it from interacting with its natural receptors and precluding its inflammatory cascade (Figure 11.1). It was developed using the linked sequence of DNA coding for the TNF receptor and Fc portion of IgG. Furthermore, etanercept is able to bind to TNF with an affinity 50–1000 times higher than its natural receptors [5–7].

CHEMISTRY AND PHARMACOKINETICS

Etanercept is supplied in 50 mg and 25 mg prefilled syringes, the 50 mg Sureclick® autoinjector, and 25 mg powder formulations. Adult dosing for psoriasis is 50 mg twice weekly for three months followed by 50 mg/week. The recommended treatment regimen for patients with PsA is two 25 mg injections weekly given at separate locations [8]. Etanercept has a mean half-life of approximately 4.3 days. Etanercept is slowly absorbed from the site of injection and reaches its peak concentration at approximately 51 ± 14 hours with a mean absolute bioavailability of 58%. Patients with increased body weight have decreased drug levels due to a larger volume of distribution. Clearance is not affected by renal, hepatic, or cardiac function [9,10]. Although there are numerous drug–drug interactions with traditional systemic agents such as

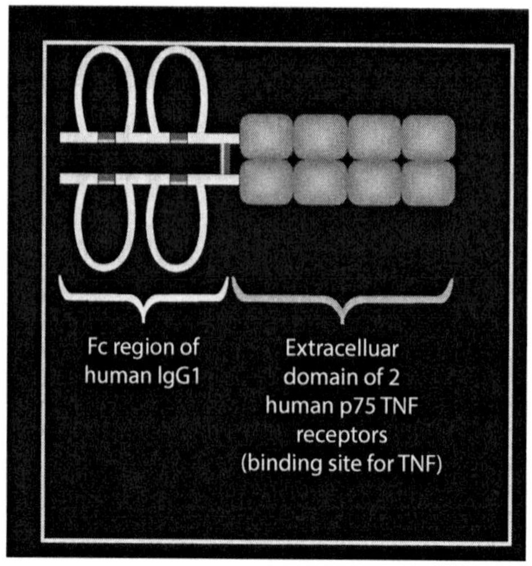

FIGURE 11.1 (See color insert.) Structure of etanercept.

cyclosporine and methotrexate, there is little concern with biologic medications; no significant interactions have been reported as yet, beyond anecdotal case reports.

No formal study has evaluated the use of etanercept during lactation. However, a case report of a lactating mother using etanercept twice weekly for rheumatoid arthritis revealed a small amount of excretion of etanercept in breast milk [11]. Although the amount transferred would more likely not be sufficient to reach significant concentrations, dermatologists and mothers should decide whether to continue lactation or discontinue etanercept therapy.

MONOTHERAPY

Plaque Psoriasis

In a 24-week, multi center phase III trial, etanercept was shown to induce clinically significant improvement in patients with chronic plaque psoriasis [12]. In this study, 583 subjects were randomized to receive 50 mg etanercept biweekly (BIW), 25 mg etanercept biweekly, or placebo for 12 weeks. After 12 weeks, all patients received etanercept 25 mg biweekly. At week 12, Psoriasis Area and Severity Index (PASI) 75 (improvement of at least 75% in the PASI score compared to baseline) was achieved by 49%, 34%, and 3% of the groups, respectively ($p < .0001$). At week 24, PASI 75 was attained by 54% of the patients originally in the 50 mg BIW group, by 45% of the patients originally in the 25 mg BIW group, and by 28% of patients originally in the placebo group (who received etanercept 25 mg twice weekly starting in week 12). Results at weeks 12 and 14 were similar to those in other phase III trials in psoriasis [13].

Another phase III, randomized, open-label extension study demonstrated the efficacy and safety of long-term treatment with etanercept. Patients ($n = 618$) were randomized to placebo or 50 mg etanercept biweekly for 12 weeks after which the placebo group also received etanercept therapy [14]. At week 12, 47% of the patients treated with etanercept achieved

PASI 75 versus 5% of those receiving placebo ($p < .0001$). By week 96, about half of all patients reached PASI 75. Exposure-adjusted rates of adverse events and infections were similar between the two groups. Nonneutralizing antibodies to etanercept were observed in 18.3% of the patients but had no discernible effect on drug efficacy or safety.

Etanercept monotherapy has been used successfully in pediatric and geriatric patients [15–16]. In a pediatric study, 57% of patients treated with etanercept 0.8 mg/kg weekly achieved PASI 75 by week 12 (vs. 11% in placebo; $p < .001$) [15]. An open-label extension continued after week 12 through week 48 during which three serious adverse events were reported. One 14-year-old girl underwent surgical removal of an ovarian cyst; etanercept was discontinued. A nine-year-old girl experienced infectious episodes of gastroenteritis and dehydration that required hospitalization; etanercept was continued. A seven-year-old asthmatic patient had serious pneumonia treated with antibiotics; etanercept was discontinued. All events resolved without sequelae. No deaths, cancers, opportunistic infections, tuberculosis, or demyelinating events were found. In the geriatric population, a retrospective study reported that greater than 80% of patients remained PASI 75 responders through 156 weeks of treatment [16].

Psoriatic Arthritis

Etanercept was also approved by the FDA for the treatment of PsA in 2002. A pivotal phase III clinical trial confirmed the safety and efficacy of etanercept. Two hundred and five patients were randomized to receive either etanercept 25 mg twice weekly or placebo for 24 weeks followed by open-label etanercept administration for 48 weeks [17]. In contrast to dermatology, clinical trials in rheumatology are usually designed to allow patients to continue methotrexate during the study. Thus, patients in both treatment groups may have also been on concomitant methotrexate. After 12 weeks, 59% of patients being treated with etanercept had achieved the American College of Rheumatology 20% improvement criteria (ACR20) compared to 15% of placebo patients ($p < .0001$). These results were maintained through weeks 24 and 48. Radiographic disease progression was also halted in the etanercept group. The mean annual rate of change in the modified total Sharp score was −0.03 units in the etanercept group as compared to 1.00 in the placebo group ($p = .0001$). In another open-label study ($n = 141$), the modified total Sharps score (higher number indicates more joint destruction) was −0.38 in patients being treated with etanercept after two years as compared to −0.22 in patients receiving placebo [18]. Thus, etanercept was shown to be well-tolerated, to have improved rheumatologic symptoms, to have reduced psoriatic lesions, and to have inhibited radiographic joint deterioration.

The majority of patients with PsA first present with skin lesions. Thus, when treating patients with psoriasis, dermatologists must be cognizant of the potential coexistence of PsA [19]. Referral to a rheumatologist for further evaluation is indicated in any psoriasis patients who complain of joint pains or prolonged morning stiffness.

In comparison to the other TNF-inhibitors, etanercept is less efficacious for psoriatic skin disease. However, the same appears not to be true for PsA; TNF-α agents may have similar efficacy in treating PsA [20].

COMBINATION THERAPY

Biologics may be used in combination with other agents including topical steroids, methotrexate, and phototherapy to enhance improvement in patients who are not well controlled with biologics alone.

Etanercept and Methotrexate

In patients where monotherapy is insufficient in disease management, combination treatment with methotrexate can be helpful [21–22]. In one study, patients with severe psoriasis who had not responded to methotrexate monotherapy were randomized to receive either concomitant etanercept or etanercept monotherapy. A physician global assessment (PGA) of "clear" or "almost clear" was achieved by 66.7% of patients in the combination therapy group as compared to 37.0% in the monotherapy group ($p = 0.025$). Adverse events were similar in both groups. Furthermore, the addition of methotrexate to etanercept treatment may allow for a reduction in dosing of etanercept with continued improvements in PASI [23].

Etanercept and Acitretin

Few studies have investigated the efficacy of acitretin in combination with etanercept. However, one potential benefit is the protective effects of acitretin against skin cancer. There is a theoretical concern that etanercept and other biologics may increase the risk of skin cancer. Therefore, use of concomitant acitretin may help to decrease this risk [24,25]. A randomized, controlled, double-blind study demonstrated the efficacy and safety of combination treatment with etanercept and acitretin [26]. Sixty patients were randomized to one of three treatment regimens: etanercept 25 mg twice weekly, oral acitretin 0.4 mg/kg daily, or etanercept 25 mg once weekly plus acitretin 0.4 mg/kg. After 24 weeks, PASI 75 was reached by 45% of the etanercept group, 30% of the acitretin group, and 44% of the combination group. Etanercept treatment either in combination with acitretin or alone was superior to acitretin monotherapy ($p = 0.001$). Administering etanercept plus acitretin once weekly is as effective as administering etanercept twice weekly. Thus, the addition of acitretin allows for a reduction in etanercept dose. Larger studies, however, are needed to confirm these results.

A retrospective review and case series have shown the safety and efficacy of etanercept combined with acitretin [27,28].

Etanercept and Narrowband Ultraviolet Light B

A single arm, open-label study examined the efficacy of etanercept 50 mg twice weekly combined with narrowband ultraviolet light B (NBUVB) three times/week [29]. After 12 weeks, 85% of patients achieved PASI 75. Although not designed as a head-to-head comparison, this appears more effective than etanercept monotherapy in the pivotal phase III clinical trial, where 49% of patients achieved PASI 75 at week 12 [12].

In another single arm, open-label study, the administration of etanercept in combination with NBUVB was shown to be an effective treatment regimen. Thirty-three patients were administered etanercept 50 mg once weekly in addition to NBUVB phototherapy three times weekly for eight weeks, followed by etanercept monotherapy until week 12. By week 8, two-thirds of the patients achieved PASI 75 [30]. However, this study was limited by small sample size, absence of an NBUVB monotherapy control, and a short follow-up period. The addition of NBUVB to etanercept also resulted in reduced epidermal immunoreactivity shown by decreased CD1a, CD4, and CD8 in lesions treated with combinational therapy versus lesions treated with etanercept only [31]. In 2012, the first randomized trial evaluated the efficacy of adding NBUVB for patients in whom etanercept monotherapy had failed to produce an adequate response [32]. Patients who did not achieve PASI 90 after 12 weeks of etanercept monotherapy were randomized to continue on etanercept monotherapy or receive additional NBUVB three times weekly. At week 24, PASI 90 was achieved in 16.2% of patients under combinational therapy as compared to 15.8% of patients under monotherapy ($p = 1.0$). Only 21.6% of the patients, however, had completed an adherence of at least 80% to NBUVB treatments. Among patients with high adherence, 42.9% in the combination group had attained PASI 90 as compared to 3.4% in the monotherapy group. The addition of NBUVB may thus be beneficial in patients that are recalcitrant to monotherapy. However, this adherence to the frequent phototherapy regimen is important in achieving therapeutic results. The treatment of psoriasis is especially challenging in obese patients given the reduced efficacy of etanercept with increased body weight. The addition of NBUVB, however, has not been shown to lead to an enhancement in achieving PASI 75 in this patient population [33].

TOXICITIES AND ADVERSE REACTIONS

Numerous clinical trials have evaluated the safety of etanercept in psoriasis, rheumatoid arthritis, and PsA. The most common side effect of etanercept administration is injection site reaction, which is generally mild and does not require treatment [34]. Patients can be counseled on rotation of injection sites to avoid this problem. There is also concern for increased incidence of upper respiratory tract infection. A series of connected trials in 108 patients with moderate to severe psoriasis evaluated the long-term safety of etanercept for up to 48 months [35]. The occurrence of adverse events and serious adverse events was not shown to increase with cumulative exposure. Nasopharyngitis and upper respiratory tract infections had the greatest rate of occurrence [35].

A five-year observational safety registry of etanercept, which enrolled 2511 patients, concluded that the occurrence of serious infections, nonmelanoma skin cancer (NMSC), malignancies not including NMSC, and lymphomas among patients treated with etanercept was not increased as compared to that of the general population [36]. The limitations of the study, however, were that there was no control group, and the study number was too small to detect rare events. An open-label study performed in pediatric patients receiving etanercept over 96 weeks determined this therapy to be safe, with the most frequent side effects being nasopharyngitis, upper respiratory infections, and streptococcal pharyngitis [37].

Cases of hepatitis B reactivation following etanercept therapy in chronic hepatitis B carriers have been reported [38]. All patients should be screened for hepatitis prior to starting etanercept. A patient who is determined to be a carrier of hepatitis B virus should then be referred to a hepatologist for evaluation [39]. Conversely, there have been no reported cases of hepatitis C exacerbation in patients on etanercept [40]. Thus, etanercept offers a safe option in treating psoriasis in patients with a history of hepatitis C.

PREGNANCY

Data on the use of etanercept during pregnancy are limited. Etanercept and other anti-TNF drugs are considered category B, and no evidence of teratogenicity or pregnancy loss have been illustrated [41,42]. According to the National Psoriasis Foundation, biologics are likely safe but must be used with caution in pregnant women.

FOLLOW-UP

A baseline and annual purified protein derivative (PPD) or γ-interferon must be obtained. If a baseline tuberculosis (TB) test is positive, treatment for latent TB infection should be started prior to starting etanercept treatment. However, the time to initiation of etanercept therapy in the setting of a latent TB infection is not completely clear. In the opinion of some dermatologists, etanercept treatment may be initiated after one to two months of prophylaxis. The Centers for Disease Control (CDC), however, advises completing the full course of TB prophylaxis prior to etanercept administration [43]. A baseline complete blood count and liver function tests are also advised. Given the possibility for reactivation of latent hepatitis B, screening for hepatitis B is also advised. Periodic history and physical exams should be performed in the appropriate clinical setting [44–46].

REFERENCES

1. Bradley JR. TNF-mediated inflammatory disease. *J Pathol* 2008;214(2):149–60.
2. Krueger JG. The immunologic basis for the treatment of psoriasis with new biologic agents. *J Am Acad Dermatol* 2002;46(1):1–23; quiz 23–6.
3. Kristensen M, Chu CQ, Eedy DJ, et al. Localization of tumour necrosis factor-alpha (TNFα) and its receptors in normal and psoriatic skin: epidermal cells express the 55 kDa but not the 75 kDa TNF receptor. *Clin J Am Acad Dermatol* 2002;46(1):1–23; quiz 23–6.
4. Ettehadi P, Greaves MW, Wallach D, et al. Elevated tumour necrosis factor-alpha (TNFα) biological activity in psoriatic skin lesions. *Clin Exp Immunol* 1994;96(1):146–51.
5. Mohler KM, Torrance DS, Smith CA, et al. Soluble tumor necrosis factor (TNF) receptors are effective therapeutic agents in lethal endotoxemia and function simultaneously as both TNF carriers and TNF antagonists. *J Immunol* 1993;151(3):1548–61.
6. Keystone EC. Safety of biologic therapies—an update. *J Rheumatol Suppl* 2005;74:8–12.
7. Spahn TW, Eugster HP, Fontana A, et al. Role of lymphotoxin in experimental models of infectious diseases: potential benefits and risks of a therapeutic inhibition of the lymphotoxin-beta receptor pathway. *Infect Immun* 2005;73(11):7077–88.
8. Zhou H. Clinical pharmacokinetics of etanercept: a fully humanized soluble recombinant tumor necrosis factor receptor fusion protein. *J Clin Pharmacol* 2005;45(5):490–7.
9. Don BR, Spin G, Nestorov I, et al. The pharmaco kinetics of etanercept in patients with end-stage renal disease on haemodialysis. *J Pharm Pharmacol* 2005;57(11):1407–13.
10. Soran O, Feldman A, Schneider V, et al. The pharmacokinetics of etanercept in patients with heart failure. *Br J Clin Pharmacol* 2001;51:191–3.
11. Ostensen M, Eigenmann GO. Etanercept in breast milk. *J Rheumatol* 2004;31:1017.
12. Papp KA, Tyring S, Lahfa M, et al. A global phase III randomized controlled trial of etanercept in psoriasis: safety, efficacy, and effect of dose reduction. *Br J Dermatol* 2005;152(6):1304–12.
13. Leonardi CL, Powers JL, MathesonRT, et al. Etanercept as monotherapy in patients with psoriasis. *N Engl J Med* 2003;349(21):2014–22.

14. Tyring S, Gordon KB, Poulin Y, et al. Long-term safety and efficacy of 50 mg of etanercept twice weekly in patients with psoriasis. *Arch Dermatol* 2007;143(6):719–26.
15. Paller AS, Siegfried EC, Langley RG, et al. Etanercept treatment for children and adolescents with plaque psoriasis. *N Engl J Med* 2008;358(3):241–51.
16. Esposito M, Giunta A, Mazzotta A, et al. Efficacy and safety of subcutaneous anti-tumor necrosis factor-alpha agents, etanercept and adalimumab, in elderly patients affected by psoriasis and psoriatic arthritis: an observational long-term study. *Dermatology* 2012;225(4):312–19.
17. Mease PJ, Kivitz AJ, Burch FX, et al. Etanercept treatment of psoriatic arthritis: safety, efficacy, and effect on disease progression. *Arthritis Rheum* 2004;50(7):2264–72.
18. Klareskog LM, Cohen SB, Kalden JR, et al. Safety and efficacy of over 10 years of continuous etanercept therapy in patients with rheumatoid arthritis in North America and Europe. Presented at the European League Against Rheumatism (EULAR) 2008: Paris, France, 11–14 June 2008.
19. Gottlieb AB, Leonardi CL, Goffe BS, et al. Etanercept monotherapy in patients with psoriasis: a summary of safety, based on an integrated multistudy database. *J Am Acad Dermatol* 2006;54(3 Suppl 2):S92–100.
20. Migliore A, Bizzi E, Broccoli S, et al. Indirect comparison of etanercept, infliximab, and adalimumab for psoriatic arthritis: mixed treatment comparison using placebo as common comparator. *Clin Rheumatol* 2012;31(1):133–7.
21. Driessen RJ, van de Kerkhof PC, de Jong EM. Etanercept combined with methotrexate for high-need psoriasis. *Br J Dermatol* 2008;159(2):460–3.
22. Zachariae C, Mørk NJ, Reunala T, et al. The combination of etanercept and methotrexate increases the effectiveness of treatment in active psoriasis despite inadequate effect of methotrexate therapy. *Acta Derm Venereol* 2008;88(5):495–501.
23. Gottlieb AB, Langley RG, Strober BE, et al. A randomized, double-blind, placebo-controlled study to evaluate the addition of methotrexate to etanercept in patients with moderate to severe plaque psoriasis. *Br J Dermatol* 2012;167(3):649–57.
24. McKenna DB, Murphy GM. Skin cancer chemoprophylaxis in renal transplant recipients: 5 years of experience using low-dose acitretin. *Br J Dermatol* 1999;140(4):656–60.
25. Gottlieb AB, Gordon KB, Giannini EH, et al. Malignancies from patients receiving etanercept across indications. [abstract] *Ann Rheum Dis* 2008;67(Suppl II):322.
26. Gisondi P, Del Giglio M, Cotena C, et al. Combining etanercept and acitretin in the therapy of chronic plaque psoriasis: a 24-week, randomized, controlled, investigator-blinded pilot trial. *Br J Dermatol* 2008;158(6):1345–9.
27. Smith EC, Riddle C, Menter MA, et al. Combining systemic retinoids with biologic agents for moderate to severe psoriasis. *Int J Dermatol* 2008;47(5):514–18.
28. Conley J, Nanton J, Dhawan S, et al. Novel combination regimens: biologics and acitretin for the treatment of psoriasis—a case series. *J Dermatol Treat* 2006;17:86–9.
29. Kircik L, Bagel J, Korman N, et al. Utilization of narrow band ultraviolet light B therapy and etanercept for the treatment of psoriasis (UNITE): efficacy, safety, and patient-reported outcomes. *J Drugs Dermatol* 2008;7(3):245–53.
30. De Simone C, D'Agostino M, Capizzi R, et al. Combined treatment with etanercept 50 mg once weekly and narrow-band ultraviolet B phototherapy in chronic plaque psoriasis. *Eur J Dermatol* 2011;21(4):568–72.
31. Gambichler T, Tigges C, Scola N, et al. Etanercept plus narrowband ultraviolet B phototherapy of psoriasis is more effective than etanercept monotherapy at 6 weeks. *Br J Dermatol* 2011;164(6):1383–6.
32. Lynde CW, Gupta AK, Guenther L, et al. A randomized study comparing the combination of nbUVB and etanercept to etanercept monotherapy in patients with psoriasis who do not exhibit an excellent response after 12 weeks of etanercept. *J Dermatol Treat* 2012;23(4):261–7.
33. Park KK, Wu JJ, Koo J. A randomized, "head-to-head" pilot study comparing the effects of etanercept monotherapy vs. etanercept and narrowband ultraviolet B (NB-UVB) phototherapy in obese psoriasis patients. *J Eur Acad Dermatol Venereol* 2013;27(7):899–906.
34. Kerensky TA, Gottlieb AB, Yaniv S, et al. Etanercept: efficacy and safety for approved indications. *Expert Opin Drug Saf* 2012;11(1):121–39.
35. Papp KA, Poulin Y, Bissonnette R, et al. Assessment of the long-term safety and effectiveness of etanercept for the treatment of psoriasis in an adult population. *J Am Acad Dermatol* 2012;66:e33–45.

36. Kimball AB, Pariser D, Yamauchi PS, et al. OBSERVE-5 interim analysis: an observational postmarketing safety registry of etanercept for the treatment of psoriasis. *J Am Acad Dermatol* 2013;68(5):756–64.
37. Paller AS, Siegfried EC, Eichenfield LF, et al. Long-term etanercept in pediatric patients with plaque psoriasis. *J Am Acad Dermatol* 2010;63:762–8.
38. Montiel PM, Solis JA, Chirinos JA, et al. Hepatitis B virus reactivation during therapy with etanercept in an HBsAg-negative and anti-HBs-positive patient. *Liver Int* 2008;28(5):718–20.
39. Abramson A, Menter A, Perrillo R. Psoriasis, hepatitis B, and the tumor necrosis factor-alpha inhibitory agents: a review and recommendations for management. *J Am Acad Dermatol* 2012;67(6):1349–61.
40. Prignano F, Ricceri F, Pescitelli L, Zanieri F, Lotti T. Tumour necrosis factor-alpha antagonists in patients with concurrent psoriasis and hepatitis B or hepatitis C: a retrospective analysis of 17 patients. *Br J Dermatol* 2011;164(3):645–7.
41. Roux CH, Brocq O, Breuil V, et al. Pregnancy in rheumatology patients exposed to anti-tumour necrosis factor (TNF)-alpha therapy. *Rheumatology (Oxford)* 2007;46(4):695–8.
42. Hyrich KL, Symmons DP, Watson KD, et al. Pregnancy outcome in women who were exposed to anti-tumor necrosis factor agents: results from a national population register. *Arthritis Rheum* 2006;54(8):2701–2.
43. Balato N, Costanzo LD, Ayala F, et al. Psoriatic disease and tuberculosis nowadays. *Clin Dev Immunol* 2012;2012:747204.
44. Hsu S, Papp KA, Lebwohl MG, et al. Consensus guidelines for the management of plaque psoriasis. *Arch Dermatol* 2012;148(1):95–102.
45. Menter A, Gottlieb A, Feldman SR, et al. Guidelines of care for the management of psoriasis and psoriatic arthritis: section 1. Overview of psoriasis and guidelines of care for the treatment of psoriasis with biologics. *J Am Acad Dermatol* 2008;58(5):826–50.
46. Doherty SD, VanVoorhees A, Lebwohl MG, et al. National Psoriasis Foundation consensus statement on screening for latent tuberculosis infection in patients with psoriasis treated with systemic and biologic agents. *J Am Acad Dermatol* 2008;59(2):209–17.

Chapter 12

Adalimumab

Maya G. Debbaneh and John Y. M. Koo

INTRODUCTION

Adalimumab (Humira®) [1] is the most widely used biologic agent for moderate to severe plaque psoriasis. It was the third tumor necrosis factor-α (TNF-α) inhibitor and first fully human monoclonal antibody to be approved by the U.S. Food and Drug Administration (FDA).

Adalimumab currently has seven FDA-approved indications. These include (in order of the oldest to the most recently approved): rheumatoid arthritis (2002), psoriatic arthritis, ankylosing spondylitis, Crohn's disease, juvenile idiopathic arthritis, psoriasis (2008), and ulcerative colitis.

Adalimumab is an immunoglobulin (Ig) G1, human monoclonal antibody with a half-life of 12–14 days [2]. This agent acts by binding to the inflammatory cytokine TNF-α and preventing its interaction with p55 and p75 cell surface TNF receptors. TNF-α is a cytokine mediator involved in normal inflammatory responses. Elevated levels of TNF-α are found in psoriatic plaques as well as in the synovial fluid of patients with rheumatoid arthritis, psoriatic arthritis, and ankylosing spondylitis.

Adalimumab is administered as a subcutaneous injection, which the patient can self-administer with a prefilled injection pen or regular syringe [2]. The dosing regimen is not the same for all indications. In the treatment of plaque psoriasis, adalimumab is administered with an 80 mg starting dose, followed by 40 mg every other week starting one week after the initial dose. For the treatment of rheumatoid arthritis, psoriatic arthritis, and ankylosing spondylitis, adalimumab is normally administered as a 40 mg injection every other week. For Crohn's disease, treatment begins with a starting dose of 160 mg at week and 0, 80 mg at week 2, and is subsequently continued at a maintenance dose of 40 mg every other week beginning at week 4. As of 2012, more than 676,000 patients worldwide are being treated with adalimumab for the aforementioned indications [3].

EFFICACY IN PSORIASIS

Phase II

The efficacy of adalimumab in the treatment of moderate to severe psoriasis has been tested in several clinical trials. In a phase II, double-blind, placebo-controlled clinical trial, adalimumab was administered in one of two dosing regimens [4]. The trial enrolled 147 adult patients with chronic plaque psoriasis who had at least 5% body surface area involvement and who had not had prior treatment with anti-TNF-α agents. Patients were randomized 1:1:1 in the following manner: the first study arm received 80 mg of adalimumab at week 0, followed by 40 mg every other week; the second arm received 80 mg of adalimumab at weeks 0 to 1,

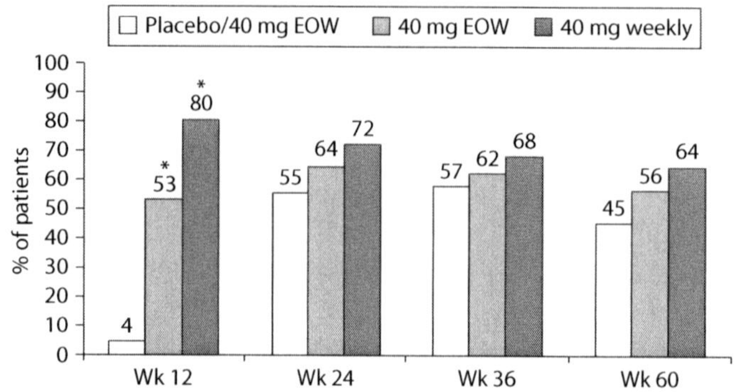

FIGURE 12.1 Percentage of patients achieving 75% improvement in the Psoriasis Aarea and Severity Index score (PASI 75) at weeks 12, 24, 36, and 60. Patients originally randomized to placebo began adalimumab treatment at week 12 (*p < 0.001 versus placebo). (Reprinted from *J Am Acad Dermatol* 55, Gordon KB et al., Clinical response to adalimumab treatment in patients with moderate to severe psoriasis: double-blind, randomized controlled trial and open-label extension study, 598–606, Copyright 2006, with permission from Elsevier.)

followed by 40 mg/ week; and the third study arm received weekly placebo. Subsequently, patients who completed this initial 12-week trial were eligible to continue in a 48-week open-label extension trial. After the initial 12 weeks of blinded therapy, patients taking adalimumab continued their same dosing regimens, and patients taking placebo were switched to 40 mg adalimumab every other week for the remaining 48 weeks. During the study, low- to mid-potency topical steroids were allowed for application to the palms, soles, groin, and face. The use of other concomitant antipsoriatic medications was prohibited.

The primary end point was percentage of patients achieving a Psoriasis Area and Severity Index (PASI) 75 response after 12 weeks of treatment [4] (Figure 12.1). Greater percentages of patients in the adalimumab treatment arms achieved PASI 75 responses as compared to placebo. Generally, patients in the adalimumab treatment arms who continued treatment throughout week 60 had a sustained response to treatment over time (Figure 12.1). Differences in PASI 75 responses and PGA scores between the two adalimumab dosing arms were not statistically significant at any time point. Thus, in subsequent phase III studies, only every other week dosing was tested.

Phase III

The randomized controlled evaluation of adalimumab dosing every other week in a moderate to severe psoriasis trial (REVEAL) was a phase III study designed to evaluate the efficacy and safety of adalimumab in the treatment of moderate to severe psoriasis [5]. This multiphase, 52-week, randomized, double-blind, placebo-controlled trial was divided into three treatment periods. Patients included in the study had moderate to severe plaque psoriasis with greater than or equal to 10% body surface area affected and a PASI of greater than or equal to 12. Patients previously taking systemic therapies or biologic medications (not including TNF antagonists) were eligible, with washout periods of 4 weeks for nonbiologic systemic therapies, 6 weeks for efalizumab, and 12 weeks for other biologic medications. The only concomitant medications allowed were low and midpotency topical steroids for the face, palms, soles, and intertriginous areas.

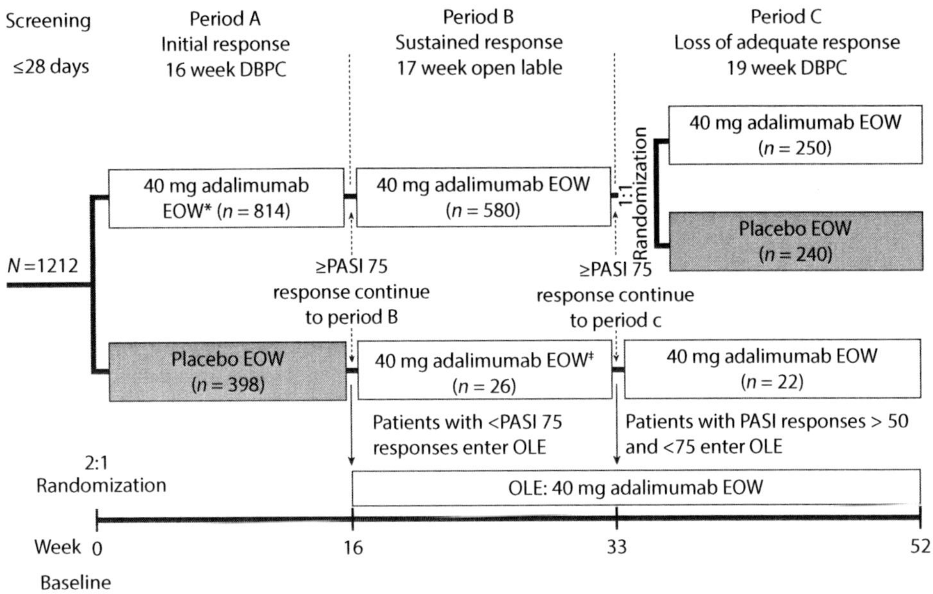

FIGURE 12.2 REVEAL study design describing periods A, B, and C. Period A evaluated initial response to treatment with adalimumab. Period B evaluated the sustained response to adalimumab. Period C evaluated loss of adequate response with adalimumab therapy. DBPC, double-blind, placebo-controlled; EOW, every other week; OLE, open-label extension; PASI 75, 75% improvement in psoriasis area and severity index. *After 80 mg at week 0 and 40 mg at week 1. ‡After 80 mg at week 16 and 40 mg at week 17. (Reprinted from *J Am Acad Dermatol* 58, Menter A et al., Adalimumab therapy for moderate to severe psoriasis: a randomized, controlled phase III trial, 106–115, Copyright 2008, with permission from Elsevier.)

Period A tested the initial response to treatment with adalimumab versus placebo over 16 weeks in 1212 patients (Figure 12.2) [5]. Patients were randomized 2:1 to receive 80 mg of adalimumab at week 0 followed by 40 mg dosing every other week or placebo injections. Those patients from either treatment arm of period A who achieved a PASI 75 response by week 16 continued into period B, a 17-week time period in which all patients received open-label adalimumab 40 mg every other week. Period B was designed to test the sustained efficacy of adalimumab. Those patients who did not achieve a PASI 75 response at the end of period A could enter a separate open-label extension with adalimumab treatment 40 mg every other week. Finally, patients who maintained a PASI 75 response at week 33 were eligible to continue into period C from week 33 through week 52. At week 33, patients who had achieved a PASI 75 response at both week 16 and week 33 were re-randomized 1:1, to receive either adalimumab or placebo. Period C was designed to examine duration of treatment effect and to compare the proportion of patients in each group who lost adequate response from week 33 forward. For this multiphase trial, primary end points included percentage of patients achieving PASI 75 after 16 weeks of therapy and the proportion of patients losing adequate response after week 33. Loss of adequate response was specifically defined as loss of PASI-50 *and* an increase in the PASI score by at least six points.

After 16 weeks of therapy (period A), 71% of patients in the adalimumab group had achieved a PASI 75 response as compared to 7% in the placebo group, respectively ($p < 0.001$) [5].

A significant number of patients achieved a PASI 75 response after only four weeks of adalimumab treatment; 19% of patients actively treated for one month achieved PASI 75 as compared to 1% in placebo group (with $p < 0.001$) [5]. In addition, at week 12, 68% of patients in the adalimumab group had achieved a PASI 75 response as compared to 5% in the placebo group ($p < 0.001$) [5]. Furthermore, after 16 weeks of adalimumab treatment, 45% of patients achieved PASI 90 and 20% of patients achieved PASI 100 versus 2% and 1% for placebo ($p < 0.001$) [5].

During the first 16 weeks of treatment, adalimumab was effective in patients across all weight quartiles [6]. Notably, the median patient weight in this study was 90.3 kg at baseline. In the heaviest weight quartile (weight range from 105 to 203.6 kg), 62% of patients achieved PASI 75 response by 16 weeks compared to 7% in the placebo group ($p < 0.001$). In addition, in the 50th to 75th percentile for weight (ranging from 90.3 to 105 kg), two-thirds of patients achieved a PASI 75 response compared to 4% in the placebo group ($p < 0.001$).

Of the initial 814 patients randomized to receive adalimumab in period A, 71% (578 patients) achieved a PASI 75 response at 16 weeks and continued adalimumab treatment at 40 mg every other week during period B [5]. For these patients actively treated from week 0 forward, mean improvement in PASI score from baseline was 92% at week 16 and 89% at week 33. Thus, in patients treated with adalimumab from week 0 through week 33, the mean improvement in PASI score was generally sustained throughout 33 weeks of therapy.

After 33 weeks of continuous treatment with adalimumab, patients achieving a PASI 75 response at week 16 and at week 33 were re-randomized 1:1 to receive adalimumab or placebo in order to evaluate loss of adequate response following discontinuation of active drug. Of the patients re-randomized to placebo at week 33 ($n = 240$), 28% experienced loss of adequate response by week 52 as compared to 5% of patients on continuous adalimumab therapy ($n = 250$; $p < 0.001$) [5].

Remarkably, for patients re-randomized to placebo at week 33, who received no active treatment for nearly five months, 43% maintained their PASI 75 response at week 52 [5]. In addition, 79% of patients actively treated with adalimumab throughout the 52-week trial maintained a PASI 75 response [6]. The REVEAL study not only demonstrated the rapid and marked efficacy of adalimumab in the treatment of moderate to severe psoriasis but also illustrated that patients typically experience a sustained response to adalimumab treatment over time.

In addition, an open-label extension study offered to patients from REVEAL provides additional efficacy and safety data for patients treated with adalimumab continuously over three years [7]. For the purposes of analysis, patients were divided into four groups. Group A failed to achieve PASI 75 at week 16; group B achieved PASI 75 at week 16 but lost the response by week 33 (but still maintained PASI 50); group C achieved PASI 75 at both week 16 and week 33 (also known as "sustained responders"); and group D included the patients randomized to placebo who then started adalimumab at week 16. Adalimumab was administered at 40 mg dose every other week. But if patients did not achieve PASI 50 by week 24 of the extension study, they were allowed to increase adalimumab dosing to 40 mg weekly. However, these patients were not involved in analysis for long-term efficacy.

Patients in groups A and B had relatively stable and similar long-term efficacies. Following more than three years of treatment with adalimumab, group A saw a 40% mean percentage improvement in PASI and group B saw 44% improvement. Group C also saw stable response rates over time; PASI 75/90/100 response rates after 100 and 160 weeks of adalimumab treatment were 83%/59%/33% and 76%/50%/31%, respectively.

Another study examined the effect of withdrawal of adalimumab and retreatment following relapse [8]. In this study, subjects (n = 285) had a sustained PGA of 0–2 for12 weeks (on 40 mg every other week dosing); 107 patients (37.5%) did not relapse within the 40-week nontreatment period, although 178 (62.4%) patients relapsed (defined as PGA of 3 or greater) within this time frame (median = 141 days). Therapy was reinitiated for patients either at time of relapse or at the end of the 40-week withdrawal period if no relapse was observed. After 16 weeks of retreatment with adalimumab, 83% of the group who relapsed achieved a PASI 75, although 93% of those who did not relapse achieved the same end point. This study suggests that retreatment after interruption of adalimumab is often effective, but patients may not achieve previous levels of psoriasis control.

Efficacy in Psoriatic Arthritis

The Adalimumab Effectiveness in Psoriatic Arthritis Trial (ADEPT) was a double-blind, randomized, placebo-controlled trial evaluating the efficacy and safety of adalimumab therapy in patients with psoriatic arthritis [9]. This phase III study included 315 adult patients with moderate to severe psoriatic arthritis, randomized 1:1 to receive treatment with 40 mg adalimumab every other week or placebo for 24 weeks. Notably, patients in this study did not receive the initial 80 mg dose of adalimumab, which is often administered in the treatment of plaque psoriasis in order to achieve a rapid steady state concentration of adalimumab in the serum.

Patients included had a history of inadequate response to nonsteroidal, anti-inflammatory drugs in the treatment of psoriatic arthritis [9]. Of note, the use of methotrexate was allowed during the study if it had been taken for at least three months and the dose was stable for at least one month. Approximately half of the patients (50.5%) enrolled in the study were receiving methotrexate at baseline, and patients were stratified according to methotrexate use. The primary end point was the American College of Rheumatology 20% improvement response (ACR20), which in this study was based on a count of tender and swollen joints. This response requires a patient to have a 20% reduction in the number of swollen or tender joints and requires a reduction of 20% in three of five parameters: patient pain assessment, C-reactive protein or erythrocyte sedimentation rate, degree of disability in health assessment questionnaire score, physician global assessment of disease, and patient global assessment of disease.

The ACR20 response rate after 12 weeks of treatment was 58% in the adalimumab group versus 14% in the placebo group (with $p < 0.001$) [6]. Similarly, after 24 weeks, the ACR20 response was 57% in the adalimumab group and 15% in placebo group ($p < 0.001$). Overall, patients in the adalimumab treatment arm demonstrated significantly higher response rates compared to patients in the placebo group. In addition, ACR20 response rates did not differ significantly for patients concomitantly using methotrexate compared to patients receiving adalimumab monotherapy; week 12 ACR20 response rates were 55% and 61% in the combination and monotherapy groups, respectively. When treating patients with psoriatic arthritis in clinical practice, adalimumab may be administered alone or in combination with disease-modifying antirheumatic drugs (DMARDs) such as methotrexate [2].

In the ADEPT study, a subset of 138 patients with psoriatic skin involvement more than or equal to 3% body surface area had their skin disease evaluated simultaneously [9]. After 24 weeks of treatment, the PASI 75 response was 59% in the adalimumab group compared to 1% in the placebo group ($p < 0.001$). Furthermore, at 24 weeks, 42% of patients in the adalimumab group achieved PASI 90, a 90% improvement in their skin disease, versus zero patients in the placebo group. After six months of treatment, approximately two-thirds of patients treated with adalimumab (67%) achieved a PGA rating of "clear" or "almost clear." In addition, PASI improvement was comparable between patients with moderate to severe psoriasis (PASI ≥10 at baseline) and patients with mild to moderate psoriasis (PASI <10 at baseline) (10). This study demonstrated the utility of adalimumab in psoriatic arthritis and psoriatic skin disease, and that it can be very effective for patients suffering from both ailments.

An open-label extension study (n = 285) was performed in which patients were given 40 mg adalimumab for up to 120 weeks following participation in the ADEPT trial [10]. Patients who failed to demonstrate improvement in certain parameters used to measure severity of psoriatic arthritis were allowed to increase the adalimumab dosage to 40 mg weekly. Most recently, two-year data from ADEPT and the open-label extension study showed that 58.7% of the patients achieved the ACR20 response at week 48 and 57.3% of patients at week 104.

In addition, radiographs were obtained at the ADEPT baseline and various time points throughout the study. After six months, 10% of patients treated with adalimumab had radiographic progression of disease compared to 30% of patients in the placebo group.

Adalimumab versus Methotrexate in Psoriasis

The efficacies of methotrexate and adalimumab in the treatment of moderate to severe psoriasis were compared in a head-to-head, placebo-controlled study (CHAMPION) [11]. This clinical trial was the first of its kind, a phase III study evaluating the efficacy and safety of a biologic versus a nonbiologic systemic medication. CHAMPION was a 16-week, multicenter clinical trial with 271 patients randomized 2:2:1 into three treatment arms (Figure 12.3). One treatment arm received 40 mg injections of adalimumab every other week after an initial 80 mg dose at week 0, along with methotrexate placebo. The second treatment arm received oral methotrexate weekly and placebo injections of adalimumab. In the third study arm, patients received placebo subcutaneous injections along with oral placebo. Because this treatment arm required patients to receive both oral placebo and placebo injection, this type of clinical trial is referred to as a double-blind, double-dummy, placebo-controlled study. All patients had at least 10% body surface area involvement and were naïve to TNF-antagonist therapy and methotrexate.

Regarding methotrexate dosing in the second study arm, patients received 7.5 mg/week from weeks 0–1, followed by 10 mg/week from weeks 2–3, and 15 mg/week from weeks 4–7 [11].

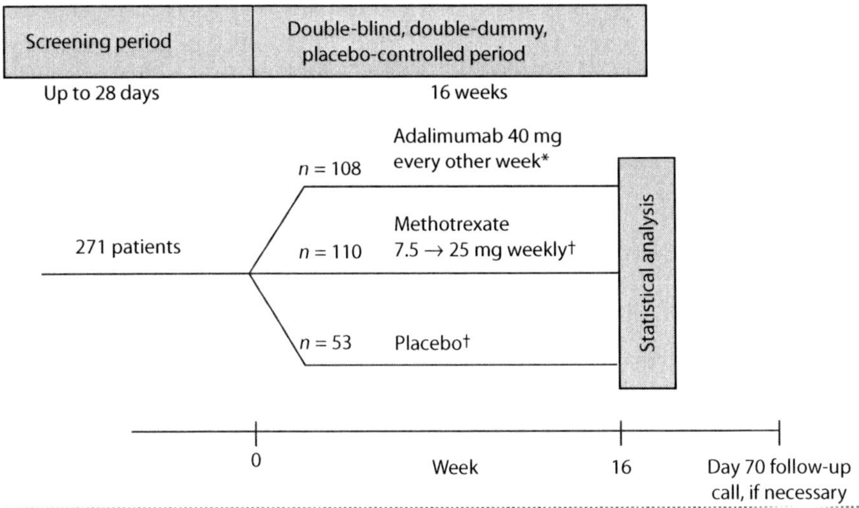

†Dosage increase of oral methotrexate/placebo					
Week	0–1	2–3	4–7	8–11†	12–15†
Maximum dosage (mg/wk)	7.5	10	15	20	25

FIGURE 12.3 CHAMPION study design including three treatment arms. *Adalimumab was administered as 80 mg subcutaneously at week 0, followed by 40 mg every other week through week 15. Matching placebo injections were administered with the same dosing regimen. †Oral methotrexate was administered as a single weekly dose, started at 7.5 mg/week at week 0. Dosage was increased to 10 mg/week at week 2 and subsequently increased to 15 mg/week at week 4 for all patients. At week 8, patients who achieved a PASI 50 response remained at their current dosage (maximum 15 mg/week) for the duration of the study. At week 8, patients who did not achieve PASI 50 had methotrexate dosage increased to 20 mg/week. Similarly, at week 12, patients who achieved less than PASI 50 at weeks 8 and 12 underwent a further increase in methotrexate dosing to 25 mg/week. Patients who did achieve a PASI 50 response at week 12 maintained their current dosage (20 mg/week maximum) throughout the study. (From Saurat JH et al., *Br J Dermatol* 158, 558–566, 2008. Reproduced with permission of Blackwell Publishing Ltd.)

From weeks 8–11, methotrexate dose was increased to 20 mg/week only if patients did not achieve a PASI 50 response. Similarly, from weeks 12–15, the methotrexate dose was increased to 25 mg/week only if patients did not achieve a PASI 50 response. The mean weekly dosage of oral medication in the methotrexate group was 18.8 mg at weeks 12 and 19.2 mg at week 15. The methotrexate dosing schedule was designed so that any patient who achieved a PASI 50 response by week 8 was maintained at a dose of 15 mg/week, instead of having the dose gradually increased, which potentially could have been more therapeutic (but also more toxic). The efficacy of methotrexate in this study may not have been fully realized because of the short 16-week evaluation and due to the insufficient titration of methotrexate. This controlled dosing regimen is a potential contributing factor in the marked difference in PASI improvement between adalimumab and methotrexate following 16 weeks of therapy.

The primary end point was percentage of patients achieving at least a 75% reduction in PASI score at week 16 (Figure 12.4) [11]. After 16 weeks of treatment, 79.6% of patients in

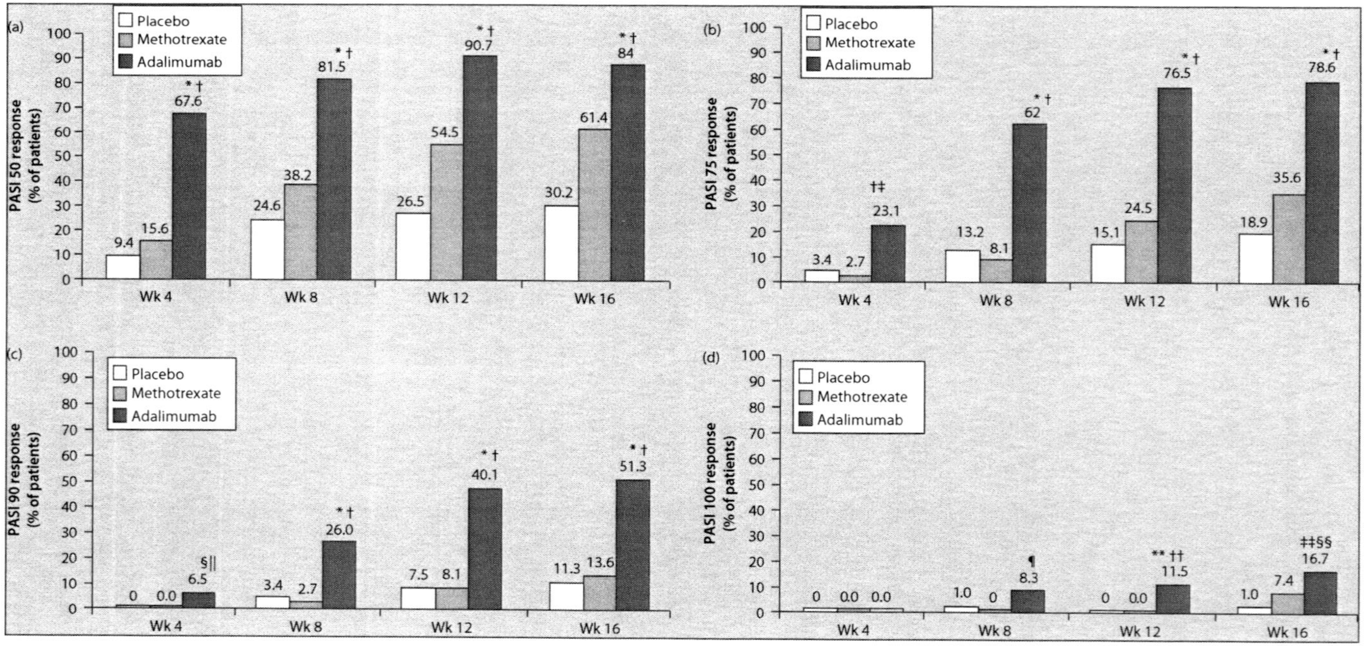

FIGURE 12.4 PASI response rates over 16 weeks. (a) Patients achieving at least 50% reduction in Psoriasis Area and Severity Index (PASI 50). (b) Patients achieving PASI 75. (c) Patients achieving PASI 90. (d) Patients achieving PASI 100, complete skin clearance. *$p < 0.001$ versus placebo; †$p < 0.001$ versus methotrexate; ‡$p = 0.001$ versus placebo; §$p = 0.10$ versus placebo; ||$p = 0.03$ versus methotrexate; ¶$p = 0.002$ versus methotrexate; **$p = 0.009$ versus placebo; ††$p = 0.001$ versus methotrexate; ‡‡$p = 0.004$ versus placebo; §§$p = 0.04$ versus methotrexate. (From Saurat JH et al., *Br J Dermatol* 158, 558–566, 2008. Reproduced with permission of Blackwell Publishing Ltd.)

the adalimumab group versus 35.5% of patients in the methotrexate group achieved a PASI 75 response ($p < 0.001$). After only eight weeks of treatment, 62% of patients in the adalimumab arm achieved PASI 75 as compared to 9.1% of patients treated with methotrexate ($p < 0.001$).

In the CHAMPION open-label extension trial, patients initially randomized to methotrexate administration were transitioned to adalimumab 40 mg every other week dosing at the end of the initial 16-week trial [12]. At the 16-week primary end point, 28% of the patients receiving methotrexate had achieved a PASI 75 response. All patients in the methotrexate treatment arm were then transitioned to the adalimumab open-label extension, and, subsequently, 75% and 73% of patients achieved a PASI 75 response after adalimumab treatment for 12 and 24 weeks, respectively. Overall, the CHAMPION study demonstrated that treatment with adalimumab resulted in more rapid and greater efficacy as compared to oral methotrexate. After approximately four months of treatment with adalimumab, one in two patients achieved a 90% improvement in their psoriasis and nearly four in five patients achieved a 75% improvement in their psoriasis. However, specific limitations of this study such as the methotrexate dosing regimen must be considered carefully when examining these data.

Dose Escalation

Although specific guidelines defining treatment failure are not specified, many open-label extension studies have offered participants every week dosing for adalimumab if clinical response is not adequate [7,8,9,10]. Leonardi et al. published the results of a six-year open-label extension study, which included eligible patients from various adalimumab phase II and III studies, including the REVEAL and CHAMPION studies ($n = 1468$). The main aim of this study was to determine the effectiveness of escalating adalimumab dosage from 40 mg every other week to 40 mg weekly in patients with a suboptimal response (less than PASI 50 response) after 24 weeks of treatment. All patients began the extension study on 40 mg adalimumab every other week. At week 24 and throughout the remainder of the study, patients who had less than a PASI 50 response could increase to weekly dosing. Those patients on weekly dosing who achieved a PASI 75 response were required to decrease the dosing frequency to every other week.

Of the 1256 patients who began with the standard every other week dose, approximately one-third (349) underwent dosing escalation at week 24. Approximately one-quarter (26.6%) of these patients achieved PASI 75 after 12 weeks of weekly dosing.

Interestingly, patients in the dosing escalation group who had at one time achieved a PASI 75 in the REVEAL study—deemed secondary nonresponders—benefitted most from dose escalation, with 35% of patients regaining a PASI 75 response at 12 weeks after dose escalation. In contrast, primary nonresponders gained little advantage from dose escalation with five of 55 patients achieving a PASI 75 response. In summary, this study suggests that dose escalation may only be helpful in a minority of patients. Those patients who initially respond to every other week dosing and then subsequently lose their response may have the most benefit from dosing escalation [13].

SAFETY AND ADVERSE EVENTS

The safety profile of adalimumab in the treatment of various autoimmune diseases, including moderate to severe psoriasis, has come from more than 12 years of clinical trial exposure involving more than 23,000 patients across six indications [14]. Adverse events including infectious events and serious adverse events will be discussed further along with warnings and contraindications.

BLACK BOX WARNINGS

Adalimumab carries two black box warnings involving fatal infections and tuberculosis that pertain to all TNF blockers, including adalimumab. Each is discussed here.

Fatal Infections

Serious and potentially fatal infections (including tuberculosis and invasive fungal and other opportunistic infections) have been reported in patients receiving TNF-blocking agents, including adalimumab. Many of the serious infections have occurred in patients on concomitant immunosuppressive therapy. Other opportunistic infections included histoplasmosis, aspergillosis, nocardiosis, legionellosis, and listeriosis. The FDA recommends the use of adalimumab with caution in patients who have resided in regions where histoplasmosis is endemic. In addition, caution should be exercised when considering the use of adalimumab in patients with chronic infection, history of recurrent infection, or predisposition to infection. TNF blocking agents should not be given to patients with an active chronic or localized infection. If a patient develops a serious infection, therapy should be discontinued.

The incidence of serious infections was 0.04/patient-year (PY) in adalimumab-treated patients versus 0.02/PY in placebo-treated patients with rheumatoid arthritis [2]. These serious infections included pneumonia, septic arthritis, prosthetic and postsurgical infections, erysipelas, cellulitis, diverticulitis, and pyelonephritis. However, in period A of the aforementioned phase III trial for psoriasis (REVEAL), in which the safety profile of adalimumab was compared head-to-head against placebo, the rate of serious infectious adverse events was 1% in the placebo group versus 0.6% in the adalimumab group following 16 weeks of therapy [5]. The rest of this trial demonstrated that of all patients exposed to at least one dose of adalimumab, totaling 540 patient-years (PYs), the rate of serious infections was 0.02 events/ PY. These infections mainly consisted of abscesses, cellulitis, and one case of tuberculosis (see following section).

The most recent long-term safety data reported by Burmester et al. included 23,458 patients who received adalimumab in 71 clinical trials over a 12-year period for the treatment of all of its currently approved indications—except ulcerative colitis—including 3010 patients with plaque psoriasis. It showed that serious infectious events were the most frequently reported serious adverse events, with the greatest rates of serious infectious events (SIEs) seen in rheumatoid arthritis or Crohn's disease. The incidence of serious infections in rheumatoid arthritis and Crohn's disease was 4.6 events/100 PYs and 6.7 events/100 PYs, respectively, while psoriasis patients had a rate of 1.7 events/100 PYs. However, the majority of patients with SIEs (70%) across all indications continued adalimumab therapy. The most common SIE in psoriasis patients was cellulitis [14].

In addition, results from the open-label extension study that examined the long-term efficacy and safety of weekly dosing of adalimumab in psoriatic patients with inadequate response to the usual every other week dosing showed rates of all adverse events, infections adverse events, and serious infectious adverse events were not increased in patients receiving weekly dosing [13].

Tuberculosis Evaluation

Tuberculosis (TB) (disseminated or extra pulmonary) has been reactivated while on adalimumab; most cases of reactivation have been reported within the first eight months of treatment. Doses higher than recommended are associated with an increased risk for tuberculosis reactivation.

TB evaluation and screening was deemed necessary after a clinical trial of adalimumab for rheumatoid arthritis revealed a tuberculosis rate of 1.3/100 PYs [15]. After implementation of TB screening, the TB rate decreased to 0.27/100 PYs in Europe and 0.08/100 PYs in North America [15]. The phase III clinical trial for psoriasis (REVEAL) had implemented TB screening, and the rate of TB in all patients exposed to adalimumab was 0.2/100 PYs [5]. There was one presumed but inconclusive case of TB. This occurred in a patient who had a positive tuberculin skin test result and a negative chest X-ray. This patient was noncompliant with isoniazid prophylactic therapy (started before adalimumab treatment) and subsequently developed clinical symptoms compatible with tuberculosis, although the patient's sputum was negative for an acid fast bacteria stain and sputum culture was negative for tuberculosis. Adalimumab therapy was promptly discontinued, and the patient was treated successfully with a multidrug antituberculosis drug regimen. In the most recent published long term safety data in patients using adalimumab over a 12-year period, incidence rates for active tuberculosis were comparable to a previous 2009 long-term safety data analysis (0.29/100 PYs) [14,16]. The rate of active TB in adalimumab clinical trials across all indications was 0.2/100 PYs, including cases from rheumatoid arthritis clinical studies prior to implementation of a tuberculin test screening program. Since latent TB infection screening and prophylaxis as implemented in 1998 and 1999, respectively, the rate has decreased from 1.5/100 PY to 0.2/100 PY [14].

Patients must be evaluated for latent tuberculosis infection with a tuberculin skin test or quantiferon gold blood test prior to therapy and, if positive, a chest radiograph should be obtained to rule out active infection. Treatment of latent tuberculosis should be initiated under guidelines by the Centers for Disease Control before beginning adalimumab therapy. To date, there is no established guideline regarding how long a patient must be receiving antituberculosis prophylactic therapy prior to initiation of adalimumab. Patients with initial negative tuberculin skin tests should receive continued monitoring for tuberculosis throughout treatment; patients who develop persistent cough, weight loss, malaise, or low-grade fever should be evaluated for active tuberculosis. Adalimumab should be used with caution in patients who have resided in regions where tuberculosis is endemic. Recommendations for monitoring are discussed here.

SIDE EFFECTS AND ADVERSE EVENTS

Injection Site Reactions

The most common adverse reaction seen with adalimumab is injection site reaction. In placebo-controlled trials of patients with rheumatoid arthritis, 20% of patients treated with adalimumab developed injection site reactions consisting of erythema, itching, hemorrhage, pain, or swelling versus 14% of patients receiving placebo [15]. In the REVEAL study, 3.2% of patients with psoriasis developed injection site reactions versus 1.8% of patients receiving placebo [5]. Most injection site reactions were described as mild and generally did not necessitate drug discontinuation.

Infections

Infections continue to be the most commonly reported serious adverse events across all six therapeutic indications according to the latest safety data, with the greatest rates of serious infectious events seen in patients with rheumatoid arthritis or Crohn's disease [14]. In the phase III trial evaluating adalimumab for treatment of psoriasis (REVEAL), the risk of infectious adverse events was slightly higher in the adalimumab treatment arm, at 28.9% in the adalimumab group versus 22.4% in the placebo group [5]. One case of non-TB opportunistic infection was reported in a patient who developed oral candidiasis, and it was treated successfully with fluconazole. (A discussion on serious infectious adverse events is described earlier in this chapter.)

Malignancies

When subjects with similar demographics were compared, the observed numbers were similar to the expected number of malignancies excluding nonmelanoma skin cancer (NMSC) and lymphomas [14]. In placebo-controlled trials of 2468 rheumatoid arthritis patients treated for an average of two years, 48 malignancies of various types were observed [15]. Ten of these patients were found to have lymphoma. Furthermore, the 12-year safety data showed similar rates to those reported in previous studies. For malignancies not including lymphoma and NMSC, rates observed were 0.7 events/100 PYs [14]. In earlier studies, the standardized incidence ratio (SIR) for patients on adalimumab (the ratio of observed rate to age-adjusted expected frequency in the general population) was 1.0 (95% CI, 0.7, 1.3) for malignancies and 5.4 (95% CI, 2.6, 10.0) for lymphomas [15]. Long-term data showed that the SIR of lymphoma in all patients with rheumatoid arthritis was 2.74 (1.83–3.93) [14]. Thus, it appears that, although the risk of lymphoma in patients with rheumatoid arthritis is increased at baseline, it may be higher in those patients on adalimumab [17,18].

However, in psoriasis, there is not sufficient evidence to suggest an increased risk of lymphoma associated with adalimumab use. The most recent long-term safety data reported the standardized incidence rate of lymphoma for psoriasis patients to be 0.63 (0.01–3.49) [14]. In two randomized, placebo-controlled studies of adalimumab in the treatment of psoriasis, namely, a phase II study by Gordon et al. and a phase III study by Menter et al. (REVEAL), no incidence of lymphoma was reported [4,5]. The phase II study (n = 147) suggests that risk of malignancy may increase with more frequent dosing evidenced by a higher incidence of malignancy among the 40 mg/week group compared to the 40 mg every other week group [4]. The more recent open-label extension study following subjects with suboptimal response that increased dosing to 40 mg/ week reported no cases of lymphoma.

The risk of NMSC was shown to be slightly elevated in patients with rheumatoid arthritis, psoriasis, and Crohn's disease (1.39; 1.10 to 1.60, 1.76; 1.26 to 2.39 and 2.29; 1.44 to 3.47), although these patients may be at an increased risk of NMSC due to their disease, other previous treatments—such as psoralen plus ultraviolet A (PUVA), or due to detection bias [14]. Finally, the SIR of melanoma for psoriasis patients (4.37, 1.89 to 8.61) suggests that use of adalimumab leads to an increased risk of melanoma. However, many of these patients were on multiple therapies such as phototherapy (including PUVA) and immunosuppressants that raise the risk of skin cancers [14]. In addition, skin cancer data are confounded by the "detection phenomenon." That is, as psoriasis is treated with adalimumab, skin cancer becomes more readily apparent and thus incidence appears higher even though the cancer may have been present before treatment was started.

The malignancies observed during use of adalimumab were breast, colon-rectum, uterine-cervical, prostate, melanoma, nonmelanoma skin cancer, gallbladder-bile ducts, and other carcinomas. The authors of this manuscript recommend that treatment with adalimumab be avoided in patients with malignancy or a history of malignancy and discontinued in patients who develop malignancy while on adalimumab therapy.

Neurologic Events

TNF blocking agents have been associated with rare cases of exacerbation of clinical symptoms and/or radiographic evidence of demyelinating disease [2]. In studies evaluating adalimumab for treatment of psoriasis, demyelinating diseases were not reported [4,5,14]. Adalimumab should not be used in patients with demyelinating diseases or in patients with first-degree relatives with multiple sclerosis [19].

Autoantibodies

A concern for development of autoantibodies is present with all biologics, and the long-term clinical effects of adalimumab on autoimmunity are unknown at this time. In placebo-controlled trials of patients with rheumatoid arthritis and negative baseline antinuclear antibody (ANA) titers, 12% of patients treated with adalimumab developed positive ANA titers versus 7% of patients on placebo [2]. Among 2334 patients in these trials, one patient developed clinical signs suggestive of new-onset lupus-like syndrome, which improved following discontinuation of therapy [2]. In studies evaluating adalimumab in the treatment of psoriasis, there were no reports of lupus-like syndromes [4,5,11,14].

Immunogenicity

A percentage of patients may develop antibodies against adalimumab while on therapy, as shown by clinical trials in patients with rheumatoid arthritis, in which less than 5% of patients developed antibodies by week 24 of treatment (n = 1062) [2]. However, a greater proportion of patients (17%) had detected antibodies after 28 weeks of treatment in another study involving 121 rheumatoid arthritis patients. Nine of the 11 patients with anti-adalimumab concentrations above 100 AU/mL were nonresponders and two were moderate responders. Of note, patients receiving concomitant methotrexate had a lower rate of antibody development than patients receiving adalimumab monotherapy (12% vs. 38%) [20]. Studies in these patients showed no correlation with adverse events; therefore, routine testing for these antibodies is not advised.

CONTRAINDICATIONS AND PRECAUTIONS

Tuberculosis Infection

Adalimumab should not be administered to a patient with active tuberculosis infection, as discussed earlier.

Immunosuppression

Because TNF-blocking agents are immunomodulators, they may negatively impact the immune system. Although adalimumab has not been tested in patients with immunosuppression, caution should be exercised when considering treatment with adalimumab.

Anaphylactic Reaction

Rare reports of anaphylactic reactions following injections of adalimumab have been reported. Therapy should be discontinued immediately and appropriate therapy started.

Hepatitis B Reactivation

Use of the TNF-blockers (including adalimumab) has been shown to reactivate hepatitis B virus (HBV) in patients who are chronic carriers. It is recommended that a hepatitis panel and liver function tests (LFTs) be performed prior to initiation of medication, and caution should be exercised in giving adalimumab to patients identified as carriers [19]. Discontinuation of anti-TNF therapy is required if reactivation occurs, and appropriate antiviral and/or supportive therapy should be initiated. Data are insufficient on whether resuming anti-TNF therapy is safe in patients whose HBV reactivation is controlled.

Congestive Heart Failure

Cases of worsening congestive heart failure (CHF) have been reported in patients on adalimumab and other TNF antagonists as well [2]. In a phase III randomized, placebo-controlled study of adalimumab therapy for psoriasis (REVEAL), Menter et al. reported one case of CHF during period A in a patient who developed ankle swelling but no shortness of breath. The patient was treated with oral furosemide; hospitalization was not necessary, and the patient was continued in the study [5]. Four serious CHF events were reported for the first time in patients with psoriasis in the most recent 12-year data, although three of the patients had two or more risk factors for CHF, including hypertension, hyperlipidemia, diabetes mellitus, myocardial ischemia, and obesity. The fourth patient developed pulmonary edema secondary to a near-drowning [14]. It is recommended that adalimumab be avoided in patients with New York Heart Association (NYHA) Class III or Class IV congestive heart failure [19]. Patients with NYHA Class I or II congestive heart failure should undergo echocardiogram testing and, if the ejection fraction is less than 50%, TNF inhibitors should be avoided [19].

Immunizations

There are no available data on anti-TNF agents with regard to live vaccinations. However, it is recommended that live vaccinations not be given concurrently with adalimumab due to the potential for poor response to the vaccination or due to the potential for secondary transmission of infection [19]. Immune response may be compromised in recombinant vaccines as well. Furthermore, it is suggested that a physician ensures vaccinations are up to date prior to initiation of adalimumab.

Pregnancy and Lactation

Adalimumab is pregnancy category B. It is not known whether adalimumab or other anti-TNF agents can cause harm to a developing fetus; thus, it should be given to pregnant women only if absolutely necessary. For lactating women, it is unknown whether adalimumab is excreted in breast milk. However, due to potential side effects in nursing infants, nursing women should not use adalimumab, or lactating women on adalimumab should not breast feed.

Drug–Drug Interactions

The combination of the immunomodulator anakinra and adalimumab is not recommended due to the theoretical class risk of serious infections, as previously seen with concurrent use of anakinra and etanercept [21]. Methotrexate has been shown to reduce the clearance of adalimumab after single and multiple dosing by 29% and 44%, respectively. However, dose adjustments are not needed for methotrexate or adalimumab when using them in combination [22].

MONITORING

Required

Required monitoring for adalimumab includes baseline and periodic tuberculosis screening, although the frequency of screening has not been specified. The authors of this chapter routinely require yearly tuberculosis screening. An explanation on management of positive tuberculosis tests can be found earlier, in the section on black box warnings.

Optional

Most practitioners check liver function tests, complete blood count, and a hepatitis profile at baseline and on a periodic basis. However, FDA labeling does not require these tests.

DISCUSSION

The efficacy of adalimumab in the treatment of moderate to severe psoriasis has been well demonstrated, with 68% of patients achieving a PASI 75 response after 12 weeks of therapy in the randomized, placebo-controlled phase III trial [5]. No head-to-head clinical trials have been conducted comparing adalimumab to other biologic agents in the management of psoriasis. However, different patients respond differently to adalimumab therapy, and safe use of this agent requires baseline screening for tuberculosis along with consideration of the aforementioned recommendations per clinician's judgment. Future clinical trials involving adalimumab are needed to evaluate its merits in combination therapy and in further sophisticated usages in the treatment of plaque psoriasis.

REFERENCES

1. IMS National Prescription Audit: Total Humira prescriptions written by dermatologists from 10/28/11 to 7/27/12 vs Enbrel, Stelara and Simponi.
2. Abbott Laboratories.2013. *Humira full prescribing information*. Revised. North Chicago, IL: Abbott Laboratories.
3. Leonardi C, Papp K, Strober B, et al. The long-term safety of adalimumab treatment in moderate to severe psoriasis: a comprehensive analysis of all adalimumab exposure in all clinical trials. *Am J Clin Dermato* 2011;12(5):321–37.
4. Gordon KB, Langley RG, Leonardi C, et al. Clinical response to adalimumab treatment in patients with moderate to severe psoriasis: double-blind, randomized controlled trial and open-label extension study. *J Am Acad Dermatol* 2006; 55(4): 598–606.
5. Menter A, Tyring SK, Gordon K, et al. Adalimumab therapy for moderate to severe psoriasis: a randomized, controlled phase III trial. *J Am Acad Dermatol* 2008; 58(1): 106–115.
6. Behrens S, Grundmann-Kollmann M, Peter RU, Kerscher M. Combination treatment of psoriasis with photochemotherapy and tazarotene gel, a receptor-selective topical retinoid. *Br J Dermatol* 1999; 141(1): 177.
7. Gordon K, Papp K, Poulin Y, et al. Long-term efficacy and safety of adalimumab in patients with moderate to severe psoriasis treated continuously over 3 years: results from an open-label extension study for patients from REVEAL. *J Am Acad Dermatol* 2012; 66(2): 241–251.
8. Papp K, Crowley J, Ortonne JP, et al. Adalimumab for moderate to severe chronic plaque psoriasis: efficacy and safety of retreatment and disease recurrence following withdrawal from therapy. *Br J Dermatol* 2011; 164(2): 434–441.
9. Mease PJ, Gladman DD, Ritchlin CT, et al. Adalimumab for the treatment of patients with moderately to severely active psoriatic arthritis: results of a double-blind, randomized, placebo-controlled trial. *Arthritis Rheum* 2005; 52(10): 3279–3289.
10. Mease PJ, Ory P, Sharp JT, et al. Adalimumab for long-term treatment of psoriatic arthritis: 2-year data from the Adalimumab Effectiveness in Psoriatic Arthritis Trial (ADEPT). *Ann Rheum Dis* 2009; 68(5): 702–709.
11. Saurat JH, Stingl G, Dubertret L, et al. Efficacy and safety results from the randomized controlled comparative study of adalimumab vs. methotrexate vs. placebo in patients with psoriasis (CHAMPION). *Br J Dermatol* 2008; 158(3): 558–566.
12. Mrowietz U, Luger T. Presented at: Winter American Academy of Dermatology Meeting; February 2008; San Antonio, TX.
13. Leonardi C, Sobell JM, Crowley JJ, et al. Efficacy, safety and medication cost implications of adalimumab 40 mg weekly dosing in patients with psoriasis with suboptimal response to 40 mg every other week dosing: results from an open-label study. *Br J Dermatol* 2012; 167(3): 658–667.
14. Burmester GR, Panaccione R, Gordon KB, et al. Adalimumab: long-term safety in 23 458 patients from global clinical trials in rheumatoid arthritis, juvenile idiopathic arthritis, ankylosing spondylitis, psoriatic arthritis, psoriasis and Crohn's disease. *Ann Rheum Dis* 2013; 72(4): 517–524.
15. Schiff MH, Burmester GR, Kent JD, et al. Safety analyses of adalimumab (HUMIRA) in global clinical trials and US postmarketing surveillance of patients with rheumatoid arthritis. *Ann Rheum Dis* 2006; 65(7): 889–894.
16. Burmester GR, Mease P, Dijkmans BA, et al. Adalimumab safety and mortality rates from global clinical trials of six immune-mediated inflammatory diseases. *Ann Rheum Dis* 2009; 68(12): 1863–1869.
17. Mellemkjaer L, Linet MS, Gridley G, et al. Rheumatoid arthritis and cancer risk. *Eur J Cancer* 1996; 32A(10): 1753–1757.
18. Baecklund E, Ekbom A, Sparen P, et al. Disease activity and risk of lymphoma in patients with rheumatoid arthritis: nested case-control study. *BMJ* 1998; 317(7152): 180–181.

19. Menter A, Gottlieb A, Feldman SR, et al. Guidelines of care for the management of psoriasis and psoriatic arthritis: section 1. Overview of psoriasis and guidelines of care for the treatment of psoriasis with biologics. *J Am Acad Dermatol* 2008; 58(5): 826–850.
20. Bartelds GM, Wijbrandts CA, Nurmohamed MT, et al. Clinical response to adalimumab: relationship to anti-adalimumab antibodies and serum adalimumab concentrations in rheumatoid arthritis. *Ann Rheum Dis* 2007; 66(7): 921–926.
21. Genovese MC, Cohen S, Moreland L, et al. Combination therapy with etanercept and anakinra in the treatment of patients with rheumatoid arthritis who have been treated unsuccessfully with methotrexate. *Arthritis Rheum* 2004; 50(5): 1412–1419.
22. Weisman MH, Moreland LW, Furst DE, et al. Efficacy, pharmacokinetic, and safety assessment of adalimumab, a fully human anti-tumor necrosis factor-alpha monoclonal antibody, in adults with rheumatoid arthritis receiving concomitant methotrexate: a pilot study. *Clin Ther* 2003; 25(6): 1700–1721.

Chapter 13

Ustekinumab

Andrew Blauvelt

INTRODUCTION

The etiology of psoriasis is unknown, although it is generally believed to be a complex T-cell-mediated inflammatory disease with a genetic basis [1,2]. Psoriasis shares immunologic and genetic features with other T-cell-mediated autoimmune inflammatory conditions, such as Crohn's disease, rheumatoid arthritis, and multiple sclerosis; CD4+ T-helper cells, called T-helper (Th) 17 cells, are important in the pathogenesis of many of these diseases [3], including psoriasis [2,4–6]. Interleukin-23 (IL-23) stimulates survival and proliferation of Th17 cells and thus serves as a key master cytokine regulator for these diseases. In psoriasis, IL-23 is overproduced by activated dermal dendritic cells, and this cytokine stimulates Th17 cells within the dermis to make IL-17A and IL-22. In turn, IL-17A and IL-22 drive keratinocyte activation and hyperproliferation in psoriasis. This chapter will focus on the role of the IL-23/Th17 inflammatory pathway in psoriasis pathogenesis and on the specific targeting of IL-12/IL-23 by ustekinumab.

BASIC BIOLOGY OF TH17 CELLS AND INTERLEUKIN-23

In 1986, Mosmann and colleagues first described Th1 and Th2 cells, distinct T-cell subsets that express a unique set of cytokines and are each involved in mediating unique immune responses to differing pathogens [7]. In 2005, a third distinct T-cell subset was defined: Th17 cells [8,9]. Naïve T cells are induced to differentiate into Th1, Th2, or Th17 based upon T-cell receptor stimulation and costimulation and the specific cytokines released by antigen presenting cells [3,10]. For example, Th17 cells develop in peripheral tissue of humans after exposure to extracellular IL-1β (Figure 13.1) [11,12]. Both IL-6 and IL-23 can amplify Th17 cell differentiation but cannot substitute for IL-1β. The intracellular transcription factors RORγt and Stat3 are also critical in the development of Th17 cells from naïve T-cell precursors (Figure 13.1) [13,14]. By contrast, Th1 cells develop from naïve T cells after exposure to IL-12 and characteristically express the transcription factor T-bet [10]. Both Th17 and Th1 cells are defined at least in part by the specific set of pro-inflammatory cytokines that they produce and secrete. Th17 cells produce IL-17A (see Chapter 16), IL-17F, IL-21, IL-22, IL-6, and tumor necrosis factor-α (TNF-α), whereas Th1 cells produce IFN-γ, IL-2, and TNF-α (Figure 13.1) [3,10].

IL-23 is the key cytokine involved in the survival and proliferation of Th17 cells (Figure 13.1) [15,16]. IL-23 is a heterodimeric protein that consists of a unique p19 subunit that is paired with a second subunit called p40 (Figure 13.2). IL-12 is a related heterodimer consisting of p40 and a unique subunit called p35, and it promotes development of Th1 cells (Figure 13.2) [3]. The IL-23 receptor is also a heterodimer consisting of IL-12Rβ1 and IL-23R subunits, whereas the IL-12 receptor is composed of IL-12Rβ1 and IL-12Rβ2 subunits (Figure 13.2).

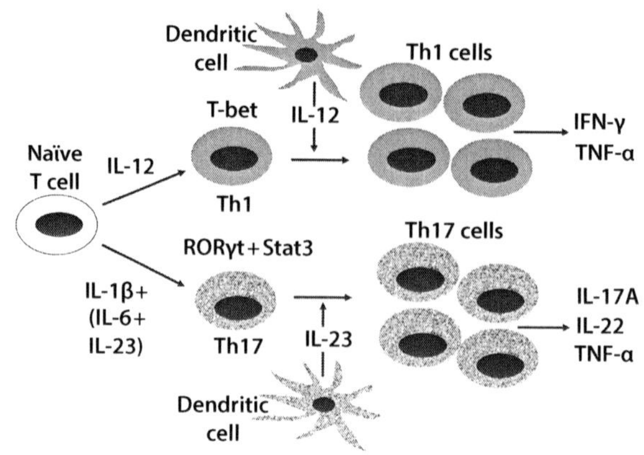

FIGURE 13.1 Schematic showing the key cytokines and transcription factors involved in the differentiation, proliferation, and effector function of Th17 cells versus Th1 cells.

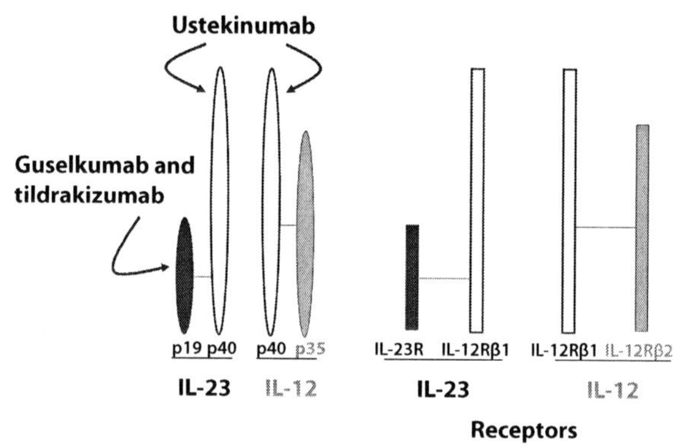

FIGURE 13.2 Schematic showing the subunits of IL-23, IL-12, and their respective receptors, including p40, the shared subunit targeted by ustekinumab.

IL-23 is produced by dendritic cells and other antigen presenting cells [15,17]. It also is produced, albeit at low levels, by keratinocytes [18].

Interestingly, dendritic cells produce IL-23 when stimulated by infection with *Candida albicans*, and this event is mediated by dectin-1, a C-type lectin receptor [19,20]. IL-23-deficient mice are susceptible to chronic *Candida* infections [21]. In addition, activation through other innate receptors can trigger IL-23 production by dendritic cells, including toll-like receptor 4 signaling induced by lipopolysaccharide from *Bordetella pertussis* and other sources [22,23]. It is unknown whether *C. albicans* and toll-like receptor ligands stimulate keratinocytes to make IL-23, although this is an intriguing possibility because microorganisms have long been postulated to be triggers for some types of psoriasis.

ROLES OF INTERLEUKIN-23 AND TH17 CELLS IN PSORIASIS PATHOGENESIS

In transgenic mice, overexpression of individual subunits of IL-23 leads to inflammation. Ubiquitous expression of p19 causes severe multiorgan inflammation, runting, infertility, high circulating levels of TNF-α and IL-1, and premature death [24]. Overexpression of p40 in basal keratinocytes induces psoriasis-like inflammatory skin disease [25]. These investigators also suggested that transgenic p40 combined with endogenous p19 to form IL-23 and causes cutaneous inflammation.

In other mouse studies, recombinant IL-23 injected into normal-appearing skin produced erythematous, thick, scaly skin, with histologic features reminiscent of psoriasis [26–28]. Recombinant IL-12, injected in a similar manner, did not [26,27]. Interestingly, acanthosis induced by injection of IL-23 is dependent upon both key Th17 cytokines: IL-17A and IL-22 [28]. When IL-23 was injected into IL-17A or IL-22 knockout mice, no keratinocyte hyperproliferation was observed [27,28]. Thus, these studies directly demonstrate that both of these cytokines are critical downstream mediators of IL-23-induced psoriasis-like inflammation in skin.

In humans, IL-23 is clearly elevated in psoriasis lesions as indicated by increased levels of both *p19* and *p40* mRNA in lesional skin as compared to nonlesional skin, whereas mRNA levels of *p35* are not elevated [12,26,29–31]. This implies that IL-23, but not IL-12, is increased in skin affected by psoriasis. Furthermore, immunohistochemical analyses have revealed p40 and p19 protein expression in dermal dendritic cells [12,31,32] and keratinocytes [33] in lesions of psoriasis. Importantly, IL-23 levels (assessed by either mRNA or protein) decrease with clinical improvement of psoriasis following effective treatment, providing a direct correlation between overproduction of IL-23 and active psoriasis [26,29–31,33–35]. Th17 cells are also significantly elevated in the blood of psoriatics and decrease during effective therapy for psoriasis [36].

The importance of IL-23 in psoriasis pathogenesis has also been strengthened by recent genetic studies. Tsunemi et al. found that a single nucleotide polymorphism in *p40* was associated with psoriasis [37]. This polymorphism was confirmed using genome-wide association studies and gene sequencing techniques in additional independent cohorts [38–40]. The association was independent of *HLA-Cw*0602*, another gene linked to psoriasis [41]. Polymorphisms in the gene encoding the IL-23-specific subunit, *p19*, are also associated with psoriasis development [38–40]. In addition, a common risk haplotype was identified for the gene encoding the receptor subunit that is specific for IL-23, *IL-23R*, with proline at amino acid 310 and arginine at amino acid 381 [38–40]. Conversely, a change in *IL-23R* at 381 from arginine to glutamine was found to be *protective* against psoriasis [38–40]. This amino acid is located in the JAK2 kinase-binding domain of IL-23R, which transmits intracellular signals that are triggered following ligation of IL-23R. This change to glutamine inhibits IL-23R signaling cascade and prevents inflammatory responses mediated by Th17 cells [42]. Of particular importance, no polymorphisms specific to IL-12 (e.g., *p35* or *IL-12Rβ2*) are associated with psoriasis susceptibility.

IL-17A mRNA is elevated in psoriatic skin when compared to nonlesional skin [12,26]. Immunohistochemical staining for IL-17A positive cells has also been reported [43,44]. These cells include Th17 cells, mast cells, and neutrophils [45]. IL-17A likely plays a role in the subcorneal accumulation of neutrophils and the marked angiogenesis that are both tissue hallmarks of psoriasis.

Large numbers of recent reports suggest that Th17 cells and IL-23 are critically involved in psoriasis pathogenesis (summarized in Table 13.1). Taken together, hypotheses can be

TABLE 13.1 IL-23/Th17 Inflammatory Pathway in Psoriasis Pathogenesis

Evidence for Role in Psoriasis[a]	IL-23/Th17 Cells	IL-12/Th1 Cells
p19 (the IL-23-specific subunit) elevated in lesional psoriatic skin	++	N/A
p40 (the subunit shared by both IL-23 and IL-23) elevated in lesional psoriatic skin	++	++
p35 (the subunit used by IL-12) not elevated in lesional psoriatic skin	N/A	–
IL-17A and IL-22 (key Th17 cytokines) elevated in lesional psoriatic skin	++	N/A
IL-17A and IL-22 elevated in psoriatic blood	++	N/A
Th17 cytokines cause angiogenesis and keratinocyte hyperproliferation	++	N/A
IFN-γ (a key Th1 cytokine) elevated in lesional psoriatic skin	N/A	++
IFN-γ elevated in psoriatic blood	N/A	++
Th1 cytokines not implicated in angiogenesis and keratinocyte hyperproliferation	N/A	–
Polymorphisms in *p19* associated with susceptibility to psoriasis	++	N/A
Polymorphisms in *p40* associated with susceptibility and protection from psoriasis, depending on the genetic change	++	++
No polymorphisms in *p35* associated with psoriasis	N/A	–
Polymorphisms in *IL-23R* (IL-23 receptor-specific subunit) associated with susceptibility and protection from psoriasis, depending on the genetic change	++	N/A
No polymorphisms in *IL-12Rβ1* (receptor subunit shared by both IL-23 and IL-12) associated with psoriasis	–	–
No polymorphisms in *IL-12Rβ2* (IL-12 receptor-specific subunit) associated with psoriasis	N/A	–
Anti-p40 monoclonal antibodies markedly efficacious in psoriasis	++	++
Anti-p19 monoclonal antibodies markedly efficacious in psoriasis	++	N/A
p19 transgenic mouse develops widespread inflammatory disease	+	N/A
p40 transgenic expression in skin causes inflammatory skin disease	+	+
IL-23 injected into mouse skin causes psoriasis-like disease	+	N/A
IL-12 injected into mouse skin does not cause psoriasis-like disease	N/A	–

Note: ++ = positive evidence for an association in humans; + = positive evidence for an association in mice; – = negative evidence for an association; N/A = not applicable.

[a] see text for specific references.

generated as to how these particular cells and cytokines could cause psoriasis. Perturbation of resident keratinocytes and dendritic cells by trauma and/or stimulation of pattern recognition receptors (e.g., dectin-1, and TLR 2 and 4) by microbes on the skin surface may trigger conditions that promote IL-23 production [19,20] and thus lead to survival and proliferation of Th17 cells within skin. Th17 cells may migrate into the skin via chemokine receptors [19,46]. CCR6, whose chemokine ligand CCL20 is secreted by keratinocytes, is found in abundance on Th17 cells; CCR4 is also expressed on Th17 cell surfaces [19,46]. Interestingly, these chemokine receptors are also characteristically found on resident skin T cells [47]. Thus, it is possible that skin preferentially recruits Th17 cells in resting or non-inflammatory states, and that perturbations that enhance local IL-23 production would allow for expansion of these cells and thus produce inflammation. CCL20 is overexpressed in psoriasis [48], and we have also demonstrated recently that IL-17A induces keratinocytes to produce CCL20 *in vitro* [44]. This may be important in maintenance of psoriasis lesions by stimulating ongoing chemotaxis of new CCR6+ Th17 cells and of CCR6+ dendritic cells from blood. Genetic alterations that augment IL-23 signaling may increase susceptibility to psoriasis [37–40]. By contrast, other mutations that result in decreased IL-23 production and receptor-mediated signaling [38,39] confer protection from psoriasis [42]. Finally, because IL-23 is now believed to be a key master cytokine in psoriasis pathogenesis (Table 13.1), it is also predicted that specific inhibition of IL-23 alone will lead to death of Th17 cells and abrogation of psoriasis.

USTEKINUMAB MECHANISM OF ACTION

Ustekinumab is a monoclonal antibody directed against p40 and thus will inhibit action of IL-23 and IL-12 (Figure 13.2). As discussed, inhibition of IL-23 is predicted to induce death of Th17 cells because these cells are dependent upon IL-23 for survival and proliferation. Blocking IL-12 is predicted to cause loss of Th1 cells because IL-12 stimulates function of these cells. Thus, although ustekinumab does not directly act upon T cells, the most likely end result of their pharmacologic action is to cause T-cell death by inhibition of two major T-cell growth factors, IL-23 and IL-12.

Apoptosis of Th17 and Th1 cells has not been directly evaluated in patients receiving either ustekinumab. If this mechanism of action is proven to be true, this would explain the prolonged clinical effects of these drugs long after they have been cleared from serum because a relatively lengthy series of immunologic events would be required to re-populate Th17 and Th1 cells into skin.

Cooper and colleagues showed that ustekinumab therapy rapidly decreased expression of a variety of proinflammatory cytokine genes in lesional psoriatic skin, including *p19*, *p40*, and *IL-17A* [30]. TNF-α blocking agents do the same, and it appears that genes associated with the IL-23/Th17 inflammatory pathway are downregulated earlier than genes associated with the IL-12/Th1 inflammatory pathway [34,49]. This finding suggests that IL-23 and Th17 cells are more primary, or earlier, targets for these biologic therapies when compared to IL-12 and Th1 cells. TNF-α is made by numerous cell types, including Th17 cells [36], and has pleiotropic inflammatory effects. Although TNF-α antagonists likely have anti-inflammatory effects on multiple cell types and tissues, recent data suggest that these agents also work, at least in part, by blocking the IL-23/Th17 inflammatory pathway.

USTEKINUMAB EFFICACY IN CHRONIC PLAQUE PSORIASIS

In early phase I clinical trials, ustekinumab use led to demonstrable clinical effects on psoriasis after intravenous and subcutaneous administration of single doses of the drug [50,51]. These early trials led to a large phase II study that produced striking clinical results [52]. In a classic dose–response manner, 52% of low-dose patients, 59% of low- to medium-dose patients, 67% of medium- to high-dose patients, and 81% of high-dose patients achieved Psoriasis Area and Severity Index (PASI) 75 at week 12, which means a reduction in the PASI of at least 75%.

These early phase studies were confirmed by three major phase III studies, PHOENIX I and II, and one etanercept comparator trial, which had a total combined enrollment of more than 3500 individuals from more than 100 sites in the United States and Europe [53–55]. These three studies evaluated doses of 45 and 90 mg of ustekinumab given subcutaneously at weeks 0 and 4 (initiation therapy) and then dosing given every 8 or 12 weeks (maintenance therapy). Psoriasis responded rapidly to ustekinumab; at week 12, PASI 75 ranged from 67% to 76% [53–55,56–59] (Table 13.2). By comparison, the etanercept response rate given at a dose of 50 mg twice weekly was 57% at week 12 [55]. Interestingly, the highest PASI 75 rates were recorded between weeks 20 and 24; they were approximately 75% with the 45 mg dose and 85% with the 90 mg dose [53,54]. The majority of patients treated with either 45 mg or 90 mg every 12 weeks maintained clinical response to ustekinumab for up to 76 weeks of therapy (Figure 13.3) [53]. When a subset of patients was switched from ustekinumab to placebo at

TABLE 13.2 PASI 75 Phase III Short- and Long-Term Efficacy Results for Ustekinumab

Conditions	PASI 75 (%)[a]	References
Week 12, 45 mg	67	56–58
Week 12, 90 mg	66–76	56–58
Weeks 20–24, 45 mg	75–76	56,57
Weeks 20–24, 90 mg	84–85	56,57
Maintenance among initial responders (> PASI 75), week 244, 45 mg	79	59
Maintenance among initial responders (> PASI 75), week 244, 90 mg	81	59
Maintenance among initial partial responders (PASI 50–PASI 75), week 244, 45 mg	58	59
Maintenance among initial partial responders (PASI 50–PASI 75), week 244, 90 mg	55	59

[a] PASI 75 = percentage of patients that improved their Psoriasis Area and Severity Index scores by at least 75% when compared to baseline index scores.

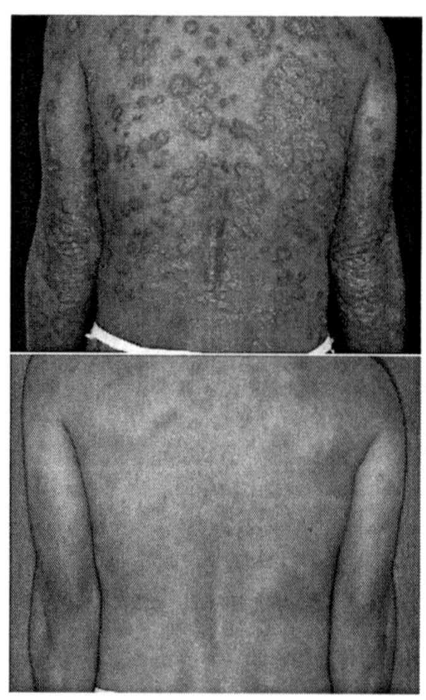

FIGURE 13.3 (See color insert.) Representative patient with severe psoriasis at baseline (top) and following 52 weeks of treatment with ustekinumab (bottom).

week 40, most individuals demonstrated long-lasting clinical effects on their psoriasis, with gradual—not abrupt—return of disease over the course of 24 weeks following discontinuation of the drug [53].

Not all psoriasis patients responded well to ustekinumab in the phase III studies. Of note, partial responders at week 28 (PASI 50–PASI 75) were compared with responders achieving more than PASI 75 in a variety of ways. Partial responders were more likely to demonstrate the following historical, clinical, or immunologic features: (1) higher body weight; (2) inadequate response to at least one biologic agent in the past; (3) longer duration of psoriasis; (4) history of psoriatic arthritis; and (5) presence of neutralizing antibodies to ustekinumab [53,54]. For the latter assay, antibodies to ustekinumab were detected in 12.7% of partial responders and in 2% of responders (i.e., at least PASI 75). Partial responders at week 28 tended to fare better when subsequently given doses of 90 mg every eight weeks than those partial responders who received either 45 mg and/or dosing every 12 weeks [54]. Thus, the ability to give ustekinumab at higher doses (90 mg instead of 45 mg) and for shorter intervals (every 8 weeks instead of every 12 weeks) may prove clinically meaningful for certain patients that do not respond well at lower and/or less frequent doses. These trials proved that regular dosing of ustekinumab over the course of 1.5 years is a highly efficacious therapy for individuals with psoriasis. Based upon these phase III results, in 2009, the U.S. Food and Drug Administration (FDA) recommended approval of ustekinumab for moderate to severe plaque psoriasis.

Importantly, the PHOENIX I and II ustekinumab trials were continued for a five-year period [60]. Sixty-nine percent of patients originally placed on ustekinumab in these phase III studies completed the entire trial. Approximately 80% of initial responders maintained PASI 75 responses over the course of five years, and approximately 55% of initial partial responders (i.e., those who first reached PASI 50–PASI 75) achieved PASI 75 by week 244 (Table 13.2) [60]. These results demonstrate that clinical efficacy of ustekinumab is robust over an extended period of time.

USTEKIMUMAB EFFICACY IN OTHER FORMS OF PSORIASIS

A variety of controlled studies, cases series, and case reports support the use of ustekinumab in other forms of psoriasis. In psoriatic arthritis, 42%–49% of patients achieved American College of Rheumatology (ACR) 20 responses at six months, with slightly greater responses observed in patients receiving 90 mg compared to those receiving 45 mg (Kavanaugh et al., American College of Rheumatology annual meeting, November 2012). ACR 20 responses were also greater at the 12-month point compared to the 6-month point, indicating that ustekinumab may require more time to achieve clinically meaningful results for psoriasis patients with joint disease. In fact, the FDA recently approved (Sept 2013) the use of ustekinumab in adult patients with active psoriatic arthritis. The medication can be used alone or in combination with methotrexate. Of note, there was a recent paradoxical report of an occurrence of new onset psoriatic arthritis in two psoriasis patients receiving ustekinumab [61].

In off-label usage, individuals with erythrodermic psoriasis [62–65], palmoplantar psoriasis [66–69], and TNF-blocker-induced psoriasis/psoriasiform dermatitis [56,57] have also been reported to respond well to ustekinumab. One common theme from these reports is that higher dosages of ustekinumab (i.e., 90 mg every eight weeks) may be necessary to treat patients with more refractory or unusual forms of disease. Although initial results are hopeful, further controlled studies are needed to assess the usefulness of ustekinumab in these conditions.

USTEKINUMAB DOSING

It should be emphasized that dosing for ustekinumab is infrequent and thus very convenient for patients with a chronic disease such as psoriasis. Currently, the FDA has approved ustekinumab for use as subcutaneous injections of 45 mg for individuals weighing less than 100 kg and of 90 mg for individuals weighing 100 kg or more. Approved dosing intervals are at weeks 0 and 4, and then every 12 weeks thereafter. In Canada and Europe, more flexible dosing is allowed if there is inadequate response to initial dosing, such as increasing the dose from 45 to 90 mg in patients less than 100 kg in weight and decreasing the long-term dosing interval from 12 to 8 weeks. Long-term dosing of ustekinumab at intervals greater than every 12 weeks is currently being explored in the PSTELLAR study (see http://www.clinicaltrials.gov/ct2/show/NCT01550744?term=PSTELLAR&rank=1.). This trial is evaluating and comparing dosing intervals of 12, 16, 20, and 24 weeks to determine optimal dosing for patients who are clear or near clear at week 28 following standard initial dosing. Results from this study may lead to even more convenient dosing intervals for a subset of psoriasis patients.

USTEKINUMAB SAFETY

Safety results from short-term [53–55] and longer-term [58,59,70,71] clinical trials are highly encouraging. Rates of infection were not higher in ustekinumab-treated patients when compared to placebo-treated patients over a 12-week period [53,54]. These rates remain very low with chronic use of ustekinumab (i.e., up to five years), and there does not appear to be any increase in infection rate with higher drug doses [53–55,58,59,70,71].

Insight on infection risk can also be gleaned from other diseases. Humans that have genetic defects in p40 or in the IL-12 receptor subunit, IL-12Rβ1, and thus either cannot produce IL-12/IL-23 or signal through the IL-12/IL-23 receptor, are susceptible to intracellular bacterial infections such as those caused by mycobacteria and *Salmonella enteritidis* [72–74]. However, there have not been cases of tuberculosis, atypical mycobacterial infection, or *Salmonella* infection reported with ustekinumab to date [53–55,58,59,70,71]. In fact, patients diagnosed with latent tuberculosis upon screening were allowed into the phase III ustekinumab trials as long as they received appropriate anti-tuberculous therapy; none of these individuals experienced worsening pulmonary disease [53,54,75]. Patients with a history of tuberculosis or those with potential to reactivate latent disease should either avoid treatment with ustekinumab or be treated with concomitant antituberculous medication [75].

Regarding the potential for ustekinumab-treated patients to develop malignancies, five-year studies show no significant signals [59,71]. In particular, the number of cases of lymphoma and squamous cell carcinomas—two cancers often associated with immunosuppression—is lower than what would be expected in the general population over a five-year period [59,71].

Although no clear cancer "signal" has yet emerged, this will be an important issue to study further with long-term ustekinumab therapy.

The roles that IL-23 and IL-12 play in the development of cancer are very controversial. Some studies have shown that these cytokines are pro-oncogenic, yet others point to an important role for these cytokines in generating anti-tumor T-cell immunity. The type of cancer seems to be important regarding the relative pro- or anti-oncogenic activity of IL-23 and IL-12 [3,76]. Making this even more confusing is that the IL-23/Th17 inflammatory pathway has mostly been shown to promote tumorigenesis [3], whereas the IL-12/Th1 inflammatory pathway is generally considered to block tumor formation [76]. Thus, it is difficult to predict whether cancer (and which type of cancer) will be promoted by blocking IL-23 and IL-12 function with ustekinumab use.

In early studies, five major adverse cardiovascular events (MACE) were reported in patients receiving ustekinumab within the first 12 weeks of therapy, whereas no cases in placebo-treated patients were noted during this time period [53,54]. These results were not statistically significant by standard methodology [77], but some have expressed concern with these numbers [78,79]. Of major importance, this possible initial signal has not been borne out in follow-up studies to date [55,70,71,79–81]. In fact, there is a suggestion from long-term studies that ustekinumab may not increase, but actually *decrease*, the likelihood of cardiovascular disease over time [71,81]. More long-term results are needed to clarify this important issue.

SUMMARY

Numerous recent studies suggest that psoriasis is a Th17-cell-mediated disease driven by IL-23 (Table 13.1). Thus, it is not surprising that therapeutic targeting of IL-23 by ustekinumab demonstrates considerable efficacy in psoriatics over a long period of time (Table 13.2). Although most scientists involved in studying psoriasis pathogenesis believe that ustekinumab principally acts through IL-23 inhibition (Table 13.1), additional research is required to prove this assertion. Indeed, testing programs of targeted drugs that block p19, and thus selectively block the IL-23/Th17 inflammatory pathway (e.g., guselkumab and tildrakizumab), are in late stages of clinical development (Figure 13.2). Thus far, these biologic therapies appear to offer the same short-term efficacy and safety when compared to ustekinumab. In summary, ustekinumab use is a major advance in the treatment of individuals with moderate to severe psoriasis based upon short-term and long-term efficacy, a reassuring safety profile with short-term and long-term use, and a convenient dosing schedule.

REFERENCES

1. Nestle FO, Kaplan DH, Barker J. Psoriasis. *N Engl J Med* 2009; 361(5): 496–509.
2. Di Cesare A, Di Meglio P, Nestle FO. The IL-23/Th17 axis in the immunopathogenesis of psoriasis. *J Invest Dermatol* 2009; 129: 1339–50.
3. Tesmer LA, Lundy SK, Sarkar S, Fox DA. Th17 cells in human disease. *Immunol Rev* 2008; 223: 87–113.
4. Blauvelt A. New concepts in the pathogenesis and treatment of psoriasis: key roles for IL-23, IL-17A and TGF-b1. *Expert Rev Dermatol* 2007; 2(1): 1–10.
5. Fitch E, Harper E, Skorcheva I, Kurtz SE, Blauvelt A. Pathophysiology of psoriasis: recent advances on IL-23 and Th17 cytokines. *Curr Rheumatol Rep* 2007; 9(6): 461–7.

6. Blauvelt A. T-helper 17 cells in psoriatic plaques and additional genetic links between IL-23 and psoriasis. *J Invest Dermatol* 2008; 128(5): 1064–7.
7. Mosmann TR, Cherwinski H, Bond MW, Giedlin MA, Coffman RL. Two types of murine helper T cell clone. I. Definition according to profiles of lymphokine activities and secreted proteins. *J Immunol* 1986; 136(7): 2348–57.
8. Harrington LE, Hatton RD, Mangan PR, Turner H, Murphy TL, Murphy KM, et al. Interleukin 17-producing CD4+ effector T cells develop via a lineage distinct from the T helper type 1 and 2 lineages. *Nat Immunol* 2005; 6(11): 1123–32.
9. Park H, Li Z, Yang XO, Chang SH, Nurieva R, Wang YH, et al. A distinct lineage of CD4 T cells regulates tissue inflammation by producing interleukin 17. *Nat Immunol* 2005; 6(11): 1133–41.
10. Murphy KM, Reiner SL. The lineage decisions of helper T cells. *Nat Rev Immunol* 2002; 2(12): 933–44.
11. Acosta-Rodriguez EV, Napolitani G, Lanzavecchia A, Sallusto F. Interleukins 1beta and 6 but not transforming growth factor-beta are essential for the differentiation of interleukin 17-producing human T helper cells. *Nat Immunol* 2007; 8(9): 942–9.
12. Wilson NJ, Boniface K, Chan JR, McKenzie BS, Blumenschein WM, Mattson JD, et al. Development, cytokine profile and function of human interleukin 17-producing helper T cells. *Nat Immunol* 2007; 8(9): 950–7.
13. Ivanov II, McKenzie BS, Zhou L, Tadokoro CE, Lepelley A, Lafaille JJ, et al. The orphan nuclear receptor RORgammat directs the differentiation program of proinflammatory IL-17+ T helper cells. *Cell* 2006; 126(6): 1121–33.
14. Nurieva R, Yang XO, Martinez G, Zhang Y, Panopoulos AD, Ma L, et al. Essential autocrine regulation by IL-21 in the generation of inflammatory T cells. *Nature* 2007; 448(7152): 480–3.
15. Oppmann B, Lesley R, Blom B, Timans JC, Xu Y, Hunte B, et al. Novel p19 protein engages IL-12p40 to form a cytokine, IL-23, with biological activities similar as well as distinct from IL-12. *Immunity* 2000; 13(5): 715–25.
16. Stockinger B, Veldhoen M. Differentiation and function of Th17 T cells. *Curr Opin Immunol* 2007; 19(3): 281–6.
17. Gerosa F, Baldani-Guerra B, Lyakh LA, Batoni G, Esin S, Winkler-Pickett RT, et al. Differential regulation of interleukin 12 and interleukin 23 production in human dendritic cells. *J Exp Med* 2008; 205(6): 1447–61.
18. Piskin G, Sylva-Steenland RM, Bos JD, Teunissen MB. *In vitro* and *in situ* expression of IL-23 by keratinocytes in healthy skin and psoriasis lesions: enhanced expression in psoriatic skin. *J Immunol* 2006; 176(3): 1908–15.
19. Acosta-Rodriguez EV, Rivino L, Geginat J, Jarrossay D, Gattorno M, Lanzavecchia A, et al. Surface phenotype and antigenic specificity of human interleukin 17-producing T helper memory cells. *Nat Immunol* 2007; 8(6): 639–46.
20. LeibundGut-Landmann S, Gross O, Robinson MJ, Osorio F, Slack EC, Tsoni SV, et al. Syk- and CARD9-dependent coupling of innate immunity to the induction of T helper cells that produce interleukin 17. *Nat Immunol* 2007; 8(6): 630–8.
21. Kagami S, Rizzo HL, Kurtz SE, Miller LS, Blauvelt A. IL-23 and IL-17A, but not IL-12 and IL-22, are required for optimal skin host defense against Candida albicans. *J Immunol* 2010; 185(9): 5453–62.
22. Re F, Strominger JL. Toll-like receptor 2 (TLR2) and TLR4 differentially activate human dendritic cells. *J Biol Chem* 2001; 276(40): 37692–9.
23. Higgins SC, Jarnicki AG, Lavelle EC, Mills KH. TLR4 mediates vaccine-induced protective cellular immunity to Bordetella pertussis: role of IL-17-producing T cells. *J Immunol* 2006; 177(11): 7980–9.
24. Wiekowski MT, Leach MW, Evans EW, Sullivan L, Chen SC, Vassileva G, et al. Ubiquitous transgenic expression of the IL-23 subunit p19 induces multiorgan inflammation, runting, infertility, and premature death. *J Immunol* 2001; 166(12): 7563–70.
25. Kopp T, Lenz P, Bello-Fernandez C, Kastelein RA, Kupper TS, Stingl G. IL-23 production by cosecretion of endogenous p19 and transgenic p40 in keratin 14/p40 transgenic mice: evidence for enhanced cutaneous immunity. *J Immunol* 2003; 170(11): 5438–44.
26. Chan JR, Blumenschein W, Murphy E, Diveu C, Wiekowski M, Abbondanzo S, et al. IL-23 stimulates epidermal hyperplasia via TNF and IL-20R2-dependent mechanisms with implications for psoriasis pathogenesis. *J Exp Med* 2006; 203(12): 2577–87.

27. Zheng Y, Danilenko DM, Valdez P, Kasman I, Eastham-Anderson J, Wu J, et al. Interleukin-22, a T(H)17 cytokine, mediates IL-23-induced dermal inflammation and acanthosis. *Nature* 2007; 445(7128): 648–51.
28. Rizzo HL, Kagami S, Phillips KG, Kurtz SE, Jacques SL, Blauvelt A. IL-23-mediated psoriasis-like epidermal hyperplasia is dependent on IL-17A. *J Immunol* 2011; 186(3): 1495–502.
29. Chamian F, Lowes MA, Lin SL, Lee E, Kikuchi T, Gilleaudeau P, et al. Alefacept reduces infiltrating T cells, activated dendritic cells, and inflammatory genes in psoriasis vulgaris. *Proc Natl Acad Sci U S A* 2005; 102(6): 2075–80.
30. Toichi E, Torres G, McCormick TS, Chang T, Mascelli MA, Kauffman CL, et al. An anti-IL-12p40 antibody down-regulates type 1 cytokines, chemokines, and IL-12/IL-23 in psoriasis. *J Immunol* 2006; 177(7): 4917–26.
31. Lee E, Trepicchio WL, Oestreicher JL, Pittman D, Wang F, Chamian F, et al. Increased expression of interleukin 23 p19 and p40 in lesional skin of patients with psoriasis vulgaris. *J Exp Med* 2004; 199(1): 125–30.
32. Lillis JV, Guo CS, Lee JJ, Blauvelt A. Increased IL-23 expression in palmoplantar psoriasis and hyperkeratotic hand dermatitis. *Arch Dermatol* 2010; 146(8): 918–19.
33. Piskin G, Tursen U, Sylva-Steenland RM, Bos JD, Teunissen MB. Clinical improvement in chronic plaque-type psoriasis lesions after narrow-band UVB therapy is accompanied by a decrease in the expression of IFN-gamma inducers—IL-12, IL-18 and IL-23. *Exp Dermatol* 2004; 13(12): 764–72.
34. Gottlieb AB, Chamian F, Masud S, Cardinale I, Abello MV, Lowes MA, et al. TNF inhibition rapidly down-regulates multiple proinflammatory pathways in psoriasis plaques. *J Immunol* 2005; 175(4): 2721–9.
35. Lowes MA, Chamian F, Abello MV, Fuentes-Duculan J, Lin SL, Nussbaum R, et al. Increase in TNF-alpha and inducible nitric oxide synthase-expressing dendritic cells in psoriasis and reduction with efalizumab (anti-CD11a). *Proc Natl Acad Sci U S A* 2005; 102(52): 19057–62.
36. Kagami S, Rizzo HL, Lee JJ, Koguchi Y, Blauvelt A. Circulating Th17, Th22, and Th1 cells are increased in psoriasis. *J Invest Dermatol* 2010; 130(5): 1373–83.
37. Tsunemi Y, Saeki H, Nakamura K, Sekiya T, Hirai K, Fujita H, et al. Interleukin-12 p40 gene (IL12B) 3'-untranslated region polymorphism is associated with susceptibility to atopic dermatitis and psoriasis vulgaris. *J Dermatol Sci* 2002; 30(2): 161–6.
38. Cargill M, Schrodi SJ, Chang M, Garcia VE, Brandon R, Callis KP, et al. A large-scale genetic association study confirms IL12B and leads to the identification of IL23R as psoriasis-risk genes. *Am J Hum Genet* 2007; 80(2): 273–90.
39. Capon F, Di Meglio P, Szaub J, Prescott NJ, Dunster C, Baumber L, et al. Sequence variants in the genes for the interleukin-23 receptor (IL23R) and its ligand (IL12B) confer protection against psoriasis. *Hum Genet* 2007; 122: 201–6.
40. Nair RP, Ruether A, Stuart PE, Jenisch S, Tejasvi T, Hiremagalore R, et al. Polymorphisms of the IL12B and IL23R genes are associated with psoriasis. *J Invest Dermatol* 2008; 128(7): 1653–61.
41. Nair RP, Stuart PE, Nistor I, Hiremagalore R, Chia NV, Jenisch S, et al. Sequence and haplotype analysis supports HLA-C as the psoriasis susceptibility 1 gene. *Am J Hum Genet* 2006; 78(5): 827–51.
42. Di Meglio P, Di Cesare A, Laggner U, Chu CC, Napolitano L, Villanova F, et al. The IL23R R381Q gene variant protects against immune-mediated diseases by impairing IL-23-induced Th17 effector response in humans. *PLoS One* 2011; 6(2): e17160.
43. Conrad C, Tonel G, Qin J, Xin H, Oldham E, Kastelein RA, et al. Functional dissection of interleukin-17 in the pathogenesis of psoriasis. *J Invest Dermatol* 2007; 127: S13.
44. Harper EG, Guo C, Rizzo H, Lillis JV, Kurtz SE, Skorcheva I, et al. Th17 cytokines stimulate CCL20 expression in keratinocytes *in vitro* and *in vivo*: implications for psoriasis pathogenesis. *J Invest Dermatol* 2009; 129: 2175–83.
45. Kryczek I, Bruce AT, Gudjonsson JE, Johnston A, Aphale A, Vatan L, et al. Induction of IL-17+ T cell trafficking and development by IFN-gamma: mechanism and pathological relevance in psoriasis. *J Immunol* 2008; 181(7): 4733–41.
46. Annunziato F, Cosmi L, Santarlasci V, Maggi L, Liotta F, Mazzinghi B, et al. Phenotypic and functional features of human Th17 cells. *J Exp Med* 2007; 204(8): 1849–61.
47. Clark RA, Chong B, Mirchandani N, Brinster NK, Yamanaka K, Dowgiert RK, et al. The vast majority of CLA+ T cells are resident in normal skin. *J Immunol* 2006; 176(7): 4431–9.

48. Homey B, Dieu-Nosjean MC, Wiesenborn A, Massacrier C, Pin JJ, Oldham E, et al. Up-regulation of macrophage inflammatory protein-3 alpha/CCL20 and CC chemokine receptor 6 in psoriasis. *J Immunol* 2000; 164(12): 6621–32.
49. Zaba LC, Cardinale I, Gilleaudeau P, Sullivan-Whalen M, Suarez Farinas M, Fuentes-Duculan J, et al. Amelioration of epidermal hyperplasia by TNF inhibition is associated with reduced Th17 responses. *J Exp Med* 2007; 204(13): 3183–94.
50. Kauffman CL, Aria N, Toichi E, McCormick TS, Cooper KD, Gottlieb AB, et al. A phase I study evaluating the safety, pharmacokinetics, and clinical response of a human IL-12 p40 antibody in subjects with plaque psoriasis. *J Invest Dermatol* 2004; 123(6): 1037–44.
51. Gottlieb AB, Cooper KD, McCormick TS, Toichi E, Everitt DE, Frederick B, et al. A phase 1, double-blind, placebo-controlled study evaluating single subcutaneous administrations of a human interleukin-12/23 monoclonal antibody in subjects with plaque psoriasis. *Curr Med Res Opin* 2007; 23(5): 1081–92.
52. Krueger GG, Langley RG, Leonardi C, Yeilding N, Guzzo C, Wang Y, et al. A human interleukin-12/23 monoclonal antibody for the treatment of psoriasis. *N Engl J Med* 2007; 356(6): 580–92.
53. Leonardi CL, Kimball AB, Papp KA, Yeilding N, Guzzo C, Wang Y, et al. Efficacy and safety of ustekinumab, a human interleukin-12/23 monoclonal antibody, in patients with psoriasis: 76-week results from a randomised, double-blind, placebo-controlled trial (PHOENIX 1). *Lancet* 2008; 371(9625): 1665–74.
54. Papp KA, Langley RG, Lebwohl M, Krueger GG, Szapary P, Yeilding N, et al. Efficacy and safety of ustekinumab, a human interleukin-12/23 monoclonal antibody, in patients with psoriasis: 52-week results from a randomised, double-blind, placebo-controlled trial (PHOENIX 2). *Lancet* 2008; 371(9625): 1675–84.
55. Griffiths CE, Strober BE, van de Kerkhof P, Ho V, Fidelus-Gort R, Yeilding N, et al. Comparison of ustekinumab and etanercept for moderate-to-severe psoriasis. *N Engl J Med* 2010; 362(2): 118–28.
56. Chu DH, Van Voorhees AS, Rosenbach M. Treatment of refractory tumor necrosis factor inhibitor-induced palmoplantar pustulosis: a report of 2 cases. *Arch Dermatol* 2011; 147(10): 1228–30.
57. Puig L, Morales-Munera CE, Lopez-Ferrer A, Geli C. Ustekinumab treatment of TNF antagonist-induced paradoxical psoriasis flare in a patient with psoriatic arthritis: case report and review. *Dermatology* 2012; 225(1): 14–17.
58. Lebwohl M, Leonardi C, Griffiths CE, Prinz JC, Szapary PO, Yeilding N, et al. Long-term safety experience of ustekinumab in patients with moderate-to-severe psoriasis (Part I of II): results from analyses of general safety parameters from pooled phase 2 and 3 clinical trials. *J Am Acad Dermatol* 2012; 66(5): 731–41.
59. Gordon KB, Papp KA, Langley RG, Ho V, Kimball AB, Guzzo C, et al. Long-term safety experience of ustekinumab in patients with moderate to severe psoriasis (Part II of II): results from analyses of infections and malignancy from pooled phase II and III clinical trials. *J Am Acad Dermatol* 2012; 66(5): 742–51.
60. Kimball AB, Papp KA, Wasfi Y, Chan D, Bissonnette R, Sofen H, et al. Long-term efficacy of ustekinumab in patients with moderate-to-severe psoriasis treated for up to 5 years in the PHOENIX 1 study. *J Eur Acad Dermatol Venereol* 2012. doi: 10.1111/jdv.12046.
61. de Souza A, Ali-Shaw T, Reddy SM, Fiorentino D, Strober BE. Inflammatory arthritis following ustekinumab treatment for psoriasis: a report of two cases. *Br J Dermatol* 2013; 168(1): 210–12.
62. Santos-Juanes J, Coto-Segura P, Mas-Vidal A, Galache Osuna C. Ustekinumab induces rapid clearing of erythrodermic psoriasis after failure of antitumour necrosis factor therapies. *Br J Dermatol* 2010; 162(5): 1144–6.
63. Wang TS, Tsai TF. Clinical experience of ustekinumab in the treatment of erythrodermic psoriasis: a case series. *J Dermatol* 2011; 38(11): 1096–9.
64. Castineiras I, Fernandez-Diaz L, Juarez Y, Lueiro M. Sustained efficacy of ustekinumab in refractory erythrodermic psoriasis after failure of antitumor necrosis factor therapies. *J Dermatol* 2012; 39(8): 730–1.
65. Buggiani G, D'Erme AM, Krysenka A, Pescitelli L, Lotti T, Prignano F. Efficacy of ustekinumab in sub-erythrodermic psoriasis: when TNF-blockers fail. *Dermatol Ther* 2012; 25(3): 283–5.
66. Gerdes S, Franke J, Domm S, Mrowietz U. Ustekinumab in the treatment of palmoplantar pustulosis. *Br J Dermatol* 2010; 163(5): 1116–18.

67. Bulai Livideanu C, Lahfa M, Mazereeuw-Hautier J, Paul C. Efficacy of ustekinumab in palmoplantar psoriasis. *Dermatology* 2010; 221(4): 321–3.
68. Au SC, Goldminz AM, Kim N, Dumont N, Michelon M, Volf E, et al. Investigator-initiated, open-label trial of ustekinumab for the treatment of moderate-to-severe palmoplantar psoriasis. *J Dermatolog Treat* 2013; 24(3): 179–87.
69. Morales-Munera C, Vilarrasa E, Puig L. Efficacy of ustekinumab in refractory palmoplantar pustular psoriasis. *Br J Dermatol* 2013; 168(4): 820–4.
70. Papp KA, Griffiths CE, Gordon K, Lebwohl M, Szapary PO, Wasfi Y, et al. Long-term safety of ustekinumab in patients with moderate-to-severe psoriasis: final results from 5 years of follow-up. *Br J Dermatol* 2013; 168(4): 844–54.
71. Papp KA, Strober B, Augustin M, Calabro S, Londhe A, Chevrier M, et al. PSOLAR: design, utility, and preliminary results of a prospective, international, disease-based registry of patients with psoriasis who are receiving, or are candidates for, conventional systemic treatments or biologic agents. *J Drugs Dermatol* 2012; 11(10): 1210–17.
72. de Jong R, Altare F, Haagen IA, Elferink DG, Boer T, van Breda Vriesman PJ, et al. Severe mycobacterial and Salmonella infections in interleukin-12 receptor-deficient patients. *Science* 1998; 280(5368): 1435–8.
73. Altare F, Lammas D, Revy P, Jouanguy E, Doffinger R, Lamhamedi S, et al. Inherited interleukin 12 deficiency in a child with bacille Calmette-Guerin and Salmonella enteritidis disseminated infection. *J Clin Invest* 1998; 102(12): 2035–40.
74. Altare F, Jouanguy E, Lamhamedi S, Doffinger R, Fischer A, Casanova JL. Mendelian susceptibility to mycobacterial infection in man. *Curr Opin Immunol* 1998; 10(4): 413–17.
75. Tsai TF, Ho V, Song M, Szapary P, Kato T, Wasfi Y, et al. The safety of ustekinumab treatment in patients with moderate-to-severe psoriasis and latent tuberculosis infection. *Br J Dermatol* 2012; 167(5): 1145–52.
76. Weiss JM, Subleski JJ, Wigginton JM, Wiltrout RH. Immunotherapy of cancer by IL-12-based cytokine combinations. *Expert Opin Biol Ther* 2007; 7(11): 1705–21.
77. Ryan C, Leonardi CL, Krueger JG, Kimball AB, Strober BE, Gordon KB, et al. Association between biologic therapies for chronic plaque psoriasis and cardiovascular events: a meta-analysis of randomized controlled trials. *JAMA* 2011; 306(8): 864–71.
78. Tzellos T, Kyrgidis A, Trigoni A, Zouboulis CC. Association of ustekinumab and briakinumab with major adverse cardiovascular events: an appraisal of meta-analyses and industry sponsored pooled analyses to date. *Dermatoendocrinol* 2012; 4(3): 320–3.
79. Dommasch ED, Troxel AB, Gelfand JM. Major cardiovascular events associated with anti-IL 12/23 agents: a tale of two meta-analyses. *J Am Acad Dermatol* 2013; 68(5): 863–5.
80. Reich K, Langley RG, Lebwohl M, Szapary P, Guzzo C, Yeilding N, et al. Cardiovascular safety of ustekinumab in patients with moderate to severe psoriasis: results of integrated analyses of data from phase II and III clinical studies. *Br J Dermatol* 2011; 164(4): 862–72.
81. Reich K, Papp KA, Griffiths CE, Szapary PO, Yeilding N, Wasfi Y, et al. An update on the long-term safety experience of ustekinumab: results from the psoriasis clinical development program with up to four years of follow-up. *J Drugs Dermatol* 2012; 11(3): 300–12.

Chapter 14

Infliximab

Ethan C. Levin, John Y. M. Koo, and Alice B. Gottlieb

INTRODUCTION

Infliximab (Remicade®) is the only intravenously infused biologic agent approved for the treatment of chronic severe plaque-type psoriasis in adults. The onset of action is very fast and thus, infliximabis also commonly used to treat emergent erythrodermic and pustular psoriasis (see Chapter 17). In addition to its use in dermatology, infliximab has been used for many years to treat other inflammatory diseases such as Crohn's disease, ulcerative colitis, rheumatoid arthritis, psoriatic arthritis, and ankylosing spondylitis.

The aim of this chapter is to familiarize the practicing dermatologist with the use of infliximab in severe plaque-type psoriasis; we will review the mechanism of action, efficacy in psoriasis, and safety profile.

MECHANISM OF ACTION

Structure

Infliximab is a chimeric immunoglobulin G1 (IgG1) kappa monoclonal antibody composed of human and murine variable regions (Figure 14.1) [1] that was developed to block tumor necrosis factor-α (TNF-α). Infliximab binds soluble and membrane-bound TNF-α, preventing it from activating its receptor. Each molecule of infliximab can bind two TNF-α molecules, while a maximum of three infliximab molecules can bind to a single TNF-α [2,3].

The Role of Tumor Necrosis Factor-α

TNF-α is a proinflammatory cytokine that is elevated in the psoriatic plaques [4] and sera in patients with psoriasis and is a key "driver" cytokine in the pathogenesis of psoriasis. The receptors for TNF-α are expressed on many cell types that are critical to psoriatic inflammation such as lymphocytes, endothelial cells, keratinocytes, and fibroblasts. Depending on the target cell, TNF-α signaling may (i) induce proinflammatory cytokines and chemokines (e.g., interleukin-1 [IL-1], IL-6, nuclear factor kappa B [NF-κB], chemokine ligand 27 [CCL27]), (ii) promote angiogenesis, (iii) induce keratinocyte proliferation, (iv) promote lymphocyte migration to the site of psoriatic inflammation, (v) activate neutrophils and eosinophils, (vi) induce acute phase reactants and tissue remodeling enzymes, or (vii) stimulate fibroblast growth. By blocking TNF-α, infliximab dampens a significant part of the inflammatory cascade that leads to the clinical appearance of psoriasis [3,5,6].

Specific Mechanisms

There are three mechanisms by which infliximab can neutralize the biologic activity of TNF-α. Infliximab can bind soluble TNF-α, preventing it from activating its cognate receptor. Infliximab may also bind TNF-α, which is already bound to its receptor, thus inactivating it.

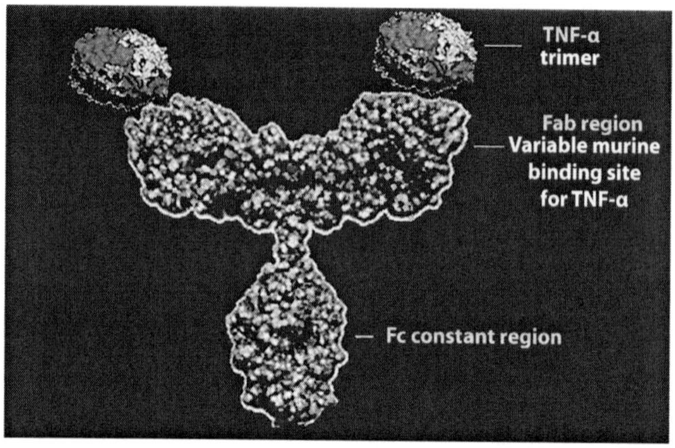

FIGURE 14.1 (See color insert.) Infliximab molecule. (Adapted from Knight DM et al., *Mol Immunol* 30, 1443–1453, 1993; Infliximab.)

Finally, infliximab may aid in complement- or antibody-mediated destruction of inflammatory cells that express the TNF-α receptor [2,5].

CLINICAL INDICATIONS AND DOSING

Infliximab is approved by the U.S. Food and Drug Administration (FDA) for adult use in many inflammatory diseases, including rheumatoid arthritis, Crohn's disease, ulcerative colitis, ankylosing spondylitis, psoriatic arthritis, and plaque psoriasis [7–17]. It is also approved for pediatric patients with Crohn's disease (older than six years of age). For treatment of severe plaque-type psoriasis, 5 mg/kg is administered at weeks 0, 2, and 6 followed by maintenance dosing every eight weeks. Clinicians may adjust the dosing frequency or amount in order to maintain the optimal therapeutic response. Maintenance dosing is sometimes administered as frequently as every four weeks. In other diseases, doses of up to 20 mg/kg have been given without any direct toxic effects [3].

When Is Infliximab Used in Psoriasis?

Infliximab is indicated for the treatment of adult patients with chronic severe (i.e., extensive and/or disabling) plaque psoriasis who are candidates for systemic therapy and when other systemic therapies are medically less appropriate. Due to its quick onset of action, infliximab is also recommended by the National Psoriasis Foundation as one of the first-line treatment options for severe erythrodermic or pustular psoriasis flares, which can be potentially life threatening (see Chapter 17) [18,19]. Any patient who starts infliximab must not have tuberculosis, active infection, or malignancy, and they will need to be closely monitored with regular follow-up visits [3].

PLACEBO-CONTROLLED CLINICAL TRIALS IN PSORIASIS: SPIRIT, EXPRESS I, AND EXPRESS II

Study Design

Prior to FDA approval of infliximab for use in severe plaque-type psoriasis, there were four randomized, double-blind, placebo-controlled studies that assessed safety and efficacy.

We will discuss the larger of the two phase II trials (SPIRIT) and both of the phase III trials (EXPRESS I and EXPRESS II) [2,20,21]. In all of these trials, key inclusion criteria were age greater than or equal to 18, plaque-type psoriasis with a body surface area (BSA) coverage of atleast 10%, and a Psoriasis Area and Severity Index (PASI) greater than or equal to 12.

No concomitant therapy was allowed. Patients who had guttate, erythrodermic, or pustular psoriasis were excluded [3].

The design of each study is simplified in a flow chart (Figure 14.2) [2,20,21] and is explained below:

- The SPIRIT study enrolled 249 patients. Patients were randomized to placebo or infliximab at 3 or 5 mg/kg. The medication was dosed at weeks 0, 2, and 6, followed by an extra dose at week 26 (only if the physician's global assessment [PGA] was more than 3). The primary end point was the percentage of patients who reached PASI 75 at week 10. The total study duration was 46 weeks [20].
- The EXPRESS I study enrolled 378 patients. Patients were randomized to placebo or infliximab 5 mg/kg. The medication was dosed at weeks 0, 2, and 6 (induction), followed by every eight weeks (maintenance). The primary end point was the percentage of patients who reached PASI 75 at week 10. The total study duration was 50 weeks [21].

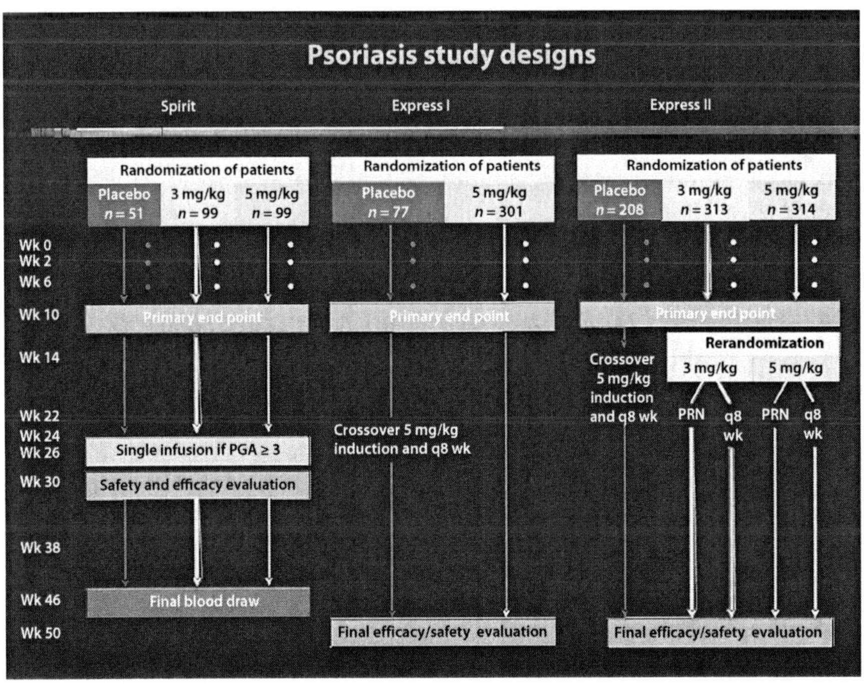

FIGURE 14.2 (See color insert.) Infliximab psoriasis clinical trial study designs. (Adapted from Menter A et al., *J Am Acad Dermatol* 56, 31.e1–15, 2007; Gottlieb AB et al., *J Am Acad Dermatol* 51, 534–542, 2004; and Reich K et al., *Lancet* 366, 1367–1374, 2005.)

- The EXPRESS II study enrolled 835 patients. Patients were randomized to placebo or infliximab at 3 or 5 mg/kg. The medication was dosed at weeks 0, 2, and 6. At week 14, those patients in either of the infliximab treatment arms were rerandomized to either every eight weeks or as needed maintenance dosing. The primary end point was the percentage of patients who reached PASI 75 at week 10. The total study duration was 50 weeks [2].

Results

In all three studies, over three-fourths of the patients in the 5 mg/kg dosing group reached PASI 75 by week 10 (vs. 2%–6% in placebo, $p < 0.001$ for all studies) (Figure 14.3) [2,20,21]. In addition, about half of patients in the 5 mg/kg dosing group reached PASI 90 by week 10 (vs. 1%–2% in placebo, $p < 0.001$ for all studies) (Figure 14.4) [2,20,21].

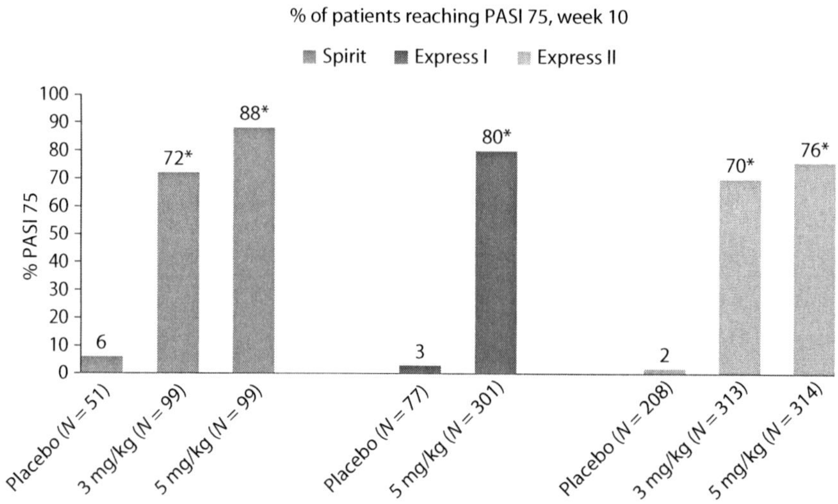

FIGURE 14.3 (See color insert.) PASI 75 responses at week 10 in infliximab psoriasis clinical trials. *$p < 0.001$ for comparison with placebo. (Adapted from Menter A et al., *J Am Acad Dermatol* 56, 31.e1–15, 2007; Gottlieb AB et al., *J Am Acad Dermatol* 51, 534–542, 2004; and Reich K et al., *Lancet* 366, 1367–1374, 2005.)

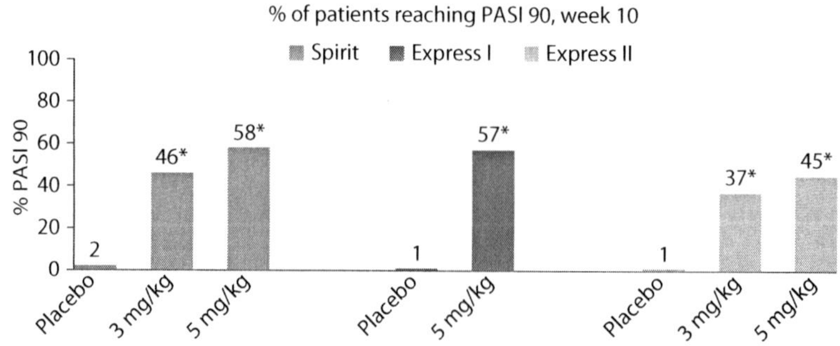

FIGURE 14.4 (See color insert.) PASI 90 responses at week 10 in infliximab psoriasis clinical trials. *$p < 0.001$ for comparison with placebo. (Adapted from Menter A et al., *J Am Acad Dermatol* 56, 31.e1–15, 2007; Gottlieb AB et al., *J Am Acad Dermatol* 51, 534–542, 2004; and Reich K et al., *Lancet* 366, 1367–1374, 2005.)

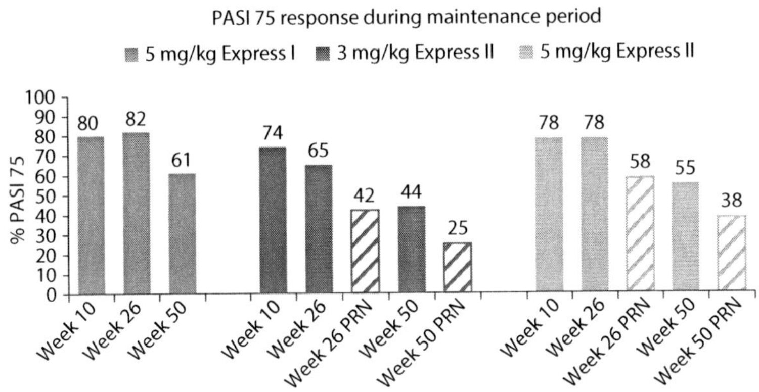

FIGURE 14.5 (See color insert.) Maintenance of clinical response: Percent of PASI 75 responders at weeks 10, 26, and 50 from EXPRESS I and II Study. *Note:* Week 10 reflects only those patients who were randomized to continue in the maintenance phase of the studies. "PRN" dosing: patients treated with infliximab if they have less than PASI 75 improvement from baseline (week 0) during monthly assessments. (Adapted from Menter A et al., *J Am Acad Dermatol* 56, 31.e1–15, 2007; Reich K et al., *Lancet* 366, 1367–1374, 2005.)

To measure durability of response, EXPRESS I and II continued to week 50 with regular maintenance dosing every eight weeks. At week 50, there were about 20% fewer patients at PASI 75 than at week 10 for both studies. This indicates that, over time, a significant percentage of patients who initially achieved PASI 75 failed to maintain their response (Figure 14.5) [2,21]. It should be noted that Figure 14.5 captures lack of efficacy and lack of tolerability (e.g., study discontinuation due to infusion reaction).

EXPRESS II was unique in that it assessed scheduled versus as needed maintenance dosing (defined as loss PASI 75). In the 3 mg/kg and 5 mg/kg dosing groups, about 15% more patients who received regular, every eight-week dosing maintained PASI 75 at week 50 compared to those that only received maintenance dosing as needed.

Safety

The safety of infliximab for severe plaque-type psoriasis is discussed at the end of the chapter with the exception of the RESTORE trial, which had to be terminated early due to safety concerns.

Summary

Phase II and III placebo-controlled clinical trials have shown that infliximab is an effective therapy for treating severe plaque-type psoriasis. In all of these studies, at least 75% of patients reached PASI 75 by week 10. Even with regular maintenance dosing, a significant number of patients may lose their response to infliximab over time (see discussion on "biologic fatigue" later in this chapter and in Chapter 15).

A Head-to-Head Study with Methotrexate, RESTORE I and II

Study Design There was one open-label phase IIIb study that compared the efficacy and safety of infliximab versus methotrexate in patients with moderate to severe plaque psoriasis

(RESTORE1) [22]. Key inclusion criteria included a PASI greater than or equal to 12 and at least 10% BSA of psoriasis. Patients were excluded if they had received any previous treatment with methotrexate or if they had received any biologic therapy within three months of the first study treatment.

The patients were randomized 3:1 to receive infliximab or methotrexate. Infliximab-treated patients received 5 mg/kg infusions at weeks 0, 2, 6, 14, and 22. Methotrexate-treated patients received 15 mg weekly for the first six weeks, with an option to increase the dose to 20 mg weekly thereafter (if PASI 25 was not reached). Patients who did not reach PASI 50 by week 16 were allowed to switch treatment groups. Treatment continued until week 26. The primary end point was PASI 75 at week 16.

At week 26, patients receiving infliximab who had reached PASI 75 were eligible to enroll in a two-and-a-half year open-label extension study in which they were assigned to continuous or intermittent infliximab therapy (RESTORE2) [23]. The continuous therapy arm received infliximab infusions every eight weeks. The intermittent therapy arm received therapy only after relapse, defined as loss of at least 50% of the total PASI improvement from baseline (i.e., PASI 50) during RESTORE1. After relapse, the patients received re-induction therapy, with up to four infliximab infusions at weeks 0, 2, 6, and 14, until the patient reached PASI 75. The primary end point of the extension study was PASI 75 at week 128.

Results Study investigators enrolled 868 patients of which 668 completed treatment; 41% of patients in the methotrexate group and 17% in the infliximab group discontinued therapy. The most common reason was crossover at week 16; 29% of patients randomized to methotrexate crossed over to infliximab therapy at week 16 (compared to 1% of patients randomized to infliximab who crossed over to methotrexate). The mean baseline characteristics were not significantly different between treatment groups and included an age of 44 years, weight of 84 kg, and PASI of 21.3.

At week 16, about twice as many patients in the infliximab group reached PASI 75 compared to patients in the methotrexate group (78% vs. 42%, $p < 0.001$).

In all, 441 patients continued into the extension study. The extension study was terminated by the sponsor after less than one year due to numerically more serious infusion related reactions in the intermittent therapy group (4%, 8/219) than the continuous therapy group (<1%, 1/222). By the time the study was terminated, about 80% of patients in the intermittent therapy group had received re-induction therapy, a median of approximately 4.5 months after the last dose of infliximab.

Safety In the base study, a similar proportion of patients in each group reported serious infections (2% in both groups). Through week 26, 12% of infliximab patients and 4% of methotrexate patients discontinued use due to adverse events. The most common reason for discontinuation in the infliximab group was infusion related reaction (11%). Of these reactions, 8% were considered moderate-or-severe (not defined).

In the extension study, the infusion reactions that resulted in study termination were considered severe, but not life threatening, and all resolved within one day. No further detail was reported. In total (including nonsevere), 15% of patients in the intermittent arm reported infusion-related reactions, of which 8% led to discontinuation; 15% of patients in the continuous arm reported infusion-related reactions, of which 5% led to discontinuation. There were more serious infections in the continuous dosing group (4%) than in the intermittent group (1%). This included one case of pulmonary tuberculosis (TB) and one case of disseminated TB.

Summary The RESTORE study was the first clinical trial that compared infliximab head-to-head with another systemic agent commonly used to treat moderate to severe psoriasis. In this study, infliximab was about twice as effective as methotrexate in achieving PASI 75 by week 16. Even though infliximab demonstrated superior efficacy, there was a significant proportion of patients who experienced an infusion reaction related to infliximab therapy. Further, infusion reactions during maintenance therapy appeared to be more likely with intermittent regimens than with continuous regimens and were most likely to occur during the second infusion of the re-induction period. Similar results were reported in a meta-analysis of inflammatory bowel disease patients treated with infliximab [24]. In this study, the formation of anti-infliximab antibodies, which are reported to be associated with infusion reactions, were three times as likely in the intermittent dosing group than in the every eight week dosing group (30% vs. 10%) [25–27].

A Study in Patients Who Failed Etanercept: PSUNRISE

Study Design The Prospective Study Using Remicade in Psoriasis Patients with an Inadequate Response to Etanercept (PSUNRISE) was a multicenter, open-label study in patients with moderate to severe plaque psoriasis with an inadequate response to etanercept [28]. Key inclusion criteria were a physician global assessment (PGA) of at least 2 on a scale of 0 to 5, prior treatment with etanercept for at least four months, and a two-week washout between last etanercept dose and first infliximab dose. Both cyclosporine and methotrexate were allowed as concomitant therapy only if started at least one month (for cyclosporine) and three months (for methotrexate) before screening and maintained at a stable dose throughout the study.

The patients were treated with infliximab 5mg/kg infusions at weeks 0, 2, 6, 14, and 22. At the end of the treatment period, the patients entered a follow-up period of four weeks. The primary end point was the percentage of patients who reached a PGA of "clear" (i.e., zero) or "minimal" (i.e., one) at week 10.

Results In all, 215 patients were enrolled and 179 completed treatment. The most common reasons for discontinuation were adverse events (n = 13) and lack of efficacy (n = 11). Seven patients (3.3%) used concomitant methotrexate and three patients used concomitant cyclosporine (1.4%). The mean baseline characteristics included an age of 44 years, weight of 94 kg, PASI of 11.6, and PGA of 2.8.

At week 10, 65% of patients reached a PGA of zero or one. Most patients maintained this response through week 26 (61%). In addition, more than half of the patients reached PASI 75 at week 10 (52%).

Summary The study investigators concluded that patients with moderate to severe plaque psoriasis and an inadequate response to etanercept may benefit from switching to infliximab therapy.

Combination Therapy: Infliximab + Methotrexate

FDA approval for the use of infliximab in moderate to severe plaque-type psoriasis came more than five years after other major inflammatory disease states such as rheumatoid arthritis and Crohn's disease. Therefore, it would be reasonable to assume that dermatologists might mimic successful therapeutic strategies commonly used in rheumatology or gastroenterology. In these specialties, infliximab is often used in combination with methotrexate to enhance and maintain the efficacy over time and to decrease the likelihood of infusion reactions.

In psoriatic arthritis, infliximab can be used with or without methotrexate. In rheumatoid arthritis, the only on-label use of infliximab is in combination with methotrexate, even in patients with early disease [29]. In fact, infliximab is the only anti-TNF biologic that is not recommended for use as monotherapy in rheumatoid arthritis. This is supported by numerous clinical trials showing superior efficacy with combination therapy [9,30,31]. Similarly, in Crohn's disease, infliximab combined with another immunosuppressant such as azathioprine or methotrexate is significantly more efficacious when compared to infliximab monotherapy [32–35]. This may be due to decreased formation of anti-infliximab antibodies when concomitant immunosuppression is used. The presence of anti-infliximab antibodies is associated with an increased risk for infusion reaction, lower post-infusion levels of infliximab, and a shorter duration of remission [25,26]. Both methotrexate and azathioprine have been shown to be equally effective in reducing the formation of anti-infliximab antibodies in inflammatory bowel disease [36]. In one study, about three-fourths of patients using infliximab monotherapy developed antibodies versus less than half of patients on combination therapy. It may be worth considering a similar regimen to treat moderate to severe psoriasis patients [37], although such a recommendation is off-label and there has never been a randomized clinical trial.

In one retrospective study, 23 cases of moderate to severe plaque psoriasis were treated with infliximab combined with either methotrexate or azathioprine [38]. The methotrexate was dosed 7.5–15 mg once weekly. Five patients could not tolerate methotrexate and instead received combination therapy with azathioprine 50 mg/day. The mean duration of follow-up was 26.5 months.

By week 14, 70% of patients had reached PASI 75. Only three patients discontinued therapy: two due to loss of efficacy and one due to a pulmonary embolism. There were no serious infections or other serious adverse events reported. There were four infusion reactions reported, only one of which led to treatment discontinuation. The other three reactions were mild and transient and included symptoms such as headache and dizziness. The treatment discontinuation rate due to serious adverse events in this study (<5%) seems favorable compared to other studies where rates range from 10% to 25% [22,23,39].

Another retrospective study on the use of infliximab for the treatment of moderate to severe psoriasis showed that concomitant methotrexate may reduce the risk of infusion reaction [40]. This study reviewed 59 patients who received a total of 858 infusions. Overall, 17% of patients had at least one infusion reaction. However, only 4% of patients treated with concomitant methotrexate were affected compared to 27% of those treated with infliximab monotherapy ($p = 0.05$).

It should be noted that the combination of infliximab and azathioprine in adolescent or young adult patients should be avoided because there have been reports of hepatosplenic T-cell lymphoma with inflammatory bowel disease in this patient demographic [41].

In summary, although combination therapy with infliximab and methotrexate may result in greater improvement in psoriasis, the greatest benefit may be in reducing the likelihood of anti-infliximab antibodies and subsequent risk of infusion reactions. These reactions are detrimental to the patient by causing the discontinuation of an effective therapy, loss of treatment efficacy, or rare anaphylactic-like reactions.

Biologic Fatigue and "Dose-Creep"

When comparing data from psoriasis clinical trials using TNF-α inhibitors (infliximab, adalimumab, etanercept), infliximab appears to have the highest number of patients who reached PASI 75 but subsequently lost their response [42]. This "biologic fatigue" may be due to the development of anti-infliximab antibodies, a hypothesis supported by studies that have reported significantly lower trough levels of infliximab in patients with anti-infliximab antibodies [43]. Furthermore, the presence of anti-infliximab antibodies are associated with loss of response to treatment [21].

Patients with elevated pretreatment anti-double-stranded DNA concentrations may be at the greatest risk for developing anti-drug antibodies and loss of response to infliximab [44]. Although the clinical trials data indicate that infliximab may have the largest loss of efficacy over time, other retrospective studies seem to contradict this finding [45].

One retrospective study of more than 800 treatment series of etanercept, adalimumab, and infliximab reviewed the four-year "retention rate" of each medication. This rate was determined by the percentage of patients who continued on each specific biologic medication over the four-year time period. The retention rate for infliximab was reported as almost twice that of the other TNF-α inhibitors (70% vs. 40% for both etanercept and adalimumab) [46]. There are a few possible explanations for this discrepancy. Most importantly, dosing in clinical trials is predetermined. Likewise, constant dosing of etanercept and adalimumab is recommended for all patients. However, infliximab is the only TNF-α inhibitor where dosing adjustments are allowed, in frequency and in absolute amount [47]. As a result, patients on infliximab often experience a "dose-creep," or an increase in dose or dose frequency in order to maintain the same response over time [48]. Therefore, although the mouse–human chimeric structure of infliximab may increase the likelihood of anti-drug antibody formation, a clear advantage of infliximab is the ability of clinicians to titrate the dose to maintain a satisfactory therapeutic response.

Safety

More than 5500 patients in clinical trials have been treated with infliximab worldwide, including more than 1500 psoriasis patients. The three aforementioned placebo-controlled clinical trials in psoriasis showed that, at week 16, the proportion of patients experiencing at least one serious adverse event (SAE) was as follows: 3.2% in the placebo group, 1.7% in the 3 mg/kg infliximab group, and 3.9% in the 5 mg/kg infliximab group. The SAEs reported in these trials were as follows: one death due to sepsis, two active cases of tuberculosis (TB), seven cases of nonmelanotic skin cancer (NMSC), and 15 cases of serum sickness or infusion reaction [3].

Black Box Warning

The most worrisome side effects noted with infliximab, given the black box warning by the FDA, are increased risk of infection, reactivation TB, and increased risk of malignancy. A brief description of each will be discussed here [3].

Increased Risk of Infection There have been fatalities secondary to infection reported in patients on infliximab, alone and in combination with other immunosuppressive agents. In psoriasis studies, the most common serious infection requiring hospitalization was abscess (skin, throat, and perirectal). Cases of bacterial sepsis were less common but more severe. For these reasons, infliximab should not be given to patients with a clinically active infection, chronic infection, or to those patients with a history of recurrent infections.

Furthermore, cases of histoplasmosis, coccidioidomycosis, listeriosis, pneumocystosis, and other bacterial, mycobacterial, and fungal infections have been observed. The FDA suggests careful consideration prior to initiation of infliximab for patients living in regions where histoplasmosis and coccidioidomycosis are endemic. As opposed to the most severe, the most common infections reported were upper respiratory and urinary tract infections [3,49].

Reactivation of Tuberculosis TB, oftentimes disseminated or extrapulmonary, has been observed in patients on infliximab. Thus, all patients should be evaluated for TB risk factors and be screened for active and latent tuberculosis *prior* to initiation of infliximab therapy. Treatment for latent infection should be initiated *prior* to infliximab use, although there is no specific recommendation for the duration of treatment prior to starting infliximab [3].

Increased Risk of Malignancy The black box warning for infliximab and increased risk of malignancy is specifically for hepatosplenic T-cell lymphoma, which is rare, aggressive, and usually fatal. The cases observed were shown to occur in adolescent and young adult patients with Crohn's disease who were on concomitant treatment with azathioprine or 6-mercaptopurine. Other malignancies associated with infliximab treatment that do not have a black box warning include other types of lymphomas and NMSC [49].

Other Side Effects

Infusion Reactions (Acute and Delayed Type Hypersensitivity) Infliximab is known to induce hypersensitivity reactions that vary in time of onset and severity. Infusion reactions can be categorized as acute (within 24 hours) or delayed (24 hours–14 days). Acute reactions can be mild to severe, with symptoms ranging from dizziness and headache to those seen in anaphylactic reactions. Delayed reactions occur 24 hours to 14 days after infusion and may include serum sickness–like symptoms, such as fever, rash, fatigue, myalgias, and arthralgia. In the event of a mild to moderate infusion reaction, the infusion should be stopped or slowed, and medications such as antihistamine, acetaminophen, or corticosteroids should be considered. If there is incomplete resolution of symptoms or new symptoms arise, the infusion should be discontinued altogether. In this case, infliximab should not be the treatment of choice in the future [50].

More severe infusion reactions have been associated with high levels of anti-infliximab antibodies, low serum concentrations of infliximab, as well as loss of efficacy of the medication. Factors that seem to reduce the incidence of infusion reactions included a regular maintenance dosing schedule (as opposed to as needed) and the addition of concomitant immunosuppressive medications, such as methotrexate [2,25,27,49]. The most severe reactions appear to occur early in treatment. In contrast, the available data suggest a potentially lower risk after 18 months of regular treatment without an infusion reaction [51].

In all completed clinical trials, 18% of patients treated with infliximab (average of six infusions per patient) reported an infusion reaction versus 5% of patients in the placebo group (average of four infusions per patient) (unpublished data, Centocor). In the three placebo-controlled psoriasis clinical trials discussed in this chapter, 23% of patients treated with infliximab experienced at least one infusion reaction versus 6% of patients in the placebo group. The increase in infusion reactions in the psoriasis studies may be due in part to the as needed maintenance dosing in the EXPRESS II trial and to the use of concomitant methotrexate in the studies of other disease states (i.e., rheumatoid arthritis). However, even with this increase, only 0.7% of patients treated with infliximab in the psoriasis trials experienced a serious infusion reaction.

With regard to the recommended infusion rate, the authors of a large British study of 858 infliximab infusions in 59 psoriasis patients recommend a two-hour infusion followed by a two-hour post-infusion monitoring period. If certain criteria are met, the infusion period may be shortened to one hour, with as little as 30 minutes of post-infusion monitoring [51].

Hepatotoxicity Infliximab-associated hepatic reactions have occurred, which in some cases were fatal or required transplantation. These included acute liver failure, jaundice, hepatitis, and/or cholestasis. In many cases, elevation in liver enzymes was not apparent prior to the hepatic injury. However, with elevations in liver enzymes greater than five times the upper limit of normal, infliximab should be discontinued. Patients should also be evaluated for signs and symptoms of liver dysfunction such as jaundice, icterus, hematuria, and abdominal pain prior to and after initiation of therapy.

Hematologic Events Infliximab has been reported to cause thrombocytopenia, leucopenia, neutropenia, and pancytopenia; thus, care should be exercised with patients who have hematologic abnormalities. Discontinuation of medication is recommended in cases of worsening blood dyscrasias.

Autoantibodies/Lupus-Like Syndrome Infliximab therapy is associated with the development of autoantibodies, including anti-nuclear (ANA), anti-double-stranded DNA (anti-dsDNA), and anti-nucleosome antibodies [52]. This has been reported in multiple disease states, including psoriasis, psoriatic arthritis, Crohn's disease, and rheumatoid arthritis [53–55]. Although many patients on infliximab develop autoantibodies, it is rarely associated with the onset of systemic lupus erythematosus (SLE) [56,57]. Moreover, anti-histone antibodies, which are often positive in drug-induced lupus, are rarely detected [58]. The clinical significance of these antibodies is not fully understood. Some studies have shown an association between the development of antinuclear antibodies and loss of response to infliximab [44,54,55]; other studies have failed to confirm this association [52].

Weight Gain TNF-α is involved in body weight homeostasis, and it is known to induce production and release of leptin, a satiety hormone. Therefore, it is possible that TNF-α inhibition could lead to decreased leptin levels, resulting in increased hunger and weight gain. This has been reported in multiple disease states treated with anti-TNF-α therapy, including psoriasis, spondyloarthropathy, and Crohn's disease [59–64]. In one retrospective study of 35 patients with psoriasis, average weight gain was 2.5 kg after one year (vs. −0.1 in control patients, $p = 0.003$) [64]. In addition, patients with a normal baseline weight experienced larger weight gain than those who were overweight or obese at baseline.

Contraindications/Precautions

Tuberculosis Infection Infliximab should not be administered to a patient with active TB infection, as discussed earlier.

Hepatitis B Infection Use of the TNF blockers (including infliximab) has been shown to reactivate hepatitis B virus (HBV) in patients who are chronic carriers. A hepatitis panel should be done prior to initiation of medication, and caution should be exercised in giving infliximab to patients identified as carriers. Discontinuation of anti-TNF therapy is required if reactivation occurs. Data are insufficient on whether concomitant use of anti-HBV agents prevents HBV reactivation.

Congestive Heart Failure The use of infliximab in patients with heart failure (class III/IV) may increase mortality rate and/or increase incidence of adverse cardiovascular events (dyspnea, angina, hypotension, and dizziness) [47]. Thus, this medication should only be used after other treatment options have been exhausted. Patients must be monitored for signs or symptoms of worsening failure and the medication discontinued if new or worsening symptoms occur.

Previous History of Malignancy It is recommended to avoid the use of infliximab and other biologic agents in patients with a history of previous malignancy or a current malignancy due to the medication's immunosuppressive effects. If it is a necessity, infliximab should be administered in close collaboration with the prescribing physician and an oncologist.

Live Vaccinations There is no available data on anti-TNF agents with regard to live vaccinations. However, it is recommended that live vaccinations not be given at the same time as infliximab treatment due to the potential for poor response of the vaccination or because of the potential for secondary transmission of infection. Furthermore, it is suggested that a physician should ensure a patient's vaccinations are up to date prior to initiation of infliximab or other biologic agents. All vaccines that are not live are acceptable to administer to a patient while undergoing treatment with infliximab [3].

Central Nervous System Disorders The initiation of infliximab (and other anti-TNF agents) should be cautiously considered in patients with preexisting central nervous system (CNS) demyelinating disorders, such as multiple sclerosis or CNS vasculitis, and in patients with new onset seizure disorder. Discontinuation of medication is recommended if CNS changes occur while on infliximab.

Drug Interactions—Anakinra The combination of anakinra and infliximab is not recommended due to the theoretical class risk of serious infections, as previously seen with concurrent use of anakinra and etanercept (another anti-TNF agent) [3].

Pregnancy/Lactation Infliximab is pregnancy category B. It is not known whether it or other anti-TNF agents can cause harm to a developing fetus; thus, it should be given to pregnant women only if absolutely needed. Lactating women should not breast-feed their infants because it is unknown whether infliximab is excreted in breast milk.

Monitoring

Required All patients need to be screened for TB with a quantiFERON® TB gold or purified protein derivative (PPD) test prior to initiating infliximab therapy. Once therapy is started, patients need to be screened yearly for TB. Patients with positive TB screening need to have a workup to rule out active TB (usually a chest X-ray or chest computerized tomography [CT] scan). If active TB is ruled out, treatment for latent infection needs to be initiated prior to infliximab use. Although the label does not indicate a specific duration of therapy, the authors recommend one to two months of treatment before starting infliximab [3,49]. After completing adequate prophylaxis, yearly chest imaging is needed to evaluate for reactivation TB.

Optional Optional monitoring should be considered based on infliximab's safety profile and that of other known anti-TNF agents. At baseline, complete blood count (CBC), liver function testing (LFT), hepatitis panel, and pregnancy testing are recommended.

With ongoing infliximab therapy, patients should be evaluated by a physician and obtain CBC and LFTs approximately every three months. LFTs are especially important to monitor for hepatotoxicity [3,49].

SUMMARY

Infliximab is an important medication in the treatment of psoriasis and other immune-mediated inflammatory diseases [3,49]. Phase II and III studies in psoriasis have shown impressive efficacy, with 76%–88% of patients reaching PASI 75 at week 10. This response is also rapid, which makes infliximab a first-line agent in treating psoriatic emergencies (see Chapter 17). Even though infliximab has a fast onset of action and is highly efficacious, the response appears to wane over time, with as many as 20% of patients losing the PASI 75 response by week 50 in Phase III studies, despite infusions every eight weeks [21]. This effect is even more pronounced when infliximab is used intermittently or on an as needed basis. Thus, due to biologic fatigue, many patients experience a "dose-creep" in order to maintain efficacy.

Infliximab's mechanism of administration via intravenous infusion is unique in dermatology, setting it apart from the other agents that have a more common form of administration—subcutaneous injection (adalimumab, etanercept, and ustekinumab). Perhaps the most unique side effect is the infusion reaction and serum sickness associated with infliximab. These reactions are seen more frequently in patients who have developed anti-infliximab antibodies, which are exacerbated by intermittent dosing [2]. Conversely, regular dosing and the use of concomitant immunomodulators, such as methotrexate, may decrease the incidence of infusion reactions [49].

CONCLUSION

There have been no comprehensive head-to-head comparisons of the ever-growing class of biologic agents. Although the British Association of Dermatology and the American Academy of Dermatology stop short of suggesting a specific biologic agent for specific types of patients, it is understood that each medication has characteristics that may make it more or less suitable for a specific situation. At the time of this writing, infliximab is the most efficacious biologic agent approved for the treatment of chronic severe psoriasis, and it has a quick onset of action. Therefore, it may be particularly useful in highly treatment-resistant cases of severe plaque-type psoriasis or in cases where response to treatment can be lifesaving, such as in an erythrodermic or pustular flare. Infliximab may be used for any patient with chronic, severe psoriasis. However, Algorithm 14.1 describes cases in which infliximab may be extra helpful.

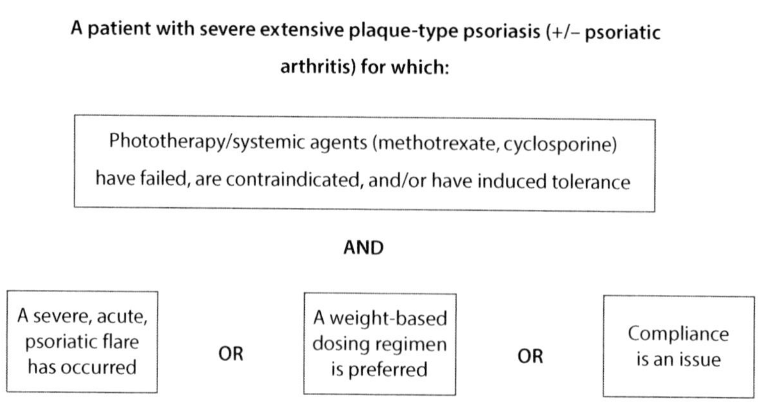

ALGORITHM 14.1 The ideal infliximab candidate.

REFERENCES

1. Knight DM, Trinh H, Le J, et al. Construction and initial characterization of a mouse-human chimeric anti-TNF antibody. *Mol Immunol* 1993; 30(16): 1443–1453.
2. Menter A, Feldman S, Weinstein GD, et al. A randomized comparison of continuous vs. intermittent infliximab maintenance regimens over one year in the treatment of moderate-to-severe plaque psoriasis (EXPRESS II). *J Am Acad Dermatol* 2007; 56(1): 31.e1–15.
3. Infliximab Full Prescribing Information [package insert]. Janssen Biotech, Inc. Horsham, PA 19044. November 2013.
4. Turbitt ML, Akhurst RJ, White SI, MacKie RM. Localization of elevated transforming growth factor-alpha in psoriatic epidermis. *J Invest Dermatol* 1990; 95(2): 229–232.
5. Gotlieb AB. Infliximab for psoriasis. *J Am Acad Dermatol* 2003; 49(2 Suppl): S112–S117.
6. Tracey D, Klareskog L, Sasso EH, et al. Tumor necrosis factor antagonist mechanisms of action: a comprehensive review. *Pharmacol Ther* 2008; 117(2): 244–279.
7. Maini R, St Clair EW, Breedveld F, et al. Infliximab (chimeric anti-tumour necrosis factor alpha monoclonal antibody) versus placebo in rheumatoid arthritis patients receiving concomitant methotrexate: a randomised phase III trial. ATTRACT Study Group. *Lancet* 1999; 354(9194): 1932–1939.
8. St Clair EW, Wagner CL, Fasanmade AA, et al. The relationship of serum infliximab concentrations to clinical improvement in rheumatoid arthritis: results from ATTRACT, a multicenter, randomized, double-blind, placebo-controlled trial. *Arthritis Rheum* 2002; 46(6): 1451–1459.
9. St Clair EW, van der Heijde DM, Smolen JS, et al. Combination of infliximab and methotrexate therapy for early rheumatoid arthritis: a randomized, controlled trial. *Arthritis Rheum* 2004; 50(11): 3432–3443.
10. Smolen JS, Van Der Heijde DM, St Clair EW, et al. Predictors of joint damage in patients with early rheumatoid arthritis treated with high-dose methotrexate with or without concomitant infliximab: results from the ASPIRE trial. *Arthritis Rheum* 2006; 54(3): 702–710.
11. Targan SR, Hanauer SB, van Deventer SJ, et al. A short-term study of chimeric monoclonal antibody cA2 to tumor necrosis factor alpha for Crohn's disease. Crohn's Disease cA2 Study Group. *N Engl J Med* 1997; 337(15): 1029–1035.
12. Hanauer SB, Feagan BG, Lichtenstein GR, et al. Maintenance infliximab for Crohn's disease: the ACCENT I randomized trial. *Lancet* 2002; 359(9317): 1541–1549.
13. Van der Heijde D, Dijkmans B, Geuses B, et al. Efficacy and safety of infliximab in patients with ankylosing spondylitis (ASSERT). *Arthritis Rheum* 2005; 52(2): 582–591.
14. Antoni CE, Kavanaugh A, Kirkham B, et al. Sustained benefits of infliximab therapy for dermatologic and articular manifestations of psoriatic arthritis (IMPACT). *Arthritis Rheum* 2005; 52(4): 1227–1236.
15. Antoni CE, Krueger GG, de Vlam K, et al. Infliximab improves signs and symptoms of psoriatic arthritis: results of the IMPACT 2 trial. *Ann Rheum Dis* 2005; 64: 1150–1157.
16. Gottlieb A, Korman NJ, Gordon KB, et al. Guidelines of the care for the management of psoriasis and psoriatic arthritis. Section 2. Psoriatic arthritis: overview and guidelines of care for treatment with an emphasis on the biologics. *J Am Acad Derm* 2008; 58: 851–864.
17. Rutgeerts P, Sandborn WJ, Feagan BG, et al. Infliximab for induction and maintenance therapy for ulcerative colitis. *N Engl J Med* 2005; 353(23): 2462–2476.
18. Robinson A, Van Voorhees AS, Hsu S, et al. Treatment of pustular psoriasis: from the Medical Board of the National Psoriasis Foundation. *J Am Acad Dermatol* 2012; 67(2): 279–288.
19. Rosenbach M, Hsu S, Korman NJ, et al. Treatment of erythrodermic psoriasis: from the medical board of the National Psoriasis Foundation. *J Am Acad Dermatol* 2010; 62(4): 655–662.
20. Gottlieb AB, Evans R, Li S, et al. Infliximab induction therapy for patients with severe plaque-type psoriasis: a randomized, double-blind, placebo controlled trial (SPIRIT). *J Am Acad Dermatol* 2004; 51: 534–542.
21. Reich K, Nestle FO, Papp K, et al. Infliximab induction and maintenance therapy for moderate-to-severe psoriasis: a phase III, multicenter, double-blind trial (EXPRESS I). *Lancet* 2005; 366: 1367–1374.
22. Barker J, Hoffmann M, Wozel G, et al. Efficacy and safety of infliximab vs. methotrexate in patients with moderate-to-severe plaque psoriasis: results of an open-label, active-controlled, randomized trial (RESTORE1). *Br J Dermatol* 2011; 165(5): 1109–1117.

23. Reich K, Wozel G, Zheng H, et al. Efficacy and safety of infliximab as continuous or intermittent therapy in patients with moderate-to-severe plaque psoriasis: results of a randomised, long-term extension trial (RESTORE2). *Br J Dermatol* 2013; 168: 1325–1334.
24. Steenholdt C, Svenson M, Bendtzen K, et al. Severe infusion reactions to infliximab: aetiology, immunogenicity and risk factors in patients with inflammatory bowel disease. *Aliment Pharmacol Ther* 2011; 34(1): 51–58.
25. Baert F, Noman M, Vermeire S, et al. Influence of immunogenicity on the long-term efficacy of infliximab in Crohn's disease. *N Engl J Med* 2003; 348(7): 601–608.
26. Farrell RJ, Alsahli M, Jeen YT, et al. Intravenous hydrocortisone premedication reduces antibodies to infliximab in Crohn's disease: a randomized controlled trial. *Gastroenterology* 2003; 124(4): 917–924.
27. Hanauer SB, Wagner CL, Bala M, et al. Incidence and importance of antibody responses to infliximab after maintenance or episodic treatment in Crohn's disease. *Clin Gastroenterol Hepatol* 2004; 2(7): 542–553.
28. Gottlieb AB, Kalb RE, Blauvelt A, et al. The efficacy and safety of infliximab in patients with plaque psoriasis who had an inadequate response to etanercept: results of a prospective, multicenter, open-label study. *J Am Acad Dermatol* 2012; 67(4): 642–650.
29. Singh JA, Furst DE, Bharat A, et al. 2012 update of the 2008 American College of Rheumatology recommendations for the use of disease-modifying antirheumatic drugs and biologic agents in the treatment of rheumatoid arthritis. *Arthritis Care Res* 2012; 64(5): 625–639.
30. Smolen JS, Han C, van der Heijde D, et al. Infliximab treatment maintains employability in patients with early rheumatoid arthritis. *Arthritis Rheum* 2006; 54(3): 716–722.
31. van der Kooij SM, le Cessie S, Goekoop-Ruiterman YP, et al. Clinical and radiological efficacy of initial vs delayed treatment with infliximab plus methotrexate in patients with early rheumatoid arthritis. *Ann Rheum Dis* 2009; 68(7): 1153–1158.
32. Arnott ID, McNeill G, Satsangi J. An analysis of factors influencing short-term and sustained response to infliximab treatment for Crohn's disease. *Aliment Pharmacol Ther* 2003; 17(12): 1451–1457.
33. Parsi MA, Achkar JP, Richardson S, et al. Predictors of response to infliximab in patients with Crohn's disease. *Gastroenterology* 2002; 123(3): 707–713.
34. Rutgeerts P, Van Assche G, Vermeire S. Review article: infliximab therapy for inflammatory bowel disease—seven years on. *Aliment Pharmacol Ther* 2006; 23(4): 451–463.
35. Vermeire S, Louis E, Carbonez A, et al. Demographic and clinical parameters influencing the short-term outcome of anti-tumor necrosis factor (infliximab) treatment in Crohn's disease. *Am J Gastroenterol* 2002; 97(9): 2357–2363.
36. Vermeire S, Noman M, Van Assche G, et al. Effectiveness of concomitant immunosuppressive therapy in suppressing the formation of antibodies to infliximab in Crohn's disease. *Gut* 2007; 56(9): 1226–1231.
37. Warren RB, Brown BC, Carmichael AJ, et al. Long-term control of recalcitrant psoriasis with combination infliximab and methotrexate. *Clin Exp Dermatol* 2009; 34(3): 415–416.
38. Dalaker M, Bonesronning JH. Long-term maintenance treatment of moderate-to-severe plaque psoriasis with infliximab in combination with methotrexate or azathioprine in a retrospective cohort. *J Eur Acad Dermatol Venereol* 2009; 23(3): 277–282.
39. Smith CH, Jackson K, Bashir SJ, et al. Infliximab for severe, treatment-resistant psoriasis: a prospective, open-label study. *Br J Dermatol* 2006; 155(1): 160–169.
40. Wee JS, Petrof G, Jackson K, et al. Infliximab for the treatment of psoriasis in the U.K.: 9 years' experience of infusion reactions at a single centre. *Br J Dermatol* 2012; 167(2): 411–416.
41. Mackey AC, Green L, Liang LC, et al. Hepatosplenic T cell lymphoma associated with infliximab use in young patients treated for inflammatory bowel disease. *J Pediatr Gastroenterol Nutr* 2007; 44(2): 265–267.
42. Noiles K, Vender R. Biologic survival. *J Drugs Dermatol* 2009; 8(4): 329–333.
43. Takahashi H, Tsuji H, Ishida-Yamamoto A, et al. Plasma trough levels of adalimumab and infliximab in terms of clinical efficacy during the treatment of psoriasis. *J Dermatol* 2013; 40(1): 39–42.
44. Hoffmann JH, Hartmann M, Enk AH, et al. Autoantibodies in psoriasis as predictors for loss of response and anti-infliximab antibody induction. *Br J Dermatol* 2011; 165(6): 1355–1358.
45. Escande H, Livideanu CB, Steiner A, et al. Incidence and risk factors for treatment failure with infliximab in psoriasis. *J Eur Acad Dermatol Venereol* 2013; 27(10): 1323–1324.

46. Gniadecki R, Kragballe K, Dam TN, et al. Comparison of drug survival rates for adalimumab, etanercept and infliximab in patients with psoriasis vulgaris. *Br J Dermatol* 2011; 164(5): 1091–1096.
47. Reich K, Griffiths C, Barker J, et al. Recommendations for the long-term treatment of psoriasis with infliximab: a dermatology expert group consensus. *Dermatology* 2008; 217(3): 268–275.
48. Mehren CR, Gniadecki R. Dose-creep of infliximab during psoriasis treatment: an observational study. *Acta Derm Venereol* 2012; 92(4): 355–357.
49. Menter A, Gottlieb A, Feldman SR, et al. Guidelines of the care for the management of psoriasis and psoriatic arthritis. Section 1. Overview of psoriasis and guidelines of care for the treatment of psoriasis with biologics. *J Am Acad Derm* 2008; 58: 826–850.
50. Cheifetz A, Smedley M, Martin S, et al. The incidence and management of infusion reactions to infliximab: a large center experience. *Am J Gastro* 2003; 98(2): 1315–1324.
51. Boehncke WH, Gottlieg AB. Therapies for psoriasis: a systematic review. *J Rheumatol* 2006; 33: 1447–1451.
52. Lora V, Bonaguri C, Gisondi P, et al. Autoantibody induction and adipokine levels in patients with psoriasis treated with infliximab. *Immunol Res* 2013; 56: 382–389.
53. Atzeni F, Talotta R, Salaffi F, et al. Immunogenicity and autoimmunity during anti-TNF therapy. *Autoimmun Rev* 2013; 12(7): 703–708.
54. Pink AE, Fonia A, Allen MH, et al. Antinuclear antibodies associate with loss of response to antitumour necrosis factor-alpha therapy in psoriasis: a retrospective, observational study. *Br J Dermatol* 2010; 162(4): 780–785.
55. Poulalhon N, Begon E, Lebbe C, et al. A follow-up study in 28 patients treated with infliximab for severe recalcitrant psoriasis: evidence for efficacy and high incidence of biological autoimmunity. *Br J Dermatol* 2007; 156(2): 329–336.
56. Caramaschi P, Biasi D, Colombatti M, et al. Anti-TNFalpha therapy in rheumatoid arthritis and autoimmunity. *Rheumatol Int* 2006; 26(3): 209–214.
57. De Bandt M, Sibilia J, Le Loet X, et al. Systemic lupus erythematosus induced by anti-tumour necrosis factor alpha therapy: a French national survey. *Arthritis Res Ther* 2005; 7(3): R545–551.
58. Shen GQ, Shoenfeld Y, Peter JB. Anti-DNA, antihistone, and antinucleosome antibodies in systemic lupus erythematosus and drug-induced lupus. *Clin Rev Allergy Immunol* 1998; 16(3): 321–334.
59. Briot K, Garnero P, Le Henanff A, et al. Body weight, body composition, and bone turnover changes in patients with spondyloarthropathy receiving anti-tumour necrosis factor {alpha} treatment. *Ann Rheum Dis* 2005; 64(8): 1137–1140.
60. Franchimont D, Roland S, Gustot T, et al. Impact of infliximab on serum leptin levels in patients with Crohn's disease. *J Clin Endocrinol Metab* 2005; 90(6): 3510–3516.
61. Gisondi P, Cotena C, Tessari G, et al. Anti-tumour necrosis factor-alpha therapy increases body weight in patients with chronic plaque psoriasis: a retrospective cohort study. *J Eur Acad Dermatol Venereol* 2008; 22(3): 341–344.
62. Renzo LD, Saraceno R, Schipani C, et al. Prospective assessment of body weight and body composition changes in patients with psoriasis receiving anti-TNF-alpha treatment. *Dermatol Ther* 2011; 24(4): 446–451.
63. Saraceno R, Schipani C, Mazzotta A, et al. Effect of anti-tumor necrosis factor-alpha therapies on body mass index in patients with psoriasis. *Pharmacol Res* 2008; 57(4): 290–295.
64. Florin V, Cottencin AC, Delaporte E, et al. Body weight increment in patients treated with infliximab for plaque psoriasis. *J Eur Acad Dermatol Venereol* 2013; 27(2): e186–190.

Chapter 15

Biologic Fatigue

Ethan C. Levin and John Y. M. Koo

INTRODUCTION

Over the past 15 years, biologic therapy has greatly enhanced the efficacy of psoriasis treatment. However, one of its main limitations is immunogenicity. Biologic molecules are seen as foreign "invaders" by the host immune system and may induce an adaptive immune response characterized by the formation of antidrug antibodies. Over time, the medication may lose effectiveness and result in clinical worsening of the patient. This is known as biologic fatigue. The prevailing hypothesis is that biologic fatigue is, at least in part, due to the development of antidrug antibodies. The presence of these antibodies is associated with lower trough levels of medication as well as a loss of response to treatment [1,2].

Although the loss of effectiveness of biologic therapy over time and the development of antidrug antibodies have been reported by many studies, the phenomenon is not fully understood. Little is known about the risk factors for biologic fatigue, and there are no standardized antidrug antibody tests available to clinicians. Further, the clinical reliability of such tests is unknown. More importantly, there is a need to develop clinical strategies that maximize the durability of response to a particular agent. In this chapter, we will review the available data on biologic fatigue for the medications approved to treat moderate to severe psoriasis. We hope to make practical recommendations to clinicians for optimally managing patients on biologic medications in order to minimize biologic fatigue.

Clinical Trials

We reviewed the longest reported phase III clinical trials for infliximab, adalimumab, etanercept, and ustekinumab in order to determine the percentage of patients who initially responded to the biologic therapy (i.e., achieved Psoriasis Area and Severity Index [PASI] 75) and then subsequently lost their response (i.e., lost PASI 75). Any reports of antidrug antibodies were noted in order to identify any other studies that may have addressed loss of response to biologic therapy due to antidrug antibodies.

Etanercept

The long-term efficacy of etanercept for the treatment of psoriasis was analyzed in a 96-week study of more than 600 patients (Table 15.1) [2–5]. In this study, the PASI 75 response rate peaked at 63% at week 48. Of the patients who reached PASI 75 at week 48, 74% of patients maintained this response at week 96. Overall 18% of patients tested positive for anti-etanercept antibodies at least once during the study. However, these antibodies were not associated with a decrease in efficacy, and thus were determined to be nonneutralizing [3].

TABLE 15.1 Summary of Loss of PASI 75 Response in Phase III Clinical Trials

	Number of Patients	Study Period	Time Period (Years)	% of Patients Losing PASI 75	Associated with Antidrug Antibodies?
Etanercept	320	Weeks 48–96	0.9	26	No[a]
Adalimumab	233	Weeks 33–160	2.4	24	Testing not performed
Ustekinumab	162[b]	Weeks 40–244	3.9	20	No
Infliximab	229	Weeks 10–50	0.8	32	Yes

Source: Reich K et al., *Lancet* 366, 1367–1374, 2005; Tyring S et al., *Arch Dermatol* 143, 719–726, 2007; Gordon K et al., *J Am Acad Dermatol* 66, 241–251, 2012; Kimball AB et al., *J Eur Acad Dermatol Venereol* 2012.

Disclaimer: These studies are not "head-to-head" comparisons. Maintenance dosing for all the studies was as per U.S. Food and Drug Administration labeling.

[a] 18% of patients tested positive for "nonneutralizing" anti-etanercept antibodies (i.e., not associated with a decrease in efficacy).

[b] 77 patients received 45 mg and 85 patients receiving 90 mg maintenance dosing every three months.

Adalimumab

The long-term efficacy of adalimumab for the treatment of psoriasis was analyzed in a 160-week (three-year) study [4]. At week 33, there were 233 patients who reached PASI 75 and were assigned to receive continuous every other week adalimumab for the duration of the study; 76% of these patients maintained PASI 75 at the final study assessment (week 160). Interestingly, the majority of patients who lost their PASI 75 response did so between weeks 33 and 52 [4]. During these weeks, twice as many week 33 responders lost their PASI 75 response compared to the following two years (weeks 52–160) (16% vs. 8%). Although this study did not report antidrug antibody testing, a one-year phase III study reported anti-adalimumab antibodies in 9% of all subjects, of which three of seven (43%) lost a response (vs. 28% of patients who were anti-adalimumab antibody negative) [6].

Ustekinumab

The long-term efficacy of ustekinumab for the treatment of psoriasis was analyzed in a 244-week (4.7-year) study [5]. At week 40, there were 162 patients who reached PASI 75 and were assigned to receive ustekinumab every three months for the duration of the study. About 80% of these patients maintained PASI 75 through the final assessment at week 244. Like adalimumab, the majority of patients who lost their response did so relatively early in the long course of the study. For patients taking ustekinumab, this occurred between weeks 40 and 76. In fact, this time period accounted for four out of every five patients who lost their response, with the remainder of patients losing response over the next 3.3 years. The study reported that loss of response was not associated with decreasing ustekinumab concentrations or with development of anti-ustekinumab antibodies (numbers not reported). Prior phase III studies of one year in length reported anti-ustekinumab antibodies in about 5% of all patients. However, the association with loss of response was not reported [7,8].

Infliximab

The long-term efficacy of infliximab for the treatment of psoriasis was analyzed in two 50-week studies [2,9]. Only the smaller study reported maintenance of response in the group of patients who achieved PASI 75 at week 10 (Table 15.1) [2]. In this study, 229 patients who reached PASI 75 at week 10 were assigned to receive infliximab every eight weeks for the duration of the study. About 68% of these patients maintained PASI 75 through week 50. The larger study, which enrolled more than twice as many patients, reported the percentage of *all* patients who achieved PASI 75 at week 50 (i.e., including those patients who were not PASI 75 responders at week 10 but achieved PASI 75 by week 50) [9]. Thus, the number reported most likely under-represents the true percentage of subjects who lost their response. This study used two different maintenance regimens—every eight weeks or as needed. In the every eight-week dosing regimen, 23% fewer patients had a PASI 75 response at week 50 compared to week 10 (55% vs. 78%). In the as needed dosing regimen, patients fared worse; 40% fewer patients had a PASI 75 response at week 50 compared to week 10 (38% vs. 78%). Both studies found the presence of anti-infliximab antibodies to be associated with loss of PASI 75 response. In the larger study, patients who were antibody positive were more than three times as likely to lose their response by week 50 than those patients who were antibody negative (61% vs. 19%) [2].

Unfortunately, longer clinical trials with infliximab have not been completed. One three-year study was designed to test continuous versus intermittent maintenance dosing but was terminated by the sponsor due to numerically more serious infusion reactions in the intermittent therapy group (4%, 8/219) than the continuous therapy group (<1%, 1/222) [10].

DISCUSSION

Overall, 20%–32% of patients lost their PASI 75 response during 0.8–3.9 years of follow-up in phase III clinical trials [2–5]. Of these, the number that can be attributed to biologic fatigue (e.g., the development of drug-neutralizing antibodies) is not clear. Antibody testing was inconsistent, and when tested, the methods were not always described. Further, not all antibodies are drug neutralizing; therefore, the presence of antibody may not correlate with a loss of clinical efficacy. The ability of antidrug antibodies to neutralize a biologic medication can also be measured by laboratory assays, although this has not been reported in psoriasis studies [11].

We cannot make any definitive conclusions regarding which medication is most likely to lose efficacy over time by comparing the studies, given that they were not performed as head-to-head trials and the length of follow-up was not consistent across the studies. However, it appears that infliximab had the largest percentage of responders who lost their response over the shortest time period, while ustekinumab had the lowest percentage of responders who lost their response over the longest time period. The human-mouse chimeric structure of infliximab is more immunogenic than the other biologic medications and may contribute to this result. Thus, the development of antidrug antibodies is thought to be the key driver of biologic fatigue. Other reasons patients may have lost their PASI 75 response include normal fluctuation in psoriatic disease severity, noncompliance, adverse events, or inability to tolerate the medication.

ANTIDRUG ANTIBODIES

The development of antidrug antibodies has been linked to the loss of response to adalimumab and infliximab (Table 15.2) [2–5,9,12,13]. In contrast, etanercept may be less vulnerable to biologic fatigue because its biologic activity is less likely be inhibited by antidrug antibodies [11,14,15]. Etanercept is a dimeric fusion protein consisting of two tumor necrosis factor-receptors (TNF-receptors) linked to the fragment crystallizable (Fc) portion of immunoglobulin G1 (IgG1). Antibodies to etanercept are likely directed against the fusion region of the dimeric protein [11,14]. When this region is bound by antibody, etanercept can still effectively bind TNF. However, antibodies to both infliximab and adalimumab most likely develop against epitopes in the variable region of the antibody, which would impair the ability to bind TNF.

There are few studies examining the impact of antidrug antibodies in the treatment of psoriasis. In one prospective study of 29 psoriasis patients treated with adalimumab for 24 weeks, 45% (13/29) tested positive for antidrug antibodies during the study (Table 15.2) [13]. All patients with high titers of antibodies to adalimumab at weeks 12 and 24 were nonresponders. Further, nonresponders had significantly lower trough levels of adalimumab ($p = 0.01$ vs. responders). Thus, as antibodies to adalimumab increased, trough levels of the medication decreased and PASI scores increased. Similar findings linking antidrug antibodies to loss of response have been reported in clinical trials using infliximab [2–5,9,12]. These studies support the hypothesis that biologic fatigue is associated with the development of antidrug antibodies, which decrease the bioavailability of the medication [1].

Another study reported that over 24 weeks of treatment, 17% (3/18) of patients treated with adalimumab, 13% (2/15) of patients treated with infliximab, and 0% (0/18) of patients treated with etanercept tested positive for antidrug antibodies [16]. However, this study was limited by a small sample size and retrospective design.

The mechanism of action by which antidrug antibodies neutralize biologic therapy has been studied most extensively in patients treated with infliximab [17]. The antidrug antibodies form complexes with infliximab, which can then be removed from the liver or spleen (Table 15.3) [13,16,18]. This can explain why patients with high antidrug antibody titers have low or undetectable trough levels of medication. By increasing the dose or frequency of infliximab, clinicians are often able to maintain the therapeutic response by overcoming the rate of antibody formation or immune-complex clearing. The need for an increased dose or dosing frequency to maintain therapeutic response with biologic therapy is known as “dose-creep” [18].

Other studies have attempted to determine which patients are at risk for developing antidrug antibodies. In one study of patients receiving infliximab for psoriasis, there was an association between elevated anti-double-stranded DNA concentrations (pretreatment) and the development of antidrug antibodies and subsequent loss of response [19]. Genetic factors are also likely to contribute to antibody formation, an area that needs further investigation [15].

TABLE 15.2 Studies Investigating Impact of Antidrug Antibodies on Biologic Therapy

Reference, Type of Study, Antibody Assay, Disease	Medication	Number of Patients	Length of Treatment	No. of Patients Testing Positive for Antidrug Antibodies	Comments
Lecluse 2010 Prospective Radio immunoassay Psoriasis	Adalimumab	29	24 weeks	13 (45%)	All patients with high titers of anti-adalimumab antibody at weeks 12 and 24 were nonresponders. Nonresponders had lower trough levels of adalimumab ($p = 0.01$ vs. responders).
Cozzani 2013 Retrospective ELISA Psoriasis	Adalimumab Infliximab Etanercept	18 15 18	24 weeks	3 (17%) 2 (13%) 0	Association of antidrug antibodies with loss of efficacy not clearly reported. Study limited by small sample size, retrospective design.
Bartelds 2011 Prospective Radio immunoassay Rheumatoid Arthritis[a]	Adalimumab	272	156 weeks	76 (28%)	Patients with anti-adalimumab antibodies were: (1) more likely to discontinue due to treatment failure ($p < 0.001$ compared to those without antibodies); (2) less often taking concomitant methotrexate ($p < 0.001$); (3) taking lower doses of methotrexate ($p = 0.005$).

[a] Listed for comparison due to small size of psoriasis studies.

TABLE 15.3 Proposed Sequence of Events Leading to Biologic Fatigue

1. Patient injected or infused with biologic medication
2. Antigen-presenting cell processes and presents the protein to naïve T cells in lymph node
3. T-cell activation
4. Activated T cells stimulate humoral immune response—B cells begin producing antidrug antibodies
5. On subsequent injections or infusions, antidrug antibodies complex with the biologic medication
6. Antibody–drug complexes are unable to bind to target cytokines or receptors and are removed in the liver or spleen by resident macrophages
7. Systemic concentration of the medication decreases correlating with a loss of clinical efficacy

Other reports speculate that production of antidrug antibody is greater when the body's immune system is in an activated state, such as during a common viral infection, bacterial infection, or a flare of psoriasis [20]. In addition, patients with the most severe, recalcitrant disease or those who have a history of developing antibodies to a previous agent may be at increased risk of biologic fatigue.

Given that there are few studies that investigate the significance of antidrug antibodies in psoriasis patients on biologics, it may be useful to examine other disease states such as rheumatoid arthritis or inflammatory bowel disease. In one study of 272 rheumatoid arthritis patients on adalimumab, 28% of patients developed antidrug antibodies during 156 weeks of follow-up [18]. Those patients with antidrug antibodies were more likely to discontinue due to treatment failure than those without antibodies (38% vs. 14%, $p < 0.001$). Further, those patients who developed antidrug antibodies were less often taking concomitant methotrexate or taking lower doses of methotrexate than those patients who did not develop antibodies ($p < 0.001$, $p = 0.005$) [18]. These findings are consistent with those in inflammatory bowel disease [21–23].

CLINICAL STRATEGIES TO COMBAT BIOLOGIC FATIGUE

Consider a Dose-Creep to Maintain Therapeutic Efficacy

Retrospective studies that measure "drug survival" demonstrate the importance of dose-creep [24] in maintaining therapeutic response to infliximab (Table 15.4) [25–27]. One study of more than 800 treatment series of etanercept, adalimumab, and infliximab reviewed the four-year "retention rate" of each medication. This rate was determined by the percentage of patients who continued on each specific biologic medication over the four-year time period. The retention rate for infliximab was reported as almost twice that of the other TNF-α (TNF-α) inhibitors (70% vs. 40% for both etanercept and adalimumab) [27].

There are a few possible explanations for this discrepancy. Most importantly, dosing in clinical trials is predetermined. Likewise, constant dosing of ustekinumab, etanercept, and adalimumab is recommended for all patients. However, infliximab is the only biologic medication where dosing adjustments are allowed, in frequency and in absolute amount [28]. As a result, patients on infliximab often experience a "dose-creep," or an increase in dose or dose frequency in order to maintain response over time [24]. Therefore, although the

TABLE 15.4 Clinical Strategies to Reduce the Impact of Biologic Fatigue

I.	Increase the dose of the biologic medication to maintain therapeutic efficacy (i.e., "dose-creep")
II.	Proactively inform patients about the risk of biologic fatigue and counsel the importance of consistent use, especially when psoriasis is under control
III.	Consider concomitant immunosuppression with methotrexate, especially in patients on infliximab or patients who have developed biologic fatigue to a previous biologic therapy

mouse–human chimeric structure of infliximab may increase the likelihood of antidrug antibody formation, a clear advantage of infliximab is the ability of clinicians to titrate the dose to maintain a satisfactory therapeutic response. In other words, there is the opportunity to overcome the capacity of the immune system to produce antibodies or to possibly induce immunologic tolerance [15].

However, when the clinician does not adjust the dose of infliximab or use concomitant immunosuppression, the retention rate decreases [26]. In a retrospective study of first-time anti-TNF-α therapy in 650 patients treated for an average of 29 months, etanercept had a better retention rate than infliximab or adalimumab (81% vs. 62% or 59%; $p < 0.0001$ for comparison to etanercept) [26]. The results of this study have limited application because infliximab doses were not increased when the initial response to the medication was lost. In real clinical practice, patients on infliximab frequently have the dosing adjusted and are often prescribed concomitant methotrexate. Further, the baseline PASI scores of the study population indicate that the patients treated with infliximab had the most severe disease.

Although dosing adjustments for all other biologic therapies are off-label, there may be merit to augmented dosing in those other than infliximab. Unfortunately, most of the clinical trials data for dose escalation are in partial responders (i.e., between PASI 50 and PASI 75) or nonresponders (i.e., less than PASI 50). We are most interested in the effect of dose escalation on PASI 75 responders who have lost their response, presumably after the development of antidrug antibodies. Further investigation is needed to determine whether dose escalation in these patients is beneficial at reestablishing response to therapy.

Counseling Consistent Use

The easiest way for a clinician to make an impact on the incidence of biologic fatigue is proactive and repeated counseling on the importance of adherence to the regular dosing schedule. Many patients assume that biologic medications can be used less consistently, especially once psoriasis is under control. Due to the high cost of biologic therapy, some patients may hoard or stockpile the medication when their skin is under control for fear of not having it available during a flare. Therefore, the clinician needs to educate the patient that "as needed" use of biologic medications may result in permanent loss of efficacy.

It is not known why intermittent therapy may speed the development of biologic fatigue. One hypothesis is that waiting until the body has an overactive immune state (i.e., during a flare of psoriasis) to administer the medication increases the likelihood of antibody formation. This may also explain why those patients with severe disease refractory to treatment may also be more likely to develop antidrug antibodies. A flare of psoriasis results in a generalized inflammatory state with a hyperactive immune system, marked by increased cytokine production, dendritic cell, and T-cell activation. These factors may contribute to the likelihood of a B-cell response to a foreign protein. Therefore, patients need to be counseled early and reminded often about the importance of adherence to the dosing schedule for maintaining drug efficacy, especially when they have come into the office with a great response to the medication.

Certain situations, such as surgery or infection, warrant that the use of the medication be temporarily interrupted. In these situations, patients should be reassured that several weeks of dosing interruption should not jeopardize their future response to the medication. Rather, it is those patients that habitually skip doses of medication for months at a time that may be at the greatest risk of losing their response.

Concomitant Immunosuppression with Methotrexate

The majority of data supporting the use of methotrexate in combination with biologic therapy is from studies using infliximab to treat Crohn's disease or rheumatoid arthritis. In these diseases, this combination is used to enhance and maintain the efficacy of infliximab and to decrease the likelihood of an infusion reaction. In fact, the use of infliximab *without* methotrexate in rheumatoid arthritis is considered off-label, even in patients with early disease [29]. This is supported by numerous clinical trials showing superior efficacy with combination therapy [30–32]. Similarly, in Crohn's disease, infliximab combined with another immunosuppressant such as azathioprine or methotrexate is significantly more efficacious when compared to infliximab monotherapy [22,33–35]. In addition, combination therapy decreases the risk of developing anti-infliximab antibodies, which are associated with an increased risk of infusion reaction, lower post-infusion levels of infliximab, and a shorter duration of remission [9,36–41]. In one study, about three-fourths of patients using infliximab monotherapy developed anti-infliximab antibodies versus less than half of patients on combination therapy [22].

It may be worth considering a similar regimen to treat moderate to severe psoriasis [42], although there has never been a randomized clinical trial. Two retrospective studies investigated the safety and efficacy of infliximab combined with methotrexate in treating psoriasis [41,43]. Although these studies are limited by their small size and retrospective design, they suggest that the addition of methotrexate to infliximab may be helpful in decreasing the likelihood of infusion reactions and biologic fatigue.

In one study, 23 cases of moderate to severe plaque psoriasis were treated with infliximab combined with either methotrexate or azathioprine [43]. The methotrexate was dosed 7.5–15 mg once weekly. Five patients could not tolerate methotrexate and instead received combination therapy with azathioprine 50 mg/day. The mean duration of follow-up was 26.5 months. By week 14, 70% of patients had reached PASI 75. Only three patients discontinued therapy: two due to loss of efficacy and one due to a pulmonary embolism. There were no serious infections or other serious adverse events reported. There were four infusion reactions reported, only one of which led to treatment discontinuation. The other three reactions were mild and transient and included symptoms such as headache and dizziness. The treatment discontinuation rate due to serious adverse events in this study (<5%) seems favorable compared to other studies where rates range from 10% to 25% [10,44,45].

Another retrospective study on the use of infliximab for the treatment of moderate to severe psoriasis showed that concomitant methotrexate might reduce the risk of infusion reaction [41]. This study reviewed 59 patients who received a total of 858 infusions. Overall, 17% of patients had a least one infusion reaction. However, only 4% of patients treated with concomitant methotrexate were affected compared to 27% of those treated with infliximab monotherapy ($p = 0.05$).

Few studies have investigated the use of methotrexate with other biologic agents for the treatment of psoriasis. There are three prospective studies in combination with etanercept [46–48], one with adalimumab [49], and none with ustekinumab. However, these studies do not report antidrug antibody testing. Although no serious adverse events were reported, less than 300 patients in total received combination therapy and most did so for six months or less. In order to adequately assess long-term safety and the effect of combination therapy on reducing biologic fatigue, larger studies over longer time periods are needed.

In summary, although combination therapy with infliximab and methotrexate may result in greater improvement in psoriasis, the greatest benefit may be in reducing the likelihood of anti-infliximab antibodies and the subsequent risk of infusion reactions and biologic fatigue. These reactions are detrimental to the patient by causing loss of efficacy or by increasing the risk for rare anaphylactic-like reactions. Given that infusion reactions (or injection site reactions) are much less of a concern with etanercept, adalimumab, and ustekinumab, it remains to be seen whether the addition of methotrexate will be similarly beneficial to patients on these medications.

CONCLUSION

In phase III clinical trials of approved biologic therapies for the treatment of psoriasis, 20%–32% of patients lost their PASI 75 response during 0.8–3.9 years of follow-up. Biologic fatigue may be most frequent in those patients using infliximab. Further studies are needed to identify risk factors associated with biologic fatigue and to develop meaningful antidrug antibody assays. Three techniques for clinicians that may be helpful in maximizing the durability of response to biologic therapy include increasing the dose or dosing frequency of the medication, counseling the patient on the importance of adherence to the dosing regimen, or adding concomitant immunosuppression with methotrexate.

REFERENCES

1. Takahashi H, Tsuji H, Ishida-Yamamoto A, et al. Plasma trough levels of adalimumab and infliximab in terms of clinical efficacy during the treatment of psoriasis. *J Dermatol* 2013; 40(1): 39–42.
2. Reich K, Nestle FO, Papp K, et al. Infliximab induction and maintenance therapy for moderate-to-severe psoriasis: a phase III, multicentre, double-blind trial. *Lancet* 2005; 366(9494): 1367–1374.
3. Tyring S, Gordon KB, Poulin Y, et al. Long-term safety and efficacy of 50 mg of etanercept twice weekly in patients with psoriasis. *Arch Dermatol* 2007; 143(6): 719–726.

4. Gordon K, Papp K, Poulin Y, et al. Long-term efficacy and safety of adalimumab in patients with moderate to severe psoriasis treated continuously over 3 years: results from an open-label extension study for patients from REVEAL. *J Am Acad Dermatol* 2012; 66(2): 241–251.
5. Kimball AB, Papp KA, Wasfi Y, et al. Long-term efficacy of ustekinumab in patients with moderate-to-severe psoriasis treated for up to 5 years in the PHOENIX 1 study. *J Eur Acad Dermatol Venereol* 2013; 27(12); 1535–1545.
6. Menter A, Tyring SK, Gordon K, et al. Adalimumab therapy for moderate to severe psoriasis: a randomized, controlled phase III trial. *J Am Acad Dermatol* 2008; 58(1): 106–115.
7. Leonardi CL, Kimball AB, Papp KA, et al. Efficacy and safety of ustekinumab, a human interleukin-12/23 monoclonal antibody, in patients with psoriasis: 76-week results from a randomised, double-blind, placebo-controlled trial (PHOENIX 1). *Lancet* 2008; 371(9625): 1665–1674.
8. Papp KA, Langley RG, Lebwohl M, et al. Efficacy and safety of ustekinumab, a human interleukin-12/23 monoclonal antibody, in patients with psoriasis: 52-week results from a randomised, double-blind, placebo-controlled trial (PHOENIX 2). *Lancet* 2008; 371(9625): 1675–1684.
9. Menter A, Feldman SR, Weinstein GD, et al. A randomized comparison of continuous vs. intermittent infliximab maintenance regimens over 1 year in the treatment of moderate-to-severe plaque psoriasis. *J Am Acad Dermatol* 2007; 56(1): 31. e31–e15.
10. Reich K, Wozel G, Zheng H, et al. Efficacy and safety of infliximab as continuous or intermittent therapy in patients with moderate-to-severe plaque psoriasis: results of a randomised, long-term extension trial (RESTORE2). *Br J Dermatol* 2013; 168: 1325–34.
11. de Vries MK, van der Horst-Bruinsma IE, Nurmohamed MT, et al. Immunogenicity does not influence treatment with etanercept in patients with ankylosing spondylitis. *Ann Rheum Dis* 2009; 68(4): 531–535.
12. Noiles K, Vender R. Biologic survival. *J Drugs Dermatol* 2009; 8(4): 329–333.
13. Lecluse LL, Driessen RJ, Spuls PI, et al. Extent and clinical consequences of antibody formation against adalimumab in patients with plaque psoriasis. *Arch Dermatol* 2010; 146(2): 127–132.
14. Mahil SK, Arkir Z, Richards G, et al. Predicting treatment response in psoriasis using serum levels of adalimumab and etanercept: a single centre, cohort study. *Br J Dermatol* 2013; 169: 306–313.
15. Wolbink GJ, Aarden LA, Dijkmans BA. Dealing with immunogenicity of biologicals: assessment and clinical relevance. *Curr Opin Rheumatol* 2009; 21(3): 211–215.
16. Cozzani E, Burlando M, Parodi A. Detection of antibodies to anti-TNF agents in psoriatic patients: a preliminary study. *G Ital Dermatol Venereol* 2013; 148(2): 171–174.
17. van der Laken CJ, Voskuyl AE, Roos JC, et al. Imaging and serum analysis of immune complex formation of radiolabelled infliximab and anti-infliximab in responders and non-responders to therapy for rheumatoid arthritis. *Ann Rheum Dis* 2007; 66(2): 253–256.
18. Bartelds GM, Krieckaert CL, Nurmohamed MT, et al. Development of antidrug antibodies against adalimumab and association with disease activity and treatment failure during long-term follow-up. *JAMA* 2011; 305(14): 1460–1468.
19. Hoffmann JH, Hartmann M, Enk AH, et al. Autoantibodies in psoriasis as predictors for loss of response and anti-infliximab antibody induction. *Br J Dermatol* 2011; 165(6): 1355–1358.
20. Matsumoto Y, Maeda T, Tsuboi R, et al. Anti-adalimumab and anti-infliximab antibodies developed in psoriasis vulgaris patients reduced the efficacy of biologics: report of two cases. *J Dermatol* 2013; 40(5): 389–392.
21. Krieckaert CL, Bartelds GM, Lems WF, et al. The effect of immunomodulators on the immunogenicity of TNF-blocking therapeutic monoclonal antibodies: a review. *Arthritis Res Ther* 2010; 12(5): 217.
22. Vermeire S, Noman M, Van Assche G, et al. Effectiveness of concomitant immunosuppressive therapy in suppressing the formation of antibodies to infliximab in Crohn's disease. *Gut* 2007; 56(9): 1226–1231.
23. Vande Casteele N, Ballet V, Van Assche G, et al. Early serial trough and antidrug antibody level measurements predict clinical outcome of infliximab and adalimumab treatment. *Gut* 2012; 61(2): 321; author reply 322.
24. Mehren CR, Gniadecki R. Dose-creep of Infliximab during psoriasis treatment: an observational study. *Acta Derm Venereol* 2012; 92(4): 355–357.
25. Escande H, Livideanu CB, Steiner A, et al. Incidence and risk factors for treatment failure with infliximab in psoriasis. *J Eur Acad Dermatol Venereol* 2013; 27(10): 1323–1324.

26. Esposito M, Gisondi P, Cassano N, et al. Survival rate of anti-TNF alpha treatments for psoriasis in routine dermatological practice: a multicenter observational study. *Br J Dermatol* 2013; 169: 666–72.
27. Gniadecki R, Kragballe K, Dam TN, et al. Comparison of drug survival rates for adalimumab, etanercept and infliximab in patients with psoriasis vulgaris. *Br J Dermatol* 2011; 164(5): 1091–1096.
28. Reich K, Griffiths C, Barker J, et al. Recommendations for the long-term treatment of psoriasis with infliximab: a dermatology expert group consensus. *Dermatology* 2008; 217(3): 268–275.
29. Singh JA, Furst DE, Bharat A, et al. 2012 update of the 2008 American College of Rheumatology recommendations for the use of disease-modifying antirheumatic drugs and biologic agents in the treatment of rheumatoid arthritis. *Arthritis Care Res* 2012; 64(5): 625–639.
30. Smolen JS, Han C, van der Heijde D, et al. Infliximab treatment maintains employability in patients with early rheumatoid arthritis. *Arthritis Rheum* 2006; 54(3): 716–722.
31. St Clair EW, van der Heijde DM, Smolen JS, et al. Combination of infliximab and methotrexate therapy for early rheumatoid arthritis: a randomized, controlled trial. *Arthritis Rheum* 2004; 50(11): 3432–3443.
32. van der Kooij SM, le Cessie S, Goekoop-Ruiterman YP, et al. Clinical and radiological efficacy of initial vs delayed treatment with infliximab plus methotrexate in patients with early rheumatoid arthritis. *Ann Rheum Dis* 2009; 68(7): 1153–1158.
33. Arnott ID, McNeill G, Satsangi J. An analysis of factors influencing short-term and sustained response to infliximab treatment for Crohn's disease. *Aliment Pharmacol Ther* 2003; 17(12): 1451–1457.
34. Parsi MA, Achkar JP, Richardson S, et al. Predictors of response to infliximab in patients with Crohn's disease. *Gastroenterology* 2002; 123(3): 707–713.
35. Rutgeerts P, Van Assche G, Vermeire S. Review article: infliximab therapy for inflammatory bowel disease—seven years on. *Aliment Pharmacol Ther* 2006; 23(4): 451–463.
36. Baert F, Noman M, Vermeire S, et al. Influence of immunogenicity on the long-term efficacy of infliximab in Crohn's disease. *N Engl J Med* 2003; 348(7): 601–608.
37. Bendtzen K, Geborek P, Svenson M, et al. Individualized monitoring of drug bioavailability and immunogenicity in rheumatoid arthritis patients treated with the tumor necrosis factor alpha inhibitor infliximab. *Arthritis Rheum* 2006; 54(12): 3782–3789.
38. Farrell RJ, Alsahli M, Jeen YT, et al. Intravenous hydrocortisone premedication reduces antibodies to infliximab in Crohn's disease: a randomized controlled trial. *Gastroenterology* 2003; 124(4): 917–924.
39. Hanauer SB, Wagner CL, Bala M, et al. Incidence and importance of antibody responses to infliximab after maintenance or episodic treatment in Crohn's disease. *Clin Gastroenterol Hepatol* 2004; 2(7): 542–553.
40. Menter A, Gottlieb A, Feldman SR, et al. Guidelines of care for the management of psoriasis and psoriatic arthritis: section 1. Overview of psoriasis and guidelines of care for the treatment of psoriasis with biologics. *J Am Acad Dermatol* 2008; 58(5): 826–850.
41. Wee JS, Petrof G, Jackson K, et al. Infliximab for the treatment of psoriasis in the U.K.: 9 years' experience of infusion reactions at a single centre. *Br J Dermatol* 2012; 167(2): 411–416.
42. Warren RB, Brown BC, Carmichael AJ, et al. Long-term control of recalcitrant psoriasis with combination infliximab and methotrexate. *Clin Exp Dermatol* 2009; 34(3): 415–416.
43. Dalaker M, Bonesronning JH. Long-term maintenance treatment of moderate-to-severe plaque psoriasis with infliximab in combination with methotrexate or azathioprine in a retrospective cohort. *J Eur Acad Dermatol Venereol* 2009; 23(3): 277–282.
44. Barker J, Hoffmann M, Wozel G, et al. Efficacy and safety of infliximab vs. methotrexate in patients with moderate-to-severe plaque psoriasis: results of an open-label, active-controlled, randomized trial (RESTORE1). *Br J Dermatol* 2011; 165(5): 1109–1117.
45. Smith CH, Jackson K, Bashir SJ, et al. Infliximab for severe, treatment-resistant psoriasis: a prospective, open-label study. *Br J Dermatol* 2006; 155(1): 160–169.
46. Driessen RJ, van de Kerkhof PC, de Jong EM. Etanercept combined with methotrexate for high-need psoriasis. *Br J Dermatol* 2008; 159(2): 460–463.
47. Gottlieb AB, Langley RG, Strober BE, et al. A randomized, double-blind, placebo-controlled study to evaluate the addition of methotrexate to etanercept in patients with moderate to severe plaque psoriasis. *Br J Dermatol* 2012; 167(3): 649–657.

48. Zachariae C, Mork NJ, Reunala T, et al. The combination of etanercept and methotrexate increases the effectiveness of treatment in active psoriasis despite inadequate effect of methotrexate therapy. *Acta Derm Venereol* 2008; 88(5): 495–501.
49. van den Reek JM, van Lumig PP, Kievit W, et al. Effectiveness of adalimumab dose escalation, combination therapy of adalimumab with methotrexate, or both in patients with psoriasis in daily practice. *J Dermatolog Treat* 2013; 24: 361–368.

Chapter 16

IL-17 and Other New Agents

Ethan C. Levin, Argentina Leon, and John Y. M. Koo

INTRODUCTION

Psoriasis was once thought to be a disease primarily mediated by the Th1 axis [1]. In 2005, Th17 cells were recognized as a distinct subtype of helper T cells (see Chapter 13) and were linked to autoimmune inflammation in murine models [2,3]. Th17 cells are defined by their ability to secrete interleukin-17 (IL-17) cytokines. These proinflammatory cytokines have increased expression in psoriatic skin and are now recognized as playing a critical role in the pathogenesis of psoriasis (Figure 16.1) [4–13]. IL-17 cytokines as well as their cell surface receptors represent promising therapeutic targets [10]. Other proinflammatory cytokines secreted by Th17 cells thought to be key players in the pathogenesis of psoriasis include tumor necrosis factor-α (TNF-α) and IL-22 (for more information on TNF-α, see Chapters 11, 12, and 14). In the skin, IL-22 primarily targets epithelial cells leading to epidermal hyperplasia [14]. Stimulation of keratinocytes with IL-22 induces proliferation and inhibits terminal differentiation. In addition, expression of antimicrobial proteins (e.g., defensins) is increased. Recently, a new subset of cells was described known as Th22 cells, which also secrete IL-22 but lack the ability to secrete IL-17 [15]. This section will focus on the role of IL-17 in the pathogenesis of psoriasis and will summarize the clinical trials data for medications that target the IL-17 inflammatory pathway.

IL-17 CYTOKINES AND RECEPTORS

The IL-17 family of cytokines includes six homodimers (IL-17A to IL-17F) [16,17], one heterodimer (IL-17A/F), and five receptors (IL-17RA to IL-17RE) [18–21]. Th17 cells secrete IL-17A, IL-17F, and IL-17A/F. These three cytokines share the same heterodimer receptor complex, two subunits of which are IL-17RA and IL-17RC (Figure 16.2) [18,22–24]. This receptor complex is expressed on many different cell types including keratinocytes, dendritic cells, fibroblasts, macrophages, and endothelial cells [25,26]. Thus, IL-17 signaling can have diverse effects depending on the target cell. In psoriasis, this can include production of inflammatory cytokines, chemokines causing neutrophil margination and homing, antimicrobial peptides, and matrix metalloproteinases (enzymes capable of remodeling the extracellular matrix) [27]. Although the Th17 cell is the predominant cell type to produce IL-17A and IL-17F, these cytokines are also expressed by other cell types, such as CD8+ T cells, gamma delta (γδ) T cells, and natural killer (NK) cells [28].

IL-17A

Of the three members of the IL-17 family secreted by the Th17 cells, IL-17A is thought to be the most potent [21,29]. IL-17A augments expression of keratinocyte genes that are involved in the innate immune response, such as the production of defensins and cathelicidin [30–32].

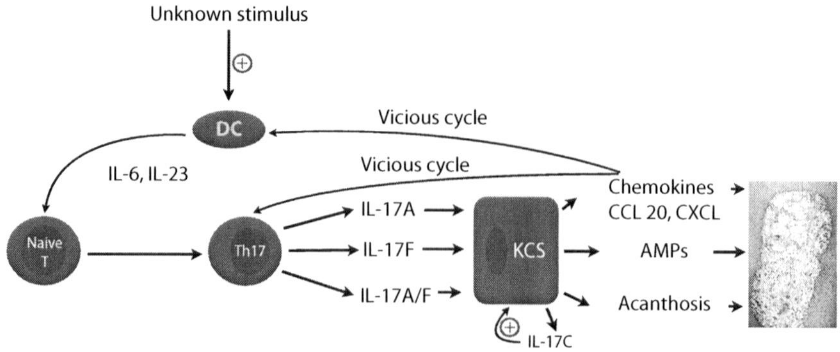

FIGURE 16.1 (See color insert.) IL-17 in psoriasis pathogenesis. An unknown stimulus leads to activation of dendritic cells (DCs). These cells produce IL-6 and IL-23, which drive differentiation of naïve T cells into Th17 cells [11,12]. Th17 cells produce IL-17A, IL-17F, and IL-17A/F, which stimulate keratinocytes (KCS) to proliferate and to produce proinflammatory antimicrobial peptides (AMPs) and chemokines (e.g., CCL20). Chemokines such as CCL20 recruit inflammatory dendritic cells and Th17 cells into the active psoriasis lesion. Other chemokines play a role in neutrophil recruitment (CXCL) and angiogenesis. Keratinocytes also produce IL-17C, which acts via an autocrine mechanism to amplify the response IL-17A. IL-17C also acts on endothelial cells to augment expression of TNF-α, which further amplifies the inflammatory pathway [13].

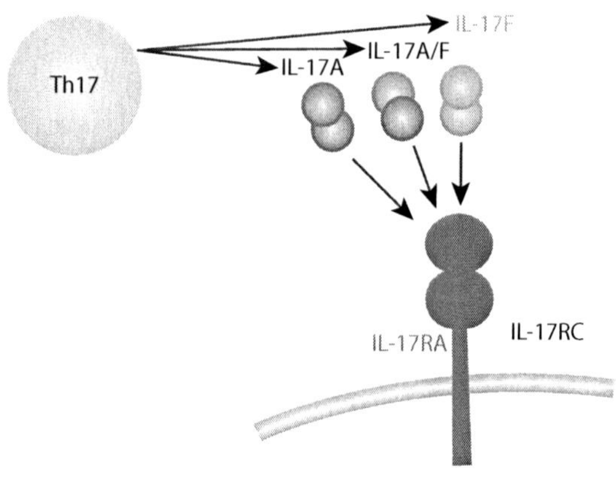

FIGURE 16.2 (See color insert.) Th17 cells secrete IL-17A, IL-17F, and IL-17A/F. These three cytokines share the same heterodimer receptor complex, two subunits of which are IL-17RA and IL-17RC.

IL-17A is also thought to drive recruitment and activation of neutrophils, inhibition of neutrophil apoptosis, and angiogenesis in psoriasis [25,33–35]. Furthermore, the combination of IL-17 with other cytokines such as TNF-α synergistically augments the proinflammatory response from keratinocytes [36,37].

Previous studies have shown that serum and lesional IL-17A levels are higher in psoriatic patients than in controls [38,39]. Moreover, there was a correlation between IL-17A levels and disease severity; those patients with generalized pustular psoriasis or those who had a

Psoriasis Area and Severity Index (PASI) score greater than 10 had the highest serum levels of IL-17A [38]. Similarly, mRNA levels of IL-17A,IL-17C, and IL-17F are elevated in psoriatic lesions [23,38,40] and may vary with disease severity. For example, the amount of IL-17A mRNA transcript in pustular psoriasis lesions was shown to be higher than in plaque-type psoriasis lesions [38].

Further evidence for the importance of IL-17A as a key "driver" cytokine of the psoriatic disease state comes from a skin biopsy study. In this study, pathologic and molecular measures of psoriasis improved within two weeks of starting ixekizumab, a monoclonal antibody that neutralizes IL-17A [32]. Histopathology showed a reduction in acanthosis, keratinocyte proliferation, and the number of lymphocytes and other inflammatory cells in the dermis. From a molecular standpoint, more than half of 1200 genes that are differentially expressed in psoriatic skin were normalized.

IL-17A is thought to not only be a driver of the skin pathology in psoriasis, but it may also contribute to the development of cardiovascular disease, for which psoriasis patients are at increased risk [41]. Patients with acute coronary syndrome show increased levels of Th17-derived cytokines [42]. In atherosclerosis, IL-17A is increased in atherosclerotic plaques and further increases at advanced stages of plaque development [43]. In murine models of atherosclerosis, mice treated with IL-17A antibodies had decreased atherosclerotic plaque size and decreased serum levels of proinflammatory cytokines, such as IL-6 [44].

IL-17F

IL-17F and IL-17A share 50% homology, more than any other members of the IL-17 family of cytokines [8]. They are secreted as disulfide linked homodimers and signal through the same receptor complex (IL-17RA/IL-17RC). However, these two cytokines have distinct biological activity. IL-17A is 10–30 times more potent than IL-17F in terms of downstream gene activation [20,45]. Thus, of the two cytokines, IL-17A is thought to be the primary contributor to the pathogenesis of psoriasis. IL-17A can also pair with IL-17F to form a heterodimer, known as IL-17A/F [21]. This heterodimer has a biologic activity intermediate between IL-17A and IL-17F [18].

IL-17C

In mucosal and epithelial cells, IL-17C is thought to play an important role in the innate immune response. Epithelial cells can detect pathogens in the microenvironment through the use of pathogen-recognition receptors such as the Toll-like receptor (TLR). These pathogen-recognition receptors can trigger the IL-17C pathway to enhance the epithelial immune response. In human epithelial cells, production of IL-17C was rapidly induced in response to stimulation with bacteria or with certain proinflammatory cytokines (IL-1β and TNF) [46–48]. Although this response was shown to be protective to the gut mucosa in a murine model of colitis, the IL-17C pathway was pathogenic in a model of psoriasis [13,46].

IL-17C is the most recently described member of the IL-17 family of cytokines that is thought to be a significant contributor to the pathogenesis of psoriasis. In biopsies of psoriatic skin,

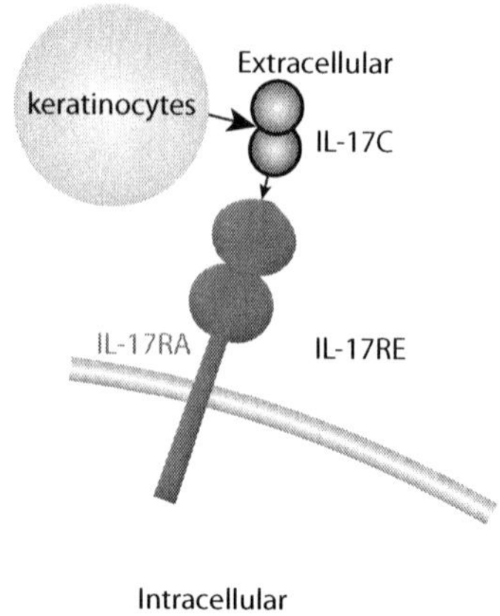

FIGURE 16.3 (See color insert.) Keratinocytes secrete IL-17C. The receptor is a heterodimer composed of IL-17RE and IL-17RA. This receptor is expressed predominantly on epithelial cells.

protein expression of IL-17C was about 125 times greater than that of IL-17A [13]. IL-17C has pro inflammatory effects similar to IL-17A; they both act synergistically with other cytokines such as TNF-α to augment the inflammatory response [13,46]. However, unlike IL-17A, which is produced by Th17 cells, IL-17C is produced by epithelial cells (e.g., keratinocytes) in response to inflammation [46].

The receptor for IL-17C is expressed predominantly on epithelial cells and is a heterodimer composed of IL-17RE and IL-17RA (Figure 16.3) [46]. Recall that the receptor for IL-17A also contains the IL-17RA subunit, which is expressed widely on many cell types. Therefore, the target cell specificity for IL-17C is determined by the IL-17RE subunit of the receptor complex. Thus, because epithelial cells express both the cytokine (IL-17C) and its receptor (IL-17RE/A complex), the IL-17C pathway has an autocrine mechanism of function.

Furthermore, IL-17C has been shown *in vitro* to act directly on endothelial cells to increase TNF-α expression, thus creating the potential for a positive feedback loop. In a disease such as psoriasis, where inflammation begets inflammation, autocrine signaling and positive feedback are critical in driving a chronic inflammatory state.

CLINICAL STUDIES TARGETING THE IL-17 PATHWAY

There are several strategies to consider when developing biologic medications to target cytokine pathways. The most straightforward approach is to develop an antibody that selectively binds the cytokine of interest, thus inhibiting interaction with its receptor (Figure 16.4). Another possibility is to antagonize the cytokine receptor with a blocking antibody. This antibody binds directly to the receptor with a greater affinity than the native cytokine, keeping the receptor in its inactive state (Figure 16.4). Other strategies include binding free cytokine with soluble receptor subunits (e.g., etanercept) or targeting the cellular assembly process of the cytokine receptor [49]. This latter strategy is protective in mouse models of inflammation but has yet to be applied in human studies [50,51].

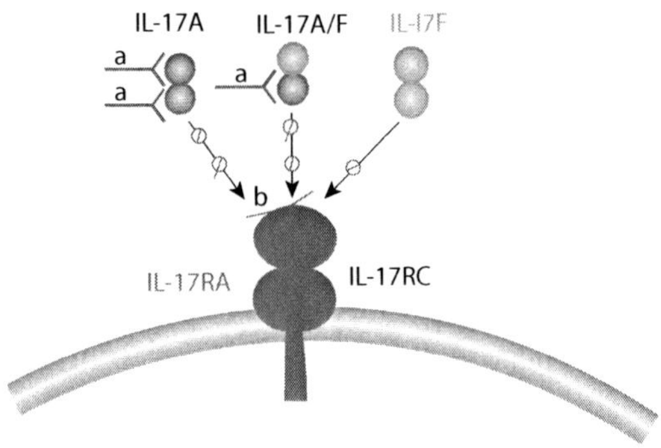

FIGURE 16.4 (See color insert.) Antibody (a) (e.g., secukinumab, ixekizumab) selectively binds IL-17A. This prevents IL-17A and IL-17A/F from interacting with its receptor. Blocking antibody (b) (e.g., brodalumab) antagonizes the receptor, keeping it in an inactive state even in the presence of IL 17A, IL 17A/F, or IL 17F.

TABLE 16.1 Biologic Medications Targeting the IL-17 Pathway with Ongoing Phase III Studies in Psoriasis

Name of Medication	Antibody Composition and Subclass	Target	Inhibited Cytokines	Company
Secukinumab (AIN457)	Human IgG1κ monoclonal antibody	IL-17A	IL-17A, IL-17A/F	Novartis
Ixekizumab (LY2439821)	Humanized IgG4κ monoclonal antibody	IL-17A	IL-17A, IL-17A/F	Eli Lilly
Brodalumab (AMG827)	Human IgG2κ monoclonal antibody	IL-17RA	IL-17A, IL-17A/F, IL-17F, IL-17E	Amgen

There are currently three biologic medications targeting the IL-17 pathway in phase III clinical trials (Table 16.1). Two of the biologics are IL-17A antibodies, and the third is an IL-17RA antagonist. In the following section, we will summarize the results of the phase II studies. All of the studies included the percent of patients that achieved PASI 75 or a physician's global assessment (PGA, also referred to as investigator's global assessment or IGA) of "clear" or "almost clear" at week 12 as either primary or secondary end points.

SECUKINUMAB

Secukinumab (AIN457) is a fully human immunoglobulin G1κ (IgG1κ) monoclonal antibody that neutralizes IL-17A. This antibody is currently being tested in psoriasis, psoriatic arthritis, rheumatoid arthritis, ankylosing spondylitis, uveitis, and multiple sclerosis. In psoriasis, the phase II studies are complete, and phase III studies are ongoing.

Study Design

There were two phase II studies in psoriasis: a dose-ranging study that focused on efficacy and safety and a dose-frequency study [52,53]. Both were randomized, double-blind, placebo-controlled, parallel-group studies. Key inclusion criteria were as follows: at least a six-month history of plaque-type psoriasis at randomization, a PASI score of at least 12, and body surface area (BSA) involvement of at least 10%. Patients were excluded from the study if they had non-plaque-type psoriasis or were being treated with other psoriasis medications including topical therapy, phototherapy, systemic agents, or other biologic agents.

Study 1: Dose-Ranging Study The patients were randomized into five treatment arms: placebo, secukinumab 25 mg once, or secukinumab 25 mg, 75 mg, or 150 mg at weeks 0, 4, and 8. At the end of the 12-week treatment period, patients entered a follow-up period of 24 weeks.

Results The study enrolled 125 patients, of which 78 completed treatment. Most of the discontinuations were in the placebo group (due to lack of efficacy) and in the single-dose group. For the key baseline characteristics of the population, refer to Table 16.2. There were no statistically significant differences in baseline characteristics between the different treatment arms. Of the 125 patients randomized, 29% (36/125) had previous exposure to biologic agents.

At week 12, 82% of patients on the 150 mg dose and 57% of patients on the 75 mg dose achieved PASI 75 (vs. 9% in placebo; $p < 0.001$ and $p = 0.002$) (Table 16.3, Figure 16.5). In addition, 52% of patients in the 150 mg arm achieved PASI 90 at week 12 (vs. 4% in placebo; $p < 0.001$). Regarding PGA, 48% of patients on the 150 mg dose were "clear" or "almost clear" at week 12 (vs. 9% in placebo, $p = 0.005$) (Table 16.4). Follow-up ended at week 36, which was more than six months since the last injection (week 8). At week 36, 26% of patients in the 150 mg arm and 19% of patients in the 75 mg arm maintained PASI 75 (vs. 4% in placebo, statistical analysis not reported).

Safety No opportunistic infections, malignancies, hypersensitivity reactions, injection-site reactions, or autoimmune reactions were observed. The most common infectious adverse events were nasopharyngitis and upper respiratory tract infection (15%–19% in the secukinumab monthly dosing groups versus 9% in placebo). There were five serious adverse events reported, two of which were in the placebo group and none that were suspected to be related to the study drug.

Study 2: Dose-Frequency Study The study was divided into a 12-week induction period followed by a 20-week maintenance period. During the induction period, patients were randomized to either placebo or one of three secukinumab 150 mg treatment arms: monthly dosing at weeks 0, 4, and 8; "early" dosing at weeks 0, 1, 2, and 4; or a single dose at week 0. At week 12, those patients who reached PASI 75 were re randomized to one of two 20-week maintenance regimens: secukinumab 150 mg at weeks 12 and 24 ("fixed-interval" group) or placebo with secukinumab 150 mg administration only at the start of relapse. Relapse was

TABLE 16.2 Key Baseline Characteristics of Patients in Dose-Ranging, Phase II Studies of Anti-IL-17 Agents

	Number of Patients	Age (Year)	Weight (kg)	PASI	Prior Systemic Therapy (%)
Secukinumab	125	46	91	21.0	62
Ixekizumab	142	46	93	17.9	35
Brodalumab	198	43	90	19.1	76

Note: Reported as averages across entire cohort.

TABLE 16.3 PASI Study End Points at Week 12 in Dose-Ranging, Phase II Studies of Anti-IL-17 Agents

	Proportion of Patients Achieving Reduction in PASI Score (No.)		
	By ≥75%	**By ≥90%**	**By 100%**
Secukinumab			
Placebo ($N = 22$)	9% (2)	4% (1)	NR
25 mg ($N = 26$)	19% (5)	8% (2)	NR
75 mg ($N = 21$)	57% (12)[a]	19% (4)	NR
150 mg ($N = 27$)	82% (22)[b]	52% (14)[b]	NR
Ixekizumab			
Placebo ($N = 26$)	8% (2)	0	0
10 mg ($N = 28$)	29% (8)	18% (5)	0
25 mg ($N = 30$)	77% (23)[b]	50% (15)[b]	17% (5)
75 mg ($N = 29$)	83% (24)[b]	59% (17)[b]	38% (11)[b]
150 mg ($N = 28$)	82% (23)[b]	71% (20)[b]	39% (11)[b]
Brodalumab			
Placebo ($N = 38$)	0	0	0
70 mg ($N = 39$)	33% (13)[b]	18% (7)[c]	10% (4)[d]
140 mg ($N = 39$)	77% (30)[b]	72% (28)[b]	38% (15)[b]
210 mg ($N = 40$)	82% (33)[b]	75% (30)[b]	62% (25)[b]
280 mg ($N = 42$)	67% (28)[b]	57% (24)[b]	29% (12)[b]

Disclaimer: These were not "head-to-head" studies.

Note: NR, not reported. Highlighted rows indicate doses chosen for Phase III studies: for ixekizumab, single dose of 80 mg being tested in Phase III and for secukinumab, a second dose of 300 mg is being tested in Phase III studies.

[a] $p = 0.002$ for the comparison with placebo.

[b] $p \leq 0.001$ for the comparison with placebo.

[c] $p < 0.01$ for the comparison with placebo.

[d] $p < 0.05$ for the comparison with placebo.

defined as the loss of one-third of the maximum PASI improvement from baseline. Those patients who did not reach PASI 75 by week 12 could chose to participate in an open-label extension and receive secukinumab 150 mg every four weeks through week 32.

Results The study enrolled 404 subjects, of which 380 completed induction. At week 12, 55% of patients in the 150 mg "early" dosing arm (weeks 0, 1, 2, and 4) and 42% of patients in the 150 mg monthly dosing arm (weeks 0, 4, and 8) achieved PASI 75 (vs. 1.5% in placebo; $p < 0.001$ for both). In the group that received a single 150 mg dose, 11% achieved PASI 75 by week 12 ($p = 0.225$ vs. placebo). During follow-up, 71% of patients in the fixed-interval group maintained PASI 75 for three months after their week 12 injection. Of the patients assigned to the open-label extension (nonresponders), 46% reached PASI 75 by week 16.

Safety Nasopharyngitis was the most commonly reported adverse event. During the induction period, nasopharyngitis was reported in a greater percentage of patients in the monthly

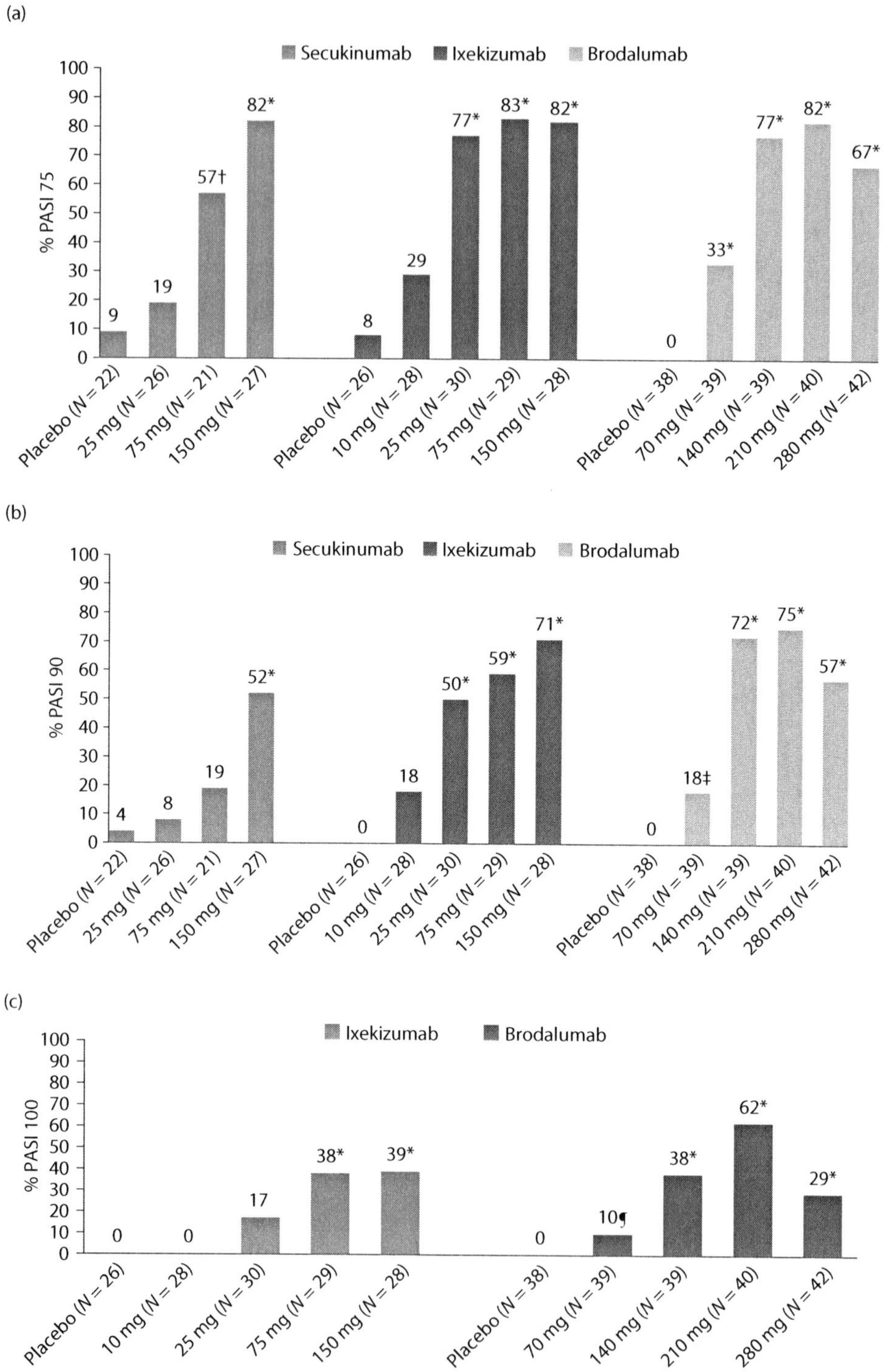

FIGURE 16.5 (See color insert.) At week 12, percentage of patients reaching: (a) PASI 75, (b) PASI 90, and (c) PASI 100. *$p \le 0.001$ for the comparison with placebo; †$p = 0.002$ for the comparison with placebo; ‡$p < 0.01$ for the comparison with placebo; ¶$p < 0.05$ for the comparison with placebo.

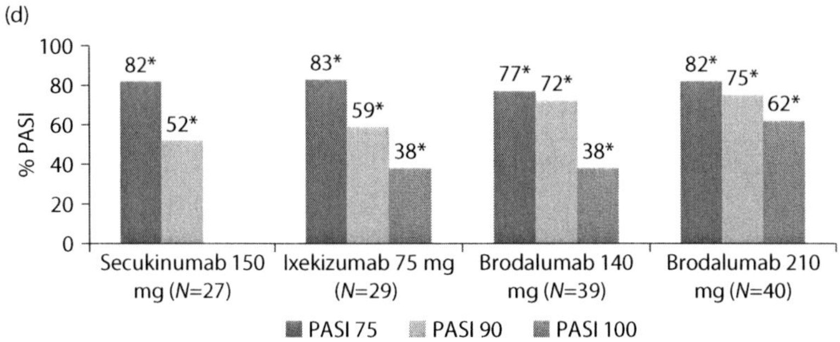

FIGURE 16.5 (*Continued*) At week 12, percentage of patients reaching (d) PASI response at week 12 for doses closest to those being tested in phase III clinical trials. *$p \leq 0.001$ for the comparison with placebo.

TABLE 16.4 PGA Study End Point at Week 12, in Dose-Ranging, Phase II Studies of Anti-IL-17 Agents

	Percent of Patients "Clear" or "Almost Clear" at Week 12 (No.)
Secukinumab	
Placebo (N = 22)	9% (2)
25 mg (N = 26)	12% (3)
75 mg (N = 21)	33% (7)
150 mg (N = 27)	48% (13)[a]
Ixekizumab	
Placebo (N = 26)	8% (2)
10 mg (N = 28)	25% (7)
25 mg (N = 30)	70% (21)[b]
75 mg (N = 29)	72% (21)[b]
150 mg (N = 28)	71% (20)[b]
Brodalumab	
Placebo (N = 38)	3% (1)
70 mg (N = 39)	26% (10)[b]
140 mg (N = 39)	85% (33)[b]
210 mg (N = 40)	80% (32)[b]
280 mg (N = 42)	69% (29)[b]

[a] $p = 0.005$ for the comparison with placebo.
[b] $p \leq 0.001$ for the comparison with placebo.
Highlighted rows indicate doses chosen for Phase III studies: for ixekizumab, single dose of 80 mg being tested in Phase III and for secukinumab, a second dose of 300 mg is being tested in Phase III studies.

(23%) and early dosing groups (23%) than in the placebo (18%) or single dosing group (12%). The overall rate of infection in the treatment groups during the induction period was similar to or less than placebo (21%, 41%, and 34% in treatment groups, 39% in placebo). Serious adverse events were reported in 3% (n = 13) and 5% (n = 18) of the patients during the induction and maintenance periods, none resulting in death. Mild neutropenia (absolute neutrophil count 1000–1500/mm^3) was reported in 5% and 8% of patients who received secukinumab during the induction and maintenance periods, respectively. However, these cases spontaneously resolved during the study and did not result in any clinically significant adverse events or result in any patients discontinuing from the study.

Ixekizumab Ixekizumab (LY2439821) is a humanized IgG4κ monoclonal antibody that neutralizes IL-17A. This antibody is currently being tested in psoriasis, psoriatic arthritis, rheumatoid arthritis, and other autoimmune conditions. In psoriasis, the phase II studies are complete and phase III studies are ongoing.

Study Design There was a single phase II, dose-ranging study designed to evaluate the safety and efficacy of ixekizumab in patients with chronic moderate to severe plaque psoriasis [54]. This study was randomized, double-blind, and placebo-controlled. Key inclusion criteria included: at least a six-month history of plaque-type psoriasis at randomization, PASI score of at least 12 and a PGA of at least three, and BSA involvement of at least 10%. Patients were excluded from the study if they had non-plaque-type psoriasis, had a clinically significant flare in the 12 weeks before randomization, or were being treated with other psoriasis medications including topical therapy, phototherapy, systemic agents, or other biologic agents.

The patients were randomly assigned to receive placebo or subcutaneous ixekizumab, at a dose of 10 mg, 25 mg, 75 mg, or 150 mg, administered at weeks 0, 2, 4, 8, 12, and 16. At the end of the treatment period, patients entered a follow-up period of four weeks.

Results The study enrolled 142 patients, and 129 completed treatment. For the key baseline characteristics of the population, refer to Table 16.2. There were no statistically significant differences in baseline characteristics between the different treatment arms.

At week 12, at least 77% of patients achieved PASI 75 in the 25 mg, 75 mg, and 150 mg dosing groups (vs. 8% in placebo, $p \leq 0.001$) (Table 16.3, Figure 16.5). Furthermore, almost 40% of patients in the 75 and 150 mg dosing groups achieved PASI 100. Regarding PGA at week 12, more than 70% of patients in the 25, 75, and 150 mg dosing groups were "clear" or "almost clear" (Table 16.4).

Safety The most common adverse events were nasopharyngitis, upper respiratory infection, injection-site reaction, and headache. None of the adverse events occurred at greater frequency in the treatment groups compared to the placebo group. There were no reported serious adverse events in any group, including death, major adverse cardiac events, or serious infections. Two of the 115 patients (1.7%) receiving ixekizumab had mild, asymptomatic neutropenia (absolute neutrophil count 1000–1500/mm^3) that spontaneously returned to baseline. There were no cases of moderate or severe neutropenia. Neutropenia was also reported in a phase I clinical trial of ixekizumab in rheumatoid arthritis patients [55]. It is not known how blocking IL-17 contributes to neutropenia. In murine models, mice deficient in IL-17 receptor have decreased neutrophil counts compared to wild-type mice [56].

In one patient in the 150 mg group ($N = 28$), two new basal cell carcinomas were diagnosed during the treatment period. However, this patient had a history of basal cell carcinoma. No other cancer was reported. Two patients in the 25 mg group ($N = 30$) had at least grade three (>5 times upper limit of normal) elevations in creatine kinase, aspartate aminotransferase, or alanine aminotransferase without associated symptoms that returned to baseline levels over time. These patients continued in the trial, and treatment was not interrupted.

Brodalumab Brodalumab (AMG827) is a human IgG2κ monoclonal antibody that binds with high affinity to IL-17RA. In other words, this antibody antagonizes the IL-17 pathway by blocking the receptor subunit, IL-17RA. The receptor has multiple ligands, including IL-17A, IL-17F, IL-17A/F heterodimer, and IL-17E (IL-25). Therefore, brodalumab is able to block signaling of multiple proinflammatory cytokines through the action of a single receptor. In addition to psoriasis, brodalumab is also being tested in psoriatic arthritis and asthma. The single phase II study in psoriasis is summarized here.

Study Design The phase II study was a randomized, double-blind, placebo-controlled, dose-ranging study designed to evaluate the safety and efficacy of brodalumab in patients with chronic moderate to severe plaque psoriasis [57]. Key inclusion criteria included: at least a six-month history of plaque-type psoriasis at randomization, PASI score of at least 12, and BSA involvement of at least 10%. Patients were excluded from the study if they had non-plaque-type psoriasis or were being treated with other psoriasis medications including topical therapy, phototherapy, systemic agents, or other biologic agents.

The patients were randomly assigned to receive placebo or subcutaneous brodalumab, at a dose of 70, 140, or 210 mg, administered at weeks 0, 1, 2, 4, 6, 8, and 10, or at a dose of 280 mg administered at weeks 0, 4, and 8.

Results The study enrolled 198 patients, and 188 completed treatment. For the key baseline characteristics of the population, refer to Table 16.2. There were no statistically significant differences in baseline characteristics among the different treatment arms.

At week 12, at least 77% of patients achieved PASI 75 in the 140 and 210 mg dosing groups (vs. 0 patients in placebo, $p < 0.001$) (Table 16.3, Figure 16.5). About 60% and 40% of patients in the 210 and 140 mg dosing groups achieved PASI 100 at week 12 (vs. 0 patients in the placebo group, $p < 0.001$ for both groups). Regarding PGA at week 12, at least 80% of patients in the 140 and 210 mg dosing groups were "clear" or "almost clear" (vs. 3% of patients in the placebo group, $p \leq 0.001$) (Table 16.4). The clinical response was rapid in all brodalumab groups; nearly all of the PASI improvement was seen by week 6. In fact, more than 75% of patients in the 210 mg dosing group achieved PASI 75 by week 6.

Safety The most common adverse events were nasopharyngitis, upper respiratory infection, arthralgia, and injection-site erythema. Of these, upper respiratory infection and injection site erythema occurred at a greater frequency in the brodalumab groups compared to the placebo group (8% vs. 5% and 6% vs. 3%). There were no deaths, major adverse cardiac events, serious infections, or cancer reported. Two of the 160 patients (1.3%) receiving brodalumab had grade three, asymptomatic neutropenia (absolute neutrophil count 500–1000/mm^3) two weeks after receiving one dose of brodalumab 210 mg. Both patients had a positive dechallenge reaction with the neutrophil counts returning to baseline after the study drug was held. One of the patients had a positive rechallenge reaction; grade three neutropenia again developed after reintroduction of the study medication. This patient was discontinued from the study, and his neutrophil count normalized 17 days later.

Of note, a phase II trial of subcutaneous brodalumab in patients with Crohn's disease was discontinued due to worsening of Crohn's disease in some patients who received the study medication. For this reason, a history of Crohn's disease is an exclusion criteria for phase III studies in psoriasis.

Other Agents

Drug development in psoriasis over the past two decades has focused primarily on biologic medications that neutralize specific cytokines critical to psoriatic inflammation. These medications are expensive and may have decreased efficacy over time. Traditionally available systemic therapies (e.g., methotrexate, cyclosporine, acitretin) have potentially serious side effects and require frequent laboratory monitoring. Therefore, treatments that are safer, less costly, or more convenient than the currently available alternatives may be useful.

Apremilast Apremilast is an orally administered small molecule inhibitor of phosphodiesterase 4 (PDE4). PDE4 is an enzyme that degrades the secondary messenger cyclic adenosine monophosphate (cAMP). Low levels of cAMP promote the production of proinflammatory mediators. Thus by inhibiting PDE4, apremilast is able to have an anti-inflammatory effect on the cell by increasing levels of cAMP [58,59]. In one phase II study in psoriasis, 352 patients were randomized to placebo or 10 mg, 20 mg, or 30 mg of apremilast twice daily. After 16 weeks of treatment, 41% of patients in the 30 mg dosing group achieved PASI 75 by week 16 (vs. 6% in placebo; $p < 0.0001$) [60]. There were not any reported treatment-related serious adverse events or any safety concerns from laboratory assessments. However, there was an increased incidence of headache, nausea, diarrhea, vomiting, and upper respiratory tract infection in those patients taking apremilast, with the highest rates in those patients taking 30 mg twice daily. In many of these patients, these side effects were associated with the initiation of therapy and subsided after one week without a closing interruption of the study medication.

Tofacitinib Tofacitinib (CP-690-550) is a small-molecule inhibitor of Janus kinase (JAK). It is currently in development in oral and topical formulations for the treatment of psoriasis. Tofacitinib inhibits JAK1 and JAK3, resulting in a decrease in proinflammatory cytokines, such as IL-6 and interferon-γ [61,62].

In a phase II study of 179 patients, patients were randomized to placebo or 2 mg, 5 mg, or 15 mg tofacitinib twice daily [63]. After 12 weeks, 67% of patients in the 15 mg dosing group and 41% of patients in the 5 mg dosing group reached PASI 75 (vs. 2% in the placebo group; $p < 0.0001$ for both comparisons) [63]. Although this study was small and not long enough to adequately assess long-term safety, adverse event rates were not higher in the tofacitinib groups than in the placebo group. There were dose-related decreases in hemoglobin and absolute neutrophil count and dose-related increases in total cholesterol, high-density lipoprotein cholesterol, and low-density lipoprotein cholesterol. These changes led to one treatment discontinuation in a patient with hypercholesterolemia in the 15 mg dosing group.

CONCLUSION

In the past fifteen years, advances in immunology have greatly enhanced our knowledge of the pathogenesis of psoriasis. There are multiple biologic medications in development targeting the IL-17 inflammatory pathway. Although the long-term safety of these medications is not known, in the short-term, they appear to be well tolerated and very effective. There are also new medications being developed that target more "upstream" regulators of inflammation, such as JAK inhibitors and phosphodiesterase type 4 (PDE-4) inhibitors. Thus, we are in the middle of an exciting and fast-evolving landscape of psoriasis therapy. Perhaps most gratifying is that psoriasis patients today have more effective and more convenient treatment alternatives than patients did as recently as 10 years ago.

REFERENCES

1. Schlaak JF, Buslau M, Jochum W, Hermann E, Girndt M, Gallati H, et al. T cells involved in psoriasis vulgaris belong to the Th1 subset. *J Invest Dermatol* 1994; 102(2): 145–9.
2. Harrington LE, Hatton RD, Mangan PR, Turner H, Murphy TL, Murphy KM, et al. Interleukin 17-producing CD4+ effector T cells develop via a lineage distinct from the T helper type 1 and 2 lineages. *Nat Immunol* 2005; 6(11): 1123–32.
3. Park H, Li Z, Yang XO, Chang SH, Nurieva R, Wang YH, et al. A distinct lineage of CD4 T cells regulates tissue inflammation by producing interleukin 17. *Nat Immunol* 2005; 6(11): 1133–41.
4. Di Cesare A, Di Meglio P, Nestle FO. The IL-23/Th17 axis in the immunopathogenesis of psoriasis. *J Invest Dermatol* 2009; 129(6): 1339–50.
5. Lowes MA, Kikuchi T, Fuentes-Duculan J, Cardinale I, Zaba LC, Haider AS, et al. Psoriasis vulgaris lesions contain discrete populations of Th1 and Th17 T cells. *J Invest Dermatol* 2008; 128(5): 1207–11.
6. Chan JR, Blumenschein W, Murphy E, Diveu C, Wiekowski M, Abbondanzo S, et al. IL-23 stimulates epidermal hyperplasia via TNF and IL-20R2-dependent mechanisms with implications for psoriasis pathogenesis. *J Exp Med* 2006; 203(12): 2577–87.
7. Raychaudhuri SP. Role of IL-17 in psoriasis and psoriatic arthritis. *Clin Rev Allergy Immunol* 2013; 44(2): 183–93.
8. Pappu R, Ramirez-Carrozzi V, Sambandam A. The interleukin-17 cytokine family: critical players in host defence and inflammatory diseases. *Immunology* 2011; 134(1): 8–16.
9. Ariza ME, Williams MV, Wong HK. Targeting IL-17 in psoriasis: from cutaneous immunobiology to clinical application. *Clin Immunol* 2013; 146(2): 131–9.
10. Martin DA, Towne JE, Kricorian G, Klekotka P, Gudjonsson JE, Krueger JG, et al. The emerging role of IL-17 in the pathogenesis of psoriasis: preclinical and clinical findings. *J Invest Dermatol* 2013; 133(1): 17–26.
11. Chu CC, Di Meglio P, Nestle FO. Harnessing dendritic cells in inflammatory skin diseases. *Semin Immunol* 2011; 23(1): 28–41.
12. McGeachy MJ, Cua DJ. Th17 cell differentiation: the long and winding road. *Immunity* 2008; 28(4): 445–53.
13. Johnston A, Fritz Y, Dawes SM, Diaconu D, Al-Attar PM, Guzman AM, et al. Keratinocyte overexpression of IL-17C promotes psoriasiform skin inflammation. *J Immunol* 2013; 190(5): 2252–62.
14. Fujita H. The role of IL-22 and Th22 cells in human skin diseases. *J Dermatol Sci* 2013; 72: 3–8.
15. Trifari S, Kaplan CD, Tran EH, Crellin NK, Spits H. Identification of a human helper T cell population that has abundant production of interleukin 22 and is distinct from T(H)-17, T(H)1 and T(H)2 cells. *Nat Immunol* 2009; 10(8): 864–71.
16. Weaver CT, Hatton RD, Mangan PR, Harrington LE. IL-17 family cytokines and the expanding diversity of effector T cell lineages. *Ann Rev Immunol* 2007; 25: 821–52.
17. Lee J, Ho WH, Maruoka M, Corpuz RT, Baldwin DT, Foster JS, et al. IL-17E, a novel proinflammatory ligand for the IL-17 receptor homolog IL-17Rh1. *J Biol Chem* 2001; 276(2): 1660–4.
18. Gaffen SL. Structure and signalling in the IL-17 receptor family. *Nat Rev Immunol* 2009; 9(8): 556–67.

19. Moseley TA, Haudenschild DR, Rose L, Reddi AH. Interleukin-17 family and IL-17 receptors. *Cytokine Growth Factor Rev* 2003; 14(2): 155–74.
20. Wright JF, Guo Y, Quazi A, Luxenberg DP, Bennett F, Ross JF, et al. Identification of an interleukin 17F/17A heterodimer in activated human CD4+ T cells. *J Biol Chem* 2007; 282(18): 13447–55.
21. Chang SH, Dong C. A novel heterodimeric cytokine consisting of IL-17 and IL-17F regulates inflammatory responses. *Cell Res* 2007; 17(5): 435–40.
22. Ely LK, Fischer S, Garcia KC. Structural basis of receptor sharing by interleukin 17 cytokines. *Nat Immunol* 2009; 10(12): 1245–51.
23. Johansen C, Usher PA, Kjellerup RB, Lundsgaard D, Iversen L, Kragballe K. Characterization of the interleukin-17 isoforms and receptors in lesional psoriatic skin. *Br J Dermatol* 2009; 160(2): 319–24.
24. Zuniga LA, Shen WJ, Joyce-Shaikh B, Pyatnova EA, Richards AG, Thom C, et al. IL-17 regulates adipogenesis, glucose homeostasis, and obesity. *J Immunol* 2010; 185(11): 6947–59.
25. Miossec P, Kolls JK. Targeting IL-17 and TH17 cells in chronic inflammation. *Nat Rev Drug Discov* 2012; 11(10): 763–76.
26. Ge D, You Z. Expression of interleukin-17RC protein in normal human tissues. *Int Arch Med* 2008; 1(1): 19.
27. Onishi RM, Gaffen SL. Interleukin-17 and its target genes: mechanisms of interleukin-17 function in disease. *Immunology* 2010; 129(3): 311–21.
28. Cua DJ, Tato CM. Innate IL-17-producing cells: the sentinels of the immune system. *Nat Rev Immunol* 2010; 10(7): 479–89.
29. Wright JF, Bennett F, Li B, Brooks J, Luxenberg DP, Whitters MJ, et al. The human IL-17F/IL-17A heterodimeric cytokine signals through the IL-17RA/IL-17RC receptor complex. *J Immunol* 2008; 181(4): 2799–805.
30. Kao CY, Chen Y, Thai P, Wachi S, Huang F, Kim C, et al. IL-17 markedly up-regulates beta-defensin-2 expression in human airway epithelium via JAK and NF-kappaB signaling pathways. *J Immunol* 2004; 173(5): 3482–91.
31. Liang SC, Tan XY, Luxenberg DP, Karim R, Dunussi-Joannopoulos K, Collins M, et al. Interleukin (IL)-22 and IL-17 are coexpressed by Th17 cells and cooperatively enhance expression of antimicrobial peptides. *J Exp Med* 2006; 203(10): 2271–9.
32. Krueger JG, Fretzin S, Suarez-Farinas M, Haslett PA, Phipps KM, Cameron GS, et al. IL-17A is essential for cell activation and inflammatory gene circuits in subjects with psoriasis. *J Allergy Clin Immunol* 2012; 130(1): 145–54. e9.
33. Laan M, Cui ZH, Hoshino H, Lotvall J, Sjostrand M, Gruenert DC, et al. Neutrophil recruitment by human IL-17 via C-X-C chemokine release in the airways. *J Immunol* 1999; 162(4): 2347–52.
34. Numasaki M, Fukushi J, Ono M, Narula SK, Zavodny PJ, Kudo T, et al. Interleukin-17 promotes angiogenesis and tumor growth. *Blood* 2003; 101(7): 2620–7.
35. Starnes T, Broxmeyer HE, Robertson MJ, Hromas R. Cutting edge: IL-17D, a novel member of the IL-17 family, stimulates cytokine production and inhibits hemopoiesis. *J Immunol* 2002; 169(2): 642–6.
36. Chiricozzi A, Guttman-Yassky E, Suarez-Farinas M, Nograles KE, Tian S, Cardinale I, et al. Integrative responses to IL-17 and TNF-alpha in human keratinocytes account for key inflammatory pathogenic circuits in psoriasis. *J Invest Dermatol* 2011; 131(3): 677–87.
37. Ruddy MJ, Wong GC, Liu XK, Yamamoto H, Kasayama S, Kirkwood KL, et al. Functional cooperation between interleukin-17 and tumor necrosis factor-alpha is mediated by CCAAT/enhancer-binding protein family members. *J Biol Chem* 2004; 279(4): 2559–67.
38. Yilmaz SB, Cicek N, Coskun M, Yegin O, Alpsoy E. Serum and tissue levels of IL-17 in different clinical subtypes of psoriasis. *Arch Dermatol Res* 2012; 304(6): 465–9.
39. Yan KX, Fang X, Han L, Zhang ZH, Kang KF, Zheng ZZ, et al. Foxp3+ regulatory T cells and related cytokines differentially expressed in plaque vs. guttate psoriasis vulgaris. *Br J Dermatol* 2010; 163(1): 48–56.
40. Harper EG, Guo C, Rizzo H, Lillis JV, Kurtz SE, Skorcheva I, et al. Th17 cytokines stimulate CCL20 expression in keratinocytes *in vitro* and *in vivo*: implications for psoriasis pathogenesis. *J Invest Dermatol* 2009; 129(9): 2175–83.
41. Armstrong AW, Schupp C, Bebo B. Psoriasis comorbidities: results from the National Psoriasis Foundation Surveys 2003 to 2011. *Dermatology* 2012; 225(2): 121–6.

42. Cheng X, Yu X, Ding YJ, Fu QQ, Xie JJ, Tang TT, et al. The Th17/Treg imbalance in patients with acute coronary syndrome. *Clin Immunol* 2008; 127(1): 89–97.
43. de Boer OJ, van der Meer JJ, Teeling P, van der Loos CM, Idu MM, van Maldegem F, et al. Differential expression of interleukin-17 family cytokines in intact and complicated human atherosclerotic plaques. *J Pathol* 2010; 220(4): 499–508.
44. Erbel C, Chen L, Bea F, Wangler S, Celik S, Lasitschka F, et al. Inhibition of IL-17A attenuates atherosclerotic lesion development in apoE-deficient mice. *J Immunol* 2009; 183(12): 8167–75.
45. McAllister F, Henry A, Kreindler JL, Dubin PJ, Ulrich L, Steele C, et al. Role of IL-17A, IL-17F, and the IL-17 receptor in regulating growth-related oncogene-alpha and granulocyte colony-stimulating factor in bronchial epithelium: implications for airway inflammation in cystic fibrosis. *J Immunol* 2005; 175(1): 404–12.
46. Ramirez-Carrozzi V, Sambandam A, Luis E, Lin Z, Jeet S, Lesch J, et al. IL-17C regulates the innate immune function of epithelial cells in an autocrine manner. *Nat Immunol* 2011; 12(12): 1159–66.
47. Chang SH, Reynolds JM, Pappu BP, Chen G, Martinez GJ, Dong C. Interleukin-17C promotes Th17 cell responses and autoimmune disease via interleukin-17 receptor E. *Immunity* 2011; 35(4): 611–21.
48. Song X, Zhu S, Shi P, Liu Y, Shi Y, Levin SD, et al. IL-17RE is the functional receptor for IL-17C and mediates mucosal immunity to infection with intestinal pathogens. *Nat Immunol* 2011; 12(12): 1151–8.
49. Deng GM, Zheng L, Chan FK, Lenardo M. Amelioration of inflammatory arthritis by targeting the pre-ligand assembly domain of tumor necrosis factor receptors. *Nat Med* 2005; 11(10): 1066–72.
50. Wang YL, Chou FC, Chen SJ, Lin SH, Chang DM, Sytwu HK. Targeting pre-ligand assembly domain of TNFR1 ameliorates autoimmune diseases – an unrevealed role in downregulation of Th17 cells. *J Autoimmun* 2011; 37(3): 160–70.
51. Deng GM, Liu L, Tsokos GC. Targeted tumor necrosis factor receptor I preligand assembly domain improves skin lesions in MRL/lpr mice. *Arthritis Rheum* 2010; 62(8): 2424–31.
52. Papp KA, Langley RG, Sigurgeirsson B, Abe M, Baker DR, Konno P, et al. Efficacy and safety of secukinumab in the treatment of moderate-to-severe plaque psoriasis: a randomized, double-blind, placebo-controlled phase II dose-ranging study. *Br J Dermatol* 2013; 168(2): 412–21.
53. Rich P, Sigurgeirsson B, Thaci DP, Ortonne JP, Paul C, Schopf RE, et al. Secukinumab induction and maintenance therapy in moderate-to-severe plaque psoriasis: a randomised, double-blind, placebo-controlled, phase II regimen-finding study. *Br J Dermatol* 2013; 168: 402–11.
54. Leonardi C, Matheson R, Zachariae C, Cameron G, Li L, Edson-Heredia E, et al. Anti-interleukin-17 monoclonal antibody ixekizumab in chronic plaque psoriasis. *N Engl J Med* 2012; 366(13): 1190–9.
55. Genovese MC, Van den Bosch F, Roberson SA, Bojin S, Biagini IM, Ryan P, et al. LY2439821, a humanized anti-interleukin-17 monoclonal antibody, in the treatment of patients with rheumatoid arthritis: a phase I randomized, double-blind, placebo-controlled, proof-of-concept study. *Arthritis Rheum* 2010; 62(4): 929–39.
56. Smith E, Stark MA, Zarbock A, Burcin TL, Bruce AC, Vaswani D, et al. IL-17A inhibits the expansion of IL-17A-producing T cells in mice through "short-loop" inhibition via IL-17 receptor. *J Immunol* 2008; 181(2): 1357–64.
57. Papp KA, Leonardi C, Menter A, Ortonne JP, Krueger JG, Kricorian G, et al. Brodalumab, an anti-interleukin-17-receptor antibody for psoriasis. *N Engl J Med* 2012; 366(13): 1181–9.
58. Houslay MD, Schafer P, Zhang KY. Keynote review: phosphodiesterase-4 as a therapeutic target. *Drug Discov Today* 2005; 10(22): 1503–19.
59. Tasken K, Aandahl EM. Localized effects of cAMP mediated by distinct routes of protein kinase A. *Physiol Rev* 2004; 84(1): 137–67.
60. Papp K, Cather JC, Rosoph L, Sofen H, Langley RG, Matheson RT, et al. Efficacy of apremilast in the treatment of moderate to severe psoriasis: a randomised controlled trial. *Lancet* 2012; 380(9843): 738–46.
61. Murray PJ. The JAK-STAT signaling pathway: input and output integration. *J Immunol* 2007; 178(5): 2623–9.
62. O'Sullivan LA, Liongue C, Lewis RS, Stephenson SE, Ward AC. Cytokine receptor signaling through the Jak-Stat-Socs pathway in disease. *Mol Immunol* 2007; 44(10): 2497–506.
63. Papp KA, Menter A, Strober B, Langley RG, Buonanno M, Wolk R, et al. Efficacy and safety of tofacitinib, an oral Janus kinase inhibitor, in the treatment of psoriasis: a phase 2b randomized placebo-controlled dose-ranging study. *Br J Dermatol* 2012; 167(3): 668–77.

Chapter 17

Erythrodermic and Pustular Psoriasis

Ethan C. Levin, Eric Y. Sako, Shannon Famenini, and Jashin J. Wu

INTRODUCTION

Erythrodermic and generalized pustular psoriasis can become dermatologic emergencies. They are the most severe forms of psoriasis, characterized by an uncontrolled, widespread, severe eruption over most of the body. Patients are at risk for developing potentially fatal complications, including sepsis, acute renal failure, high-output congestive heart failure, and acute respiratory distress syndrome [1–9]. Therefore, the dermatologist must quickly start the most effective and aggressive treatment. In this chapter, we will review the clinical presentation, epidemiology, and management of erythrodermic and generalized pustular psoriasis.

CLINICAL PRESENTATION AND EPIDEMIOLOGY

Erythrodermic psoriasis presents as an intense, bright-red, inflammatory dermatitis involving at least 75% of the body surface area (Figure 17.1) [10]. It is rare, with an estimated prevalence of 1%–2.25% among psoriasis patients, and can occur *de novo* or in patients with preexisting psoriasis [11]. Patients may appear ill—with fever, chills, and malaise [11]. The course of erythrodermic psoriasis varies from acute and rapidly progressive to prolonged and chronic, which may follow a relapsing-remitting pattern.

Psoriasis is the most common cause of erythroderma and represents about 25% of cases. Other causes of erythroderma include cutaneous lymphoma, pityriasis rubra pilaris, severe eczema, and drug eruptions [12–14]. Thus, biopsy may be useful in distinguishing erythrodermic psoriasis from these other causes of erythroderma.

Pustular psoriasis has been historically classified into two forms: localized and generalized. Generalized pustular psoriasis can be further divided based on the acuity of presentation and natural history of disease. Annular pustular psoriasis usually follows a chronic, more benign course. In contrast, the von Zumbusch type is often a more severe presentation, characterized by the rapid onset of widespread sterile pustules on a background of erythema (Figure 17.2) [15]. Like erythrodermic psoriasis, preexisting psoriasis vulgaris may or may not be present [16]. Initially, pustules may be located at the periphery of psoriatic plaques, where inflammation is the most active. However, once the disease becomes generalized, it can develop on any involved skin [17]. Confluence of these pustules may form irregular "lakes of pus" over part or all of the body. The patient may appear toxic, with fever, chills, pain, and intense pruritus [18]. Other possible findings include a geographic or fissured tongue, scaly lips with superficial ulcerations, and ocular involvement (e.g., conjunctivitis, uveitis, or iritis).

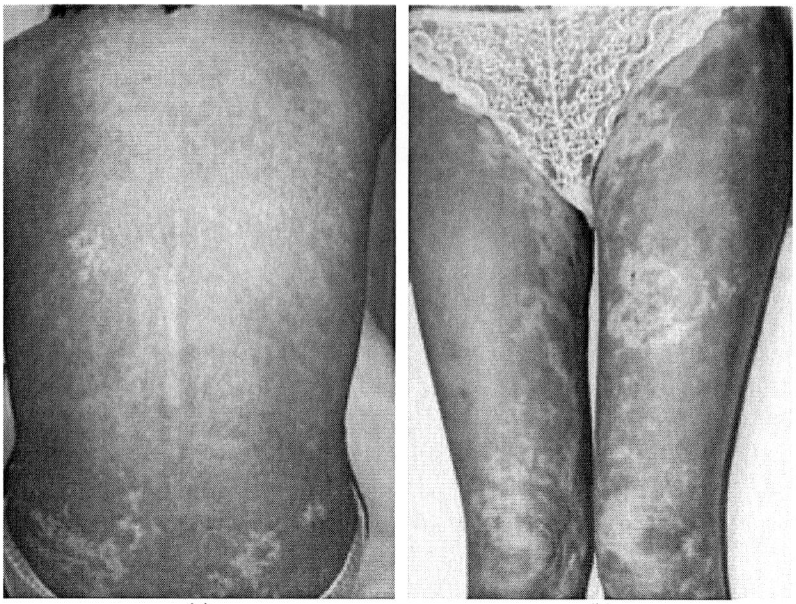

(a) (b)

FIGURE 17.1 (See color insert.) Erythrodermic psoriasis. (a) Erythematous, diffuse, confluent plaque covering most of the back with few islands of sparing. (b) Large, coalescing erythematous patches with islands of sparing involving the bilateral lower extremities. (Reprinted from Santos-Juanes J et al.: Ustekinumab induces rapid clearing of erythrodermic psoriasis after failure of antitumor necrosis factor therapies. *Br J Dermatol.* 2010. 162, 1144–6. Copyright Wiley-VCH Verlag GmbH & Co. KGaA. Reproduced with permission.)

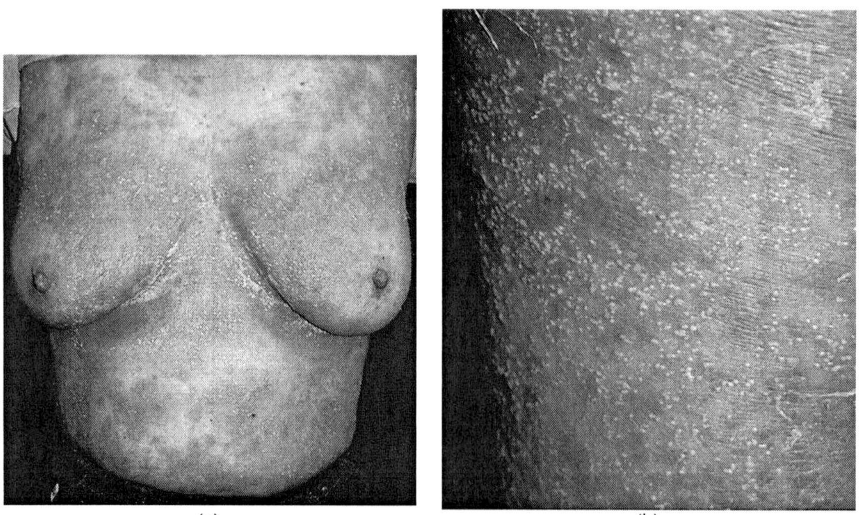

(a) (b)

FIGURE 17.2 (See color insert.) Generalized pustular psoriasis. (a) Extensive erythematous plaques with multiple pustules distributed over the upper trunk, breasts and abdomen. There is adherent scale along the underside of the breasts. (b) Numerous sterile pustules on a deeply erythematous plaque. (Wu MC, Lee JY: Generalized flare of pustular psoriasis induced by PEGylated interferon-alpha2b therapy for chronic hepatitis C. *Aust J Dermatol.* 2012. 53, e69–72. Copyright Wiley-VCH Verlag GmbH & Co. KGaA. Reproduced with permission.)

Histopathological examination is characterized Kogoj's spongiform pustules, a subcorneal neutrophilic infiltrate with damaged or swollen keratinocytes as well as the classic histologic findings of psoriasis (i.e., parakeratosis, hyperkeratosis, elongated rete ridges, Munro's microabscesses, and superficial perivascular lymphocytic infiltrate). The inflammation and edema are more severe than in the other subtypes of psoriasis [18].

Although the cause of erythrodermic psoriasis and generalized pustular psoriasis is often idiopathic, potential triggers include withdrawal of antipsoriatic therapy (e.g., systemic steroids) [19–21], infection, or medications (e.g., lithium, calcium channel blockers). There have been a number of case reports of new pustular psoriasis arising after treatment with a tumor necrosis factor-α (TNF-α) inhibitor in patients with Crohn's disease, rheumatoid arthritis, or psoriasis [22–24].

There are hereditary forms of generalized pustular psoriasis. These patients possess a mutation in the interleukin-1 (IL-1) or IL-36 receptor antagonist genes. A deficiency of either of these anti-inflammatory proteins leads to unopposed activity of proinflammatory signaling pathways, such as nuclear factor kB (NF-kB) and mitogen-activated protein (MAP) kinases [25]. In some patients, pustular dermatitis is part of a systemic inflammatory syndrome of skin and bone that has a neonatal onset [26]. This syndrome is called either deficiency of interleukin-1 receptor antagonist (DIRA) or deficiency of IL-36 receptor antagonist (DITRA) depending on the affected gene [25].

Both erythrodermic psoriasis and generalized pustular psoriasis are associated with severe and sometimes fatal complications. The loss of epidermal integrity may predispose to sepsis from skin pathogens, especially *Staphylococcus aureus* [27]. Cutaneous fluid loss can lead to shock and acute renal failure [28]. Derangements in the distribution of blood may cause high-output congestive heart failure [9]. Patients may also be at risk for acute respiratory distress syndrome [8]. Thus, it is important that the clinician quickly distinguishes these potentially fatal subtypes of psoriasis from other conditions so that therapy can be started immediately.

TRIAGING PATIENTS WITH ERYTHRODERMIC AND GENERALIZED PUSTULAR PSORIASIS

Erythrodermic psoriasis and generalized pustular psoriasis are two of the rare clinical emergencies with which a dermatologist may be confronted. Therefore, it is important to be able to recognize which of these patients require immediate hospitalization due to high risk of deterioration or mortality. We recommend considering inpatient admission for patients that are systemically ill with fevers, chills, shortness of breath, or changes in mental status. Inpatient admission should also be considered for elderly patients or for those with comorbidities that place them at high risk for deterioration or development of complications. These comorbidities include a history of congestive heart failure, renal insufficiency, diabetes, or immunodeficiency. Those patients who do not have multiple medical problems and are not systemically ill may be managed in an outpatient setting. The treatments discussed in this chapter apply to erythrodermic psoriasis and to generalized pustular psoriasis patients in both inpatient and outpatient settings.

TABLE 17.1 Recommended Internal Agents for Erythrodermic Psoriasis and Generalized Pustular Psoriasis

Adults, First Line	Pregnancy, First Line	Pediatric, First Line
Infliximab[a], cyclosporine[a], acitretin, methotrexate	Infliximab[a], cyclosporine[a], oral prednisone	Cyclosporine[a], acitretin, methotrexate, etanercept
Second Line	**Second Line**	**Second Line**
Etanercept, ustekinumab, adalimumab, anakinra[b]	Etanercept, ustekinumab, adalimumab, phototherapy	Infliximab, ustekinumab, adalimumab, anakinra[b]

[a] Most appropriate for acute or severe presentations.
[b] Only for pustular psoriasis.

ORAL MEDICAL MANAGEMENT

The most effective and rapid control of erythrodermic or generalized pustular psoriasis is achieved with high-dose of cyclosporine (Neoral®) or through infusions of infliximab (Remicade®) (Table 17.1). Acitretin (Soriatane®) also has a reputation for being efficacious, more so than when used for plaque-type psoriasis. Methotrexate is also a valid alternative. However, neither acitretin nor methotrexate is as effective or as fast at improving psoriatic skin inflammation as cyclosporine or infliximab (as will be discussed later in this chapter).

CYCLOSPORINE

When faced with erythrodermic psoriasis or generalized pustular psoriasis, it is critical to use the maximum dermatologic dose of cyclosporine, 5 mg/kg/day divided into two or three doses. The exception to this rule is if the patient is obese, in which case the ideal body weight is used to calculate the initial dose. However, if the dose calculated through ideal body weight proves inadequate, we recommend considering higher doses in order to promptly bring the intensity of generalized inflammation under control.

Common side effects from short-term cyclosporine use include gastrointestinal discomfort, temperature hypersensitivity, and electrolyte abnormalities. The risk of more severe side effects from cyclosporine relates to the duration of use as opposed to the absolute dosage used [29]. When cyclosporine is used in transplant patients, there is no dosing limit. During the critical initial phase after transplantation, whatever dose is needed to prevent organ rejection is used and is generally well tolerated by the patient. In other words, even though 5 mg/kg/day is generally adequate for even the most intense bright-red skin inflammation, a rare situation may require a dose higher than the U.S. Food and Drug Administration (FDA)–recommended limit for dermatologic use. It is the opinion of the authors that, if 5 mg/kg/day is not adequate, the clinician should increase the dose. The risk of a higher dose of cyclosporine is likely to be less than the risk of sepsis or other serious consequences of uncontrolled, whole-body inflammation. Moreover, the occurrence of catastrophic side effects from very short-term cyclosporine use would be highly unusual. Whenever cyclosporine is used in high doses, it is important to make sure that the patient is well hydrated to prevent renal hypoperfusion.

When using cyclosporine at 5 mg/kg/day in divided doses, there should be notable improvement in the intensity of erythema within a few days. If no improvement in erythema or pustulation is observed in five to seven days, the clinician may consider checking compliance. If the patient is compliant, consider increasing the dose of cyclosporine to bring the intensity of inflammation under control promptly. In cases refractory to high doses of cyclosporine, alternative diagnoses such as erythroderma of cutaneous lymphoma should be considered, and a skin biopsy may be performed.

Once the intensity of inflammation is under control, it is important not to discontinue or decrease the dose of cyclosporine prematurely. Intense inflammation has "momentum." The rapidity of skin improvement on cyclosporine can easily deceive a clinician into decreasing the dose of cyclosporine prematurely. Erythrodermic psoriasis generally requires weeks to months of treatment before the underlying "momentum" of intense inflammation finally weakens. Otherwise, the disease may recur or rebound when discontinuing the cyclosporine. A slow tapering off of the dosage is recommended rather than an abrupt discontinuation.

ACITRETIN

If the patient is not pregnant, acitretin can be added to cyclosporine as a second medication to further enhance the efficacy and rapidity of the onset of action. Moreover, the presence of acitretin in the highest tolerable dose for the patient will facilitate the tapering of cyclosporine. If there are no contraindications, we recommend starting both agents simultaneously or within the first few days, especially if the patient is at serious risk for sepsis or other immediate complications. Because erythrodermic psoriasis and generalized pustular psoriasis are dermatological emergencies, this is one rare instance where acitretin has a recommended starting dose of 50–100 mg/day, rather than 25 mg/day or less typically used for long-term control of plaque-type psoriasis. The use of acitretin in conjunction with cyclosporine is widely practiced in the transplant population to decrease skin cancer or verrucae risk [30–33].

Serious side effects from acitretin, such as pseudotumor cerebri and/or acute hypertriglyceridemia causing pancreatitis, are extremely rare [34,35]. When acitretin is used in high doses of up to 100 mg/day, the patient may be at increased risk for these unusual, but serious, side effects and should be monitored closely. However, the fear of these rare complications should not discourage the clinician from using the most appropriate dose of acitretin for rapid control. Other side effects from high-dose acitretin include alopecia and periungual lesions that resemble pyogenic granulomas [36]. Both of these side effects are reversible and dose dependent. When the acitretin dose is reduced or discontinued, normal hair growth will resume in almost all cases. The periungual lesions can be unsightly and somewhat uncomfortable for the patient. The patient can be reassured that the lesions usual resolve when the dose of acitretin is decreased to approximately 25 mg/day or less.

METHOTREXATE

Methotrexate is a valid alternative for the acute treatment of erythrodermic psoriasis or generalized pustular psoriasis. However, there are some key concerns with the use of methotrexate as compared to cyclosporine or acitretin. One major difficulty is the possibility of acute catastrophic side effects such as pancytopenia, fulminant hepatitis, or pneumonitis [37–43]. Therefore, even in times of dermatologic emergency, it is still recommended to do a methotrexate test-dose for the patient's safety. This one-week period during the test-dose could delay adequate treatment, possibly to the detriment of the patient. For this reason, cyclosporine and acitretin are more readily employable for erythrodermic or pustular psoriatic emergencies.

PHOTOTHERAPY

Psoralen plus ultraviolet A (PUVA) or ultraviolet B (UVB) phototherapy may be second-line options for controlling the chronic form of erythrodermic or generalized pustular psoriasis. Due to the intensity of inflammation in the acute setting, phototherapy may exacerbate the condition. Thus, all forms or phototherapy should be avoided in the acute setting and employed only after the skin has had a chance to "cool down" through the use of other agents [16]. Even after the intensity of inflammation has decreased, an extra cautious approach to the dosimetry of ultraviolet light can help decrease the chance of aggravating psoriatic skin, which has just recovered from erythroderma or pustulation.

BIOLOGIC MANAGEMENT OF ERYTHRODERMIC AND GENERALIZED PUSTULAR PSORIASIS

Although cyclosporine, acitretin, and methotrexate are effective medications, they each have specific limitations. Some patients find these medications ineffective, or they must discontinue therapy due to side effects. Acitretin and methotrexate are contraindicated in patients with severely impaired hepatic function and in pregnancy. Cyclosporine is contraindicated in patients with kidney disease and in patients with uncontrolled hypertension. In contrast, TNF-α inhibitors and other biologic medications have no absolute contraindications in patients with renal disease, hepatic disease, or in pregnancy.

During the past 10–15 years, the use of biologic medications for the treatment of refractory cases of erythrodermic or pustular psoriasis has increased. Infliximab (Remicade®) has been shown to induce a rapid improvement in erythrodermic and pustular psoriasis [44]. Infliximab is a chimeric TNF-α monoclonal antibody that can neutralize soluble and membrane-bound TNF-α. The medication is infused intravenously and, as a result, has an extremely fast onset of action. In fact, some case series report significant improvement in erythroderma and pustulation as well as resolution of fevers and laboratory abnormalities within 24–72 hours [45–47]. As a result, use of infliximab has been shown to greatly reduce the amount of time a patient stays in the hospital with each erythrodermic or pustular flare [48].

Although initial efficacy is robust, over a period of months to years, up to half of the initial responders may develop tachyphylaxis to infliximab, also known as "biologic fatigue" (see Chapter 15) [49]. This may be due in part to the development of anti-infliximab antibodies [50]. Although a similar problem can occur with other biologic medications, it occurs with greater frequency in infliximab because of its mouse–human chimeric structure. Further, use of infliximab is associated with the risk of an infusion reaction. These reactions pose a rare but serious risk of anaphylaxis and result in a small but significant number of patients who have to stop the medication. In order to decrease the likelihood of biologic fatigue and infusion reactions, some practitioners routinely use concomitant immunosuppression with

TABLE 17.2 Summary of Reported Cases of Biologic Use in Erythrodermic and Pustular Psoriasis

Erythrodermic Psoriasis	Total Number of Cases Reported	Number of Cases Where Patient Showed Improvement[a]
Infliximab	52	36
Etanercept	17	11
Ustekinumab	15	8
Adalimumab	8	6
Pustular Psoriasis		
Infliximab	30	30
Etanercept	10	9
Ustekinumab	7	7
Adalimumab	6	6
Anakinra	2	2

[a] Improvement defined by achieving Psoriasis Area and Severity Index (PASI) 50, PASI-75, physician's global assessment of "clear" or "almost clear," or by subjective report of the investigator.

methotrexate [45,48,50–54]. Thus, although infliximab is an extremely effective rescue medication, we recommend transitioning to another agent for maintenance therapy.

As with systemic medications, there are no placebo-controlled or head-to-head clinical trials data for the treatment of erythrodermic or generalized pustular psoriasis with biologic agents. In fact, most clinical trials for biologic agents exclude these subtypes of psoriasis. There are case reports and case series that show successful use of infliximab, adalimumab (Humira®), etanercept (Enbrel®), and ustekinumab (Stelara®) in treating erythrodermic and generalized pustular psoriasis (Table 17.2) [44–48,10,50–82]. Anakinra may also be useful in cases of generalized pustular psoriasis [50]. Thus, in addition to infliximab, these biologic medications are viable options if a patient fails one of the primary treatments for erythrodermic or pustular psoriasis.

TOPICAL MANAGEMENT OF ERYTHRODERMIC AND PUSTULAR PSORIASIS

Although prompt initiation of systemic therapy is critical in managing an erythrodermic or pustular flare, one should not forget the helpfulness of a topical "cooling procedure." This procedure provides immediate relief to the painful, inflamed skin while the systemic therapy takes effect. In order to cool down whole-body, "beef-red" skin inflammation, we recommend applying superpotent topical corticosteroids, such as clobetasol 0.05% ointment, to the entire body surface area. The skin should then be covered with an occlusive dressing, such as plastic wrap or a whole-body occlusive suit. Impermeable gloves can be used to occlude the hands, shower caps inside of socks for the feet, and a shower cap for the scalp if needed. The patient should remain occluded for at least two to three hours, twice daily. Repeat the cooling procedure until the erythema is significantly reduced, which can take anywhere from 3 to 14 days.

Although liberal use of superpotent topical corticosteroids is not recommended for long-term management due to the risk of hypothalamic–pituitary–adrenal (HPA) axis suppression, skin atrophy, and possible rebound, use for less than two weeks has not been shown to be associated with any clinical signs or symptoms of these side effects [83].

MANAGEMENT IN PREGNANCY

For management of generalized pustular psoriasis (i.e., impetigo herpetiformis) or erythrodermic psoriasis in pregnancy, cyclosporine, infliximab, and oral steroids are the first-line agents recommended by the National Psoriasis Foundation (Table 17.1) [16]. Despite being pregnancy category C, cyclosporine use during pregnancy is not associated with an increased risk of birth defects. This is supported by several decades of registry data in transplant patients [84,85]. The use of cyclosporine in patients with erythrodermic or generalized pustular psoriasis is limited to case reports [86,87]. Unlike cyclosporine, all biologic therapies (including infliximab) are pregnancy category B. Given this difference, it is reasonable to expect biologic use to become more widespread among pregnant patients with erythrodermic or generalized pustular psoriasis [78]. Oral prednisone at doses of 30–40 mg/day is also effective. Topical therapy with steroids should be instituted along with systemic management.

MANAGEMENT IN CHILDREN

First-line internal therapy for erythrodermic or generalized pustular psoriasis in pediatric patients includes acitretin, methotrexate, cyclosporine, and etanercept (Table 17.1) [65,73,88–93]. Acitretin at doses less than 1 mg/kg/day is recommended due to the potential for skeletal toxicity. In addition, this medication is relatively contraindicated in girls of reproductive age. Low-dose methotrexate (0.2–0.4 mg/kg/day) or low-dose cyclosporine (1–3 mg/kg/day) may also be effective with fewer side effects than other agents. Second-line agents include adalimumab, infliximab, and UVB phototherapy (only after an adequate "cool down" procedure) [58,94,95].

CONCLUSION

Erythrodermic and generalized pustular psoriasis are rare psoriatic emergencies that require immediate treatment to avoid the development of catastrophic complications. Clinicians may strongly consider hospitalization for those patients who appear systemically ill or who have comorbidities such as congestive heart failure, renal insufficiency, diabetes mellitus, or old age. Therapy is determined by the severity of illness. Those patients who are most severely affected should be treated promptly with cyclosporine 5 mg/kg/day or an infliximab infusion of 5 mg/kg. For long-term management, these patients can be transitioned to acitretin, methotrexate, or any of the biologic agents approved for the treatment of plaque psoriasis. In order to assess the comparative efficacy and safety of the different medications available to treat erythrodermic or generalized pustular psoriasis, controlled studies are needed.

REFERENCES

1. Abou-Samra T, Constantin JM, Amarger S, Mansard S, Souteyrand P, Bazin JE, et al. Generalized pustular psoriasis complicated by acute respiratory distress syndrome. *Br J Dermatol* 2004; 150(2): 353–6.
2. Doval IG, Peteiro C, Toribio J. Acute respiratory distress syndrome and generalized pustular psoriasis: another case report. *Arch Dermatol* 1998; 134(1): 103.

3. Griffiths MR, Porter W, Fergusson-Wood LA, Adriaans B. Generalized pustular psoriasis complicated by acute respiratory distress syndrome. *Br J Dermatol* 2006; 155(2): 496–7.
4. Handfield-Jones SE, Garvey M, McGibbon DH, Black MM. Capillary leak syndrome in generalized pustular psoriasis. *Br J Dermatol* 1992; 127(1): 64.
5. Matsubara M, Komori M, Koishi K, Yasuno H, Ueda K, Seto Y, et al. Generalized pustular psoriasis and bacteremia. *J Dermatol* 1983; 10(6): 525–9.
6. McGregor JM, Barker JN, MacDonald DM. Pulmonary capillary leak syndrome complicating generalized pustular psoriasis: possible role of cytokines. *Br J Dermatol* 1991; 125(5): 472–4.
7. O'Donnell PG, Hughes JR, Higgins EM, Groves RW, Pembroke AC. A fatal case of capillary leak syndrome in erythrodermic psoriasis. *Br J Dermatol* 1995; 132(1): 160–1.
8. Sadeh JS, Rudikoff D, Gordon ML, Bowden J, Goldman BD, Lebwohl M. Pustular and erythrodermic psoriasis complicated by acute respiratory distress syndrome. *Arch Dermatol* 1997; 133(6): 747–50.
9. Voigt GC, Kronthal HL, Crounse RG. Cardiac output in erythrodermic skin disease. *Am Heart J* 1966; 72(5): 615–20.
10. Santos-Juanes J, Coto-Segura P, Mas-Vidal A, Galache Osuna C. Ustekinumab induces rapid clearing of erythrodermic psoriasis after failure of antitumour necrosis factor therapies. *Br J Dermatol* 2010; 162(5): 1144–6.
11. Rosenbach M, Hsu S, Korman NJ, Lebwohl MG, Young M, Bebo BF, Jr, et al. Treatment of erythrodermic psoriasis: from the medical board of the National Psoriasis Foundation. *J Am Acad Dermatol* 2010; 62(4): 655–62.
12. Botella-Estrada R, Sanmartin O, Oliver V, Febrer I, Aliaga A. Erythroderma. A clinicopathological study of 56 cases. *Arch Dermatol* 1994; 130(12): 1503–7.
13. Hasan T, Jansen CT. Erythroderma: a follow-up of fifty cases. *J Am Acad Dermatol* 1983; 8(6): 836–40.
14. Sigurdsson V, Toonstra J, Hezemans-Boer M, van Vloten WA. Erythroderma. A clinical and follow-up study of 102 patients, with special emphasis on survival. *J Am Acad Dermatol* 1996; 35(1): 53–7.
15. Wu MC, Lee JY. Generalized flare of pustular psoriasis induced by PEGylated interferon-alpha2b therapy for chronic hepatitis C. *Aust J Dermatol* 2012; 53(4): e69–72.
16. Robinson A, Van Voorhees AS, Hsu S, Korman NJ, Lebwohl MG, Bebo BF, Jr, et al. Treatment of pustular psoriasis: from the Medical Board of the National Psoriasis Foundation. *J Am Acad Dermatol* 2012; 67(2): 279–88.
17. James WD, Berger T, Elston DM. *Andrews' Diseases of the Skin: Clinical Dermatology*, 11th ed. Philadelphia, PA: Saunders; 2011.
18. Umezawa Y, Ozawa A, Kawasima T, Shimizu H, Terui T, Tagami H, et al. Therapeutic guidelines for the treatment of generalized pustular psoriasis (GPP) based on a proposed classification of disease severity. *Arch Dermatol Res* 2003; 295(Suppl 1): S43–54.
19. De Silva BD, Benton EC, Tidman MJ. Generalized pustular psoriasis following withdrawal of oral cyclosporin treatment for palmo-plantar pustulosis. *Clin Exp Dermatol* 1999; 24(1): 10–13.
20. Elston GE, Charles-Holmes R, Carr RA. Precipitation of generalized pustular psoriasis by prednisolone. *Clin Exp Dermatol* 2006; 31(1): 133–4.
21. Georgala S, Koumantaki E, Rallis E, Papadavid E. Generalized pustular psoriasis developing during withdrawal of short-term cyclosporin therapy. *Br J Dermatol* 2000; 142(5): 1057–8.
22. Cohen JD, Bournerias I, Buffard V, Paufler A, Chevalier X, Bagot M, et al. Psoriasis induced by tumor necrosis factor-alpha antagonist therapy: a case series. *J Rheumatol* 2007; 34(2): 380–5.
23. Thurber M, Feasel A, Stroehlein J, Hymes SR. Pustular psoriasis induced by infliximab. *J Drugs Dermatol* 2004; 3(4): 439–40.
24. Ubriani R, Van Voorhees AS. Onset of psoriasis during treatment with TNF-{alpha} antagonists: a report of 3 cases. *Arch Dermatol* 2007; 143(2): 270–2.
25. Marrakchi S, Guigue P, Renshaw BR, Puel A, Pei XY, Fraitag S, et al. Interleukin-36-receptor antagonist deficiency and generalized pustular psoriasis. *N Engl J Med* 2011; 365(7): 620–8.
26. Jesus AA, Osman M, Silva CA, Kim PW, Pham TH, Gadina M, et al. A novel mutation of IL1RN in the deficiency of interleukin-1 receptor antagonist syndrome: description of two unrelated cases from Brazil. *Arthritis Rheum* 2011; 63(12): 4007–17.
27. Green MS, Prystowsky JH, Cohen SR, Cohen JI, Lebwohl MG. Infectious complications of erythrodermic psoriasis. *J Am Acad Dermatol* 1996; 34(5 Pt 2): 911–14.

28. Takedai T, Yamamoto I, Tokeshi J. Acute generalized pustular psoriasis presenting with erythroderma associated with shock and acute renal failure. *Hawaii Med J* 2003; 62(12): 278–81.
29. Koo J, Lee J. Cyclosporine: what clinicians need to know. *Dermatol Clin* 1995; 13(4): 897–907.
30. George R, Weightman W, Russ GR, Bannister KM, Mathew TH. Acitretin for chemoprevention of non-melanoma skin cancers in renal transplant recipients. *Aust J Dermatol* 2002; 43(4): 269–73.
31. Yuan ZF, Davis A, Macdonald K, Bailey RR. Use of acitretin for the skin complications in renal transplant recipients. *N Z Med J* 1995; 108(1002): 255–6.
32. Bavinck JN, Tieben LM, Van der Woude FJ, Tegzess AM, Hermans J, ter Schegget J, et al. Prevention of skin cancer and reduction of keratotic skin lesions during acitretin therapy in renal transplant recipients: a double-blind, placebo-controlled study. *J Clin Oncol* 1995; 13(8): 1933–8.
33. McKenna DB, Murphy GM. Skin cancer chemoprophylaxis in renal transplant recipients: 5 years of experience using low-dose acitretin. *Br J Dermatol* 1999; 140(4): 656–60.
34. Katz HI, Waalen J, Leach EE. Acitretin in psoriasis: an overview of adverse effects. *J Am Acad Dermatol* 1999; 41(3 Pt 2): S7–S12.
35. Roenigk HH, Jr, Callen JP, Guzzo CA, Katz HI, Lowe N, Madison K, et al. Effects of acitretin on the liver. *J Am Acad Dermatol* 1999; 41(4): 584–8.
36. Badri T, Hawilo AM, Benmously R, Fenniche S, Mokhtar I. Acitretin-induced pyogenic granuloma. *Acta Dermatovenerol Alp Panonica Adriat* 2011; 20(4): 217–18.
37. Abel EA, Farber EM. Pancytopenia following low-dose methotrexate therapy. *JAMA* 1988; 259(24): 3612.
38. Groenendal H, Rampen FH. Methotrexate and trimethoprim-sulphamethoxazole—a potentially hazardous combination. *Clin Exp Dermatol* 1990; 15(5): 358–60.
39. Gutierrez-Urena S, Molina JF, Garcia CO, Cuellar ML, Espinoza LR. Pancytopenia secondary to methotrexate therapy in rheumatoid arthritis. *Arthritis Rheum* 1996; 39(2): 272–6.
40. Phillips TJ, Jones DH, Baker H. Pulmonary complications following methotrexate therapy. *J Am Acad Dermatol* 1987; 16(2 Pt 1): 373–5.
41. Searles G, McKendry RJ. Methotrexate pneumonitis in rheumatoid arthritis: potential risk factors. Four case reports and a review of the literature. *J Rheumatol* 1987; 14(6): 1164–71.
42. Shupack JL, Webster GF. Pancytopenia following low-dose oral methotrexate therapy for psoriasis. *JAMA* 1988; 259(24): 3594–6.
43. Sostman HD, Matthay RA, Putman CE, Smith GJ. Methotrexate-induced pneumonitis. *Medicine* 1976; 55(5): 371–88.
44. Torii H, Nakagawa H. Long-term study of infliximab in Japanese patients with plaque psoriasis, psoriatic arthritis, pustular psoriasis and psoriatic erythroderma. *J Dermatol* 2011; 38(4): 321–34.
45. Routhouska SB, Sheth PB, Korman NJ. Long-term management of generalized pustular psoriasis with infliximab: case series. *J Cutan Med Surg* 2008; 12(4): 184–8.
46. Trent JT, Kerdel FA. Successful treatment of Von Zumbusch pustular psoriasis with infliximab. *J Cutan Med Surg* 2004; 8(4): 224–8.
47. Weisenseel P, Prinz JC. Sequential use of infliximab and etanercept in generalized pustular psoriasis. *Cutis* 2006; 78(3): 197–9.
48. Heikkila H, Ranki A, Cajanus S, Karvonen SL. Infliximab combined with methotrexate as long-term treatment for erythrodermic psoriasis. *Arch Dermatol* 2005; 141(12): 1607–10.
49. Levin EC, Gupta R, Brown G, Malakouti M, Koo J. Biologic Fatigue in psoriasis. *J Dermatolog Treat* 2013. [Epub ahead of print].
50. Viguier M, Pages C, Aubin F, Delaporte E, Descamps V, Lok C, et al. Efficacy and safety of biologics in erythrodermic psoriasis: a multicentre, retrospective study. *Br J Dermatol* 2012; 167(2): 417–23.
51. Benoit S, Toksoy A, Brocker EB, Gillitzer R, Goebeler M. Treatment of recalcitrant pustular psoriasis with infliximab: effective reduction of chemokine expression. *Br J Dermatol* 2004; 150(5): 1009–12.
52. Elewski BE. Infliximab for the treatment of severe pustular psoriasis. *J Am Acad Dermatol* 2002; 47(5): 796–7.
53. Lisby S, Gniadecki R. Infliximab (Remicade) for acute, severe pustular and erythrodermic psoriasis. *Acta Derm Venereol* 2004; 84(3): 247–8.
54. Varma R, Cantrell W, Elmets C, Elewski B. Infliximab for the treatment of severe pustular psoriasis: 6 years later. *J Eur Acad Dermatol Venereol* 2008; 22(10): 1253–4.
55. Alvarez AC, Rodriguez-Nevado I, De Argila D, Rubio FP, Rovira I, Torrelo A, et al. Recalcitrant pustular psoriasis successfully treated with adalimumab. *Pediatr Dermatol* 2011; 28(2): 195–7.

56. Andrulonis R, Ferris LK. Treatment of severe psoriasis with ustekinumab during pregnancy. *J Drugs Dermatol* 2012; 11(10): 1240.
57. Buggiani G, D'Erme AM, Krysenka A, Pescitelli L, Lotti T, Prignano F. Efficacy of ustekinumab in sub-erythrodermic psoriasis: when TNF-blockers fail. *Dermatol Ther* 2012; 25(3): 283–5.
58. Callen JP, Jackson JH. Adalimumab effectively controlled recalcitrant generalized pustular psoriasis in an adolescent. *J Dermatolog Treat* 2005; 16(5–6): 350–2.
59. Castineiras I, Fernandez-Diaz L, Juarez Y, Lueiro M. Sustained efficacy of ustekinumab in refractory erythrodermic psoriasis after failure of antitumor necrosis factor therapies. *J Dermatol* 2012; 39(8): 730–1.
60. Chandran NS, Chong WS. A dramatic response to a single dose of infliximab as rescue therapy in acute generalized pustular psoriasis of von Zumbusch associated with a neutrophilic cholangitis. *Aust J Dermatol* 2010; 51(1): 29–31.
61. Dauden E, Santiago-et-Sanchez-Mateos D, Sotomayor-Lopez E, Garcia-Diez A. Ustekinumab: effective in a patient with severe recalcitrant generalized pustular psoriasis. *Br J Dermatol* 2010; 163(6): 1346–7.
62. Esposito M, Mazzotta A, Casciello C, Chimenti S. Etanercept at different dosages in the treatment of generalized pustular psoriasis: a case series. *Dermatology* 2008; 216(4): 355–60.
63. Esposito M, Mazzotta A, de Felice C, Papoutsaki M, Chimenti S. Treatment of erythrodermic psoriasis with etanercept. *Br J Dermatol* 2006; 155(1): 156–9.
64. Fiehn C, Andrassy K. Case number 29: hitting three with one strike: rapid improvement of psoriatic arthritis, psoriatic erythroderma, and secondary renal amyloidosis by treatment with infliximab (Remicade). *Ann Rheum Dis* 2004; 63(3): 232.
65. Fraga NA, Paim Mde F, Follador I, Ramos AN, Rego VR. Refractory erythrodermic psoriasis in a child with an excellent outcome by using etanercept. *An Bras Dermatol* 2011; 86(4 Suppl 1): S144–7.
66. Jordan J, Bieber T, Wilsmann-Theis D. Adalimumab: safe and successful in severe pustular psoriasis. *J Eur Acad Dermatol Venereol* 2009; 23(5): 592–3.
67. Kimura U, Kinoshita A, Sekigawa I, Takamori K, Suga Y. Successful treatment with adalimumab in a patient with psoriatic arthritis and generalized pustular psoriasis. *J Dermatol* 2012; 39(12): 1071–2.
68. Lewis TG, Tuchinda C, Lim HW, Wong HK. Life-threatening pustular and erythrodermic psoriasis responding to infliximab. *J Drugs Dermatol* 2006; 5(6): 546–8.
69. Lo Schiavo A, Brancaccio G, Puca RV, Caccavale S. Etanercept in the treatment of generalized annular pustular psoriasis. *Ann Dermatol* 2012; 24(2): 233–4.
70. Mikhail M, Weinberg JM, Smith BL. Successful treatment with etanercept of von Zumbusch pustular psoriasis in a patient with human immunodeficiency virus. *Arch Dermatol* 2008; 144(4): 453–6.
71. Newland MR, Weinstein A, Kerdel F. Rapid response to infliximab in severe pustular psoriasis, von Zumbusch type. *Int J Dermatol* 2002; 41(7): 449–52.
72. O'Quinn RP, Miller JL. The effectiveness of tumor necrosis factor alpha antibody (infliximab) in treating recalcitrant psoriasis: a report of 2 cases. *Arch Dermatol* 2002; 138(5): 644–8.
73. Pereira TM, Vieira AP, Fernandes JC, Antunes H, Basto AS. Anti-TNF-alpha therapy in childhood pustular psoriasis. *Dermatology* 2006; 213(4): 350–2.
74. Poulalhon N, Begon E, Lebbe C, Liote F, Lahfa M, Bengoufa D, et al. A follow-up study in 28 patients treated with infliximab for severe recalcitrant psoriasis: evidence for efficacy and high incidence of biological autoimmunity. *Br J Dermatol* 2007; 156(2): 329–36.
75. Richetta AG, Maiani E, Carlomagno V, Carboni V, Mattozzi C, Giancristoforo S, et al. Treatment of erythrodermic psoriasis in HCV+ patient with adalimumab. *Dermatol Ther* 2009; 22(Suppl 1): S16–18.
76. Rongioletti F, Borenstein M, Kirsner R, Kerdel F. Erythrodermic, recalcitrant psoriasis: clinical resolution with infliximab. *J Dermatolog Treat* 2003; 14(4): 222–5.
77. Schmick K, Grabbe J. Recalcitrant, generalized pustular psoriasis: rapid and lasting therapeutic response to antitumour necrosis factor-alpha antibody (infliximab). *Br J Dermatol* 2004; 150(2): 367.
78. Sheth N, Greenblatt DT, Acland K, Barker J, Teixeira F. Generalized pustular psoriasis of pregnancy treated with infliximab. *Clin Exp Dermatol* 2009; 34(4): 521–2.
79. Takahashi MD, Castro LG, Romiti R. Infliximab, as sole or combined therapy, induces rapid clearing of erythrodermic psoriasis. *Br J Dermatol* 2007; 157(4): 828–31.

80. Wang TS, Tsai TF. Clinical experience of ustekinumab in the treatment of erythrodermic psoriasis: a case series. *J Dermatol* 2011; 38(11): 1096–9.
81. Weishaupt C, Metze D, Luger TA, Stander S. Treatment of pustular psoriasis with infliximab. *J Dtsch Dermatol Ges* 2007; 5(5): 397–9.
82. Zangrilli A, Papoutsaki M, Talamonti M, Chimenti S. Long-term efficacy of adalimumab in generalized pustular psoriasis. *J Dermatolog Treat* 2008; 19(3): 185–7.
83. Castela E, Archier E, Devaux S, Gallini A, Aractingi S, Cribier B, et al. Topical corticosteroids in plaque psoriasis: a systematic review of risk of adrenal axis suppression and skin atrophy. *J Eur Acad Dermatol Venereol* 2012; 26(Suppl 3): 47–51.
84. Armenti VT, Ahlswede KM, Ahlswede BA, Jarrell BE, Moritz MJ, Burke JF. National transplantation pregnancy registry—outcomes of 154 pregnancies in cyclosporine-treated female kidney transplant recipients. *Transplantation* 1994; 57(4): 502–6.
85. Armenti VT, Jarrell BE, Radomski JS, McGrory CH, Gaughan WJ, Moritz MJ. National Transplantation Pregnancy Registry (NTPR): cyclosporine dosing and pregnancy outcome in female renal transplant recipients. *Transplant Proc* 1996; 28(4): 2111–12.
86. Edmonds EV, Morris SD, Short K, Bewley SJ, Eady RA. Pustular psoriasis of pregnancy treated with ciclosporin and high-dose prednisolone. *Clin Exp Dermatol* 2005; 30(6): 709–10.
87. Finch TM, Tan CY. Pustular psoriasis exacerbated by pregnancy and controlled by cyclosporin A. *Br J Dermatol* 2000; 142(3): 582–4.
88. Al-Shobaili H, Al-Khenaizan S. Childhood generalized pustular psoriasis: successful treatment with isotretinoin. *Pediatr Dermatol* 2007; 24(5): 563–4.
89. Dogra S, Kumaran MS, Handa S, Kanwar AJ. Methotrexate for generalized pustular psoriasis in a 2-year-old child. *Pediatr Dermatol* 2005; 22(1): 85–6.
90. Ergin S, Ersoy-Evans S, Sahin S, Ozkaya O. Acitretin is a safe treatment option for infantile pustular psoriasis. *J Dermatolog Treat* 2008; 19(6): 341–3.
91. Juanqin G, Zhiqiang C, Zijia H. Evaluation of the effectiveness of childhood generalized pustular psoriasis treatment in 30 cases. *Pediatr Dermatol* 1998; 15(2): 144–6.
92. Kilic SS, Hacimustafaoglu M, Celebi S, Karadeniz A, Ildirim I. Low dose cyclosporin A treatment in generalized pustular psoriasis. *Pediatr Dermatol* 2001; 18(3): 246–8.
93. Xiao T, Li B, He CD, Chen HD. Juvenile generalized pustular psoriasis. *J Dermatol* 2007; 34(8): 573–6.
94. Kim HS, Kim GM, Kim SY. Two-stage therapy for childhood generalized pustular psoriasis: low-dose cyclosporin for induction and maintenance with acitretin/narrowband ultraviolet B phototherapy. *Pediatr Dermatol* 2006; 23(3): 306–8.
95. Kopp T, Karlhofer F, Szepfalusi Z, Schneeberger A, Stingl G, Tanew A. Successful use of acitretin in conjunction with narrowband ultraviolet B phototherapy in a child with severe pustular psoriasis, von Zumbusch type. *Br J Dermatol* 2004; 151(4): 912–16.

Chapter 18

Pediatric Psoriasis

Lauren Becker, Kelly M. Cordoro, and Amy S. Paller

Psoriasis is one of several papulosquamous diseases that represent 10% of all cutaneous disorders seen in a busy pediatric dermatology clinic [1] and accounts for 4% of all dermatoses seen in patients younger than 16 years [2]. The overall incidence of pediatric psoriasis has increased since 1970 and is now in the range of 62.7/ 100,000 [3]. In childhood, psoriasis may vary from a life-threatening neonatal pustular or exfoliative dermatosis to an entity of almost subclinical impact. Psoriasis in children can profoundly impact quality of life [4,5].

EPIDEMIOLOGY

For adults with psoriasis, 31%–45% have the onset of the disease during the first two decades of life [6–8]. To some extent, the incidence estimates have been hampered by the unclear definitions of childhood psoriasis, particularly the question of whether psoriatic diaper rash is true psoriasis, and by underrecognition by primary care physicians. In children, there is evidence that there is no sex preference [3,9] or a slight female predominance with a female-to-male ratio of 1.13:1 [10] to 1.25:1 [6,11]. As in adult populations, white children develop psoriasis more commonly than African American children, who in turn develop it more commonly than Native Americans and Asians [11,12]. Although Farber and Nall noted that 2% of all patients with psoriasis had the initial onset of disease by two years of age [7], a survey of 1262 Australian children with psoriasis, including diaper region psoriasis, found that 16% of the patients were younger than one year and 27% were younger than two years [10]. Neonatal and congenital onsets of psoriasis have been reported.

The origin of psoriasis appears to be multifactorial, with genetic and environmental factors playing major roles. A positive immediate family history of psoriasis has been found in approximately 30% of pediatric patients [13].

Twin studies have demonstrated an eight-fold increased risk of psoriasis relative to the general population if a monozygotic twin is affected, and a four-fold increased risk if a dizygotic twin is affected [14]. Swanbeck et al. investigated the first-degree relatives of more than 3000 patients with psoriasis and showed a lifetime risk of inheriting psoriasis if no parent, one parent, and two parents had psoriasis of 4%, 28%, and 65%, respectively [15]. Human leukocyte antigen (HLA) types Cw6 and DR7 are linked to early-onset psoriasis (younger than 40 years) [16]. Tiilikainen et al. noted the prevalence of HLA-Cw6 (PSORS1) in 72.7% of patients with the guttate form of psoriasis and in 45.9% of patients overall with the medium-to-large plaque form (vs. 7.4% of the general population of Finland) [17].

Genome-wide association studies (GWAS) have thus far identified 36 loci that have been associated with psoriasis; these genes are involved with skin barrier functions (LCE3A and LCE3C), interleukin-23 (IL-23) signaling (IL23A, IL23R, and IL12B), nuclear factor-kB and interferon signaling (NFKBIA, REL, TYK2, IRIH1, IL28RA, TNIP1, TNFAIP3, CARD14, and CARM1), interferon-mediated antiviral responses (DDX58), macrophage activation (ZCH12C), IL-17 cellular responses (TRAF3IP2, TYK2, and IL23R), regulation of T cell function (RUNX3, TAGAP, and STAT3), and the aforementioned HLA-C gene [18–20].

Psoriasis susceptibility locus 2 (PSORS2) on chromosome 17q25.3 has been associated with psoriasis and psoriatic arthritis [21] and is now known to reflect changes in caspase recruitment domain family, member 14 (CARD14), an activator of NF-kB, which upregulates genes of chemokines involved in psoriasis (IL8 and CCL20) [21]. CARD14 mutations cause familial psoriasis and autosomal-dominant pityriasis rubra pilaris [22].

Generalized pustular psoriasis has now been linked to mutations in IL36RN (DITRA, deficiency of IL-36 receptor antagonist), leading to increased expression of this IL-1 family protein and activation of proinflammatory signaling pathways, including NF-kB [23,24].

MANIFESTATIONS OF PEDIATRIC PSORIASIS

In general, the diagnosis of psoriasis in children is based on clinical features. Biopsy confirmation is rarely necessary and should be avoided unless important to the diagnosis, such as in pustular psoriasis. In children, the most commonly involved areas are elbows (Figure 18.1) and knees [3,7]. However, psoriasis in the flexural areas, known as inverse psoriasis, is more common in children than adults [25]. Psoriasis may take on several presentations in the pediatric population. Most common is the medium-to-large plaque type (34%–84%) [8,10,26]. Compared to adults, children typically have smaller plaques with finer and softer scale (Figure 18.2). In dark-skinned children, the scale may be so subtle that the lesions appear to be areas of hypopigmentation, with the scale becoming obvious only

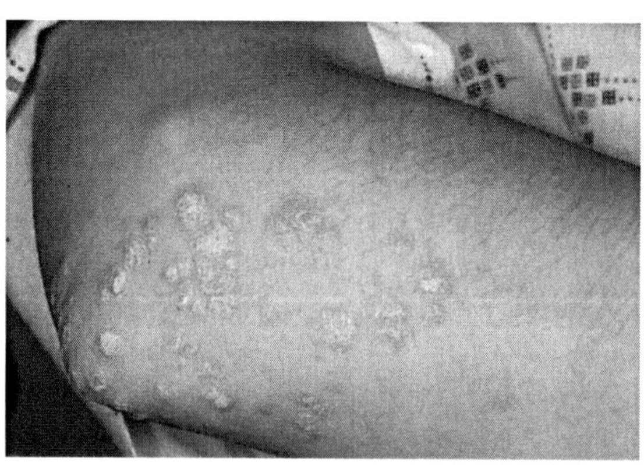

FIGURE 18.1 (See color insert.) Extensor surfaces of knees and elbows are the most commonly involved areas in children. This older child has involvement of the right elbow with round to oval erythematous plaques with overlying silver scale.

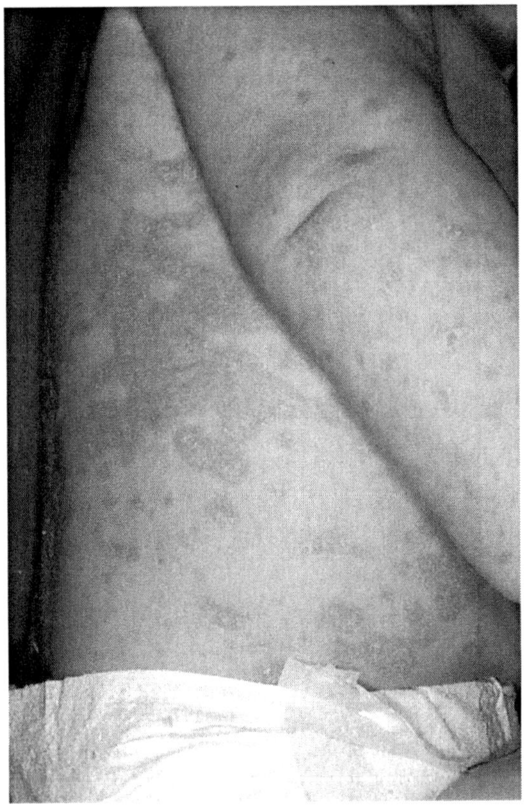

FIGURE 18.2 (See color insert.) Small coalescing plaques on the right side of the trunk of an infant. In comparison with the psoriatic plaques in the older child in Figure 18.1, the scale on these plaques is thinner and finer.

when the lesions are scratched. The appearance of psoriatic lesions after skin injury (Koebner phenomenon) has been described in 50% of pediatric patients, in contrast to 39% of adults [6]. A characteristic Auspitz sign, with pinpoint bleeding after mechanical removal of the scales, reflects the increased vascularity of lesions.

The small plaques of guttate (or teardrop-shaped) psoriasis are the presenting manifestation in 6.4%–44% of patients [8,10,27]. The 1–3 mm guttate lesions are most commonly distributed on the trunk and proximal extremities (Figure 18.3). There is a well-known association between guttate psoriasis and recent streptococcal infection (usually one to three weeks earlier), particularly of the throat or perianal area [8,28]. In a questionnaire study of 5600 patients, 17% of patients nine years of age and younger and 32% of patients between 10 and 19 years of age reported a recent throat infection as an initial trigger of their psoriasis [7]. In a separate retrospective study, 21.3% of children had a positive throat culture for group A β-hemolytic streptococcus [29]. The incidence of guttate psoriasis in a given population may reflect the frequency and form of streptococcal infection. Although the probability of developing chronic psoriasis after an episode of guttate psoriasis is only about 33% [30], a recent study showed evidence of greater psoriatic severity in children whose psoriasis had started as guttate versus plaque type [31].

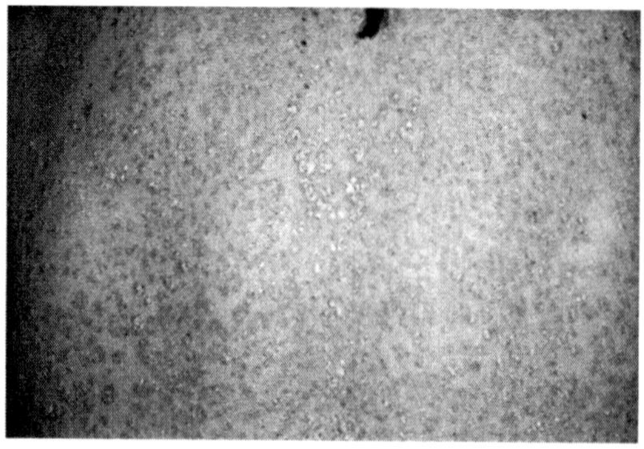

FIGURE 18.3 (See color insert.) The small guttate plaques of psoriasis, most common on the trunk, are frequently the presenting feature of pediatric psoriasis, especially following streptococcal infection. Note that the patient shows peripheral residual postinflammatory hypopigmentation at sites of resolution.

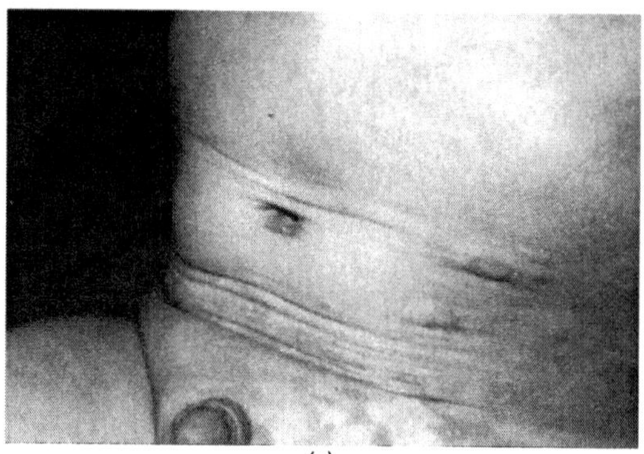

(a)

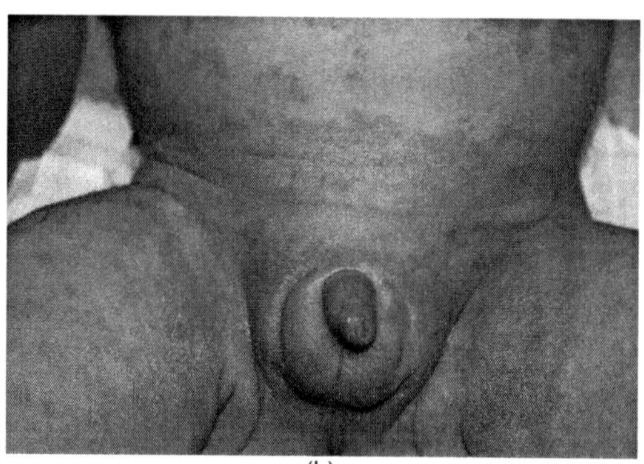

(b)

FIGURE 18.4 (See color insert.) Diaper area psoriasis shows brightly erythematous, well-demarcated plaques. (a) Well demarcated plaques on the lateral diaper area. (b) Frontal view of diaper area shows brightly erythematous, well demarcated plaques.

Morris et al. have proposed that psoriatic diaper rash (Figure 18.4), with or without dissemination, should be considered psoriasis or at least a precursor to psoriasis in some children. In their recent series, 13% of children presented with psoriatic diaper rash with dissemination and 4% with localized psoriatic diaper rash [10]. The major difficulty with this classification lies in differentiating it from infantile seborrheic dermatitis, and the diagnosis is often obscured because scale is commonly absent in the moist diaper area. However, the sharp definition, bright erythema, shininess, and larger and drier scale of psoriasis plaques help to differentiate it from seborrheic dermatitis [32–37]. The frequency of diaper area psoriasis in infants likely reflects the Koebner phenomenon, triggered by the trauma from exposure to stool and urine. Biopsy of lesions at this age is usually unwarranted, and the diagnosis should be based strictly on clinical grounds. Psoriatic diaper rash with dissemination is the most common form of psoriasis in infancy, yet several of these infants have later shown other forms of psoriasis [10]. Involvement of the inguinal area more commonly persists into childhood and adolescence in boys, (Figure 18.5) but psoriasis may also involve the inguinal area in older females as well. In young girls presenting with a complaint in the vulvar region, psoriasis is the diagnosis 17% of the time [38]. Lesions may present as well-demarcated, red, nonscaling, symmetrical plaques involving the vulva, perineum, and often the natal cleft, but never the vagina.

Facial involvement has been described more commonly in children than in adults (Figure 18.6). A rash on the face is the sole manifestation in 4%–5% of patients [10,39], although 38%–46% have facial involvement in addition to other affected areas [8,10,40]. Psoriatic lesions tend to be more clearly demarcated than patches of atopic dermatitis, are less itchy, and commonly

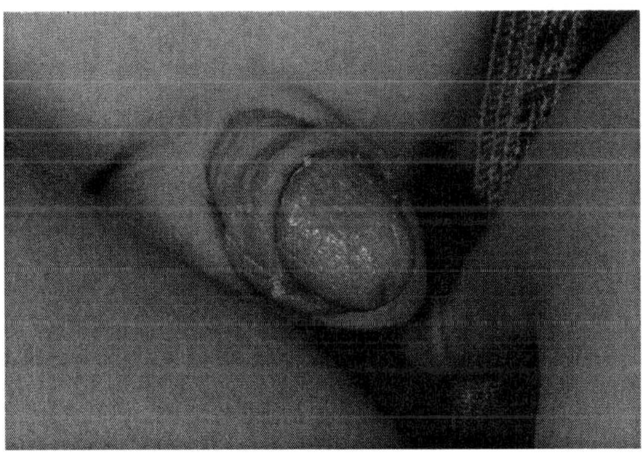

FIGURE 18.5 (See color insert.) Penile psoriasis with erythema and scaling.

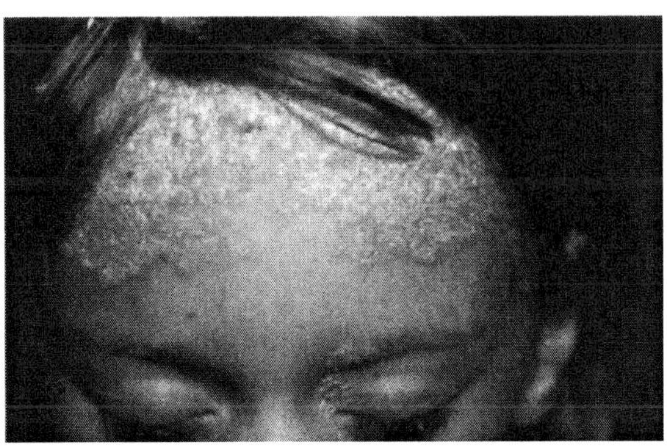

FIGURE 18.6 (See color insert.) Facial psoriasis is more common in children than in adults.

have an annular configuration. Involvement of the periorbital area is particularly common, although distribution in the nasolabial folds and perioral area is also not uncommon. Lesions may range in intensity from subtle to florid. In one series, facial involvement was noted in 98% of children with psoriatic diaper rash with dissemination [10].

Psoriasis of the scalp is the most common presenting feature for many children—in several studies, it is the site of onset for 40%–60% of patients prior to 20 years of age [40,41]. Scalp involvement has been reported more commonly in girls [31]. Scalp psoriasis is usually characterized by discrete patches of erythema with overlying scale, but many authors consider pityriasis amiantacea (tinea amiantacea) to be a form of psoriasis or a precursor to it. The classic sign of pityriasis amiantacea is the mica-like scale adherent to the hair and large plates of scale attached to the scalp (Figure 18.7). Focal hair loss and secondary infection may be associated. Pityriasis amiantacea usually begins during the teenage years and occasionally progresses to clear psoriasis (2.5%–15% of patients after a mean of six to eight years) [42,43]. Localized scalp psoriasis may also occur at the nape of the neck overlying a salmon patch in young children.

Several of the cutaneous variants of psoriasis seen in adults occur rarely in children. These include pustular, acropustular, erythrodermic, and follicular forms. Linear psoriasis is often first noted during childhood [44]. Geographic tongue may also represent a form of psoriasis in children. Pustular psoriasis has been described in more than 300 children. Five clinical patterns of sterile pustules have been noted: generalized or von Zumbusch form, annular, exanthematic, localized, and a mixed variant with features of both the generalized and annular patterns. Of these, the annular form is the most common in children (60% of the pustular psoriasis in children) [45,46]. Pattern types in children are not stagnant; initial localized presentation (particularly on the neck in infants) may progress to a more generalized pattern [47]. The mean age of onset is six years of age; however, pustular psoriasis has been described as early as first week of life [46,48]. Diagnosis should be confirmed by biopsy, which shows spongiotic pustules and Munro's abscesses, in addition to the classic parakeratosis and elongated ridges of psoriasis. Associated fever, malaise, and anorexia may be severe. All forms can have a recurrent course over years to decades, although the episodes

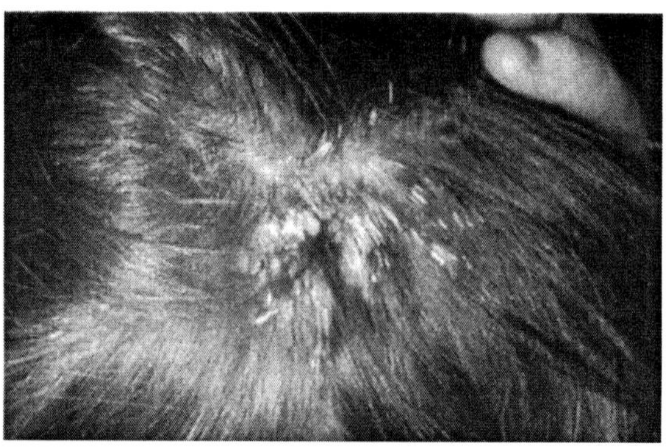

FIGURE 18.7 (See color insert.) Pityriasis amiantacea is characterized by plaques of mild to moderate erythema and scalp scaling with distinct scale that encases and is adherent to the hair shaft.

are usually less severe in the annular and mixed forms than in the generalized form. Lytic bone lesions may be associated [48,49], and when present in infants with pustular lesions, it should raise consideration of deficiency of IL-1 receptor antagonist (DIRA) [50]. DIRA, an autosomal recessive disorder with a higher prevalence in individuals of Puerto Rican descent, responds to administration of anakinra. In contrast to the occurrence of pustular psoriasis after a history of psoriasis vulgaris in adults, the occurrence of pustular psoriasis in a child is not uncommonly the presenting sign of psoriasis. The erythrodermic form is quite rare. It is characterized by erythema involving more than 90% of the total body surface and with less scaling than in the plaque type of psoriasis. Patients with erythrodermic or extensive pustular psoriasis usually require hospitalization, and courses are not uncommonly complicated by bacterial septicemia [46].

Approximately 5% of pediatric patients show an eczema/psoriasis overlap [10]. These patients may either have typical plaques of psoriasis and features of eczema or may show scaling erythematous patches with features intermediate between eczema and psoriasis. Most children with the latter initially show typical nummular dermatitis. Almost all patients with the overlap have a family history of atopic disease and psoriasis. In addition, the morphology of psoriasis may mimic atopic dermatitis, leading to a challenging diagnosis from a health professional with inexperience in pediatric dermatology [51].

Nail psoriasis occurs in up to 40% of patients younger than 18 years with psoriasis (Figure 18.8), and it occurs more frequently in boys [8,31,40,52,133,134]. Nail pitting has also been observed at birth in a neonate who developed diaper area psoriasis at two weeks of age [52]. The nail changes seen in children are similar to those seen in adults. Most common is nail pitting, caused by tiny psoriatic lesions of the nail matrix. Discoloration, onycholysis (separation of the distal and lateral nail plate edges), and subungual hyperkeratosis (lifting of the nail plate with nail thickening) are also commonly seen in children with nail involvement. Secondary bacterial, candidal, or occasionally dermatophyte infections occur with increased frequency.

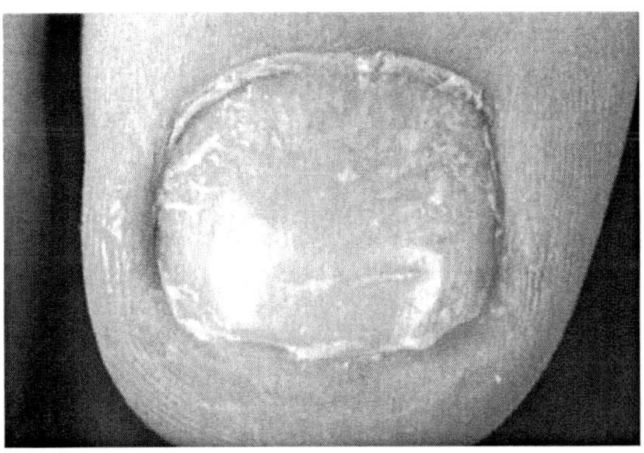

FIGURE 18.8 (See color insert.) Nail psoriasis is more common in adolescents than in young children and is characterized by nail pitting, discoloration, onycholysis, and/or subungual hyperkeratosis.

The primary noncutaneous features of childhood psoriasis are psoriatic arthritis and obesity. Juvenile psoriatic arthritis, a form of juvenile idiopathic arthritis [53,54,135], occurs in 10%–10.5% of pediatric psoriatic patients in the United States [27,55]. Either the skin disease or the arthritis may develop initially, and in most patients, flares of joint and skin disease and their severity are not correlated. Current criteria for making the diagnosis (International League of Associations for Rheumatology or ILAR criteria) are more stringent than the previous "Vancouver" criteria [56]. Psoriatic arthritis is clinically heterogeneous with more severe, recalcitrant disease in younger children, peaking at two years of age, and a milder form that peaks in incidence during adolescence [53]. Early-onset psoriatic arthritis has a female predominance, whereas older patients do not have a gender preference yet do have more axial joint involvement and enthesitis [54]. Rheumatoid factor is always negative, but antinuclear antibody is positive in 50%–63% of affected patients, especially in affected girls having more severe disease [57]. Psoriatic arthritis is considered a relatively common form of chronic arthropathy that differs clinically, genetically, and serologically from juvenile ankylosing spondylitis and juvenile rheumatoid arthritis [53]. Up to 50% of patients with psoriatic arthritis have a family history of psoriasis. Most patients have pauciarticular disease (involvement of a single joint) at onset, typically involving the knee, but the arthritis progresses to asymmetrical polyarthritis in 64% of patients [58]. Those with oligoarticular onset of psoriatic arthritis typically have small joint and wrist involvement, nail pits, as well as a positive family history of psoriasis [54]. Psoriatic uveitis, an asymmetrical anterior uveitis, is found in 14%–17% of children with juvenile psoriatic arthritis [53,58]. The outcome of the joint disease does not correlate with either the presence of a positive antinuclear antibody or uveitis. Although HLA B27 was found in 53% of children with definite psoriatic arthritis and a positive family history, but in only 5% without a family history of psoriasis [57], no such association has been described in other studies, in contrast to the documented relationship in adults with psoriatic arthritis [53,59].

The most common comorbidity in children and adolescents with psoriasis is increased and central adiposity. The clear relationship between psoriasis and metabolic syndrome (characterized by insulin resistance/glucose intolerance, hypertension, dyslipidemia, and central obesity) and myocardial infarction has been well described in adults [60–64] and correlates with severity. The correlation between psoriasis and the metabolic syndrome in children is less studied. In a small cohort, 4 out of 12 psoriasis patients met the criteria for metabolic syndrome diagnosis, compared to zero controls [65]. It has also been found that pediatric psoriasis patients have a lower high-density lipoprotein (HDL) than controls [65]. Cytokines that contribute to psoriasis and the metabolic syndrome include tumor necrosis factor-a, IL-6, adiponectin, and leptin [66]. In an international, cross-sectional study of 614 children, Paller et al. confirmed the relationship of childhood psoriasis and excess adiposity. Nationally and internationally, it was found that pediatric psoriatic patients had higher body mass index percentile ($p = 0.001$), larger waist circumference ($p < 0.001$), and larger waist to height ratio ($p = 0.02$) versus controls [27]. In a large prospective study of female nurses, Setty et al. found that increased adiposity was an independent risk factor for psoriasis [67]. Research is undergoing to determine the extent of systemic involvement of pediatric psoriatic patients. However, due to the association of increased adiposity and psoriasis at such an early age, practitioners caring for pediatric psoriatic patients should be vigilant about healthy lifestyle management as early as possible, focusing on family-centered efforts.

IMPORTANT HISTORICAL INFORMATION

Evaluation of the pediatric patient always takes longer than that of the adult patient because of the time needed to gain the trust of the child and to establish a rapport. In taking the history of a pediatric patient with a scaly inflammatory disease suspected to be psoriasis, there are several useful questions:

1. Is there a family history of psoriasis?
2. Is the eruption periodic?
3. Do new lesions appear in areas where he or she has been bruised, scratched, burned, or otherwise traumatized?
4. Is there a family history of arthritis?
5. What time of year did the eruption begin? (Psoriasis onset is more common in fall or winter than in summer.)
6. Is there a specific time of year when the eruption gets better? Is there a benefit from sunlight?
7. Has there been a recent or chronic history of sore throat or streptococcal infection?
8. Has there been a stressful life event in the past year? (Relationship problems with parents, siblings, peers, and teachers, and being diagnosed with a psychiatric disease have been associated with childhood psoriasis.) [68]
9. Is the child exposed to tobacco smoke at home? (Tobacco smoke exposure has been associated with childhood psoriasis.) [68]

PSYCHOSOCIAL ASPECTS

Psoriasis inflicts an emotional toll on affected children and their families. The highly visible disorder has an impact on one's self-esteem, psychosocial development, and ability to function socially [69,70]; it has also been associated with depression [71]. As with any visible and chronic skin disorder, the embarrassment and effect on social relationships can affect patients and families differently, based on the individual's personality and sensitivity to the opinions of others. However, teenagers and older children need to become well educated about psoriasis in order to face the disorder in a healthy manner (Table 18.1). In addition, parents of children with psoriasis need to become involved in their child's diagnosis to encourage healthy psychosocial development and effective therapy (Table 18.2). The National Psoriasis Foundation (NPF) has a youth program specifically designed for children and teenagers, their parents, and caregivers. It includes educational booklets, Web site activities, and other information that encourages dealing with the psoriasis through education and emotional support (www.psoriasis.org). The NPF also has a special page dedicated to children, (www.psoriasis.org/kids) that has kid-friendly teaching tools, forums related to kids and psoriasis, and information about where kids can meet other kids with psoriasis.

TABLE 18.1 Tips for Teens and Older Children

Become educated about psoriasis.
Develop responses to questions about the psoriasis and practice them; make sure to impart that psoriasis is not contagious or self-inflicted but a medical condition.
Be open about the disorder—do not try to hide it; however, you may choose to wear long sleeves, for example, to make coping in public easier.
Use your therapy as directed but seek guidance from your physician if the results are not satisfactory.
Check out the NPF's Web site: message boards, live chat, and educational web casts. Request one of the free booklets for kids, youth, and teens. Become a member and receive regular mailings with columns and information just for kids.
Seek support on a personal level with your doctor, other adults, and peers; discuss your feelings; remember that real friends want to know about psoriasis and want to help.
Expect some negative experiences but have the resolve to get past them.
Acknowledge that confusion and anger are normal reactions; seek help if you feel sad or depressed.
Focus on positive experiences—with family, friends, hobbies, travel, and sports; there is more to life than the skin condition.
Decide to be happy and have fun— and then do it; you are in control, not your psoriasis.

TABLE 18.2 Tips for Parents

Learn about psoriasis; if you are educated, you can teach others.
Explain to the child that the more people understand psoriasis, the better; encourage your child to practice telling you about the psoriasis as if you were a friend or teacher; make sure that the child can impart that the psoriasis is not self-inflicted or contagious but a medical condition of skin cells that grow too fast, and it is associated with inflammation.
Listen to your child and try to elicit feelings about the psoriasis and how it affects him or her; always acknowledge the feelings and that having psoriasis is not easy; encourage your child to ask for support.
Help the child find friends with whom he or she can identify, who can see beyond the psoriasis.
Dealing with psoriasis in a child can be time-consuming but recognize the potential impact on the entire family; spend equal time with other children and encourage their involvement in care of the disorder.
Find the right doctor who can educate, be supportive, and provide optimal care for this chronic disorder.
Set up a "treatment center" in the home and show the commitment to the treatment regimen that sets the example for your child in developing future responsibility.
Use games when applying treatments so that the interaction becomes pleasant and the kids are engaged in the treatment.
As the child gets older, encourage him or her to share in the responsibility of therapy and making appropriate choices; responsibility fosters independence and a sense of control over the condition; by the age of six to seven years, most children can participate in the application of moisturizers or topical medications.
Always be positive and hopeful because your attitude affects your child and sets the example.
Contact the NPF and get current information, support from other parents, and many resources to help your child, including Web activities, message boards, educational booklets, and more. Call (800) 723-9166, email getinfo@psoriasis.org, or visit www.psoriasis.org.

DISORDERS THAT RESEMBLE PSORIASIS

Psoriasis is often misdiagnosed in pediatric patients, especially by primary care providers; in fact, only 9.4% of children with psoriasis were correctly diagnosed by a referring physician [51]. Psoriasis is most commonly misdiagnosed as dermatitis, especially when the lesions are located on the face, hands, or feet. Psoriasis in children or adolescents with guttate psoriasis may be confused with pityriasis rosea or parapsoriasis (including parapsoriasis lichenoides et varioliformis acuta and parapsoriasis lichenoides chronica). Pityriasis rubra pilaris is the hardest to differentiate, especially when largely involving the palms, soles, elbows, and knees. The follicular accentuation, focal areas of sparing, and the sometimes more salmon coloration of pityriasis rubra pilaris can help to differentiate the conditions clinically; biopsy sections of pityriasis rubra pilaris may show perifollicular inflammation. In addition, widespread chronic eczematous dermatosis, lichen planus, drug eruption, or widespread dermatophytosis may also be confused with psoriasis (Table 18.3). When scaling plaques of psoriasis affect the sun-exposed areas of the face, they must be differentiated from lesions of discoid lupus erythematosus; nasolabial and periauricular involvement in the affected adolescent patient may resemble seborrheic dermatitis. Diaper area psoriasis is often confused with candidal diaper dermatitis with or without an id reaction, seborrheic dermatitis, or irritant contact dermatitis. Scalp psoriasis may be mistaken for tinea capitis or, if more widespread, severe seborrheic dermatitis. The differential diagnosis of psoriasis of the nail includes nail changes after trauma, onychomycosis, and lichen planus, the latter being the least common in a child. Pustular psoriasis may be misdiagnosed as infection (impetigo, staphylococcal folliculitis or staphylococcal-scalded skin syndrome, candidal pustulosis, or widespread herpes simplex infection) or, when exfoliative, as toxic epidermal necrolysis. Erythrodermic psoriasis may be confused with extensive pityriasis rubra pilaris and ichthyotic disorders, particularly congenital ichthyosiform erythroderma and erythrokeratodermia variabilis.

TABLE 18.3 Disorders to Be Differentiated from Psoriasis in Children

Parapsoriasis (e.g., parapsoriasis lichenoides et varioliformis acuta and parapsoriasis lichenoides chronica)
Pityriasis rubra pilaris
Pityriasis rosea
Lichen planus
Dermatophytosis
Diaper area
Irritant or atopic dermatitis
Candidal dermatitis
Nail
Onychomycosis
Trachyonychia
Scalp
Tinea capitis
Seborrheic dermatitis
Other: drug eruption, pityriasis rubra pilaris, secondary syphilis, T-cell lymphoma (adolescent)
Hands/feet: dermatitis (atopic, dyshidrotic), contact dermatitis, severe tinea pedis

THERAPY

Education is a key component of psoriasis therapy. Patients and parents must understand the chronicity of the disorder and the tendency for spontaneous remissions, particularly in the pediatric population [6]. In addition, the Koebner phenomenon, or the concept that injury to skin may exacerbate psoriasis, should be conveyed (Table 18.4). Other trigger factors should also be considered, including infection (especially streptococcal) and medications (e.g., systemic steroids, lithium, antimalarials, and β-blockers). Above all, therapy should be conservative and appropriate for the type and severity of the psoriasis, and parents must realize the potential side effects of prescribed therapy.

Topical Therapy

The most commonly used topical therapies in children include topical corticosteroids, calcipotriene, salicylic acid, ketoconazole, tar preparations, and anthralin (short-contact therapy). The most commonly prescribed topical corticosteroids are betamethasone dipropionate, fluocinonide, and fluocinolone acetonide [9]. Emollients are used as adjunctive agents to decrease the associated scaling and dryness but should not replace anti-inflammatory medications.

In plaque stage psoriasis, corticosteroid preparations remain the mainstay of treatment (Table 18.5). Most commonly, application of class II–IV midpotency topical steroids up to twice daily is most useful for lesions on the trunk and extremities. Use of halogenated steroids, however, should be avoided in the diaper area, intertriginous areas, and on the face. Topical steroid options for these sensitive areas should never be stronger than nonhalogenated low- to medium-strength preparations, such as hydrocortisone acetate (1.0%–2.5%), desonide, aclometasone dipropionate, hydrocortisone butyrate, or prednicarbate. Topical calcipotriene and tacrolimus ointment are steroid-sparing alternatives (see later in this chapter).

Once the acute lesions are under control, treatment can be tapered to lower-potency steroids and/or emollients. If individual thick plaques fail to respond, higher-potency topical steroid preparations can be used but should be limited to no longer than a two-week course. As in adults, weekend therapy with class I steroids can be used in adolescents with severe

TABLE 18.4 Prevention of Psoriasis in Pediatric Patients

Location	Intervention
Face	Avoid overexposure to ultraviolet light and irritating soaps
Creases and folds	Avoid irritating underarm deodorants
Genital and perianal regions	Avoid irritation from accumulation of feces and urine and from tight garments
Hands and feet	Avoid contact with irritating soaps or other substances
	Avoid tight shoes and accumulation of moisture, including sweat, on the feet
Scalp	Avoid vigorous combing, picking, or scratching of the scalp
Nails	Avoid long fingernails or toenails, trauma to nails in play situations, or wearing tight shoes

TABLE 18.5 Treatment of Psoriasis in Children

	Use in children	Potential side effects
Topical preparations		
Emollients	Useful in mild disease; adjunct	None
Topical steroids	First-line therapy: all types of psoriasis	Tachyphylaxis Local side effects: atrophy, striae Systemic side effects: impaired growth, adrenal suppression, cataracts
Tar/anthralin	Thicker plaques; short-contact anthralin	Irritation, staining
Calcipotriene	Limited plaques	Irritation
Tazarotene gel	Limited plaques	Irritation
Tacrolimus	Face, intertriginous areas	Burning with first applications
Phototherapy		
Ultraviolet B	Widespread plaques	Cost, inconvenience, premature aging, skin cancer
Psoralens-UVA	Rarely indicated	As for UVB/risk of later skin aging and cancer may be higher; cataracts with systemic psoralens
Systemic therapy		
Methotrexate	Recalcitrant extensive plaques, erythrodermic, pustular psoriasis, psoriatic arthritis	Bone marrow and hepatotoxicity
Cyclosporine	Recalcitrant severe psoriasis	Renal and hepatic toxicity, hypertrichosis, immunosuppression, UVB-induced skin cancer
Acetretin	Especially for pustular psoriasis	Cheilitis, hyperlipidemia, musculoskeletal pain, hair loss, skin fragility, bone toxicity if used long term
Etanercept	Recalcitrant moderate to severe psoriasis	Increased risk of serious infection, including mycobacteria

disease, but steroid use must be monitored carefully [72]. It should be noted that the preadolescent/adolescent population is particularly at risk for developing striae from the use of the superpotent steroids. Use of keratolytic agents to enhance penetration, such as 6% salicylic acid compounded into steroid ointment or at a separate time (e.g., Keralyt gel), occlusion, or steroid-impregnated tapes are alternative treatments for more hyperkeratotic, resistant lesions. Salicylate intoxication via transcutaneous poisoning is rare; however, the case reports have been limited to young children with either psoriasis or ichthyosis [73]. Selected resistant lesions may respond to the use of intralesional triamcinolone (diluted to 3–5 mg/mL). Intralesional injections are rarely used in pediatric patients because of the associated discomfort. However, the availability of topical anesthetic creams (e.g., eutectic mixture of lidocaine and prilocaine—EMLA® or ElamaxQ®) may prove helpful in diminishing the discomfort of injections, especially in younger children.

Tar and Anthralin Preparations

Tar preparations, especially when used in association with daily incremental outdoor ultraviolet light, are a time-honored and effective adjunct to the topical treatment of psoriasis. Tar (in the form of 1%–10% crude coal tar or liquor carbonis detergens) can be compounded into preparations or used alone—either at bedtime and left on overnight or applied for 30 minutes before ultraviolet light exposure (Goeckerman regimen). Tar may also be administered in the form of a tar bath. Tar preparations, however, stain skin and clothing and have an odor that is often objectionable to children and adolescents.

Anthralin preparations provide an alternative to tar treatment. Short-contact anthralin therapy led to remission in 81% of children with plaque psoriasis, treated for 30 minutes with up to 1% anthralin cream [74]. Short-contact anthralin therapy can be applied in the form of a 1% anthralin cream (Drithocreme, Psoriatec), a microencapsulated form that results in marked reduction in discoloration of skin or clothing [75,76]. This medication is formulated in a temperature-sensitive vehicle that releases the active medication at the skin surface temperature; the medication must be washed out with cold water to avoid release of the anthralin from the vehicle during washing [72]. Short-contact anthralin application should start with five-minute applications of 1% anthralin (the only concentration currently available commercially). It can be increased in duration every other day as tolerated and needed for efficacy, limiting the duration of application to no more than one hour. If the 1% anthralin causes too much irritation, it can be diluted. Bland emollient or protective paste can be applied on the normal skin surrounding the area of psoriasis to minimize the risk of irritation of noninvolved skin. Contact with face, eyes, and mucous membranes should be avoided. Triethanolamine, marketed as CuraStain, markedly reduces the minimal staining and irritation of anthralin when sprayed on skin or fabrics before and after cleaning.

Vitamin D_3 Derivatives

Calcipotriene, an analog of vitamin D_3, has been formulated as a 0.005% cream that is most effective when combined with topical steroids, but it serves as a steroidsparing agent and has been efficacious in children as monotherapy as well [77,78]. However, care must be taken to ensure compatibility of the calcipotriene ointment and the topical steroid. For example, calcipotriene can be mixed directly with halobetasol ointment for so-called weekend therapy but is destabilized by hydrocortisone valerate ointment or ammonium lactate, lotion, and it is completely inactivated by salicylic acid. A compounded formulation of betamethasone dipropionate (0.05%) and calcipotriene (0.005%) cream is now commercially available. Calcipotriene is best applied twice daily, but the onset of action is slow with maximal response reached at six to eight weeks. Calcipotriene is also available as a solution for scalp psoriasis. Irritant dermatitis, particularly on the face and intertriginous areas, occurs in up to 20% of patients. Patients may react to the propylene glycol in the solution or ointment forms; it is absent in the cream.

Tazarotene

The topical retinoid tazarotene gel is available in 0.05% and 0.1% strengths and can serve as a steroid-sparing agent. Because it is quite irritating as monotherapy, tazarotene is best applied once a day in combination with a medium to potent topical steroid applied at another time during the day. Even with the combination therapy, use of tazarotene may not be tolerated in children.

Tacrolimus Ointment

Tacrolimus ointment is frequently used in the treatment of atopic dermatitis for adults and children. Tacrolimus is a calcineurin inhibitor, which blocks the release of inflammatory cytokines by a mechanism that differs from that of topical corticosteroids. It is devoid of the potential local side effects of corticosteroids, particularly atrophy and ocular effects. Twice-daily application of tacrolimus 0.1% ointment is effective for facial and intertriginous psoriatic plaques in the majority of children [79]. It often leads to improvement in plaques elsewhere because the psoriatic plaques in children tend to be thinner than those of adults.

TOPICAL SCALP AND NAIL CARE

Scalp

Psoriatic scalp lesions are a frustrating and sometimes recalcitrant component of psoriasis. Several techniques and forms of medication are available. Topical corticosteroids may be applied in the form of oils, solutions, or foams. For example, a fluocinolone in peanut oil solution (DermaSmoothe-FS®) under shower cap occlusion can be applied for a few hours or overnight to the wet, affected scalp, followed by shampooing with a tar-containing or steroid-containing shampoo. As an alternative, a phenol and saline solution with a shower cap for occlusion can be applied overnight. In the morning, one can wash with a keratolytic and/or tar shampoo and gentle massage, followed by application of a steroid solution. Foam preparations of betamethasone valerate and clobetasol are also available to allow delivery of steroids without greasiness.

Nails

Psoriatic nail lesions can be difficult to treat because of the poor penetration of topical agents through the nail plate. Instillation of steroid preparations into the subproximal nail fold area can be successful, but nightly application of flurandrenolide-impregnated tape to the base of the nail for approximately six months yields better results and is not painful, in contrast to steroid injections. An alternative is topical tazarotene gel applied nightly to the base of the nail [80]. Parents must understand that response to therapy is measured in terms of months and that there is no instant gratification. For adolescents, the use of psoralen plus ultraviolet A (PUVA) in a hand/foot box has proven effective in many patients. Methotrexate or biologic therapy is the most effective means of treatment but only occasionally indicated for isolated nail changes. The development of nail psoriasis can be partially prevented by hydration of nails before trimming, keeping nails trimmed, avoidance of manipulation of the cuticles, and wearing shoes that fit properly.

Ultraviolet Light

Indications for phototherapy in children with psoriasis include: (i) disease that is refractory to combination topical therapies or too widespread for management with topical therapy (generally >15% body surface area); (ii) contraindications to systemic therapy; and/or

(iii) debilitating palmoplantar involvement. Three types of ultraviolet (UV) light are used for phototherapy: narrowband ultraviolet B (NB-UVB, 311–313 nm), broadband UVB (BB-UVB, 290–320 nm), and ultraviolet A (UVA, 320–400 nm). Of these, NB-UVB has emerged as the treatment of choice because of its safety and ease of administration. Narrowband UVB has a higher ratio of therapeutic to toxic wavelengths [81,136]. To minimize the risk of adverse events, children should receive phototherapy at centers staffed by personnel with experience treating pediatric patients. Once patients and parents know how to increase the dosages of UV light gradually, judge the effects of the daily treatment, and practice preventive eye care, home light box therapy can be initiated. Home light boxes are ultimately less invasive to the activities of a family and more cost-effective than treatment administered away from home. Nevertheless, ongoing contact with the family and intermittent follow-up are critical to assure safe and effective care.

In children, the initial exposure and then incremental dosing are usually based on Fitzpatrick skin type/established protocols [82,83]. Initial dosing may also be calculated based on a percentage (50%–80%) of the predetermined minimal erythema dose (MED) established by phototesting. In the clearing phase of phototherapy, the dose is increased based on clinical response and any observed adverse effects (erythema, burn, or pruritus). Once clear, the maintenance phase begins. The dose from the clearing phase is maintained, and the frequency of treatments is decreased [84]. Importantly, dosing protocols are not interchangeable among different wavelengths of light or equipment from different manufacturers. NB-UVB has proved effective for moderate to severe psoriasis in children across all skin types [82,83,85,86]. Guttate psoriasis responds best, but thin plaques will also respond. Clearance or near clearance is achieved in most patients after 15–20 treatments. Two to three treatments/week are most feasible and often adequate for children. In very refractory cases of plaque or pustular psoriasis, systemic acitretin combined with NB-UVB may decrease the time to clearance and the overall exposure to both agents [87,88].

Potential acute side effects of NB-UVB therapy include xerosis, erythema, pruritus, and photoactivation of herpes simplex virus. Suberythemogenic regimens should be used to minimize these risks. Long-term effects may include premature photoaging and skin cancer, though the precise long-term risks in children are unavailable [89]. Limiting treatment to children with darker skin types is preferable because fair-skinned patients face a lifetime of cumulative sun exposure and greater risk of cutaneous carcinogenesis.

Photochemotherapy with PUVA is an option for children with severe psoriasis but is rarely necessary given the availability and greater feasibility of NB-UVB. If used, oral psoralen should be restricted to children who are at least 12 years old or who weigh at least 100 pounds. Psoralen is taken 90 minutes before therapeutic UVA exposure. Short-term effects of oral PUVA include nausea, vomiting, headache, keratitis, hepatotoxicity, and generalized photosensitization requiring 24 hours of photoprotection. Long-term risks of PUVA include premature photoaging, cutaneous malignancy, and cataracts [90,137]. Topical PUVA is a good choice for recalcitrant palmoplantar psoriasis, though its long-term carcinogenicity in children is unknown [91,92].

Phototherapy can be challenging to administer to young children. Parents may accompany smaller children in the light unit. A radio or iPod with earphones can be used to distract the child during treatment. Protective eyewear and clothing (as appropriate) must be worn by patients receiving ultraviolet light treatments.

SYSTEMIC THERAPY

Most children with moderate to severe psoriasis will respond to treatment with combination topical therapy or phototherapy. In some cases, however, additional therapies may be necessary. Treatment with systemic or biologic agents is reserved for refractory, widespread, or incapacitating disease, for pustular or erythrodermic forms, and for psoriatic arthritis. Systemic treatments used for severe psoriasis in children include acitretin, methotrexate, cyclosporine, and biologics (largely etanercept and adalimumab). None are U.S. Food and Drug Administration (FDA) labeled for this indication in children, and only etanercept has undergone the scrutiny of a randomized controlled trial in the pediatric population [55].

The choice of treatment in children with severe disease is determined by the primary morphology, speed of progression, patient age, presence of comorbidities such as psoriatic arthropathy, impact on quality of life, and the level of disability. All systemic therapies used in children require close clinical and laboratory monitoring, as in adults. A recently published manuscript details the mechanism of action, pediatric dosing, adverse effects, and laboratory monitoring for each of the available systemic and biologic agents [93]. As a rule, systemic corticosteroids should be avoided. Although oral corticosteroids may be temporarily effective, withdrawal may precipitate severe flares, particularly of pustular psoriasis. Further, chronic use of oral corticosteroids carries significant risks in children.

When evaluating a child with new-onset or flaring psoriasis, especially of guttate morphology, consider the potential role of pharyngeal or perianal streptococcal infection. The association of group A β-hemolytic streptococci and psoriasis is well established. Streptococci organisms express M-protein superantigens that bypass normal immunological pathways and stimulate the activation of T lymphocytes. Further, streptococcal antigens stimulate IL-17 production and epidermal cell activation that are key to the development of psoriasis [94]. Patients with guttate or a significant flare of plaque-type psoriasis without an obvious sore throat or history of recent streptococcal infection may be carriers for streptococcal organisms that can be grown by culture. Although the use of systemic antibiotic therapy for unconfirmed cases is controversial, treatment is indicated if culture demonstrates streptococcal infection of the pharynx or perianal area [95–97]. Penicillin, erythromycin, and amoxicillin are most commonly used. The duration of therapy beyond treating the acute infection is unclear and must be individualized. One should consider the addition of rifampin if a carrier state is suspected.

The role of tonsillectomy for patients with chronic, recurrent, severe psoriasis remains to be fully defined because data regarding its benefit and duration of response are mixed. Although uncontrolled studies have suggested that tonsillectomy is superior to antibiotic administration in the clearance of psoriasis in children [98,99], two reviews assessed the evidence for such interventions in the management of childhood psoriasis and concluded that available evidence does not support the efficacy of oral antibiotics or tonsillectomy [100,101]. More recently, however, the mechanism and potential benefit of tonsillectomy were highlighted in a molecular study in adults showing improvement of psoriasis after tonsillectomy is associated with a reduced number of circulating T cells that recognize streptococcal determinants and homologous skin determinants [102]. Given the controversy, tonsillectomy should be considered only in select patients with documented recurrent streptococcal pharyngitis.

Methotrexate

Methotrexate (MTX) is a folic acid analog that reversibly inhibits dihydrofolate reductase, resulting in interference with DNA synthesis and effects on T cells [103]. Methotrexate has been used safely and successfully in children from 2 to 16 years of age with erythrodermic, plaque, and pustular psoriasis, and psoriatic arthritis [4]. Methotrexate treatment in children is similar to that in adults [104,105]. After appropriate screening tests, oral methotrexate is initiated at a test dosage of 2.5 mg followed in six days with a complete blood count (CBC). If the CBC is normal, dosing commences at a range from 0.2 to 0.6 mg/kg/week, up to 25 mg/week, depending on weight. Concurrent administration of folic acid 1–5 mg/day ameliorates the risk of nausea, mucosal ulcerations, and macrocytic anemia [106]. Screening tests and complications are the same as for adults, with the most common side effects being nausea, fatigue, headaches, and anorexia. The most significant is bone marrow suppression. Liver function should be monitored by blood tests but liver biopsy is unnecessary in children, and hepatic toxicity is rare. Live, attenuated vaccines—such as those for measles, mumps, and rubella (MMR) and poliovirus—may not be given to a child taking weekly methotrexate. (In the latter case, a killed polio vaccine can be substituted.) Long-term oncogenic risks in children taking methotrexate are of concern but have not been clearly delineated. An option for those who cannot tolerate oral methotrexate is weekly subcutaneously administered methotrexate. Marked improvement is generally seen within 12 weeks after initiation of treatment. Time to clearance depends on disease severity and speed of progression to optimal dosage. Once clearing is achieved, the methotrexate dosage should be gradually lowered (e.g., 2.5 mg/months) during the subsequent months until a maintenance level is achieved.

Retinoids

Retinoids are nonimmunosuppressive vitamin A analogues that bind to nuclear receptors and normalize epidermal differentiation. In general, retinoids tend to be less effective than methotrexate or cyclosporine for treating plaque-type psoriasis but can be quite effective for guttate, pustular, and palmoplantar psoriasis [107,108]. Response may be apparent in as little as three weeks or less. Retinoids and NB-UVB phototherapy (RE-NB-UVB) are synergistic and work well to treat severe generalized pustular psoriasis [109]. Dose range is 0.3–1.0 mg/kg/day and should be titrated based on patient response and laboratory results to the most effective dose [104]. Complications related to acitretin therapy in children are the same as for adults. Teratogenicity is a well-known and serious toxicity of retinoids, and these agents must be avoided in girls of childbearing potential. Isotretinoin, although not as effective for psoriasis, clears from the system in one month, as opposed to three years for acitretin, and may be used in severe cases of pustular psoriasis in adolescent females provided appropriate contraceptive counseling and control measures are in place [110]. The risk of skeletal toxicity (premature epiphyseal closure and hyperostosis) is rare at doses of 1 mg/kg/day or less for durations less than one year [111]. Children on or expected to be on long-term therapy must be monitored by radiographic evaluations during infancy, childhood, and puberty [108–113]. Otherwise, screening tests are the same as for adults [104].

Cyclosporine

Cyclosporine (CSA) is effective and well tolerated in most children with severe unresponsive plaque and pustular psoriasis and exfoliative erythrodermas [104,114]. Oral doses range from 1.5 mg/kg/day up to 5 mg/kg/ day, and CSA is often used in combination with topical agents and occasionally with acitretin [114–118]. Its mechanism of action involves inhibition of cytokine production by T lymphocytes. Among systemic therapy for psoriasis, CSA has the greatest potential toxicity, especially with long-term use, and is ideally used as a rapidly acting agent to gain control of severe disease, followed by gradual downward titration and discontinuation. The most important adverse effects of CSA are nephrotoxicity and hypertension. Close laboratory and blood pressure monitoring is necessary to detect serious dose-related side effects. More common side effects include nausea, diarrhea, anorexia, and headaches. Myalgias, arthralgias, paresthesias, gingival hyperplasia, and hypertrichosis are rare in doses used for psoriasis in contrast to the high doses used in transplant patients. Long-term risks of malignancy, skin cancer, and lymphoproliferative disorders are a concern in children; however, evidence suggests that the risk is minimal if using 5 mg/kg/ day or less in patients who are not on concomitant immunosuppressive medications [119]. Live-attenuated vaccines must be avoided during treatment. CSA is metabolized by the hepatic cytochrome P450 system, and drug levels may be influenced by medications that induce and inhibit these enzymes. Potential drug interactions should be considered before initiating therapy with CSA.

Biologics

Biologic medications target specific components of the inflammatory cascade involved in psoriasis pathogenesis. Biologic therapies are attractive options for treating psoriasis in children because they offer the convenience of less frequent dosing and less laboratory monitoring than traditional systemic agents. Further, biologics lack many of the potential end-organ toxicities of traditional agents. However, biologic therapies have not yet accumulated adequate long-term safety data, specifically in children with psoriasis, to deem them completely safe. There has been only one randomized, double-blind trial in the United States [55]; all other reports in children are case series, case reports, and anecdote. Importantly, the decision to pursue biologic therapy in a child with psoriasis must be individualized after a detailed discussion with the parents regarding the known and unknown benefits and risks. Similar to the other systemic agents, none of the biologics are approved for psoriasis in patients less than 18 years old. Because of lack of data, no formalized guidelines exist for dosing and laboratory monitoring in pediatric patients. Before initiation of therapy, children should undergo tuberculosis screening and immunization updates, followed by regularly scheduled clinical surveillance for adverse events, particularly infections.

Of all the biologics, etanercept has accumulated the most data in pediatric psoriasis. Etanercept is approved by the FDA for children with juvenile idiopathic arthritis but has yet to receive approval for psoriasis or psoriatic arthritis despite a phase III double-blind, randomized controlled trial demonstrating the safety and efficacy of the drug in the treatment of moderate to severe plaque psoriasis in children and adolescents [55]. This study compared etanercept 0.8 mg/kg weekly to placebo in 211 pediatric patients aged 4–17 years over the course of 48 weeks. No deaths, cancers, opportunistic infections, tuberculosis, or demyelination events were reported in the study. Furthermore, the children's dermatology life quality index (CDLQI) response was assessed, and the mean improvement in quality of life from baseline was significantly higher in the treatment group than in the placebo group (52% vs. 18%). Data at the 96-week point of the ongoing 264-week open-label extension of this study showed continued efficacy, tolerability, and safety of etanercept in 140 patients [120,138].

Uncontrolled data are available for successful treatment of pediatric plaque and pustular psoriasis with other tumor necrosis factor inhibitors including infliximab and adalimumab [121–123]. Infliximab was FDA approved in 2006 for the treatment of Crohn's disease in children aged six years and older. Infliximab is a chimeric monoclonal antibody with potent activity against tumor necrosis factor-α (TNF-α), although its documented use in pediatric psoriasis is limited to case reports and anecdotal experience. When used for refractory plaque and generalized pustular psoriasis in children, intravenously administered infliximab has been observed to be uniformly effective at doses of 3.3–5 mg/kg administered at weeks 0, 2, 6, and every seven to eight weeks thereafter. Time to onset of effect has been as rapid as hours to days [4,121,122,124,125]. Adalimumab received FDA approval in 2008 for the treatment of juvenile idiopathic arthritis (JIA) in patients four years of age and older [126], and it is currently being used off-label for pediatric inflammatory bowel disease (IBD), uveitis, and psoriasis. Adalimumab is a fully human monoclonal antibody against TNF-α and is administered subcutaneously every two weeks. To date, there have been no randomized controlled trials performed in the United States evaluating adalimumab in pediatric psoriasis. There are two case reports in the literature detailing the successful use of adalimumab for recalcitrant pustular psoriasis in adolescent girls after failure of other systemic and biologic agents [127,128]. Outside of the United States, a manufacturer-sponsored, multicenter, randomized, double-blind study evaluating the efficacy and safety of adalimumab versus methotrexate in pediatric patients aged 4–17 years with chronic plaque psoriasis is underway [129].

TNF-α inhibitors carry a black box warning for increased risk of lymphoma and other malignancies in the pediatric population. Thus far, no cases of lymphoma have been identified in children treated for psoriasis, and a clear causal relationship between the use of TNF blockers and malignancy in children has not been established [130].

The newest biologic agent, an anti-IL 12/23 monoclonal antibody (ustekinumab) [139] was recently approved for the treatment of moderate to severe plaque psoriasis in adults. To date, there is one published case report detailing the use of ustekinumab in a 14-year-old male with plaque psoriasis [131]. A phase III multicenter, randomized, double-blind, placebo-controlled trial evaluating the efficacy and safety of ustekinumab in the treatment of adolescent patients with moderate to severe plaque psoriasis (CADMUS) is underway outside of the United States [132].

CONCLUSIONS

Psoriasis occurs in almost 1% of children, but the diagnosis is often missed. The highly visible lesions in more severely affected children can significantly affect a child's quality of life, and pediatric psoriasis is now clearly established to be linked to obesity, as has been described in adults. The treatment of psoriasis in children most commonly involves a conventional topical therapeutic regimen of emollients, steroids, calcipotriene, tars, and keratolytics. On the other hand, more severe unresponsive psoriasis, exfoliative erythrodermas, and pustular psoriasis may require ultraviolet light therapy or treatment with systemic agents, such as methotrexate, acitretin, cyclosporine, and biologic agents.

REFERENCES

1. Schachner L, Ling MS, Press S. A statistical analysis of a pediatric dermatology clinic. *Pediatr Dermatol* 1983; 1: 157–164.
2. Beylot C, Puissant A, Bioulac P, et al. Particular clinical features of psoriasis in infants and children. *Acta Derm Venereol Suppl (Stockh)* 1979; 87: 95–97.
3. Tollefson MM, Crowson CS, McEvoy MT, et al. Incidence of psoriasis in children: a population-based study. *J Am Acad Dermatol* 2010; 62(6): 979–987.
4. de Jager ME, de Jong EM, van de Kerkhof PC, et al. Efficacy and safety of treatments for childhood psoriasis: a systematic literature review. *J Am Acad Dermatol* 2010; 62(6): 1013–1030.
5. Oostveen AM, de Jager ME, van de Kerkhof PC, et al. The influence of treatments in daily clinical practice on the Children's Dermatology Life Quality Index in juvenile psoriasis: a longitudinal study from the Child-CAPTURE patient registry. *Br J Dermatol* 2012; 167(1): 145–149.
6. Raychaudhuri SP, Gross J. A comparative study of pediatric onset psoriasis with adult onset psoriasis. *Pediatr Dermatol* 2000; 17: 174–178.
7. Farber EM, Nall ML. The natural history of psoriasis in 5600 patients. *Dermatologica* 1974; 109: 207–211.
8. Nyfors A, Lemholt K. Psoriasis in children. A short review and a survey of 245 cases. *Br J Dermatol* 1975; 92: 437–442.
9. Vogel SA, Yentzer B, Davis SA, et al. Trends in pediatric psoriasis outpatient health care delivery in the United States. *Arch Dermatol* 2012; 148(1): 66–71.
10. Morris A, Rogers M, Fischer G, et al. Childhood psoriasis: a clinical review of 1262 cases. *Pediatr Dermatol* 2001; 18: 188–198.
11. Wu JJ, Black MH, Smith N, et al. Low prevalence of psoriasis among children and adolescents in a large multiethnic cohort in southern California. *J Am Acad Dermatol* 2011; 65(5): 957–964.
12. Kinney JA. Psoriasis in the American black. In: Farber EM, Cox AJ, eds. *Psoriasis: Proceedings of the International Symposium, Stanford University*. Stanford, CA: Stanford University Press; 1971, pp. 49–52.
13. Paller AS, Mercy K, Kwasny MJ, et al. Association of pediatric psoriasis severity with excess and central adiposity: an international cross-sectional study. *JAMA Dermatol* 2013; 149: 166–176.
14. Lonnberg AS, Skov L, Skytthe A, et al. Heritability of psoriasis in a large twin sample. *Br J Dermatol* 2013; 169: 412–416.
15. Swanbeck G, Inerot A, Martinsson T, et al. Genetic counseling in psoriasis: empirical data on psoriasis among first-degree relatives of 3095 psoriatic probands. *Br J Dermatol* 1997; 137: 939–942.
16. Henseler T. The genetics of psoriasis. *J Am Acad Dermatol* 1997; 37: S1–S11.
17. Tiilikainen A, Lassus A, Karvonen J, et al. Psoriasis and HLA-Cw6. *Br J Dermatol* 1980; 192: 179–184.

18. Elder JT, Bruce AT, Gudjonsson JE, et al. Molecular dissection of psoriasis: integrating genetics and biology. *J Invest Dermatol* 2010; 130(5): 1213–1226.
19. Oka A, Mabuchi T, Ozawa A, et al. Current understanding of human genetics and genetic analysis of psoriasis. *J Dermatol* 2012; 39(3): 231–241.
20. Tsoi LC, Spain SL, Knight J, et al. Identification of 15 new psoriasis susceptibility loci highlights the role of innate immunity. *Nat Genet* 2012; 44(12): 1341–1348.
21. Jordan CT, Cao L, Roberson ED, et al. PSORS2 is due to mutations in CARD14. *Am J Hum Genet* 2012; 90(5): 784–795.
22. Fuchs-Telem D, Sarig O, van Steensel MA, et al. Familial pityriasis rubra pilaris is caused by mutations in CARD14. *Am J Hum Genet* 2012; 91(1): 163–170.
23. Marrakchi S, Guigue P, Renshaw BR, et al. Interleukin-36-receptor antagonist deficiency and generalized pustular psoriasis. *N Engl J Med* 2011; 365(7): 620–628.
24. Onoufriadis A, Simpson MA, Pink AE, et al. Mutations in IL36RN/IL1F5 are associated with the severe episodic inflammatory skin disease known as generalized pustular psoriasis. *Am J Hum Genet* 2011; 89(3): 432–437.
25. Benoit S, Hamm H. Childhood psoriasis. *Clin Dermatol* 2007; 25(6): 555–562.
26. Menter MA, Whiting DA, McWilliams J. Resistant childhood psoriasis: an analysis of patients seen in a day-care center. *Pediatr Dermatol* 1984; 2: 8–12.
27. Paller AS, Mercy K, Kwasny MJ, et al. Association of pediatric psoriasis severity with excess and central adiposity: an international cross-sectional study. *JAMA Dermatol* 2013; 149(2): 166–176.
28. Patrizi A, Costa AM, Fiorillio L, et al. Perianal streptococcal dermatitis associated with guttate psoriasis and/or balanoposthitis. *Pediatr Dermatol* 1994; 11(2): 168–171.
29. Seyhan M, Coskun BK, Saglam H, et al. Psoriasis in childhood and adolescence: evaluation of demographic and clinical features. *Pediatr Int* 2006; 48(6): 525–530.
30. Martin BA, Chalmers RJ, Telfer NR. How great is the risk of further psoriasis following a single episode of acute guttate psoriasis? *Arch Dermatol* 1996; 132(6): 717–718.
31. Mercy K, Kwasny M, Cordoro KM, et al. Clinical manifestations of pediatric psoriasis: results of a multicenter study in the United States. *Pediatr Dermatol* 2013; 30: 424–428.
32. Andersen S, La C, Thomsen K. Psoriasiform napkin dermatitis. *Br J Dermatol* 1971; 84: 316–319.
33. Neville EA, Finn OA. Psoriasiform napkin dermatitis—a follow up study. *Br J Dermatol* 1975; 92: 279–285.
34. Rasmussen HB, Hagdrup JI, Schmidt H. Psoriasiform napkin dermatitis. *Acta Dermatol Venereol (Stockh)* 1986; 66: 534–536.
35. Thomsen K. Seborrhoeic dermatitis and napkin dermatitis. *Acta Dermatol Venereol (Stockh)* 1981; 95: 40–42.
36. Menni S, Piccino R, Baietta S, et al. Infantile seborrheic dermatitis: seven year follow-up and some prognostic criteria. *Pediatr Dermatol* 1989; 6: 13–15.
37. Rattet J, Headley J, Barr R. Diaper dermatitis with psoriasiform id eruption. *Int J Dermatol* 1981; 20: 122–125.
38. Fischer G, Rogers M. Vulvar disease in children: a clinical audit of 130 cases. *Pediatr Dermatol* 2000; 17: 1–6.
39. Farber EM. Facial psoriasis. *Cutis* 1992; 50: 25–28.
40. Nanda A, Kaur S, Kaur I, et al. Childhood psoriasis: an epidemiologic survey of 112 patients. *Pediatr Dermatol* 1990; 7: 19–21.
41. Farber EM, Nall L. Natural history and treatment of scalp psoriasis. *Cutis* 1992; 49(6): 396–400.
42. Hersle K, Lindholm A, Mobacken H, et al. Relationship of pityriasis amiantacea to psoriasis: a follow-up study. *Dermatologica* 1979; 159: 245–250.
43. Hansted B, Lindskov R. Pityriasis amiantacea and psoriasis. *Dermatologica* 1983; 166: 314–315.
44. Atherton DJ, Kahan M, Russell-Jones R. Naevoid psoriasis. *Br J Dermatol* 1989; 120: 837–841.
45. Liao PB, Rubinson R, Howard R, et al. Annular pustular psoriasis—most common form of pustular psoriasis in children: report of three cases and review of the literature. *Pediatr Dermatol* 2002; 19: 19–25.
46. Zelickson BD, Muller SA. Generalized pustular psoriasis in childhood. *J Am Acad Dermatol* 1991; 24: 186–194.
47. Bellet JS, Chamlin SL, Yan AC, et al. Intertriginous pustular psoriasis. *J Am Acad Dermatol* 2009; 60(4): 679–683.

48. Ivker RA, Grin-Jorgensen CM, Vega VK, et al. Infantile generalized pustular psoriasis associated with lytic lesions of the bone. *Pediatr Dermatol* 1993; 10: 277–282.
49. Prose NS, Fahrner LJ, Miller CR, et al. Pustular psoriasis with chronic recurrent multifocal osteomyelitis and spontaneous fractures. *J Am Acad Dermatol* 1994; 31(2 Pt 2): 376–379.
50. Aksentijevich I, Masters SL, Ferguson PJ, et al. An autoinflammatory disease with deficiency of the interleukin-1-receptor antagonist. *N Engl J Med* 2009; 360(23): 2426–2437.
51. Kapila S, Hong E, Fischer G. A comparative study of childhood psoriasis and atopic dermatitis and greater understanding of the overlapping condition, psoriasis-dermatitis. *Aust J Dermatol* 2012; 53(2): 98–105.
52. Farber EM, Nall L. Nail psoriasis. *Cutis* 1992; 50: 174–178.
53. Stoll ML, Lio P, Sundel RP, et al. Patients with juvenile psoriatic arthritis comprise two distinct populations. *Arthr Rheum* 2008; 59: 51–58.
54. Stoll ML, Nigrovic PA, Gotte AC, et al. Clinical comparison of early-onset psoriatic and non-psoriatic oligoarticular juvenile idiopathic arthritis. *Clin Exp Rheumatol* 2011; 29(3): 582–588.
55. Paller AS, Langley RG, Gottlieb AB, et al. Etanercept treatment for children and adolescents with plaque psoriasis. *N Engl J Med* 2008; 358(3): 241–251.
56. Shore A, Ansell BM. Juvenile psoriatic arthritis: an analysis of 60 cases. *J Pediatr* 1982; 100: 529–535.
57. Stoll ML, Zurakowski D, Nigrovic LE, et al. Patients with juvenile psoriatic arthritis comprise two distinct populations. *Arthr Rheum* 2006; 56: 3564–3572.
58. Southwood TR, Petty RE, Malleson PN, et al. Psoriatic arthritis is children. *Arthritis Rheum* 1989; 32: 1007–1013.
59. Hamilton ML, Gladman DD, Shore A, et al. Juvenile psoriatic arthritis and HLA arthritis. *Ann Rheum Dis* 1990; 49: 694–697.
60. Hensler T, Christopher E. Disease concomitance in psoriasis. *J Am Acad Dermatol* 1995; 32: 982–986.
61. McGowan JW, Pearce DJ, Chen J, et al. The skinny on psoriasis and obesity. *Arch Dermatol* 2005; 141: 160–162.
62. Sterry W, Strober BE, Menter A. Obesity in psoriasis: the metabolic, clinical and therapeutic implications. Report of an interdisciplinary conference and review. *Br J Dermatol* 2007; 157: 649–655.
63. Sommer DM, Jenisch S, Suchan M, et al. Increased prevalence of the metabolic syndrome in patients with moderate to severe psoriasis. *Arch Dermatol Res* 2006; 298: 321–328.
64. Langan SM, Seminara NM, Shin DB, et al. Prevalence of metabolic syndrome in patients with psoriasis: a population-based study in the United Kingdom. *J Invest Dermatol* 2012; 132(3 Pt 1): 556–562.
65. Volf EM, Levine DE, Michelon MA, et al. Assessor-blinded study of the metabolic syndrome and surrogate markers of increased cardiovascular risk in children with moderate-to-severe psoriasis compared with age-matched population of children with warts. *J Drugs Dermatol* 2011; 10(8): 900–901.
66. Alikasifoglu A, Gonc N, Ozon ZA, et al. The relationship between serum adiponectin, tumor necrosis factor-alpha, leptin levels and insulin sensitivity in childhood and adolescent obesity: adiponectin is a marker of metabolic syndrome. *J Clin Res Pediatr Endocrinol* 2009; 1(5): 233–239.
67. Setty AR, Curhan G, Choi HK. Obesity, waist circumference, weight change, and the risk of psoriasis in women: nurses' health study II. *Arch Intern Med* 2007; 167(15): 1670–1675.
68. Ozden MG, Tekin NS, Gurer MA, et al. Environmental risk factors in pediatric psoriasis: a multicenter case-control study. *Pediatr Dermatol* 2011; 28(3): 306–312.
69. Leary MR, Rapp SR, Herbst KC, et al. Interpersonal concerns and psychological difficulties of psoriasis patients: effects of disease severity and fear of negative evaluation. *Health Psychol* 1998; 17: 530–536.
70. Gupta MA, Gupta AK. Depression and suicidal ideation in dermatology patients with acne, alopecia areata, atopic dermatitis, and psoriasis. *Br J Dermatol* 1998; 139: 846–850.
71. Gupta MA, Schork NJ, Gupta AK, et al. Suicidal ideation in psoriasis. *Int J Dermatol* 1993; 32: 188–190.
72. Lebwohl M, Ali S. Treatment of psoriasis. Part 1. Topical therapy and phototherapy. *J Am Acad Dermatol* 2001; 45: 487–498.

73. Chiaretti A, Schembri Wismayer D, Tortorolo L, et al. Salicylate intoxication using a skin ointment. *Acta Paediatr* 1997; 86(3): 330–331.
74. Zvulonov A, Anisfeld A, Metzker A. Efficacy of short-contact therapy with dithranol in childhood psoriasis. *Int J Dermatol* 1994; 38: 808–810.
75. Lowe NJ, Ashton RE, Koudsi H, et al. Anthralin for psoriasis: short-contact anthralin therapy compared with topical steroid and conventional anthralin. *J Am Acad Dermatol* 1984; 10: 69–72.
76. Harris DR. Old wine in new bottles: the revival of anthralin. *Cutis* 1998; 62: 201–203.
77. Darley CR, Cunliffe WJ, Green CM, et al. Safety and efficacy of calcipotriol ointment (Dovonex) in treating children with psoriasis vulgaris. *Br J Dermatol* 1996; 135: 390–393.
78. Oranje AP, Marcoux D, Svensson A, et al. Topical calcipotriol in childhood psoriasis. *J Am Acad Dermatol* 1997; 36: 203–208.
79. Brune A, Miller DW, Lin P, et al. Tacrolimus ointment is effective for psoriasis on the face and intertriginous areas in pediatric patients. *Pediatr Dermatol* 2007; 24(1): 76–80.
80. de Vries AC, Bogaards NA, Hooft L, et al. Interventions for nail psoriasis. *Cochrane Database Syst Rev* 2013; 1: CD007633.
81. Barbagallo J, Spann CT, Tutrone WD, et al. Narrowband UVB phototherapy for the treatment of psoriasis: a review and update. *Cutis* 2001; 68: 345–347.
82. Tay YK, Morelli JG, Weston WL. Experience with UVB phototherapy in children. *Pediatr Dermatol* 1996; 13: 406–409.
83. Jain VK, Aggarwal K, Jain K, et al. Narrow-band UV-B phototherapy in childhood psoriasis. *Int J Dermatol* 2007; 46: 320–322.
84. McClelland PB. Fundamentals of phototherapy. In: National Psoriasis Foundation, ed. *Guide to Phototherapy*. San Francisco, CA: National Psoriasis Foundation 2008.
85. al-Fouzan AS, Nanda A. UVB phototherapy in childhood psoriasis. *Pediatr Dermatol* 1995; 12: 66.
86. Pasić A, Ceović R, Lipozencić J, et al. Phototherapy in pediatric patients. *Pediatr Dermatol* 2003; 20: 71–77.
87. Spuls PI, Rozenblit M, Lebwohl M. Retrospective study of the efficacy of narrowband UVB and acitretin. *J Dermatolog Treat* 2003; 14(Suppl 2): 17–20.
88. Kim HS, Kim GM, Kim SY. Two-stage therapy for childhood generalized pustular psoriasis: low-dose cyclosporin for induction and maintenance with acitretin/narrowband ultraviolet B phototherapy. *Pediatr Dermatol* 2006; 23: 306–308.
89. Diffey BL, Farr PM. The challenge of follow-up in narrowband ultraviolet B phototherapy. *Br J Dermatol* 2007; 157: 344–349.
90. Wolff K. Side-effects of psoralen photochemotherapy (PUVA). *Br J Dermatol* 1990; 122(Suppl 36): 117–125.
91. Spuls PI, Hadi S, Rivera L, et al. Retrospective analysis of the treatment of psoriasis of the palms and soles. *J Dermatolog Treat* 2003; 14(Suppl 2): 21–25.
92. Delrosso G, Bornacina C, Farinelli P, et al. Bath PUVA and psoriasis: is a milder treatment a worse treatment? *Dermatology* 2008; 216: 191–193.
93. Marqueling AL, Cordoro KM. Systemic treatments for severe pediatric psoriasis: a practical approach. *Dermatol Clin* 2013; 31(2): 267–288.
94. Ferran M, Galván AB, Rincón C, et al. Streptococcus induces circulating CLA(+) memory T-cell-dependent epidermal cell activation in psoriasis. *J Invest Dermatol* 2013; 133(4): 999–1007.
95. Owen CM, Chalmers RJG, O'Sullivan T, et al. Antistreptococcal interventions for guttate and chronic plaque psoriasis. *Cochrane Database Syst Rev* 2000; (2): CD001976.
96. Vincent F, Ross JB, Dalton M, et al. A therapeutic trial of the use of penicillin V or erythromycin with or without rifampin in the treatment of psoriasis. *J Am Acad Dermatol* 1992; 26: 458–461.
97. Honig PJ. Guttate psoriasis associated with perianal streptococcal disease. *J Pediatr* 1988; 113: 1037–1039.
98. Hone SW, Donnelly MJ, Powell F, et al. Clearance of recalcitrant psoriasis after tonsillectomy. *Clin Otolaryngol Allied Sci* 1996; 21: 546–547.
99. Nyfors A, Rasmussen PA, Lemholt K, et al. Improvement of recalcitrant psoriasis vulgaris after tonsillectomy. *J Laryngol Otol* 1976; 90: 789–794.
100. Wilson JK, Al-Suwaidan SN, Krowchuk D, et al. Treatment of psoriasis in children: is there a role for antibiotic therapy and tonsillectomy? *Pediatr Dermatol* 2003; 20(1): 11–15.
101. Owen CM, Chalmers RJ, O'Sullivan T, Griffiths CE. A systematic review of antistreptococcal interventions for guttate and chronic plaque psoriasis. *Br J Dermatol* 2001; 145(6): 886–890.

102. Thorleifsdottir RH, Sigurdardottir SL, Sigurgeirsson B, et al. Improvement of psoriasis after tonsillectomy is associated with a decrease in the frequency of circulating T cells that recognize streptococcal determinants and homologous skin determinants. *J Immunol* 2012; 188(10): 5160–5165.
103. Cronstein BN. The mechanism of action of methotrexate. *Rheum Dis Clin North Am* 1997; 23: 739–755.
104. Lebwohl M, Ali S. Treatment of psoriasis. Part 2. Systemic therapies. *J Am Acad Dermatol* 2001; 45: 649–661.
105. Bright RD. Methotrexate in the treatment of psoriasis. *Cutis* 1999; 64: 332–334.
106. Duhra P. Treatment of gastrointestinal symptoms associated with methotrexate therapy for psoriasis. *J Am Acad Dermatol* 1993; 288: 466–469.
107. Shelnitz LS, Esterly NB, Honig PJ. Etretinate therapy for generalized pustular psoriasis in children. *Arch Dermatol* 1987; 123: 230–233.
108. Orfanos CE. Treatment of psoriasis with retinoids: present status. *Cutis* 1999; 64: 347–353.
109. Kopp T, Karlhofer F, Szepfalusi Z, et al. Successful use of acitretin in conjunction with narrowband ultraviolet B phototherapy in a child with severe pustular psoriasis, von Zumbusch type. *Br J Dermatol* 2004; 151: 912–916.
110. Al-Shobaili H, Al-Khenaizan S. Childhood generalized pustular psoriasis: successful treatment with isotretinoin. *Pediatr Dermatol* 2007; 24: 563–564.
111. Halverstam CP, Zeichner J, Lebwohl M. Lack of significant skeletal changes after long-term, low-dose retinoid therapy: case report and review of the literature. *J Cutan Med Surg* 2006; 10: 291–299.
112. Lacour M, Mehta-Nikhar B, Atherton DJ, et al. An appraisal of acitretin therapy in children with inherited disorders of keratinization. *Br J Dermatol* 1996; 134: 1023–1029.
113. Halkier-Sorensen L, Laurberg G, Andresen J. Bone changes in children on long-term treatment with etretinate. *J Am Acad Dermatol* 1987; 16: 999–1006.
114. Pereira TM, Vieira AP, Fernandes JC, et al. Cyclosporin A treatment in severe childhood psoriasis. *J Eur Acad Dermatol Venereol* 2006; 20: 651–656.
115. Perrett CM, Ilchyshyn A, Berth-Jones J. Cyclosporin in childhood psoriasis. *J Dermatolog Treat* 2003; 14: 113–118.
116. Alli N, Gungor E, Karakayali G, et al. The use of cyclosporin in a child with generalized pustular psoriasis. *Br J Dermatol* 1998; 139: 754–755.
117. Mahe E, Bodemer C, Pruszkowski A, et al. Cyclosporine in childhood psoriasis. *Arch Dermatol* 2001; 137: 1532–1533.
118. Sebnem Kilic S, Hacimustafaoglu M, Celebi S, et al. Low dose cyclosporin A treatment: generalized pustular psoriasis. *Pediatr Dermatol* 2001, 18. 246–248.
119. Ellis CN. Safety issues with cyclosporine. *Int J Dermatol* 1997; 36(Suppl 1): 7–10.
120. Paller AS, Siegfried EC, Eichenfield LF, et al. Long-term etanercept in pediatric patients with plaque psoriasis. *J Am Acad Dermatol* 2010; 63: 762–768.
121. Farnsworth N, George SJ, Hsu S. Successful use of infliximab following a failed course of etanercept in a pediatric patient. *Dermatol Online J* 2005; 11(3): 11.
122. Menter MA, Cush JM. Successful treatment of pediatric psoriasis with infliximab. *Pediatr Dermatol* 2004; 21: 87–88.
123. Luu M, Cordoro KM. The evolving role of biologics in the treatment of pediatric psoriasis. *Skin Therapy Lett* 2013; 18(2): 1–4.
124. Pereira TM, Vieira AP, Fernandes JC, et al. Anti-TNF-alpha therapy in childhood pustular psoriasis. *Dermatology* 2006; 213(4): 350–352.
125. Weishaupt C, Metze D, Luger TA, et al. Treatment of pustular psoriasis with infliximab. *J Dtsch Dermatol Ges* 2007; 5(5): 397–399.
126. HUMIRA (adalimumab) full prescribing information. Revised: September 2012. Abbott Laboratories. Available at: www.rxabbott.com/pdf/humira.pdf (Accessed December 16, 2012).
127. Alvarez AC, Rodriguez-Nevado I, De Argila D, et al. Recalcitrant pustular psoriasis successfully treated with adalimumab. *Pediatr Dermatol* 2011; 28(2): 195–197.
128. Callen JP, Jackson JH. Adalimumab effectively controlled recalcitrant generalized pustular psoriasis in an adolescent. *J Dermatolog Treat* 2005; 16(5–6): 350–352.
129. A multicenter, randomized, double-dummy, double-blind study evaluating two doses of adalimumab versus methotrexate (MTX) in pediatric subjects with chronic plaque psoriasis. In: ClinicalTrials.gov, Identifier: NCT01251614. Last updated October 26, 2012. Available at: http://www.clinicaltrials.gov/ct2/show/NCT01251614 (Accessed December 16, 2012).

130. Diak P, Siegel J, La Grenade L, et al. Tumor necrosis factor alpha blockers and malignancy in children: forty-eight cases reported to the Food and Drug Administration. *Arthritis Rheum* 2010; 62(8): 2517–2524.
131. Fotiadou C, Lazaridou E, Giannopoulou C, et al. Ustekinumab for the treatment of an adolescent patient with recalcitrant plaque psoriasis. *Eur J Dermatol* 2011; 21(1): 117–118.
132. Centocor, Inc. A phase 3 multicenter, randomized, double-blind, placebo-controlled study evaluating the efficacy and safety of ustekinumab in the treatment of adolescent subjects with moderate to severe plaque-type psoriasis (CADMUS). In: ClinicalTrials.gov, Identifier: NCT01090427. Last updated December 10, 2012. Available at: http://clinicaltrials.gov/ct2/show/NCT01090427 (Accessed December 16, 2012).
133. Barth JH, Dawber RPR. Diseases of nails in children. *Pediatr Dermatol* 1987; 4: 275–290.
134. Farber EM, Jacobs AH. Infantile psoriasis. *Am J Dis Child* 1977; 131: 1266–1269.
135. Hafner R, Michels H. Psoriatic arthritis in children. *Curr Opin Rheumatol* 1996; 8: 467–472.
136. Atherton DJ, Cohen BL, Knobler E, et al. Phototherapy for children. *Pediatr Dermatol* 1996; 13: 415–426.
137. Stern RS, Nichols KT. Therapy with orally administered methoxsalen and ultraviolet A radiation during childhood increases the risk of basal cell carcinoma. The PUVA Follow-up Study. *J Pediatr* 1996; 129: 915–917.
138. Lewis-Jones MS, Finlay AY. The Children's Dermatology Life Quality Index (CDLQI): initial validation and practical use. *Br J Dermatol* 1995; 132: 942–949.
139. Kimball AB, Gordon KB, Langley RG, et al. Safety and efficacy of ABT-874, a fully human interleukin 12/23 monoclonal antibody, in the treatment of moderate to severe chronic plaque psoriasis: results of a randomized, placebo-controlled, phase 2 trial. *Arch Dermatol* 2008; 144: 200–207.

Chapter 19

Psoriatic Arthritis

Dafna D. Gladman

EPIDEMIOLOGICAL EVIDENCE

The occurrence of arthritis in patients with psoriasis has been recognized since the 19th century. However, psoriatic arthritis (PsA) was identified as a distinct entity primarily as a consequence of the efforts of the late Verna Wright of Leeds, England, and his colleague John Moll of Sheffield, England [1]. Epidemiological studies have noted that among patients with psoriasis, arthritis has a higher prevalence than in the general population [2]. The frequency of inflammatory arthritis in the general population is estimated to 3%–5%, whereas among patients with psoriasis, 7%–42% have been identified as having PsA. Likewise, psoriasis occurs in a higher frequency among patients with arthritis (7%) than among the general population (1%–3%). Although there are individuals who disagree with the identification of PsA as a distinct entity [3], it is now widely accepted that there is a specific form of arthritis associated with psoriasis [4].

CLINICAL DEFINITION AND CLASSIFICATION

Based on their observations, Moll and Wright defined PsA as an inflammatory arthritis associated with psoriasis, usually seronegative for rheumatoid factor. Inflammatory-type arthritis presents with pain, swelling, and stiffness in the affected joints. The pain and stiffness are usually worse when at rest and are alleviated with activity, and patients complain of morning stiffness usually for more than 45 minutes in duration. Any of the peripheral joints may be affected. The larger the number of joints affected, the more likely it is to be in a symmetrical distribution. In addition to the peripheral joint disease, inflammation of the sacroiliac and apophyseal joints of the spine also occurs in almost half the patients with PsA. Approximately 40% of patients with PsA carry the human leukocyte allele B*27 (HLA-B*27).

Because of the presence of spondyloarthritis in 40%–50% of the patients, the usual absence of rheumatoid factor, and the association with HLA-B*27, PsA has been classified among the seronegative, HLA-B*27-associated spondyloarthropathies (SpA).

Until 2006, there were no validated and widely agreed upon classification criteria for PsA. However, Taylor et al. [5] published the results of an international study on the classification of psoriatic arthritis (CASPAR) based on a group of 588 patients with PsA and 536 patients with other forms of inflammatory arthritis, mostly rheumatoid arthritis (70%). Using a classification and regression tree analysis and logistic regression, the CASPAR group developed classification criteria (Table 19.1). The criteria may be applied to patients with inflammatory joint, spinal, or entheseal disease, and include the presence of psoriatic skin lesions (which, if current, provide two points, but if by personal history or family history, provide only one

TABLE 19.1 CASPAR Criteria for PsA

Inflammatory musculoskeletal disease (joint, spine, or entheseal) with three or more of the following:		
1. Evidence of psoriasis (one of a, b, c)	a. Current psoriasis[a]	Psoriatic skin or scalp disease present today as judged by a dermatologist or rheumatologist
	b. Personal history of psoriasis	A history of psoriasis that may be obtained from patient, family doctor, dermatologist, or rheumatologist
	c. Family history of psoriasis	A history of psoriasis in a first or second degree relative according to patient report
2. Psoriatic nail dystrophy		Typical psoriatic nail dystrophy including onycholysis, pitting, and hyperkeratosis observed on current physical examination
3. A negative test for rheumatoid factor		By any method except latex but preferably by ELISA or nephelometry, according to the local laboratory reference range
4. Dactylitis either a or b	a. Current Dactylitis	Swelling of an entire digit
	b. History of Dactylitis	Recorded by a rheumatologist
5. Radiological evidence of juxta-articular new bone formation		Ill-defined ossification near joint margins (but excluding osteophyte formation) on plain X-rays of hand or foot

Source: Taylor WJ, et al., *Arthritis Rheum* 54, 2665–2673, 2006.

[a] Current psoriasis gets two points, others each get one point.

point); nail lesions, a negative rheumatoid factor; either current or previous dactylitis documented by a rheumatologist (this is important because a recent study has shown that dermatologists are not as reliable in documenting dactylitis) [6]; and the presence of fluffy periosteal reaction. In the context of inflammatory musculoskeletal disease, if a patient achieves three of the six possible points, they may be classified as having PsA with 91.4% sensitivity and 98.7% specificity. It is expected that the CASPAR criteria will facilitate the diagnosis of PsA because they have been shown to be sensitive in early PsA [7] and sensitive and specific in a family medicine clinic [8,9].

CLINICAL PATTERNS

Moll and Wright described five clinical patterns of the disease: distal arthritis, involving primarily the distal interphalangeal (DIP) joints of the hands and feet; oligoarthritis, in which four or fewer joints were affected often in an asymmetrical distribution; polyarthritis, in which five or more joints are affected, often indistinguishable from rheumatoid arthritis (RA); arthritis mutilans, which is a destructive form of arthritis; and a spondyloarthropathy with inflammation in the spine and sacroiliac joints [1].

Since the observations of Moll and Wright, several cohorts of patients with PsA have been described, and it has become clear that there was no consensus as to the frequency of the specific patterns. Moreover, although these patterns may be defined at presentation, they tend to change over time, as more joints accrue in some patients and some joints settle in others. As the disease progresses, there often is an increasing number of joints involved, and the disease becomes more symmetrical [10,11]. The variation of the clinical patterns with time, as well as the fact that PsA is generally less tender than RA, has made it difficult to create widely accepted classification criteria for the disease. However, as pointed out earlier, the CASPAR criteria seem to overcome these problems. Indeed, the CASPAR criteria allow the diagnosis of PsA in patients who are rheumatoid factor positive and in patients who only have spondylitis or enthesitis, without the documentation of peripheral arthritis. It has also become clear that dactylitis, or inflammation of the whole digit, is an important feature of PsA, occurring in 48% of the patients [12]. Currently, physicians and investigators refer to the five domains of PsA, which include peripheral arthritis, axial disease, dactylitis, enthesitis, and skin and nail lesions rather than the five patterns originally described by Moll and Wright [13].

EXTRA-ARTICULAR MANIFESTATIONS

In addition to psoriasis and nail lesions, patients with PsA have other extra-articular manifestations that help to identify the correct diagnosis. These include iritis, mucous membrane lesions, urethritis, bowel symptoms, and aortic dilatation. These features are common to the other SpA (Table 19.2).

DIFFERENTIATING BETWEEN PsA AND OTHER ARTHROPATHIES

Not all patients with psoriasis and arthritis have PsA. Despite the variation in disease presentation, there are distinct features of PsA that differentiate it from RA, osteoarthritis (OA), and other SpA (Table 19.2).

Features That Differentiate PsA from RA

PsA commonly affects the DIP joints, which are uncommonly affected in RA. PsA tends to be asymmetrical compared to RA, and the joints tend to be affected in a ray distribution; all the joints of a single digit are involved, but the same digit on the opposite limb is spared. This contrasts with the symmetrical distribution of RA, in which the same joints on hands or feet are affected. The affected joints in PsA tend to have a purplish discoloration compared to RA. The degree of tenderness in patients with PsA is less than that of RA [14]. Almost half the patients with PsA may have spondyloarthritis, which is distinctly uncommon in RA. Enthesitis, the inflammation at tendon insertion into bone, is uncommon in RA but is a classic feature of PsA. Dactylitis, the inflammation and swelling of a whole digit, is also a distinct feature of PsA and does not occur in RA. The extra-articular manifestations of PsA are also different from those of RA. Psoriasis in a patient presenting with joint symptoms should certainly alert the physician to the presence of PsA. Nail lesions are thought to be specific differentiating features. In a study comparing patients

TABLE 19.2 Comparison of PsA and Other Arthropathies

Features	Arthritic Condition						
	PsA	**RA**	**OA**	**AS**	**ReA**	**IBD**	**Gout**
Gender distribution	Equal	F ≥ M	Equal	M ≥ F	M ≥ F	M ≥ F	M ≥ F
Age at onset (years)	35–45	20–50	≥50	20–30	20–30	30–40	≥30
Peripheral joints	Common	Common	Common	Uncommon	Common	Common	Common
Distal joints	Common	Rare	Common	Uncommon	Uncommon	Uncommon	Common
Distribution	Asymmetrical	Symmetrical	Symmetrical	Asymmetrical	Asymmetrical	Asymmetrical	Asymmetrical
Red-hot joints	Yes	No	No	No	Yes	No	Yes
Dactylitis	Yes	No	No	No	Yes	No	No
Back involvement (%)	40–50	Rare	Common	100	100	30	Rare
Nodules	No	Common	No	No	No	No	Tophi
Psoriasis	Yes	No	No	No	No	No	No
Nail lesions	Yes	No	No	No	Yes	No	No
Enthesitis	Yes	No	No	Yes	Yes	Yes	No

with PsA to patients with uncomplicated psoriasis, nail involvement was the only clinical feature that was significantly different, occurring in 87% of patients with PsA and 40% of patients with psoriasis [15]. Subsequent studies have confirmed that patients with PsA are more likely to have nail lesions [16,17]. Other specific extra-articular features of PsA include iritis, urethritis, aortic root dilatation and—at times—gut involvement. On the other hand, the presence of rheumatoid nodules is an exclusion criterion for the diagnosis of PsA because it occurs only in patients with RA. Patients with RA tend to have conjunctivitis, lung nodules or interstitial lung disease, pericarditis or myocarditis, and compression neuropathies or mononeuritis multiplex. Skin involvement in RA is usually in the form of nail-fold infarcts, periungual erythema, or leg ulcers that are typical of Felty's syndrome. It should be noted that the co-occurrence of RA and psoriasis is possible. Because psoriasis occurs in 1%–3% of the population, and RA occurs in close to 1% of the population, the likelihood of a coexistence of the two conditions in the same patient may reach 1:10,000. The features noted earlier should help identify whether the patient has PsA or psoriasis with RA.

The changes in joint distribution described clinically may also be noted in the assessment of radiographs from patients with PsA compared to RA. Although joint erosions occur in PsA and RA [10,18], the radiological changes specific to PsA include extensive joint lysis with pencil-in-cup change, as well as ankylosis (Figure 19.1). In addition, periosteal reaction is a feature of PsA not seen in patients with RA. Indeed, fluffy periostitis was the only radiological

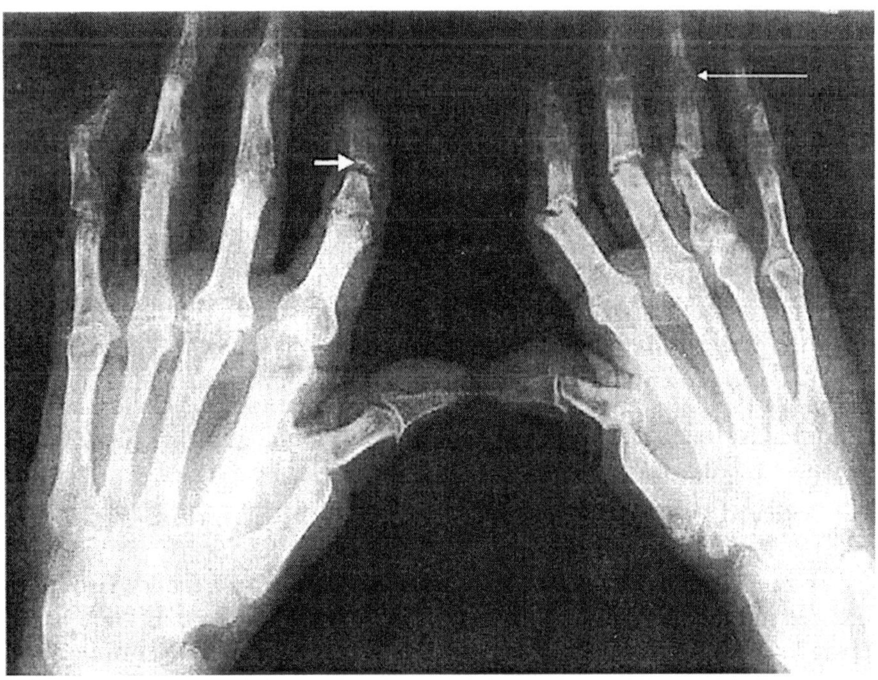

FIGURE 19.1 Radiograph of a patient with PsA demonstrates pencil-in-cup (short arrow) and ankylosing (long arrow) features.

feature included in the CASPAR criteria [5]. The presence of sacroiliitis and syndesmophytes is also typical for PsA and does not occur in RA.

Features That Differentiate PsA from OA

The DIP joints are classically affected in patients with OA. OA is the most common rheumatic disease; therefore, its association with psoriasis is expected. DIP involvement in OA usually presents with pain, which is usually noninflammatory in nature (not associated with prolonged morning stiffness and aggravated by activity rather than rest), whereas the DIP involvement in PsA patients is typically inflammatory. Moreover, on physical examination, OA presents with bony overgrowth that is recognized clinically as Heberden's nodes on the DIP joints and Bouchard's nodes on the proximal interphalangeal (PIP) joint, whereas in PsA, the joints are often swollen on palpation. Radiographs further help to differentiate the two conditions: the erosions seen in PsA are marginal as opposed to the cartilage changes seen in OA. In the spine, OA presents with degenerative disc and apophyseal joint disease and with traction osteophytes, compared with the syndesmophytes seen in PsA. Sacroiliitis is not a feature of OA. The back disease in OA is of the mechanical type as opposed to the inflammatory features of back involvement in PsA.

Features That Differentiate PsA from Other SpA

The spondyloarthritis of PsA can be differentiated from that of other SpA, particularly ankylosing spondylitis (AS), by the presence of the peripheral arthritis, the asymmetrical nature of the syndesmophytes, and the sacroiliac involvement. In addition, the spondyloarthritis of PsA tends to be less symptomatic than that of AS [19]. However, as a member of the seronegative HLA-B*27 spondyloarthritis group, PsA shares many of the extra-articular features with other conditions in the group, including AS, reactive arthritis, and the arthritis of inflammatory bowel disease.

Features That Differentiate PsA from Crystal-Induced Arthritis

Another condition that needs to be differentiated from PsA is crystal-induced arthritis, particularly gout. Gout presents as an acute monoarthritis with a red hot swollen toe (podagra) or a swollen knee or ankle. These are joints commonly involved in PsA. Because patients with psoriasis may have an increased uric acid concentration in their plasma, they are often misdiagnosed as having gout. It is important to aspirate the joint and look for crystals to ascertain the diagnosis. If there are no uric acid crystals in the fluid, it is most likely the acute onset of PsA. This is another reason why patients with psoriasis who present to their dermatologist with joint complaints should be referred to a rheumatologist.

PREVALENCE AMONG PATIENTS WITH PSORIASIS

The exact prevalence of PsA in the general population is unknown. Estimates reported in the literature vary from 0.1% at the Mayo Clinic to 1.4% in the Faroe Islands. A survey by the National Psoriasis Foundation estimated a prevalence of psoriasis in the United States of 2.1%, and of PsA at 0.5% [20]. The reported prevalence of PsA among patients with psoriasis has been variable from 7% to 42%. The value of 7% was reported from a hospital study including only patients with polyarthritis in Sweden in 1948, and the higher value was from an outpatient facility in South Africa. The difficulty in obtaining accurate information has been the lack of widely accepted classification criteria and the fact that many patients with PsA do not complain of pain. Therefore, their disease may be unnoticed until they have clear deformities. Moreover, even rheumatologists do not always make the correct diagnosis [21]. Among patients seen in dermatology clinics, the University of Toronto identified 30% of patients with psoriasis as having PsA [22]. Two studies from dermatology clinics in Germany documented a prevalence of PsA in 20% of the patients with psoriasis, with a large proportion of the patients not having been diagnosed before [23,24]. A study from Leeds reported a prevalence of 24% where as a study from Dublin identified 29% of patients with psoriasis as having PsA, and an even higher prevalence was detected in psoriasis patients in Newfoundland, Canada [25–27]. These studies all included a rheumatology assessment of patients attending dermatology clinics.

As will be noted later in this chapter, correct and early diagnosis is crucial for appropriate therapy for patients with PsA. Therefore, it is important for dermatologists to identify patients with psoriasis who have any joint complaints and to refer them to a rheumatologist, and it is important for a rheumatologist to look for skin and nail changes in patients with inflammatory arthritis and refer the patient to a dermatologist for the correct diagnosis of the skin lesion.

In order to identify patients with PsA early on, several groups have developed screening questionnaires [28]. The psoriasis and arthritis questionnaire (PAQ) is a 12-item questionnaire, which predicted PsA with a sensitivity of 0.85 and a specificity of 0.88 for a score of 7 (out of 12) or higher. However, this questionnaire was not found to be as sensitive in a larger study in Sweden that determined a best cutoff of 4 (of 8), providing a sensitivity of 0.60 and a specificity of 0.62. Two additional screening tools are based on the PAQ. The Psoriasis Epidemiology Screening Trial (PEST) developed in Leeds, England, and the Psoriatic Arthritis Screening Questionnaire (PASQ) developed in St. John's, Newfoundland [27]. These have included a homunculus or a picture depicting the joint areas involved and also questions on back pain. Both have shown high sensitivity and specificity (97% and 75%, 97% and 79%, respectively). The Psoriatic Arthritis Screening and Evaluation (PASE) questionnaire was developed in Boston primarily as a screening tool for dermatologists to identify patients with PsA because it was recognized that to have every patient with psoriasis evaluated by a rheumatologist would be impossible. PASE consists of two subscales, a symptom subscale and a function subscale. Patients with PsA had higher scores than patients with psoriasis and OA. Patients with more severe PsA had higher scores than those with milder disease. PASE scores ranged from 28 to 63. A cutoff of 47 proved to be optimal for differentiating patients with PsA from those without. Using this cutoff, the sensitivity of PASE for PsA was 82% and the specificity was 73%. The Toronto Psoriasis and Arthritis Screen (ToPAS) was designed as a screening tool for PsA regardless of whether or not a patient was followed for psoriasis [22]. It was found to be highly sensitive and specific in all groups of patients in whom it was tested, with overall sensitivity and specificity of 89% and 86%, respectively. It differs from the other questionnaires in that it includes pictures of psoriasis and nail lesions.

Unfortunately, because these questionnaires are being tested in other centers, they have proved less sensitive and specific than in the development phase [25,26]. Further work is therefore required to identify the ideal screening tool that will have high sensitivity (which is what is required of a screening questionnaire) but that will maintain high specificity as well.

JOINT ASSESSMENT OF PATIENTS WITH PsA

Although the dermatologist is not expected to perform a joint assessment, it is important that the dermatologist asks the patient about the presence of joint symptoms, including joint pain, joint stiffness, or swelling, and identifies the presence of joint changes during the skin examination. From a rheumatologist's perspective, a detailed history looking for extra-articular features suggesting another condition is important. It is also important to note whether the patient has extra-articular features of PsA, which include iritis and mucous membrane lesions. The joint assessment should include an evaluation of the number of actively inflamed and damaged joints [29], assessment of function by the grip strength, and assessment of back involvement. Evaluation of so-called sausage digits or dactylitis and attention to the sites of tendon insertion into bones (entheses) such as the Achilles tendon or the plantar fascia is important. In addition to the clinical evaluation, a laboratory assessment is usually performed including a test for rheumatoid factor and antinuclear factor. These are usually done to rule out other rheumatological disorders such as systemic lupus erythematosus (which may present with a psoriasiform rash and arthritis) and RA (which may coexist with psoriasis). Radiographs are then requested to help make the correct diagnosis and to evaluate the extent of the arthritis. Although the pain is not much of an issue for patients with PsA, they may have joint destruction that has gone unnoticed. Moreover, the only way to determine the presence of the spondyloarthropathy is through radiological assessment [30]. The assessment of skin disease should be performed by a dermatologist. Preferably, the body surface area affected and Psoriasis Area and Severity Index (PASI) score should be determined and followed. The International Multi-Center Psoriasis and Psoriatic Arthritis Reliability Trial (GRAPPA-IMPART) documented the ability of dermatologists to detect tender joints in a reliable manner and of rheumatologists to score the PASI and nail changes reliably. Dermatologists, however, were not as good at identifying dactylitis [6]. The Group for Research and Assessment of Psoriasis and Psoriatic Arthritis (GRAPPA) has developed a training video for skin and joint assessment in patients with psoriasis and PsA (www.grappanetwork.org).

RELATIONSHIP BETWEEN SKIN AND JOINTS IN PsA

The relationship between skin and joint manifestations in PsA is not uniform. Recent epidemiological studies suggest that the extent of psoriasis is an important factor in the susceptibility to PsA [24,26,31]. However, 15% of PsA patients develop their arthritis prior to the diagnosis of psoriasis. Although it is possible that the diagnosis of psoriasis was missed because patients were not undressed or questioned about the condition [21], it certainly suggests that the psoriasis was not extensive. Recent studies support the notion that there is no direct relationship between the severity of skin and joint manifestations. In a cross-sectional study, no relationship between skin and joint severity was found [32]. In an observational study, there was no statistical association between the severity of skin and joint manifestations, although it was noted that, in patients who presented with skin and joint manifestations simultaneously, there tended to be a relation between [33].

PROGNOSIS

Several studies reported in the past 20 years document that the prognosis of PsA is more serious than previously thought. Approximately 20% of patients with PsA may develop a destructive form of arthritis that can be devastating to them and their families [10]. These patients have more than five totally damaged joints and, consequently, they have a reduced quality of life and function. Moreover, it has been demonstrated that patients with PsA are at an increased risk of death compared to the general population [34]. Although the causes of death are similar to those noted in the general population, the predictive factors for mortality include active and severe disease at presentation—factors similar to those predictive of progressive joint damage [35,36]. Although the mortality risk seems to have decreased over the decades (the number of years lost is only three), patients with PsA are still at risk compared to the general population [37,38]. Early diagnosis provides an advantage in terms of damage progression [39]. It has therefore been suggested that early diagnosis and aggressive therapy may prevent these adverse outcomes in patients with PsA. Not all patients with PsA fare poorly. Some 18% of patients sustained periods of remission lasting an average of 2.5 years [40]. Male patients, and those with a smaller number of affected joints at presentation, are more likely to achieve periods of remission.

MANAGEMENT

Despite the fact that there is no direct relationship between the skin and joint manifestations in PsA, the two components of the disease require consideration when planning patients' management. The management plan begins with educating the patient that the condition is chronic, inflammatory in nature, and that consistent therapy. Patients should also be instructed to maintain a healthy lifestyle because many patients with PsA have risk factors for coronary artery disease [41]. In this chapter, only the treatment of the joint disease will be considered. Specific therapy is tailored to individual patients [42].

Nonsteroidal Anti-Inflammatory Drugs

When the joint disease is mild, nonsteroidal anti-inflammatory drugs (NSAIDs) are used. NSAIDs have analgesia and mild anti-inflammatory activity. In many patients, NSAIDs are sufficient to control the inflammatory joint disease. There are many preparations, and none is considered superior to the others. The cycloxygenase-2 (COX-2) selective inhibitors may be less harmful to the gastrointestinal tract, but they are not superior to the traditional NSAIDs in terms of anti-inflammatory activity. It should be noted that, on occasion, NSAIDs have caused an exacerbation of the psoriasis, which is why patients need to be evaluated by both a dermatologist and a rheumatologist [43].

Slow-Acting Antirheumatic Drugs

Patients who continue to demonstrate persistent inflammatory activity or who have erosive disease detected on radiographs usually deserve treatment with slow-acting antirheumatic drugs (SAARDs). However, NSAIDs remain important therapy for patients with severe PsA. The majority of patients require NSAIDs even while taking other medications. Studies have shown that active inflammation, manifested by tender and/or swollen joints, leads to global damage progression as well as in the individual joint [44,45]. Therefore, patients with significant joint disease should be treated aggressively early on, even if their skin disease is mild.

SAARDs or disease-modifying antirheumatic drugs (DMARDs) typically take several weeks to months to reach therapeutic effect. The latter definition has been replaced with the former because none of the drugs to date have actually demonstrated the ability to modify the disease process. None of the drugs were developed specifically for PsA. The majority of these drugs were borrowed from the treatment of RA. Initially, medications such as antimalarials, gold, and penicillamine were prescribed. Because these medications are hardly used any more for patients with PsA, they will not be reviewed here although they have been reviewed in the past. Medications reviewed include sulfasalazine, methotrexate, cyclosporine A, and leflunomide [46].

Sulfasalazine

Three double-blind, controlled studies of sulfasalazine support its role in the treatment of PsA [47–49]. However, the therapeutic effect has been modest at best. One of the difficulties encountered in clinical trials of PsA is the lack of established criteria for improvement. Investigators have used the response criteria for RA, which are defined as a 20% improvement in actively inflamed joint count, effusion count, the Health Assessment Questionnaire, and a reduction in either erythrocyte sedimentation rate (HSR) or C-reactive protein (CRP). However, patients with PsA do not always have an elevated erythrocyte sedimentation rate (ESR), and if it is elevated, it is difficult to discern whether this is due to skin or joint disease. Clegg and colleagues [49] defined improvement as a 30% improvement in the absence of deterioration (a worsening of 30%) in two of the following four items: actively inflamed joint count, swollen joint count, patient global assessment, and physician global assessment. At least one of the two had to be an objective joint assessment. Using these criteria, these investigators enrolled 220 patients in a double-blind, randomized, placebo-controlled trial of sulfasalazine in PsA [49]. They demonstrated a very small difference: 54% improvement in the active treatment group compared to 45% in the placebo group. Although this was statistically significant (at the $p \leq 0.05$ level), it does not seem to be a clinically important difference. Indeed, the effect size for sulfasalazine was determined to be 0.12, much lower than the value of 0.20, which is deemed clinically important [50].

Although few individual patients may benefit from sulfasalazine, in a clinical setting, many patients were unable to tolerate sulfasalazine (with a withdrawal rate of 44%), and the drug did not provide long-term protection from disease progression [51].

Methotrexate

Methotrexate (MTX) has been considered the drug of choice for the treatment of PsA since 1964 because it works for skin and joint manifestations of the disease [52,53]. A meta-analysis of therapies used in PsA demonstrated that parenteral methotrexate and sulfasalazine were the only drugs effective for PsA but noted that the effect was modest, and a systematic review identified its low effect size [46,50]. Methotrexate has also not been found to be helpful in preventing progression of joint destruction [54]. The aforementioned studies suffered from small sample sizes and low drug doses. A recent randomized controlled trial of 221 patients comparing methotrexate 15 mg/week to placebo over six months demonstrated no disease modifying effect, with only patient and physician global assessments showing a significant drug effect [55]. Although this study has a larger sample size, it still used a dose of methotrexate that is lower than that used in clinical practice, which may be as high as 25 mg per week—often via parenteral administration. Thus, physicians continue to use methotrexate in clinical practice.

Methotrexate may be given orally, intramuscularly, or subcutaneously. Patients can self-administer parenteral methotrexate [56]. Both patients and physicians are reluctant to use methotrexate because of potential liver toxicity, hair loss, predisposition to infection, and the fact that it is unsafe for use during pregnancy. Most jurisdictions require the use of methotrexate prior to consideration of biologic therapy.

Cyclosporine A

Cyclosporine A has also been used to treat patients with PsA. There are no published placebo-controlled trials of cyclosporin A in PsA, but a randomized controlled trial comparing cyclosporin to methotrexate demonstrated both to be effective for the treatment of PsA [57]. A study comparing cyclosporin A to sulfasalazine demonstrated that the former was more effective for the treatment of peripheral arthritis [58]. Cyclosporine is less well tolerated than methotrexate, with many patients discontinuing it because of hypertension and renal toxicity [59].

Leflunomide

The efficacy of leflunomide was evaluated in one randomized clinical trial (RCT) with modest benefit over placebo. In this study of 188 PsA patients, the PsA response criteria (PsARC) response was achieved by 59% of leflunomide-treated patients compared with 29.7% of placebo-treated patients ($p < 0.0001$). American College of Rheumatology (ACR) 20 response was achieved by 36.3% and 20%, respectively ($p = 0.01$). PASI 75 response was seen in 17.4% and 7.8%, respectively ($p = 0.048$). Leflunomide was found to be an effective and well tolerated option for PsA in daily clinical practice, with beneficial effects on peripheral arthritis and on other PsA manifestations, including pain, fatigue, dactylitis, and skin disease [60]. Unfortunately, radiographs were not included in the study; therefore, the effect of leflunomide on progression of joint damage has not been studied. Leflunomide may cause high blood pressure, liver toxicity, hair loss, and peripheral neuropathy. Toxicity monitoring for leflunomide is similar to that for MTX.

Other Medications That May Control Skin and Joint Disease in PsA

If skin and joint manifestations of PsA are severe, a common approach is taken. Systemic medications are likely required, and medications that treat skin and joint disease are preferred. These include, in addition to methotrexate and cyclosporine A, retinoids [61] and psoralen and ultraviolet A (PUVA) [62]. These latter medications have demonstrated efficacy in the treatment of psoriasis, but their effect in PsA has not been impressive. Moreover, these medications are toxic, and physicians have been reluctant to use them.

NEW THERAPIES BASED ON PATHOGENESIS

Based on recent insights into the pathogenesis of PsA, this millennium has provided a new era of therapy for PsA. Although the exact causes and pathogenesis of PSA are unknown, genetic, environmental, and immunological factors are considered important contributors.

Genetic Factors

It is well recognized that a family history of psoriasis or PsA may be obtained from some 40% of patients. A family investigation performed in 1973 identified a strong familial predisposition [63], with 5.5% of the relatives of patients with PsA having PsA compared to its estimated prevalence in the U.K. population of 0.1%. Thus, the risk ($\lambda 1$) for PsA among first-degree family members using current methodology is 55 [64]. Similarly, a Canadian study, which included 100 consecutive families of probands with PsA, the $\lambda 1$ was 30 and the λs was 33 [65]. Genome scans identified a number of genetic regions associated with psoriasis [66], as well as PsA. Although the Major Histocompatibility complex (MHC) has been recognized as the strongest region associated with psoriasis and PsA, HLA-B*27 is more common among patients with PsA than those without arthritis, whereas HLA-C*06 is associated with psoriasis [31]. Other genes within the MHC have also been associated with PsA. These include the MHC class I–related chain (MIC) A [67] and tumor necrosis factor (TNF) genes [68]. However, with regard to therapy, at the present time it is unlikely that we can change the genetic makeup of a patient in an attempt to modify his or her disease.

Environmental Factors

Environmental factors thought to contribute to the susceptibility of PsA include trauma and infection [69]. These are also not modifiable by specific therapy.

Immunological Factors

Immunological abnormalities have been suspected in patients with PsA because of the inflammatory nature of the joint and skin lesions. The role of T cells has been clearly recognized. In particular, a clonal expansion of cluster of differentiation (CD)8+ cells has been identified [70]. T-cell antigen receptor β-chain variable-gene repertoires in skin and synovium are similar, suggesting that there may be a common antigen triggering the disease. T cell activation may lead to the increased levels of cytokines noted in the synovial tissues in patients with PsA [71]. In particular, the increased TNF levels have been important therapeutically [72]. Because levels of TNF are elevated, and there appears to be a specific polymorphism for the TNF promoter gene among patients with PsA, it is likely that TNF plays an important role in the pathogenesis of the disease. The IL-17/IL-23 pathway has also been recognized as important in the pathogenesis of PsA and has provided another therapeutic target.

NEW BIOLOGICAL AGENTS

Based on similar pathogenic considerations, several agents have been tried in the treatment of RA as well as in psoriasis. These include anti-TNF agents, anti-CD4 agents, cytotoxic lymphocyte associated protein 4 (CTLA4-Ig), and anti-IL-12/23. In addition, small molecules have also been tested.

Anti-TNF Agents

Etanercept In the past few years, several anti-TNF agents have been developed and have proven effective in the treatment of RA. Etanercept (Enbrel®) is a human dimeric fusion protein consisting of the extracellular portion of two TNF receptors (p75) connected to the fragment crystallizable (Fc) portion of human immunoglobulin G1 (IgG1). Two double-blind, controlled trials have now been completed in PsA [73,74]. The first included 60 patients from a single center: half were randomized to etanercept while the others received placebo. Within each group, half the patients took methotrexate while the remainder received etanercept as monotherapy. Response in joint disease was determined at three months by the American College of Rheumatology (ACR) 20 response (which is borrowed from RA studies) and the PsARC, which were modified from criteria developed for PsA by Clegg et al. [49]. Response in skin disease was determined by a reduction in the PASI score as well as target lesion assessment. There was a remarkable improvement in joint and skin manifestations, with only injection site reactions being a major untoward effect. An extension of this study in which patients originally treated with etanercept were continued on it, while those initially taking placebo were given the active drug, demonstrated a similar degree of improvement [75]. The magnitude of improvement (73% of the patients) noted in these studies is unparalleled in the literature.

The second study was a phase 3 multicenter trial including 205 patients, which was similar in design to the first trial [74]. This trial also demonstrated remarkable improvement in joint and skin manifestations of PsA. Moreover, this study demonstrated the ability of etanercept to prevent progression of radiological changes [74,75]. Etanercept (Enbrel) has now been approved for treatment of patients with PsA.

Although neither of the aforementioned studies included assessment of enthesitis and dactylitis, the Psoriasis Randomized Etanercept Study in Subjects with Psoriatic Arthritis (PRESTA) trial evaluated the effect of 50 mg twice a week in comparison to 50 mg once a week for 12 weeks followed by 50 mg weekly in groups in psoriasis and PsA [76]. Although the 50 mg twice weekly produced a more rapid and higher response in psoriasis, there was no difference between the two dosing schedules, which both worked similarly in PsA. Both dose schedules also worked to reduce enthesitis and dactylitis.

Infliximab Infliximab is a chimeric monoclonal antibody, composed of human constant and murine variable regions, that binds specifically to human TNF. It has also been used effectively for the treatment of RA and is currently approved for that indication. Two double-blind, randomized controlled trials demonstrated the efficacy of infliximab for the joint and skin manifestations of PsA. The first study included 105 patients from about eight centers and demonstrated a remarkable improvement in ACR 20 as well as PASI scores [77]. The second trial included 200 patients and was multicentered. It also demonstrated the efficacy of infliximab for the joint and skin manifestations of PsA [78]. In addition, this drug worked well in both studies for other manifestations of the disease including dactylitis and enthesitis. Infliximab has also been shown to prevent progression of radiological damage in PsA [77,78].

The humanized anti-TNF agent adalimumab has also been proven effective for PsA. In a large, multicenter, randomized controlled trial of 305 patients, the superiority of adalimumab 40 mg every other week over placebo was clearly demonstrated for joint and skin manifestations [79]. This drug also prevented progression of radiological damage [80]. Although there was no statistically significant improvement in dactylitis and enthesitis during this trial, subsequent observational studies have shown its efficacy for these features as well.

Golimumab Golimumab, a human monoclonal antibody against TNF, was recently proven effective in PsA [81]. In a study of 405 patients, golimumab at doses of 50 or 100 mg once a month demonstrated improvement in all aspects of PsA—peripheral joint disease, dactylitis, enthesitis, skin disease, and nail disease.

Certolizumab Certolizumab (CZP), a PEGylated Fab fragment of a humanized TNF inhibitor monoclonal antibody, was tested in 409 patients with PsA. Patients were randomized 1:1:1 to placebo or 400 mg CZP at week loading dose at weeks 0, 2, and 4 followed by either 200 mg CZR every two weeks or 400 mg every four weeks. ACR20 response at week 12 was significantly higher in both certolizumab doses compared to placebo and was sustained through week 24 [82]. Although this drug is still not approved for PsA, it has been approved (for a number of years) for rheumatoid arthritis.

All five anti-TNF agents were shown to improve quality of life and function documented by improvement in the 36 item short-form health survey (SF-36) physical function component as well as the Health Assessment Questionnaire (HAQ) [73–82].

Other Biologicals

Anti-Interleukin-12/23 Ustekinumab Two phase 3 randomized controlled trials of ustekinumab, an anti-IL-12/23 monoclonal antibody, were recently completed [83,84]. The first trial (PSUMMIT 1) included 615 patients with active disease (≥5 swollen and ≥5 tender joints and CRP ≥ 0.3mg/dL despite DMARD and/or NSAID therapy). Patients were randomized to ustekinumab 45 mg, 90 mg, or placebo at weeks 0, 4, and every 12 weeks thereafter. At week 16, patients with less than 5% improvement in tender and swollen joint counts entered blinded early escape. Those who had taken the placebo were started on 45 mg ustekinumab and those on ustekinumab were given 90 mg using the same scheduling as noted here. Stable concomitant MTX use was permitted but not mandated, but prior anti-TNF therapy was an exclusion [83]. Significant improvement in signs and symptoms of PsA was noted with both doses of ustekinumab at 24 weeks, as well as in dactylitis, enthesitis, and skin disease. The improvement was sustained through week 52 with a magnitude similar to anti-TNF agents. Similar responses were noted for patients treated with methotrexate as those without. There were no safety signals.

In the second trial (PSUMMIT 2) [84], 312 patients with inadequate response (five tender and five swollen joints and CRP >0.3) to DMARDs and/or anti-TNF agents were randomized to receive either placebo or one of two doses (45 mg or 90 mg) of ustekinumab at 0, 4, and then every 12 weeks. Similar rules for early escape were followed as in the first trial. As in PSUMMIT 1, significant improvements in signs and symptoms of PsA were noted with both doses of ustekinumab compared to placebo at 12 and 24 weeks. Improvement in dactylitis, enthesitis, and HAQ scores was also significant in favor of the drug. No safety issues were noted.

T-Cell Inhibition

Abatacept Abatacept is a soluble, fully human fusion protein consisting of the extracellular domain of CTLA-4 linked to a modified Fc portion of human IgG1. Abatacept selectively inhibits T-cell activation via competitive binding to CD80 or CD86 and decreases serum levels of cytokines and inflammatory proteins implicated in the pathogenesis of PsA [85]. A phase 2 trial in PsA was conducted on 170 patients with PsA who had a target psoriasis lesion of at least 2 cm and who had failed either DMARDs or anti-TNF agents (three tender and three swollen joints). Abatacept was tested in two doses (3 mg/kg and 10 mg/kg intravenously every two weeks for the first month and then monthly) against placebo. At doses of 10 mg/kg, there was significantly higher improvement in signs and symptoms of PsA compared to placebo. Similarly the quality of life and function was improved, and there was an improvement in magnetic resonance imaging (MRI) of affected joints. Thus, abatacept provides an additional potential therapy for patients with PsA. A phase 3 trial is planned.

Two other T-cell inhibitors, namely alefacept and efalizumab, have been studied in PsA but have been taken off the market and will therefore not be reviewed.

Anti-B Cell Therapy Rituximab, a CD20 antibody, was tested in a pilot study in PsA but did not prove particularly effective [86].

Enzyme Inhibitors Apremilast, an oral phosphodiesterase 4 inhibitor, was recently tested in PsA. A phase 2 trial of 204 patients randomized to receive either 20 mg twice daily or 40 mg once daily for 12 weeks demonstrated better improvement among patients treated with twice daily dosing. Diarrhea was the main side effect [86]. A phase 3 trial with apremilast was recently completed [87]. It included 504 patients randomized to receive either apremilast 20 mg bid or 30 mg bid or placebo. It was a 24-week trial but at 16 weeks placebo patients who did not achieve at least a 20% reduction in inflamed joint count were rerandomized to either dose of the active drug. This study also demonstrated efficacy of both apremilast doses compared to placebo. It was noted that patients who were biologic naïve or who received apremilast monotherapy had higher responses than those on previous therapy. Higher responses also occurred among patients treated with the higher dose, but that dose was slightly more toxic, although no major safety issues were raised.

Although these new medications are efficacious for patients with PsA, it is disappointing that none of the medications work for all patients, suggesting that the pathogenesis is indeed multifactorial, and that perhaps combination therapy may be required for some patients.

Who Should Be Treated with New Therapies?

Although the new medications provide added hope for patients with PsA, they are very expensive. Anti-TNF agents have been shown to reduce progression of joint damage, but not all new medications have been studied for disease modifying effect. Although, at present, the anti-TNF agents appear safe, with the major side effects being injection site reactions and allergic reactions as well as infections, their long-term adverse event profile is unknown. However, if these drugs are proven to modify the course of PsA by preventing joint damage, providing better control of the psoriasis, achieving better quality of life for the patients, and preventing the development of comorbidities, then it would be important to include them early in the management plan. It would be advantageous if we had markers for disease expression that would allow us to identify those patients who require these drugs, so that we can avoid putting patients with mild disease at risk. Initial studies suggest that patients with HLA-B*27 in the presence of HLA-DRB1*07, patients with HLA-B*39, and patients with HLA-DQB1*03 in the absence of HLA-DRB1*07 are predictive of progression in clinical damage, while HLA-B*22 is protective [52]. Studies are currently underway to address this issue further.

Management of PsA Requires a Team Effort

The best way for patients with PsA to be managed is through a team effort, including the rheumatologist and the dermatologist. Such collaborative effort exists in our Psoriatic Arthritis Program at the University of Toronto. All our patients are reviewed by their dermatologists at regular intervals, and communication with them allows us to use appropriate therapies. A combined clinic has now been established as well.

SUMMARY

Over the past two decades, PsA has been recognized as a more severe form of arthritis than initially described. The course and prognosis of the disease suggest that early diagnosis and more aggressive treatment are important. Although several clinical and HLA markers for disease progression have been identified, further work in this area is required. Therefore, it is important for dermatologists to recognize the features of the arthritis, and it is important for rheumatologists to look for evidence of psoriasis in patients with arthritis. The management of patients with PsA is best performed with a team effort so that both aspects of the disease are dealt with. There are new and exciting treatments that should be available to these patients.

REFERENCES

1. Wright V, Moll JMH, eds. *Seronegative Polyarthritis*. Amsterdam, Netherlands: North Holland Publishing Company; 1976, pp. 169–223.
2. O'Neill T, Silman A. Psoriatic arthritis. Historical background and epidemiology. *Baillieres Clin Rheumatol* 1994; 8: 245–261.
3. Cats A. Psoriasis and arthritis. *Cutis* 1990; 46: 323–329.
4. Gladman DD. Psoriatic arthritis. *Baillières Clin Rheumatol* 1995; 9: 319–329.
5. Taylor WJ, Gladman DD, Helliwell PS, et al. Classification criteria for psoriatic arthritis: development of new criteria from a large international study. *Arthritis Rheum* 2006; 54: 2665–2673.
6. Chandran V, Gottlieb AB, Cook RJ, et al. International multi-centre psoriasis and psoriatic arthritis reliability trial (GRAPPA-IMPART): assessment of skin, joints, nails and dactylitis. *Arthritis Rheum* 2009; 61: 1235–1242.
7. Chandran V, Schentag CT, Gladman DD. Sensitivity of the classification of psoriatic arthritis (CASPAR) criteria in early psoriatic arthritis. *Arthritis Rheum* 2007; 57: 1560–1563.
8. Chandran V, Schentag CT, Gladman DD. Sensitivity and specificity of the CASPAR criteria for psoriatic arthritis when applied to patients attending a family medicine clinic. *J Rheumatol* 2008; 35: 2069–2070. (Letter).

9. Eder L, Gladman DD. Psoriatic arthritis: phenotypic variance and nosology. *Curr Rheumatol Rep* 2013; 15: 316.
10. Gladman DD. The natural history of psoriatic arthritis. *Baillières Clin Rheumatol* 1994; 8: 379–394.
11. Helliwell PS, Hetthen J, Sokoll K, et al. Joint symmetry in early and late rheumatoid and psoriatic arthritis: comparison with a mathematical model. *Arthritis Rheum* 2000; 43: 865–871.
12. Brockbank J, Stein M, Schentag CT, et al. Dactylitis in psoriatic arthritis (PsA): a marker for disease severity? *Ann Rheum Dis* 2005; 62: 188–190.
13. Ritchlin CT, Kavanaugh A, Gladman DD, et al. Treatment recommendations for psoriatic arthritis. *Ann Rheum Dis* 2009; 68: 1387–1394.
14. Buskila D, Langevitz P, Gladman DD, et al. Patients with rheumatoid arthritis are more tender than those with psoriatic arthritis. *J Rheumatol* 1992; 19: 1115–1119.
15. Gladman DD, Anhorn KB, Schachter RK, et al. HLA antigens in psoriatic arthritis. *J Rheumatol* 1986; 13: 586–592.
16. Wilson FC, Icen M, Crowson CS, et al. Incidence and clinical predictors of psoriatic arthritis in patients with psoriasis: a population-based study. *Arthritis Rheum* 2009; 61: 233–239.
17. Griffiths CE, Barker JN. Pathogenesis and clinical features of psoriasis. *Lancet* 2007; 370: 263–271.
18. Rahman P, Gladman DD, Cook RJ, et al. Radiological assessment in psoriatic arthritis. *Br J Rheumatol* 1998; 37: 760–765.
19. Gladman DD. Clinical aspects of spondyloarthropathies. *Am J Med Sci* 1998; 316: 234–238.
20. Stern RS, Nijsten T, Feldman SR, et al. Psoriasis is common, carries a substantial burden even when not extensive, and is associated with widespread treatment dissatisfaction. *J Investig Dermatol Symp Proc* 2004; 9: 136–139.
21. Gorter S, van der Heijde DM, van Der LS, et al. Psoriatic arthritis: performance of rheumatologists in daily practice. *Ann Rheum Dis* 2002; 61: 219–224.
22. Gladman DD, Schentag CT, Tom BD, et al. Development and initial validation of a screening questionnaire for psoriatic arthritis: the Toronto Psoriatic Arthritis Screen (ToPAS). *Ann Rheum Dis* 2009; 68: 497–501.
23. Reich K, Kruger K, Mossner R, et al. Epidemiology and clinical pattern of psoriatic arthritis in Germany: a prospective interdisciplinary epidemiological study of 1511 patients with plaque-type psoriasis. *Br J Dermatol* 2009; 160: 1040–1047.
24. Christophers E, Barker JN, Griffiths CE, et al. The risk of psoriatic arthritis remains constant following initial diagnosis of psoriasis among patients seen in European dermatology clinics. *J Eur Acad Dermatol Venereol* 2010; 24: 548–554.
25. Coates LC, Aslam T, Al BF, et al. Comparison of three screening tools to detect psoriatic arthritis in patients with psoriasis (CONTEST study). *Br J Dermatol* 2013; 168: 802–807.
26. Haroon M, Kirby B, Fitzgerald O. High prevalence of psoriatic arthritis in patients with severe psoriasis with suboptimal performance of screening questionnaires. *Ann Rheum Dis* 2013; 72: 736–740.
27. Khraishi M, Chouela E, Bejar M, et al. High prevalence of psoriatic arthritis in a cohort of patients with psoriasis seen in a dermatology practice. *J Cutan Med Surg* 2012; 16: 122–127.
28. Dominguez P, Gladman DD, Helliwell P, et al. Development of screening tools to identify psoriatic arthritis. *Curr Rheumatol Rep* 2010; 12: 295–299.
29. Gladman DD, Farewell VT, Buskila D, et al. Reliability of measurements of active and damaged joints in psoriatic arthritis. *J Rheumatol* 1990; 17: 62–64.
30. Khan M, Gladman D, Schentag C. Clinical and radiological changes during psoriatic arthritis disease progression: working toward classification criteria. *J Rheumatol* 2002; 29: 1569.
31. Eder L, Chandran V, Pellet F, et al. Human leukocyte antigen risk alleles for psoriatic arthritis among psoriasis patients. *Ann Rheum Dis* 2012; 71: 50–55.
32. Cohen MR, Reda DJ, Clegg DO. Baseline relationships between psoriasis and psoriatic arthritis: analysis of 221 patients with active psoriatic arthritis. Department of Veterans Affairs Cooperative Study Group on Seronegative Spondyloarthropathies. *J Rheumatol* 1999; 26: 1752–1756.
33. Elkayam O, Ophir J, Yaron M, et al. Psoriatic arthritis: interrelationships between skin and joint manifestations related to onset, course and distribution. *Clin Rheumatol* 2000; 19: 301–305.
34. Wong K, Gladman DD, Husted J, et al. Mortality studies in psoriatic arthritis. Results from a single centre. I. Risk and causes of death. *Arthritis Rheum* 1997; 40: 1868–1872.

35. Gladman DD, Farewell VT, Husted J, et al. Mortality studies in psoriatic arthritis. Results from a single centre. II. Prognostic indicators for mortality. *Arthritis Rheum* 1998; 41: 1103–1110.
36. Gladman DD, Farewell VT. Progression in psoriatic arthritis: role of time varying clinical indicators. *J Rheumatol* 1999; 26: 2409–2413.
37. Gladman DD. Mortality in psoriatic arthritis. *Clin Exp Rheumatol* 2008; 26(Suppl 5): s62–s65.
38. Ali Y, Tom BDM, Schentag CT, et al. Improved survival in psoriatic arthritis (PsA) with calendar time. *Arthritis Rheum* 2007; 56: 2708–2714.
39. Gladman DD, Thavaneswaran A, Chandran V, et al. Do patients with psoriatic arthritis who present early fare better than those presenting later in the disease? *Ann Rheum Dis* 2011; 70: 2152–2154.
40. Gladman DD, Ng Tung Hing E, Schentag CT, et al. Remission in psoriatic arthritis. *J Rheumatol* 2001; 28: 1045–1048.
41. Eder L, Jayakar J, Pollock R, et al. Serum adipokines in patients with psoriatic arthritis and psoriasis alone and their correlation with disease activity. *Ann Rheum Dis* 2013;72:1956–1961.
42. Tillett W, McHugh N. Treatment algorithms for early psoriatic arthritis: do they depend on disease phenotype? *Curr Rheumatol Rep* 2012; 14: 334–342.
43. Griffiths CE. Therapy for psoriatic arthritis: sometimes a conflict for psoriasis. *Br J Rheumatol* 1997; 36: 409–410.
44. Bond SJ, Farewell VT, Schentag CT, et al. Predictors for radiological damage in psoriatic arthritis. Results from a Single centre. *Ann Rheum Dis* 2007; 66: 370–376.
45. Cresswell L, Chandran V, Farewell VT, et al. Inflammation in an individual joint predicts damage to that joint in psoriatic arthritis. *Ann Rheum Dis* 2011; 70: 305–308.
46. Jones G, Crotty M, Brooks P. Interventions for psoriatic arthritis. *Cochrane Database Syst Rev* 2000: CD000212.
47. Gupta AK, Grober JS, Hamilton TA, et al. Sulfasalazine therapy for psoriatic arthritis: a double blind, placebo controlled trial. *J Rheumatol* 1995; 22: 894–898.
48. Dougados M, vam der Linden S, Leirisalo-Repo M, et al. Sulfasalazine in the treatment of spondylorthropathy. A randomized, multicenter, double-blind, placebo-controlled study. *Arthritis Rheum* 1995; 38: 618–627.
49. Clegg DO, Reda DJ, Mejias E, et al. Comparison of sulfasalazine and placebo in the treatment of psoriatic arthritis. A Department of Veterans Affairs Cooperative Study. *Arthritis Rheum* 1996; 39: 2013–2020.
50. Soriano ER, McHugh NJ. Therapies for peripheral joint disease in psoriatic arthritis. A systematic review. *J Rheumatol* 2006; 33: 1422–1430.
51. Rahman P, Gladman DD, Zhou Y, et al. The use of sulfasalazine in psoriatic arthritis: a clinic experience. *J Rheumatol* 1998; 25: 1957–1961.
52. Black RL, O'Brien WM, Van Scott EJ, et al. Methotrexate therapy in psoriatic arthritis. Double blind study on 21 patients. *JAMA* 1964; 189: 743–747.
53. Chang DJ. A survey of drug effectiveness and treatment choices in psoriatic arthritis. *Arthritis Rheum* 1999; 42(Suppl 9): S372.
54. Abu-Shakra M, Gladman DD, Thorne JC, et al. Longterm methotrexate therapy in psoriatic arthritis: clinical and radiologic outcome. *J Rheumatol* 1995; 22: 241–245.
55. Kingsley GH, Kowalczyk A, Taylor H, et al. A randomized placebo-controlled trial of methotrexate in psoriatic arthritis. *Rheumatology (Oxford)* 2012; 51: 1368–1377.
56. Arthur AB, Klinkhoff AV, Teufel A. Safety of self-injection of gold and methotrexate. *J Rheumatol* 1999; 26: 302–305.
57. Spadaro A, Riccieri V, Sili-Scavalli A, et al. Comparison of cyclosporin A and methotrexate in the treatment of psoriatic arthritis: a one-year prospective study. *Clin Exp Rheumatol* 1995; 13: 589–593.
58. Salvarani C, Macchioni P, Olivieri I, et al. A comparison of cyclosporine, sulfasalazine and symptomatic therapy in the treatment of psoriatic arthritis. *J Rheumatol* 2001; 28: 2274–2283.
59. Spadaro A, Taccari E, Mohtadi B, et al. Life-table analysis of cyclosporin A treatment in psoriatic arthritis: comparison with other disease-modifying antirheumatic drugs. *Clin Exp Rheumatol* 1997; 15: 609–614.
60. Behrens F, Finkenwirth C, Pavelka K, et al. Leflunomide in psoriatic arthritis: results from a large European prospective observational study. *Arthritis Care Res (Hoboken)* 2013; 65: 464–470.
61. Klinkhoff AV, Gertner E, Chalmers A, et al. Pilot study of etretinate in psoriatic arthritis. *J Rheumatol* 1989; 16: 789–791.

62. Perlman SG, Gerber LH, Roberts M, et al. Photochemotherapy and psoriatic arthritis. A prospective study. *Ann Intern Med* 1979; 91: 717–722.
63. Moll JM, Wright V. Familial occurrence of PsA. *Ann Rheum Dis* 1973; 32: 181–201.
64. Risch N. Linkage strategies for genetically complex traits. 1. Multilocus model. *Am J Hum Genet* 1990; 46: 222–228.
65. Chandran V, Schentag CT, Brockbank J, et al. Familial aggregation of psoriatic arthritis. *Ann Rheum Dis* 2009; 68: 664–667.
66. Chandran V. The genetics of psoriasis and psoriatic arthritis. *Clin Rev Allergy Immunol* 2013; 44: 149–156.
67. Pollock R, Chandran V, Barrett J, et al. Differential MICA allele associations with skin and joint manifestations of psoriatic disease. *Tissue Antigens* 2011; 77: 554–561.
68. Rahman P, Siannis F, Butt C, et al. TNF-α polymorphisms and risk of psoriatic arthritis in Caucasian populations. *Ann Rheum Dis* 2006; 65: 919–923.
69. Eder L, Law T, Chandran V, et al. The association between environmental factors and onset of psoriatic arthritis in patients with psoriasis. *Arthritis Care Res* 2011; 63: 1091–1097.
70. Haroon M, Fitzgerald O. Pathogenetic overview of psoriatic disease. *J Rheumatol Suppl* 2012; 89: 7–10.
71. Ritchlin CT. Psoriatic disease—from skin to bone. *Nat Rev Rheumatol* 2007; 3: 698–706.
72. Nograles KE, Brasington RD, Bowcock AM. New insights into the pathogenesis and genetics of psoriatic arthritis. *Nat Clin Pract Rheumatol* 2009; 5: 83–91.
73. Mease PJ, Goffe BS, Metz J, et al. Etanercept in the treatment of psoriatic arthritis and psoriasis: a randomised trial. *Lancet* 2000; 356: 385–390.
74. Mease PJ, Kivitz AJ, Burch FX, et al. Etanercept treatment of psoriatic arthritis: safety, efficacy, and effect on disease progression. *Arthritis Rheum* 2004; 50: 2264–2272.
75. Mease PJ, Kivitz AJ, Burch FX, et al. Continued inhibition of radiographic progression in patients with psoriatic arthritis following 2 years of treatment with etanercept. *J Rheumatol* 2006; 33: 712–721.
76. Sterry W, Ortonne JP, Kirkham B, et al. Comparison of two etanercept regimens for treatment of psoriasis and psoriatic arthritis: PRESTA randomised double blind multicentre trial. *BMJ* 2010; 340: c147.
77. Antoni CE, Kavanaugh A, Kirkham B, et al. Sustained benefits of infliximab therapy for dermatologic and articular manifestations of psoriatic arthritis: results from the infliximab multinational psoriatic arthritis controlled trial (IMPACT). *Arthritis Rheum* 2005; 52: 1227–1236.
78. Antoni C, Krueger GG, de Vlam K, et al. Infliximab improves signs and symptoms of psoriatic arthritis: results of the IMPACT 2 trial. *Ann Rheum Dis* 2005; 64: 1150–1157.
79. Mease PJ, Gladman DD, Ritchlin CT, et al. Adalimumab in the treatment of patients with moderately to severely active psoriatic arthritis: results of the ADEPT trial. *Arthritis Rheum* 2005; 52: 3279–3289.
80. Gladman DD, Mease PJ, Ritchlin CT, et al. Adalimumab for long-term treatment of psoriatic arthritis: 48-week data and subanalysis from ADEPT. *Arthritis Rheum* 2007; 56: 476–488.
81. Kavanaugh A, McInnes I, Mease P, et al. Golimumab, a new, human, TNF-alpha antibody administered as a monthly subcutaneous injection in psoriatic arthritis: 24-week efficacy and safety results of the randomized, placebo-controlled GO-REVEAL study. *Arthritis Rheum* 2009; 60: 976–986.
82. Mease PJ, Fleischmann R, Deodhar A, et al. Effect of certolizumab pegol on signs and symptoms in patients with psoriatic arthritis: 24 week results of a phase 3 double blind randomized placebo-controlled study (RAPID-PsA). *Ann Rheum Dis* 2012; 71(Suppl3): 150.
83. Kavanaugh A, McInnes IB, Gottlieb AB, et al. Ustekinumab improves arthritis-related and skin-related quality of life in patients with active psoriatic arthritis: patient reported outcomes from randomized and double blinded phase III summit I trial. *Arthritis Rheum* 2012; 64(Suppl 10): S248.
84. Ritchlin CR, Gottlieb AB, McInnes IB, et al. Ustekinumab in active psoriatic arthritis including patients previously treated with anti-TNF agents: results of a phase 3, multicenter, double-blind, placebo-controlled study. *Arthritis Rheum* 2012; 64(Suppl 10): S1080.
85. Mease P, Genovese MC, Gladstein G, et al. Abatacept in the treatment of patients with psoriatic arthritis: results of a double-blind, randomized, placebo-controlled phase II trial. *Arthritis Rheum* 2011; 63: 939–948.

86. Schett G, Wollenhaupt J, Papp K, et al. Oral apremilast in the treatment of active psoriatic arthritis: results of a multicenter, randomized, double-blind, placebo-controlled study. *Arthritis Rheum* 2012; 64: 3156–3167.
87. Kavanaugh A, Mease PJ, Gomez-Reino JJ, et al. Apremilast, an oral phosphodiesterase 4 inhibitor, in patients with psoriatic arthritis: results of a phase 3, randomized, controlled trial. *Arthritis Rheum* 2012; 64: 4172.

Chapter 20

Special Patient Populations

Daniel C. Butler, Faranak Kamangar, Ethan C. Levin, John Y. M. Koo, and Anne L. S. Chang

INTRODUCTION

The diversity of psoriasis is rooted in its association with a variety of complex medical issues and comorbid conditions. The management of psoriasis patients can be challenging. However, adequate knowledge of the unique needs and considerations of each patient population can help clinicians tailor an effective treatment regimen while maintaining the safety of their patients.

THE GERIATRIC POPULATION

The geriatric population of the United States is rapidly growing, and estimates indicate that it will comprise one-fourth of the total population by the year 2025 [1]. Such an increase will undoubtedly contribute to a greater prevalence of geriatric patients with psoriasis. One U.S. study showed that the 60- to 69-year-old age group is most vulnerable to psoriasis [2]. Thus, current and future treating clinicians should be fully knowledgeable and comfortable in dealing with the geriatric population. Physiologic changes, concurrent comorbidities, and polypharmacy can all complicate a clinician's treatment approach and can lead to inadequate management or undertreatment [3]. However, there are safe and effective options for elderly psoriasis patients.

Topical Steroids

Topical corticosteroids are the first-line and likely the safest option for treating psoriasis patients. However, the use of topical steroids in geriatric patients poses additional concerns. The risks of increased skin fragility, atrophy, purpura, steroid rebound, skin infections, and telangiectasias are apparent in all ages, but these risks are pronounced in older patients because of the physiologic changes of aging skin [4–6]. Therefore, although the use of topical steroids is recommended as the first-line treatment for elderly individuals by the National Psoriasis Foundation, topical steroids should be prescribed with caution, and clinicians should consider following-up with their patients at least once every three months [7].

Problems with compliance can further complicate the prescription of topical steroids in the geriatric population. With the time and difficulty of application involved because of physical limitations, patients may struggle with regular use. Prior to prescribing, clinicians should therefore ensure that patients are capable of applying topical agents or that they receive necessary assistance. One proven option is combined calcipotriol and betamethasone dipropionate, which is applied once a day and has been proven safe and effective, especially in elderly patients [8].

Phototherapy

Phototherapy is safe and is recommended for geriatric patients. Important considerations include the patient's ability to travel to a phototherapy center three times/week as well as physical limitations that may make standing in a phototherapy booth difficult [7]. These issues should be directly addressed prior to initiating treatment.

Prior to an initial phototherapy session, as well as in subsequent visits, clinicians should conduct a thorough review of the patient's medication list to evaluate for any potentially photosensitizing agent [7,9]. Phototherapy staff should be reminded to review this list before treatment, paying special attention to any new medications.

Traditional Systemics

Response to internal medication can be quite variable in geriatric patients because age-dependent changes in normal physiology alter responses, reactions, and metabolism; organs gradually lose functional capacity, homeostatic mechanisms become slow, fat content increases, and water volume decreases [10]. For traditional systemics, the general rule is to start at a low dose and then titrate slowly on the basis of the therapeutic response. Frequent follow-up is recommended to assess adverse effects and degrees of response.

Methotrexate

Methotrexate can be used safely in elderly patients, but the predominant concern is its use with concurrent age-related impaired renal function. Creatinine clearance decreases with age and thus may lead to increased serum concentrations of the medication if dosing is not adjusted by kidney function [11]. For this reason, methotrexate should be initiated at a lower dose than that used for younger psoriasis patients [12]. In addition, elderly patients on methotrexate should be reminded to stay well hydrated. Because these patients have an increased risk of dehydration, methotrexate blood levels may increase to toxic levels.

An additional concern with using methotrexate is the potential for life-threatening myelosuppression. Elderly individuals are often myelosuppressed at baseline, putting them at great risk for these rare but serious adverse events [13]. Typically, a 5 mg "test" dose of methotrexate is given before regular dosing is started. Laboratory evaluations, including liver function testing and blood counts, are performed before and after the test dose.

Methotrexate can interact with a variety of medications. The most dangerous of these interactions is that with the antibiotic trimethoprim, which can result in a fatal reaction [14]. A thorough evaluation of potential interactions with concurrent medications is required for any patient who is starting on a treatment regimen.

Acitretin

Acitretin is the only internal medication that does not have immunosuppressive qualities and is thus ideal for the geriatric population. In addition, oral retinoids may discourage neoplasm by enhancing cell maturation and differentiation [15]. The tendency of retinoids to elevate triglycerides and cholesterol can be dangerous for patients at risk for coronary disease.

The development of hypertriglyceridemia secondary to acitretin use often takes years to develop, so the short-term use of acitretin is likely safe in the geriatric population. Although not life threatening, the skin drying effects of acitretin can be particularly alarming in elderly patients who already have a tendency to develop xerosis [7].

The experience of one of this chapter's authors (John Koo) has been that low-dose acitretin (10–25 mg/day) is more effective in geriatric psoriasis patients as compared to younger patients. However, it still takes months to realize this more complete clearing on low-dose acitretin in the elderly.

Cyclosporine

As with the younger population, the main concern of using cyclosporine in the elderly population is hypertension and nephrotoxicity [16]. Given that elderly patients have less renal and cardiac reserve, these side effects may be less tolerated. Thus, cyclosporine use in geriatric patients should be reserved mainly for the most severe, recalcitrant cases [7]. Trough levels are recommended in the geriatric subgroup if the medication is used in the long term at greater than 3 mg/kg daily; the medication is contraindicated in any patient with an abnormal baseline glomerular filtration rate [17].

Biologics

Because biologic medications are immune-modulating proteins, they are less likely to have the end-organ and drug–drug interactions of traditional systemic medications. These medications are dosed less frequently than the oral systemic therapies, which can help compliance. However, as individuals age, so does their immune system, and there is concern that therapeutic immunosuppression in younger patients can become pathologic in the elderly. Due to this immunosenescence, there is increased concern for infection and malignancy that can develop under a compromised protective system. Studies on this topic are lacking. Nonetheless, the U.S. Food and Drug Administration (FDA) package inserts for infliximab, ustekinumab, and etanercept do not report any safety issues specific to the geriatric population [18–20]. However, some practitioners avoid using ustekinumab in patients with heart disease due to a controversial and unproven concern for increased cardiovascular risk [21]. Only the FDA package insert for adalimumab warns against a high incidence of serious infections and malignancies in elderly patients [22].

Specific studies on alefacept, adalimumab, and etanercept detail their safe and effective use in elderly patients [23–25]. One study that examined etanercept in a cohort of more than 4000 patients with rheumatoid arthritis, psoriatic arthritis, and ankylosing spondylitis failed to find a higher incidence of serious adverse events (eg., infectious events or malignancies) in people over 65 years old compared with those under 65 years of age [26]. Conversely, a different cohort of more than 3000 patients from the British Biologics registry found an increased risk of serious infection for geriatric patients who are taking biologics [27]. Although a definitive answer on the absolute safety of biologics remains uncertain, biologics can be recommended to elderly patients as long as appropriate caution is taken regarding screening and follow-up.

PREGNANCY AND LACTATION

Women with psoriasis or who will develop psoriasis are particularly vulnerable during pregnancy [28]. Research has shown an association between preexisting moderate to severe psoriasis and the development of adverse outcomes, including spontaneous abortions, low-birth-weight infants, and premature rupture of membranes [29,30]. This fact necessitates adequate management with effective therapeutics, which ensures the safety of mother and child.

The literature shows that close to 50% of pregnant psoriasis patients show improvement during pregnancy, but 10%–20% become worse throughout pregnancy [31–33]. Moreover, pustular psoriasis, a severely painful and dangerous form of the disease, has a unique predilection for pregnant females and is often considered under a special category of "dermatoses of pregnancy." Postpartum is another important concern because studies show that 50% of women have flare-ups during this critical period, most often associated with breastfeeding [31].

Topical Agents

The use of high-potency topical corticosteroids during pregnancy has been associated with low birth weight, so low to moderate potency medications are preferable in nonacute settings [34,35]. The observed fetal growth restriction typically corresponds with the use of more than 300 g of topical corticosteroids [34,36]. As a general rule, topical agents are considered safe because the likelihood of fetal exposure is minimal. However, tazarotene is a retinoid agent that is absolutely contraindicated during pregnancy [37].

Topical agents are considered safe during lactation but should be used only on local areas of involvement. If the nipple area needs to be treated, it should be wiped clean before feeding the infant. High-potency topical steroids should be avoided on the nipple.

Phototherapy

Narrowband ultraviolet B (UVB) and broadband UVB are safe to use during pregnancy. The major concern with the treatment is the potential for folate depletion, which can theoretically lead to neural tube defects. Although pathologic folate depletion from phototherapy is exceedingly rare, mothers should be started or continued on folate supplementation during the first trimester [38–40].

Oxsoralen and psoralen ultraviolet A (PUVA) are controversial, and their oral form is contraindicated during pregnancy because of the risk of malformation and infant death [41,42]. Topical forms are likely safer than oral forms, but because oxsoralen is a known mutagen and teratogen, it is not recommended [43]. However, systemic absorption from "bath" PUVA is negligible [44].

Traditional Systemics

Methotrexate and acitretin are labeled category X by the FDA and should never be used in pregnant patients. Moreover, these medications should be avoided in women of childbearing age to prevent any potential inadvertent exposure [43,45].

Literature on cyclosporine use during pregnancy comes from transplant patients who take higher doses than are typically required for psoriasis. In these patients, cyclosporine appears to be relatively safe based on decades of data gathered from a cyclosporine pregnancy registry [46,47]. Low birth weight and premature birth have been reported in the literature, and cyclosporine can exacerbate maternal hypertension, but it does not appear to be associated with any type of fetal malformation [46,48]. A follow-up study of children throughout childhood who were exposed to cyclosporine in utero did not show any long-term effects [49,50]. Although the literature is reassuring, cyclosporine should be used only for severe cases that are unresponsive to UVB phototherapy.

Methotrexate and acitretin also should be avoided while breastfeeding. Cyclosporine use is safe during lactation. It is transferred in small amounts through breast milk; however, the exposure is miniscule and unlikely to adversely affect the developing child [51].

Biologics

Biologic medications are pregnancy category B. All currently approved biologic medications for psoriasis are monoclonal antibodies that contain an Fc receptor and thus can theoretically cross into the placenta. Studies suggesting the safe use of tumor necrosis factor-α inhibitors (TNF-α inhibitors) during pregnancy continue to increase [43,52]. However, controversy remains because one group noted a possible increase in vertebrae, anus, trachea, esophagus, and renal (VATER) syndrome abnormalities, which consist of vertebral anomalies, anal atresia, cardiac anomalies, tracheoesophageal fistula, esophageal atresia, renal abnormalities, and limb anomalies [53,54].

There have been rare case reports of spontaneous abortion associated with the use of etanercept, adalimumab, and ustekinumab [55–57]. In addition, live vaccines should be avoided during the first six months of an infant's life because the medication can remain active in the child's serum for months after exposure. Premature vaccination in an infant exposed to biologics has resulted in death because of disseminated tuberculosis secondary to Bacille Calmette–Guerin (BCG) vaccination [58].

Investigation shows minimal to no transfer of biologics into breast milk. Case reports indicate that etanercept and infliximab have been used safely during lactation [43,59]. Moreover, infants' digestive enzymes are hypothesized to likely break down the protein medication and thus significantly limit the bioavailability of the medication.

HISTORY OF HEPATITIS B, C, AND HUMAN IMMUNODEFICIENCY VIRUS INFECTION

Psoriasis is seen concurrently with chronic infectious states, and interestingly, it can be worsened by the disease itself or by its therapeutic medications [60,61]. In these cases, the long-term safety of patients is paramount when making treatment decisions regarding psoriasis. Hepatologists and infectious disease specialists should be consulted for hepatitis and human immunodeficiency virus (HIV), respectively, to ensure that the infections are appropriately evaluated, and that antiviral therapy is considered.

Topical agents remain the first line of treatment. Although safe and effective, they may prove inadequate for those suffering from moderate to severe disease. Other options must be considered when topical agents alone are insufficient to control the psoriasis.

HEPATITIS B

The phases of hepatitis B infection reflect the replication activity of the virus and the immune response of the body. Serologic findings help dermatologists and hepatologists determine the status of the infection to assist in making an educated decision on psoriasis treatment [62].

Phototherapy

Ultraviolet B is the safest way to avoid internal immunosuppression and risk of reactivation. The risk of hepatic injury is minimal to nonexistent, and ultraviolet B can be supplemented with an aggressive topical regimen as well.

PUVA therapy has been reported to result in liver injury, but pre- and post-PUVA liver biopsies failed to show histologic differences in patients without hepatitis [63,64]. Topical PUVA does minimize systemic effects and thus should be preferentially used.

Traditional Systemics

Methotrexate has been associated with reactivation and subsequent hepatic failure in patients with a history of hepatitis B [65,66]. In addition to its reactivation potential, it is hepatotoxic and should be avoided in patients with hepatitis B [67].

Acitretin lacks immunosuppressive effects and thus is unlikely to cause reactivation. It does, however, possess hepatotoxic effects, although such an occurrence is rare with low dose usage [68]. Liver enzymes may become elevated, but cumulative toxicity is not a concern [69].

The potent immunosuppressive effects of cyclosporine put patients at risk of hepatitis reactivation [70]. Literature in the specific population is lacking, but experts recommend avoiding cyclosporine for hepatitis B patients [71].

Biologics

The decision to initiate TNF therapy for hepatitis B patients is controversial and should be made in conjunction with a hepatologist [72,73]. If the patient is surface antigen positive with chronic inactive hepatitis, the recommendation is to begin antiviral prophylaxis two to four weeks before TNF therapy. For those patients with a low risk of reactivation, such as those who are hepatitis B core-antibody positive but who lack hepatitis B surface antibodies, prophylaxis with antiviral therapy may not be necessary [73]. In either case, liver enzymes and viral load should be monitored closely with recommendations of monthly or bimonthly checks for the first six months [62,73,74].

HEPATITIS C

Similar to hepatitis B, the primary concern with hepatitis C is disease reactivation; UVB phototherapy is recommended as the first line of treatment, followed by cautious use of internal medications [62].

In the largest reported retrospective study, 25 patients with either hepatitis C virus ($n = 20$) or hepatitis B virus ($n = 5$) were treated with at least one biologic agent (etanercept, 21 treatments; adalimumab, 4; ustekinumab, 4; infliximab, 2) for more than eight weeks [75]. The follow-up period for patients with hepatitis C virus and hepatitis B virus was 15 and 25 months, respectively. The majority of all patients did not show increases in viral load or liver function tests. In the patients with hepatitis C virus treated with etanercept, disease-related events were reported in five patients, including significant elevation of liver function tests from baseline ($n = 1$), viral load increases ($n = 2$), and hepatocellular carcinoma ($n = 2$). No other disease-related events were reported.

Interestingly, there are also reports that etanercept may be helpful in hepatitis C infection when used in combination with antiretroviral agents [76]. One randomized trial that compared etanercept or placebo in combination with interferon and ribavirin showed that patients on etanercept were more likely to clear hepatitis C [76]. This has also been observed *in vitro* with cyclosporine [77,78]. However, even though a patient may benefit from these immune-modulating agents, there is concern that once the medication is stopped, viral replication may rebound to high levels.

HUMAN IMMUNODEFICIENCY VIRUS

The paramount concern in the management of HIV patients is the control of their HIV infection. Doing so entails aggressive treatments for psoriasis, as well as antiretroviral therapy, which has been proven successful in completely or partially improving psoriasis lesions [79]. The literature shows a clear association between the two diseases in that HIV patients are more likely to have severe disease than non-HIV patients, and psoriasis can be the initial presentation of HIV [61,80]. As the prevalence of HIV grows in aging individuals due to improved therapeutics, the clinical coexistence of the two diseases will become increasingly apparent.

Phototherapy

Avoiding internal immunologic modulation makes phototherapy the first line of treatment for HIV patients [81]. Although *in vitro* studies have shown the activation of HIV by UVB light, case studies in humans suggest that both UVB and PUVA are not associated with worsening of HIV infection [82–84].

Traditional Systemics

Acitretin is the preferred second-line therapy because it does not immunosuppress. Some studies report that the medication worsens psoriasis in this population, but the cause is unknown [62,85]. Although case reports have detailed the successful use of traditional systemics in HIV patients, methotrexate and cyclosporine are immunosuppressive agents and are not recommended [86,87]. They should only be used in cases of most severe, recalcitrant, and desperate disease [80]. John Koo considers methotrexate and cyclosporine to be contraindicated in HIV patients and, if they are to be used, thorough informed consent must be obtained. Trough levels should be monitored when cyclosporine is used in conjunction with protease inhibitors [80,88].

Biologics

The decision to initiate biologic therapy should be made in conjunction with infectious disease specialists who regularly assess viral load and cell counts. With limited studies addressing the long-term safety of biologic therapy, a patient's immune status is of utmost concern. Case reports have detailed the safe use of TNF agents, as well as ustekinumab [89–92]. In one case, multiple infections were seen in a patient taking etanercept, so the medication was discontinued. With a low risk of medication interaction, antiviral therapy is recommended concurrently with biologics to avoid infections and normalize immune function [61,80].

CANCER

Many of the systemic treatments for moderate-to-generalized psoriasis, such as biologics, are classified as immunosuppressants and thus raise the concern for malignancy. The cytokines blocked by biologics, such as TNF-a, interleukin-12 (IL-12), and IL-23, may play an important role in immunosurveillance. There is concern that medications that block these cytokines may increase the risk of cancer, including skin cancer. Most studies report equivocal findings regarding the overall cancer risk with biologic therapies [93–95]. However, this may not be the case with nonmelanoma skin cancers (NMSC). Immunosuppression is a known risk factor for the development of skin cancers, and this has been documented in HIV and transplant populations [95,96]. Therefore, the use of immunomodulators in patients with previous NMSC should be done under close observation.

Traditional Systemics

Prebiologic immunomodulators have also been associated with increased risk of skin cancer. Cyclosporine at dermatological doses of 3–5 mg/kg/day has not been demonstrated to have increased risk of serious complications of internal malignancy or serious infection in an evidence-based approach (i.e., a statistically significant increase over the placebo or general public comparator group), but increased rates of skin cancer were reported in a five-year cohort, especially in individuals with previous PUVA therapy [97,98]. Conversely, cyclosporine (used in the setting of transplants in an ill population and at high doses for a long duration of time) has many potential serious associated side effects [99–101]. The varying clinical sequelae observed with different doses of cyclosporine serve as a good example that the immune activity within an individual is a spectrum. At dermatologic doses of cyclosporine, even though the rates of internal side effects are low, an increased risk of cutaneous cancer exists. Skin cancer may thus be an early signal, similar to a cautionary road sign, of approaching the threshold of clinically relevant immunosuppression.

Biologics

Biologic therapies are used in various medical conditions. They were introduced in dermatology for the treatment of psoriasis vulgaris and for off-label use in other dermatological diseases, such as hidradenitis suppurativa. The increasing use of biologic medications may reflect their generally high efficacy rates, relatively good safety profiles, demonstrated improvement in quality of life, and the need for long-term treatment with a much lower risk for cumulative major organ toxicity than traditional oral agents [102–106]. However, biologic medications are classified as immunosuppressants and thus carry the potential side effects of increased risk of malignancy.

Multiple meta-analyses of randomized clinical trials of all TNF inhibitors (etanercept, adalimumab, infliximab) in psoriasis patients and rheumatoid arthritis patients have demonstrated an increased detection of NMSC risk [93–95,107,108]. This case is especially true in patients with risk factors of previous skin cancer or actinic damage or with concurrent or a history of immunosuppressive therapies or therapies known to increase skin cancer risk (i.e., cyclosporine and phototherapy, especially PUVA) [98,109].

With regard to TNF-α antagonists and melanoma, Gottlieb et al. [107] analyzed 49 trials that used etanercept in 13,977 patients, with up to 18,262 patient years (PY), and they found no increase in melanoma [110]. Wolfe and Michaud analyzed 13,001 rheumatoid arthritis (RA) patients with 49,000 PY and found an increased risk of melanoma with infliximab at an odds ratio (OR) of 2.6 [1.0–6.7] and with etanercept at an OR of 2.4 [1.0–5.8] but no increased risk with adalimumab [95]. Leombruno et al. [108] analyzed 18 randomized control trials (RCTs) with RA patients on anti-TNF therapies and reported no increased risk of melanoma with a regular dosing of biologics. However, at high doses of adalimumab and infliximab, the risk of melanoma trended toward significance ($p = 0.06$). Some cases of melanoma development while on anti-TNF therapy were also reported [111–113].

In regard to IL12/23 inhibitors, up to five years of follow-up results in clinical trials did not demonstrate a significant increase in NMSC when compared to matched controls [114]. Published literature, not specific to ustekinumab, has shown that mice treated with IL-12/IL-23 p40 antibody exhibited decreased defense against tumors, and mice genetically manipulated to be deficient in both IL-12 and IL-23 or IL-12 alone developed UV-induced skin cancers earlier and more frequently than wild-type mice [115]. The relevance of these experimental findings in mouse models for malignancy risk in humans is still unknown.

Performing skin checks on patients prior to starting biologic therapies and increased vigilance for skin cancer surveillance during treatment are important. Patients with psoriasis can experience delays in skin cancer diagnosis due to clinical similarities in presentation. Thus, these thorough examinations are especially essential in patients with known risk factors, such as old age, history of previous skin cancers or actinic damage, family history of skin cancers, and previous immunosuppressive therapy or phototherapy.

REFERENCES

1. Bureau UC. *Projected Resident Population of the United States as of July 1, 2025, Middle Series.* Washington, DC: Population Division; 2002.
2. Bell LM, Sedlack R, Beard CM, et al. Incidence of psoriasis in Rochester, Minn, 1980–1983. *Arch Dermatol* 1991; 127(8): 1184–1187.
3. Wong JW, Koo JY. The safety of systemic treatments that can be used for geriatric psoriasis patients: a review. *Dermatol Res Pract* 2012; 2012: 367475.
4. Coskey RJ. Adverse effects of corticosteroids: I. Topical and intralesional. *Clin Dermatol* 1986; 4(1): 155–160.
5. du Vivier A, Stoughton RB. Tachyphylaxis to the action of topically applied corticosteroids. *Arch Dermatol* 1975; 111(5): 581–583.

6. Singh G, Singh PK. Tachyphylaxis to topical steroid measured by histamine-induced wheal suppression. *Int J Dermatol* 1986; 25(5): 324–326.
7. Grozdev IS, Van Voorhees AS, Gottlieb AB, et al. Psoriasis in the elderly: from the Medical Board of the National Psoriasis Foundation. *J Am Acad Dermatol* 2011; 65(3): 537–545.
8. Parslew R, Traulsen J. Efficacy and local safety of a calcipotriol/betamethasone dipropionate ointment in elderly patients with psoriasis vulgaris. *Eur J Dermatol* 2005; 15(1): 37–39.
9. Gould JW, Mercurio MG, Elmets CA. Cutaneous photosensitivity diseases induced by exogenous agents. *J Am Acad Dermatol* 1995; 33(4): 551–573; quiz 574–556.
10. Bressler R, Bahl JJ. Principles of drug therapy for the elderly patient. *Mayo Clin Proc* 2003; 78(12): 1564–1577.
11. Turnheim K. Drug dosage in the elderly. Is it rational? *Drugs Aging* 1998; 13(5): 357–379.
12. Flammiger A, Maibach H. Drug dosage in the elderly: dermatological drugs. *Drugs Aging* 2006; 23(3): 203–215.
13. Boffa MJ. Methotrexate for psoriasis: current European practice. A postal survey. *J Eur Acad Dermatol Venereol* 2005; 19(2): 196–202.
14. Evans WE, Christensen ML. Drug interactions with methotrexate. *J Rheumatol Suppl* 1985; 12(Suppl 12): 15–20.
15. Bhutani T, Koo J. A review of the chemopreventative effects of oral retinoids for internal neoplasms. *J Drugs Dermatol* 2011; 10(11): 1292–1298.
16. Falck P, Asberg A, Byberg KT, et al. Reduced elimination of cyclosporine A in elderly (>65 years) kidney transplant recipients. *Transplantation* 2008; 86(10): 1379–1383.
17. Heydendael VM, Spuls PI, Ten Berge IJ, et al. Cyclosporin trough levels: is monitoring necessary during short-term treatment in psoriasis? A systematic review and clinical data on trough levels. *Br J Dermatol* 2002; 147(1): 122–129.
18. Infliximab. *(package Insert).* Toronto, Canada2010.
19. Ustekinumab. *(package insert).* Horsham, Pa2011.
20. Etanercept. *(package insert).* Thousand Oaks, Ca1998-2011.
21. Reich K, Langley RG, Lebwohl M, et al. Cardiovascular safety of ustekinumab in patients with moderate to severe psoriasis: results of integrated analyses of data from phase II and III clinical studies. *Br J Dermatol* 2011; 164(4): 862–872.
22. Adalimumab. *(package insert).* North Chicago, Ill2002.
23. Gottlieb AB, Boehncke WH, Darif M. Safety and efficacy of alefacept in elderly patients and other special populations. *J Drugs Dermatol* 2005; 4(6): 718–724.
24. Militello G, Xia A, Stevens SR, et al. Etanercept for the treatment of psoriasis in the elderly. *J Am Acad Dermatol* 2006; 55(3): 517–519.
25. Menter A, Gordon KB, Leonardi CL, et al. Efficacy and safety of adalimumab across subgroups of patients with moderate to severe psoriasis. *J Am Acad Dermatol* 2010; 63(3): 448–456.
26. Fleischmann R, Baumgartner SW, Weisman MH, et al. Long term safety of etanercept in elderly subjects with rheumatic diseases. *Ann Rheum Dis* 2006; 65(3): 379–384.
27. Galloway JB, Hyrich KL, Mercer LK, et al. Anti-TNF therapy is associated with an increased risk of serious infections in patients with rheumatoid arthritis especially in the first 6 months of treatment: updated results from the British Society for Rheumatology Biologics Register with special emphasis on risks in the elderly. *Rheumatology (Oxford)* 2011; 50(1): 124–131.
28. Barker JN. Genetic aspects of psoriasis. *Clin Exp Dermatol* 2001; 26(4): 321–325.
29. Yang YW, Chen CS, Chen YH, et al. Psoriasis and pregnancy outcomes: a nationwide population-based study. *J Am Acad Dermatol* 2011; 64(1): 71–77.
30. Cohen-Barak E, Nachum Z, Rozenman D, et al. Pregnancy outcomes in women with moderate-to-severe psoriasis. *J Eur Acad Dermatol Venereol* 2011; 25(9): 1041–1047.
31. Dunna SF, Finlay AY. Psoriasis: improvement during and worsening after pregnancy. *Br J Dermatol* 1989; 120(4): 584.
32. Murase JE, Chan KK, Garite TJ, et al. Hormonal effect on psoriasis in pregnancy and post partum. *Arch Dermatol* 2005; 141(5): 601–606.
33. Boyd AS, Morris LF, Phillips CM, et al. Psoriasis and pregnancy: hormone and immune system interaction. *Int J Dermatol* 1996; 35(3): 169–172.
34. Chi CC, Lee CW, Wojnarowska F, et al. Safety of topical corticosteroids in pregnancy. *Cochrane Database Syst Rev* 2009; (3): CD007346.

35. Chi CC, Kirtschig G, Aberer W, et al. Evidence-based (S3) guideline on topical corticosteroids in pregnancy. *Br J Dermatol* 2011; 165(5): 943–952.
36. Mahe A, Perret JL, Ly F, et al. The cosmetic use of skin-lightening products during pregnancy in Dakar, Senegal: a common and potentially hazardous practice. *Trans R Soc Trop Med Hyg* 2007; 101(2): 183–187.
37. Schaefer C, Peters PWJ, Miller RK. *Drugs During Pregnancy and Lactation: Treatment Options and Risk Assessment*, 2nd ed. Boston, MA: Elsevier Academic Press; 2007.
38. El-Saie LT, Rabie AR, Kamel MI, et al. Effect of narrowband ultraviolet B phototherapy on serum folic acid levels in patients with psoriasis. *Lasers Med Sci* 2011; 26(4): 481–485.
39. Juzeniene A, Stokke KT, Thune P, et al. Pilot study of folate status in healthy volunteers and in patients with psoriasis before and after UV exposure. *J Photochem Photobiol B* 2010; 101(2): 111–116.
40. Park KK, Murase JE. Narrowband UV-B phototherapy during pregnancy and folic acid depletion. *Arch Dermatol* 2012; 148(1): 132–133.
41. Stern RS, Lange R. Outcomes of pregnancies among women and partners of men with a history of exposure to methoxsalen photochemotherapy (PUVA) for the treatment of psoriasis. *Arch Dermatol* 1991; 127(3): 347–350.
42. Gunnarskog JG, Kallen AJ, Lindelof BG, et al. Psoralen photochemotherapy (PUVA) and pregnancy. *Arch Dermatol* 1993; 129(3): 320–323.
43. Bae YS, Van Voorhees AS, Hsu S, et al. Review of treatment options for psoriasis in pregnant or lactating women: from the Medical Board of the National Psoriasis Foundation. *J Am Acad Dermatol* 2012; 67(3): 459–477.
44. von Kobyletzki G, Hoffmann K, Kerscher M, et al. Plasma levels of 8-methoxypsoralen following PUVA-bath photochemotherapy. *Photodermatol Photoimmunol Photomed* 1998; 14(3–4): 136–138.
45. Nguyen C, Duhl AJ, Escallon CS, et al. Multiple anomalies in a fetus exposed to low-dose methotrexate in the first trimester. *Obstet Gynecol* 2002; 99(4): 599–602.
46. Armenti VT, Ahlswede KM, Ahlswede BA, et al. National transplantation pregnancy registry—outcomes of 154 pregnancies in cyclosporine treated female kidney transplant recipients. *Transplantation* 1994; 57(4): 502–506.
47. Armenti VT, Jarrell BE, Radomski JS, et al. National Transplantation Pregnancy Registry (NTPR): cyclosporine dosing and pregnancy outcome in female renal transplant recipients. *Transplantat Proc* 1996; 28(4): 2111–2112.
48. Armenti VT, Radomski JS, Moritz MJ, et al. Report from the National Transplantation Pregnancy Registry (NTPR): outcomes of pregnancy after transplantation. *Clin Transpl* 2005: 69–83.
49. Bar Oz B, Hackman R, Einarson T, et al. Pregnancy outcome after cyclosporine therapy during pregnancy: a meta-analysis. *Transplantation* 2001; 71(8): 1051–1055.
50. Nulman I, Sgro M, Barrera M, et al. Long-term neurodevelopment of children exposed in utero to ciclosporin after maternal renal transplant. *Paediatr Drugs* 2010; 12(2): 113–122.
51. Nyberg G, Haljamae U, Frisenette-Fich C, et al. Breast-feeding during treatment with cyclosporine. *Transplantation* 1998; 65(2): 253–255.
52. Verstappen SM, King Y, Watson KD, et al. Anti-TNF therapies and pregnancy: outcome of 130 pregnancies in the British Society for Rheumatology Biologics Register. *Ann Rheum Dis* 2011; 70(5): 823–826.
53. Carter JD, Valeriano J, Vasey FB. Tumor necrosis factor-alpha inhibition and VATER association: a causal relationship. *J Rheumatol* 2006; 33(5): 1014–1017.
54. Carter JD, Ladhani A, Ricca LR, et al. A safety assessment of tumor necrosis factor antagonists during pregnancy: a review of the Food and Drug Administration database. *J Rheumatol* 2009; 36(3): 635–641.
55. Vasiliauskas EA, Church JA, Silverman N, et al. Case report: evidence for transplacental transfer of maternally administered infliximab to the newborn. *Clin Gastroenterol Hepatol* 2006; 4(10): 1255–1258.
56. Chambers C, Koren G, Tutuncu ZN, et al. Are new agents used to treat rheumatoid arthritis safe to take during pregnancy? Organization of Teratology Information Specialists (OTIS) study. *Can Fam Physician* 2007; 53(3): 409–412.
57. Fotiadou C, Lazaridou E, Sotiriou E, et al. Spontaneous abortion during ustekinumab therapy. *J Dermatol Case Rep* 2012; 6(4): 105–107.

58. Cheent K, Nolan J, Shariq S, et al. Case report: fatal case of disseminated BCG infection in an infant born to a mother taking infliximab for Crohn's disease. *J Crohns Colitis* 2010; 4(5): 603–605.
59. Murashima A, Watanabe N, Ozawa N, et al. Etanercept during pregnancy and lactation in a patient with rheumatoid arthritis: drug levels in maternal serum, cord blood, breast milk and the infant's serum. *Ann Rheum Dis* 2009; 68(11): 1793–1794.
60. Frankel AJ, Van Voorhees AS, Hsu S, et al. Treatment of psoriasis in patients with hepatitis C: from the Medical Board of the National Psoriasis Foundation. *J Am Acad Dermatol* 2009; 61(6): 1044–1055.
61. Menon K, Van Voorhees AS, Bebo BF, Jr, et al. Psoriasis in patients with HIV infection: from the medical board of the National Psoriasis Foundation. *J Am Acad Dermatol* 2010; 62(2): 291–299.
62. Armstrong AW. Treatent selection for moderate to severe plaque psoriasis in special populations. In: Duffin KC, ed. *UpToDate*. Waltham, MA: UpToDate; 2013.
63. Pariser DM, Wyles RJ. Toxic hepatitis from oral methoxsalen photochemotherapy (PUVA). *J Am Acad Dermatol* 1980; 3(3): 248–250.
64. Stephens RB, Cooper A. Hepatitis from 5-methoxypsoralen occurring in a patient with previous flucloxacillin hepatitis. *Aust J Dermatol* 1999; 40(4): 217–219.
65. Watanabe K, Takase K, Ohno S, et al. Reactivation of hepatitis B virus in a hepatitis B surface antigen-negative patient with rheumatoid arthritis treated with methotrexate. *Mod Rheumatol* 2012; 22(3): 470–473.
66. Gwak GY, Koh KC, Kim HY. Fatal hepatic failure associated with hepatitis B virus reactivation in a hepatitis B surface antigen-negative patient with rheumatoid arthritis receiving low dose methotrexate. *Clin Exp Rheumatol* 2007; 25(6): 888–889.
67. King LE. Letter: complications during methotrexate therapy for psoriasis. *Arch Dermatol* 1975; 111(1): 131.
68. Katz HI, Waalen J, Leach EE. Acitretin in psoriasis: an overview of adverse effects. *J Am Acad Dermatol* 1999; 41(3 Pt 2): S7–S12.
69. Roenigk HH, Jr, Callen JP, Guzzo CA, et al. Effects of acitretin on the liver. *J Am Acad Dermatol* 1999; 41(4): 584–588.
70. Sandrini S, Callea F, Cristinelli L, et al. Viral hepatitis in HBsAg-positive renal transplant patients treated with cyclosporin and steroids. *Nephrol Dial Transplant* 1990; 5(7): 525–530.
71. Strober B, Berger E, Cather J, et al. A series of critically challenging case scenarios in moderate to severe psoriasis: a Delphi consensus approach. *J Am Acad Dermatol* 2009; 61(1 Suppl 1): S1–S46.
72. Vigano M, Degasperi E, Aghemo A, et al. Anti-TNF drugs in patients with hepatitis B or C virus infection: safety and clinical management. *Expert Opin Biol Ther* 2012; 12(2): 193–207.
73. Abramson A, Menter A, Perrillo R. Psoriasis, hepatitis B, and the tumor necrosis factor-alpha inhibitory agents: a review and recommendations for management. *J Am Acad Dermatol* 2012; 67(6): 1349–1361.
74. Hsu S, Papp KA, Lebwohl MG, et al. Consensus guidelines for the management of plaque psoriasis. *Arch Dermatol* 2012; 148(1): 95–102.
75. Navarro R, Vilarrasa E, Herranz P, et al. Safety and effectiveness of ustekinumab and antitumour necrosis factor therapy in patients with psoriasis and chronic viral hepatitis B or C: a retrospective, multicentre study in a clinical setting. *Br J Dermatol* 2013; 168(3): 609–616.
76. Zein NN, Etanercept Study Group. Etanercept as an adjuvant to interferon and ribavirin in treatment-naive patients with chronic hepatitis C virus infection: a phase 2 randomized, double-blind, placebo-controlled study. *J Hepatol* 2005; 42(3): 315–322.
77. Liu JP, Ye L, Wang X, et al. Cyclosporin A inhibits hepatitis C virus replication and restores interferon-alpha expression in hepatocytes. *Transpl Infect Dis* 2011; 13(1): 24–32.
78. Watashi K, Hijikata M, Hosaka M, et al. Cyclosporin A suppresses replication of hepatitis C virus genome in cultured hepatocytes. *Hepatology* 2003; 38(5): 1282–1288.
79. Duvic M, Crane MM, Conant M, et al. Zidovudine improves psoriasis in human immunodeficiency virus-positive males. *Arch Dermatol* 1994; 130(4): 447–451.
80. Morar N, Willis-Owen SA, Maurer T, et al. HIV-associated psoriasis: pathogenesis, clinical features, and management. *Lancet Infect Dis* 2010; 10(7): 470–478.
81. Meola T, Soter NA, Ostreicher R, et al. The safety of UVB phototherapy in patients with HIV infection. *J Am Acad Dermatol* 1993; 29(2 Pt 1): 216–220.
82. Cavard C, Zider A, Vernet M, et al. *In vivo* activation by ultraviolet rays of the human immunodeficiency virus type 1 long terminal repeat. *J Clin Invest* 1990; 86(4): 1369–1374.

83. Fotiades J, Lim HW, Jiang SB, et al. Efficacy of ultraviolet B phototherapy for psoriasis in patients infected with human immunodeficiency virus. *Photodermatol Photoimmunol Photomed* 1995; 11(3): 107–111.
84. Pechere M, Yerly S, Lemonnier E, et al. Impact of PUVA therapy on HIV viremia: a pilot study. *Dermatology* 1997; 195(1): 84–85.
85. Buccheri L, Katchen BR, Karter AJ, et al. Acitretin therapy is effective for psoriasis associated with human immunodeficiency virus infection. *Arch Dermatol* 1997; 133(6): 711–715.
86. Maurer TA, Zackheim HS, Tuffanelli L, et al. The use of methotrexate for treatment of psoriasis in patients with HIV infection. *J Am Acad Dermatol* 1994; 31(2 Pt 2): 372–375.
87. Tourne L, Durez P, Van Vooren JP, et al. Alleviation of HIV-associated psoriasis and psoriatic arthritis with cyclosporine. *J Am Acad Dermatol* 1997; 37(3 Pt 1): 501–502.
88. Rosmarin DM, Lebwohl M, Elewski BE, et al. Cyclosporine and psoriasis: 2008 National Psoriasis Foundation Consensus Conference. *J Am Acad Dermatol* 2010; 62(5): 838–853.
89. Sellam J, Bouvard B, Masson C, et al. Use of infliximab to treat psoriatic arthritis in HIV-positive patients. *Joint Bone Spine* 2007; 74(2): 197–200.
90. Cepeda EJ, Williams FM, Ishimori ML, et al. The use of anti-tumour necrosis factor therapy in HIV-positive individuals with rheumatic disease. *Ann Rheum Dis* 2008; 67(5): 710–712.
91. Lee ES, Heller MM, Kamangar F, et al. Long-term etanercept use for severe generalized psoriasis in an HIV-infected individual: a case study. *J Drugs Dermatol* 2012; 11(3): 413–414.
92. Paparizos V, Rallis E, Kirsten L, et al. Ustekinumab for the treatment of HIV psoriasis. *J Dermatolog Treat* 2012; 23(6): 398–399.
93. Askling J, Fahrbach K, Nordstrom B, et al. Cancer risk with tumor necrosis factor alpha (TNF) inhibitors: meta-analysis of randomized controlled trials of adalimumab, etanercept, and infliximab using patient level data. *Pharmacoepidemiol Drug Saf* 2011; 20(2): 119–130.
94. Askling J, Fored CM, Brandt L, et al. Risks of solid cancers in patients with rheumatoid arthritis and after treatment with tumour necrosis factor antagonists. *Ann Rheum Dis* 2005; 64(10): 1421–1426.
95. Wolfe F, Michaud K. Biologic treatment of rheumatoid arthritis and the risk of malignancy: analyses from a large US observational study. *Arthritis Rheum* 2007; 56(9): 2886–2895.
96. Clifford GM, Polesel J, Rickenbach M, et al. Cancer risk in the Swiss HIV Cohort Study: associations with immunodeficiency, smoking, and highly active antiretroviral therapy. *J Natl Cancer Inst* 2005; 97(6): 425–432.
97. Paul CF, Ho VC, McGeown C, et al. Risk of malignancies in psoriasis patients treated with cyclosporine: a 5 y cohort study. *J Invest Dermatol* 2003; 120(2): 211–216.
98. Naldi L. Malignancy concerns with psoriasis treatments using phototherapy, methotrexate, cyclosporin, and biologics: facts and controversies. *Clin Dermatol* 2010; 28(1): 88–92.
99. Penn I. Post-transplant malignancy: the role of immunosuppression. *Drug Saf* 2000; 23(2): 101–113.
100. Nelson RP, Jr, Ballow M. 26. Immunomodulation and immunotherapy: drugs, cytokines, cytokine receptors, and antibodies. *J Allergy Clin Immunol* 2003; 111(2 Suppl): S720–743.
101. Penn I. Overview of the problem of cancer in organ transplant recipients. *Ann Transplant* 1997; 2(4): 5–6.
102. Gottlieb A, Korman NJ, Gordon KB, et al. Guidelines of care for the management of psoriasis and psoriatic arthritis: section 2. Psoriatic arthritis: overview and guidelines of care for treatment with an emphasis on the biologics. *J Am Acad Dermatol* 2008; 58(5): 851–864.
103. Castelo-Soccio L, Van Voorhees AS. Long-term efficacy of biologics in dermatology. *Dermatol Ther* 2009; 22(1): 22–33.
104. Menter A. The effect of psoriasis on patients' quality of life and improvements associated with alefacept therapy. *J Cutan Med Surg* 2004; 8(Suppl 2): 20–25.
105. Katugampola RP, Lewis VJ, Finlay AY. The Dermatology Life Quality Index: assessing the efficacy of biological therapies for psoriasis. *Br J Dermatol* 2007; 156(5): 945–950.
106. Gisondi P, Girolomoni G. Biologic therapies in psoriasis: a new therapeutic approach. *Autoimmun Rev* 2007; 6(8): 515–519.
107. Chakravarty EF, Michaud K, Wolfe F. Skin cancer, rheumatoid arthritis, and tumor necrosis factor inhibitors. *J Rheumatol* 2005; 32(11): 2130–2135.
108. Leombruno JP, Einarson TR, Keystone EC. The safety of anti-tumour necrosis factor treatments in rheumatoid arthritis: meta and exposure-adjusted pooled analyses of serious adverse events. *Ann Rheum Dis* 2009; 68(7): 1136–1145.

109. Hannuksela-Svahn A, Pukkala E, Laara E, et al. Psoriasis, its treatment, and cancer in a cohort of Finnish patients. *J Invest Dermatol* 2000; 114(3): 587–590.
110. Gottlieb AB, Gordon K, Giannini EH, et al. Clinical trial safety and mortality analyses in patients receiving etanercept across approved indications. *J Drugs Dermatol* 2011; 10(3): 289–300.
111. Fulchiero GJ, Jr, Salvaggio H, Drabick JJ, et al. Eruptive latent metastatic melanomas after initiation of antitumor necrosis factor therapies. *J Am Acad Dermatol* 2007; 56(5 Suppl): S65–67.
112. Katoulis AC, Kanelleas A, Zambacos G, et al. Development of two primary malignant melanomas after treatment with adalimumab: a case report and review of the possible link between biological therapy with TNF-alpha antagonists and melanocytic proliferation. *Dermatology* 2010; 221(1): 9–12.
113. Kowalzick L, Eickenscheidt L, Komar M, et al. Long term treatment of psoriasis with TNF-alpha antagonists. Occurrence of malignant melanoma. *Hautarzt* 2009; 60(8): 655–657.
114. Papp KA, Griffiths CE, Gordon K, et al. Long-term safety of ustekinumab in patients with moderate-to-severe psoriasis: final results from 5 years of follow-up. *Br J Dermatol* 2013; 168(4): 844–854.
115. Langowski JL, Zhang X, Wu L, et al. IL-23 promotes tumour incidence and growth. *Nature* 2006; 442(7101): 461–465.

Chapter 21

Current and Potential Applications of Pharmacogenetics and Pharmacogenomics

Rishu Gupta, Wilson Liao, John Y. M. Koo, and Jashin J. Wu

INTRODUCTION

Psoriasis is a common, chronic skin disease affecting approximately 2%–3% of American adults [1]. The disease not only affects the physical health of patients but can also lead to substantial impairment of psychosocial well-being and overall quality of life. Furthermore, psoriasis represents a significant financial cost for patients and the overall health care system; the annual healthcare costs related to psoriasis are estimated to be US$11.3 billion [2]. The treatment options for psoriasis are manifold; however, none have proven to be universally remittive [3]. Why certain therapeutics are effective in some patients and ineffective in others is a question that has led some researchers to turn to the field of pharmacogenetics. Pharmacogenetic studies may identify genetic polymorphisms that can affect drug efficacy and/or toxicity among individuals.

PSORIASIS DISEASE-ASSOCIATED GENES

The development of psoriasis is multifactorial, including genetic and environment factors. Environmental triggers include group A streptococcal infection, hormonal changes, stress, alcohol, cigarette smoking, physical trauma (i.e., the Koebner phenomenon), and medications (e.g., β-blockers, lithium, antimalarials, interferon) [4]. Although the inheritance pattern of psoriasis has not been entirely elucidated, there is clearly a genetic component to the development of the disease and to the disease's severity. Approximately one-third of psoriasis patients report a family member with the disease, and the risk to first-degree relatives is estimated to be 8%–23% [5]. A concordance of 70% has been reported in monozygotic twins in comparison to a 23% concordance in dizygotic twins in the United States [6]. The heritability for psoriasis is estimated to be between 60% and 90% [7].

Recently, much progress has been made in uncovering the genes likely involved in the pathogenesis of psoriasis. Genetic linkage studies have identified and mapped several psoriasis susceptibility (*PSORS*) loci. Nevertheless, the specific location of these genes is not clear. The general consensus, however, is that psoriasis susceptibility 1 (*PSORS1*), the major genetic determinant of psoriasis, is located in the major histocompatibility complex on chromosome 6p21 [8–10]. Various reports have identified the gene encoding human leukocyte antigen (HLA) class I antigen *HLA-Cw6* as the primary susceptibility locus, especially in early-onset disease [9,11–13]. Guttate psoriasis, a clinical variant characterized by small, scattered papules, has been associated with the *HLA-Cw*0602* allele [14,15]. *HLA-Cw*0602* positive patients have also been reported to have more severe disease with more extensive plaques on the arms, legs, and trunk [14]. Recently, mutations in the interleukin-36RN (*IL-36RN*) gene have been implicated in development of generalized pustular psoriasis [16,17].

Although the finding of an association with *HLA-Cw6* was significant, only 10%–15% of *HLA-Cw6* positive individuals develop psoriasis [14]. The low penetrance rate suggests that there must be other genes, genetic combinations (a multilocus model), or required environmental factors necessary in the pathogenesis of psoriasis. For example, rare cases have been reported in which multiple members of a family develop psoriasis and genetic testing has identified the Zinc Finger Protein 750 (*ZNF750*) gene located at chromosome 17q25 within the *PSORS2* locus [18–20]. In these cases, psoriasis is inherited as an autosomal dominant disease with high penetrance. Furthermore, published studies have associated *PSOR2* with mutations in Caspase-Associated Recruitment Domain 14 (*CARD14*), which amplify the inflammatory cell recruitment cascade linked to the pathogenesis of psoriasis [21,22].

Genetic studies have identified variants in the IL-23 receptor and *IL-12B* that predispose to the development of psoriasis [23,24]. Recently, studies have also reported a strong association of multiple IL-17 related genes to the pathogenesis of psoriasis [25]. Other promising gene candidates for psoriasis include *β-defensin*, a disintegrin and metalloprotease 33 (*ADAM33*), Protein tyrosine phosphatase, non-receptor type 22 (*PTPN22*), and *ZNF313*. Large genome-wide association studies have identified more than 36 psoriasis variants to date, yielding additional clues regarding the genetic basis of psoriasis [9,26–29].

Local Therapies

Coal Tar Polymorphisms in the metabolic breakdown of coal tar have potentially harmful clinical consequences. Approximately 50% of European Caucasians have glutathione S-transferase mu 1-null (*GSTM1*-null) genotype, resulting in low or absent glutathione S-transferase activity, an enzyme involved in the detoxification of carcinogenic derivatives of coal tar [30]. As a result, these individuals have twice as much 1-hydroxypyrene, a biomarker of polyaromatic hydrocarbon exposure, in their urine after topical application of 2% coal tar compared to individuals with normal enzyme activity [30]. These individuals would therefore have a higher total body burden of mutagenic compounds. *GSTM1* genotype also was shown to influence the accumulation of the p53 protein in the stratum basale. High levels of the p53 protein may prevent the onset of carcinogenesis [31]. In another study, investigators observed an association between a polymorphism in the *myeloperoxidase* gene and altered accumulation of carcinogenic byproducts of tar [32]. However, these pharmacogenetic studies may not necessarily translate to adverse clinical events because studies, including one with 13,200 patients, did not observe an increased risk of cutaneous or noncutaneous malignancy in psoriasis and eczema patients treated with coal tar [33,34]. Furthermore, the carcinogenic effects of coal tar were reported to be lower when used on psoriatic skin compared to healthy skin [35].

Vitamin D_3 The vitamin D derivative 1,25-$(OH)_2$ D_3 is commonly used as a topical treatment for psoriasis; 1,25-$(OH)_2$ D_3 is an effective drug for the treatment of psoriasis. However, skin lesions show considerable variation in their responsiveness to treatment [36]. The effectiveness of vitamin D analogues is thought to arise from activation of the vitamin D receptor (VDR), leading to antiproliferative and prodifferentiation effects on keratinocytes as well as the overall immunosuppression via inhibition of Th1 lymphocytes [37]. Treatment response to vitamin D analogues is correlated with keratinocyte VDR mRNA expression [38]. A number of restriction fragment length polymorphisms in the VDR gene, marked by Apa1, Bsm1, Taq1, and Fok1, were initially investigated in several pharmacogenetic studies. However, the studies reported contradictory conclusions and have not yet identified a significant polymorphism [38,39]. The studies did have relatively small cohorts and were also underpowered, making it difficult to interpret the true validity of the results. However, larger studies have suggested a significant association for disease response with three polymorphisms in the VDR gene: Fok1F allele, Taq1 allele, and A-1012G A allele [40–42].

Light Interestingly, even a patient's potential response to light therapy may have a genetic component. Practitioners have recognized that, within their patient population, some patients improve with exposure to light, some show no response, and some have worsening of their symptoms. HLA-Cw*602 patients more often have a favorable response to sunlight [14]. Earlier studies have reported that phototherapy, such as narrowband ultraviolet B (NB-UVB), affects vitamin D status during the clearance of psoriasis. Therefore, variable response to light exposure may also be a factor of genetic polymorphisms in VDR. Studies have demonstrated an increased risk of melanoma associated with specific variants of VDR, although others appear to be protective [43]. In a recent study, investigators reported that even though none of the studied polymorphisms of the VDR receptor (APA1, Taq1, Bsm1, Fok1, rs4516035) affected clearance of the psoriasis, the Taq1 polymorphism was predictive of duration of remission after clearance of psoriasis [44]. The light-induced production of vitamin D, specifically the 1,25-$(OH)_2$ D_3 metabolite (which has antiproliferative and prodifferentiative effects), likely plays a role in the mechanism of therapeutic response of psoriasis to UV light; polymorphisms in the VDR would understandably alter the clinical response. Published articles have also observed that specific GSTM1 genotypes significantly affected erythema sensitivity to treatment of NB-UVB and that specific melanocortin 1 receptor (MC1R) genotypes influenced sensitivity to PUVA [45,46]. These findings may be significant because GST and MC1R genotypes have been associated with an increased risk of melanoma and nonmelanoma skin cancers [47–49].

Systemics

Methotrexate Methotrexate is an effective immunosuppressive agent that is used in a number of dermatologic conditions, including psoriasis. Years ago, many considered methotrexate to be the gold standard treatment for moderate to severe psoriasis as well as psoriatic arthritis. However, significant and potentially lethal toxicities associated with methotrexate, such as myelosuppression and hepatoxicity, may limit the long-term use of this medication. Furthermore, although methotrexate is highly effective in the majority of patients, approximately 20% show moderate-to-poor response, and approximately 30% must discontinue the medication as a result of the side effects [50,51].

Methotrexate reversibly inhibits dihydrofolate reductase, disrupting the folate metabolic pathway and resulting in a blockade in the synthesis of the purine nucleotides and thymidylate, ultimately interfering with DNA synthesis, repair, and cellular replication [52]. Although the pharmacogenetics of methotrexate have not been studied extensively with respect to psoriasis, there has been an abundance of research in patients with rheumatoid arthritis. Several polymorphisms have been identified in methylenetetrahydrofolate reductase (MTHFR), a critical enzyme in the folate pathway [53]. In a study by van Ede et al., patients with the polymorphism C677T, either homozygous or heterozygous for the variant, were found to have increased risk of experiencing elevation of liver enzymes severe enough to warrant discontinuation of the medication [54]. Another polymorphism in MTHFR, A1298C, has been discovered that also leads to an altered form of MTHFR but not to the extent that C677T disrupts the enzyme function [55]. Single-nucleotide polymorphisms (SNPs) in solute carrier family 19 (SLC19A1), which is a folate carrier controlling the influx of methotrexate in cells, have also been implicated in the increased risk of adverse events and discontinuation of methotrexate secondary to toxicity in rheumatoid arthritis patients [56].

In addition, thymidylate synthase (TYMS), an enzyme involved in DNA synthesis and repair, has been shown to have multiple polymorphisms that may potentially influence the effectiveness of methotrexate. One such polymorphism, a triplet repeat allele in the promoter region of the TYMS gene, has been associated with patients requiring a higher dose of methotrexate to achieve clinical response in rheumatoid arthritis patients [57]. Campalani et al. discovered a polymorphism in reduced folate carrier (RFC) 80A allele (which controls the influx of methotrexate in cells) and a 6 bp deletion in the 3'-untranslated region (UTR) of TYMS associated with an increased incidence of methotrexate toxicity in psoriasis patients. They also found RFC 80A and 5-aminoimidazole-4-carboxamide ribonucleotide transformylase (ATIC) 347G were associated with methotrexate discontinuation. The TYMS 5'-UTR 3R allele was associated with poor therapeutic response to methotrexate [58].

In a cohort of 374 psoriasis patients, investigators reported that SNPs in two efflux transporter proteins (three in ABCC1 and two in ABCG2) influenced the efficacy of methotrexate possibly by resulting in the intracellular retention of methotrexate. In the same study, six SNPs were also associated with the increased risk of methotrexate toxicity [59].

In another study, investigators formulated a model to predict response probability with methotrexate therapy in rheumatoid arthritis patients. The model incorporated scoring based on clinical features including disease severity as well as identification of specific polymorphisms associated with methotrexate efficacy and toxicity. Using the model on 38 patients, the investigators determined that the model was able to positively and negatively predict the response to therapy in approximately 70% of the patients [60]. Although further prospective studies are needed to assess the validity of the model, the study served as an excellent example of the potential application of a clinical pharmacogenetic index and how the application of the index can be beneficial in the treatment of psoriasis.

Cyclosporine Cyclosporine is a commonly prescribed immunosuppressive, which has long been used in the prevention and treatment of organ transplant rejection and of graft versus host disease. It has been employed in a number of dermatologic conditions, including psoriasis and eczema. Cyclosporine is likely successful in psoriasis as a result of its ability to suppress T cells. Similar to methotrexate, the pharmacogenetics of cyclosporine have not been investigated in psoriasis but instead in transplant patients. Although cyclosporine is highly effective, it also has a narrow therapeutic index with significant risk of nephrotoxicity [61]. Consequently, polymorphisms involved in the absorption, distribution, and metabolism of cyclosporine are particularly noteworthy and clinically relevant.

Cyclosporine is metabolized by the cytochrome P450 family, specifically CYP3A4 and CYP3A5, and serves as a substrate for the P-glycoprotein product of the multidrug resistance 1 (MDR 1) gene [62]. Both CYP3A4 and CYP3A5 have polymorphic variants [62,63]. Individuals with CYP3A5*3/*3 genotype have been reported to have significantly lower levels of expression of CYP3A5. Correlating the expression of CYP3A5 with the dosing of cyclosporine has been controversial because some studies have found a significant correlation, but others have not [62,64–67]. In contrast, C3435T polymorphisms in the MDR1 gene have been shown to predict cyclosporine drug levels *in vivo* [68]. Foote et al. found that the T allele in this position is inversely related to cyclosporine levels, such that each additional T allele present in an individual led to a decrease in drug exposure by 15% decrements in renal transplant patients [68]. Tacrolimus, another calcineurin inhibitor, is reported to be affected by polymorphisms in CYPA4 and CYP3A5, which can predict the necessity of either higher or reduced dosing to achieve therapeutic concentrations. Oral tacrolimus, however, is not widely used for the treatment of psoriasis [69]. It is unclear if the significance of specific polymorphisms warrants an individualized tailored drug dosing for cyclosporine in clinical practice because the evidence is limited and contradictory. However, cyclosporine is associated with serious adverse events, making it favorable for the future investigation of the possible beneficial implications of pharmacogenetics on cyclosporine dosing.

Retinoids Systemic retinoids are vitamin A derivatives frequently used in the treatment of severe psoriasis. Acitretin is the only oral retinoid currently approved in the United States for use in psoriasis. Acitretin is often an effective treatment; however, individual patient response is variable. The precise mechanism of action of retinoids in the treatment of psoriasis remains unclear, though the mechanism is likely related to their ability to alter epidermal proliferation and differentiation. Retinoids also appear to block vascular endothelial growth factor (VEGF) production [70]. Keratinocyte-derived cytokines such as VEGF promote angiogenesis and are commonly elevated in a number of inflammatory diseases, including psoriasis [70–73]. A recent study by Young et al. examined two VEGF polymorphisms, +405 and −460, located at chromosome 6p.21 and known to be associated with early-onset psoriasis. These polymorphisms are near the functional protein-1 site (+419) where retinoids are known to exert their anti-VEGF function [74]. This study found that the VEGF-460 genotype was predictive of nonresponsiveness to acitretin. Individuals homozygous for the −460 allele were twice as likely to fail systemic retinoid therapy as heterozygotes or individuals homozygous for the +405 allele [74]. The identification of this genetic predisposition to fail retinoid therapy may be used in the future to avoid unnecessarily exposing a patient with a high likelihood of nonresponsiveness to the adverse effects associated with retinoids such as teratogenicity and hepatotoxicity.

Apolipoprotein E (ApoE) gene polymorphisms have been increasingly linked with the development of psoriasis along with psoriasis severity [75]. ApoE variants have also been associated with hypertriglyceridemia, a common side effect of acitretin. Investigators prospectively studied the disease response to acitretin in relation to these polymorphisms but were unable to find a significant association with allelic variants of ApoE and acitretin response [75].

Furthermore, polymorphisms have been identified in retinoid X receptors (RXRs), the direct target for the retinoid therapy [76]. All-trans-retinoic acid and RXRs are each encoded by the three separate and distinct genes [76]. Polymorphisms identified in these genes may serve as susceptibility genes for the development of psoriasis, including an increased frequency of the AA allele of the RXR A39526 polymorphism in men with psoriasis and a higher incidence of the AA and TT genotypes of the RXRB 3'+ 140A/T polymorphism in women with guttate psoriasis [76]. However, RXR polymorphisms have not been specifically studied in relation to the response to any therapies, including acitretin. Identification of these polymorphisms and their relation to specific subtypes of psoriasis may be used as a means to target specific pharmacotherapy according to the patient's RXR genetic profile.

Biologics

The recognition of psoriasis as a T-cell-mediated disease has led to the development of new therapeutic agents that target specific inflammatory molecules. The biologics currently in use are the anti-tumor necrosis factor (anti-TNF) agents (etanercept, infliximab, and adalimumab) and anti-IL-12/23 agents (ustekinumab.) So far, clinical trials have shown the biologics to be safe and effective alternatives to traditional systemic therapy for moderate to severe psoriasis, but these agents are still relatively new and the dangers of long-term immunosuppression and possibly increased risk of infection and cancer remain to be seen. Furthermore, these agents are expensive and can present a formidable financial burden for patients.

Tumor Necrosis Factor Antagonists: Etanercept, Adalimumab, and Infliximab Etanercept, a recombinant human fusion protein consisting of a dimer of the extracellular portion of p75 TNF-receptor linked to the Fc portion of human immunoglobulin G1 (IgG1); infliximab, a chimeric monoclonal antibody; and adalimumab, a human monoclonal antibody, competitively inhibit TNF and effectively break the cascade of inflammatory cytokines in psoriasis [77]. Researchers are beginning to identify TNF polymorphisms, which can predict responsiveness to TNF antagonists. Seitz et al. identified a polymorphism at position -308 in the promoter of the TNF gene that appears to foretell therapeutic response to TNF blockers in rheumatoid arthritis, psoriatic arthritis, or ankylosing spondylitis. In the Seitz et al. study, subjects with a TNF-308 G/G genotype showed far better response to TNF antagonists than the A/A or A/G genotypes [78]. Furthermore, Miceli-Richard et al. published a pharmacogenetic study investigating the effect of TNF gene polymorphisms on patient response to adalimumab in rheumatoid arthritis. Their study suggests that the ancestral haplotype of the TNF promoter, Guanine Guanine Cytosine (GGC), in the homozygous form, is associated with a decreased response to adalimumab [79]. Tejasvi et al. found a nominally significant association with TNF-238 G/A polymorphisms and psoriasis. The authors conducted another study to investigate additional genetic loci including TNF-α-induced-protein 3 (TNFAIP3), which plays a role in the negative feedback inhibitor of TNF signaling. The TNFAIP3 gene has been associated with psoriasis in multiple published articles [80,81]. In the study by Tejasvi et al., the investigators found that polymorphisms in TNFAIP3 were correlated with response to anti-TNF agents. Specifically, positive response to all the TNF blockers was associated with the dosage of the G allele of TNFAIP3 polymorphism (rs610604), which also is a psoriasis susceptibility allele [80,82].

In addition to polymorphisms in the TNF gene, polymorphisms in the Fc receptor affect the efficacy of TNF inhibitors by enhancing or diminishing affinity for immunoglobulin binding. In a study on rheumatoid arthritis and psoriatic arthritis, Tutuncu et al. found that clinical response to TNF blockers correlated with the Fc-γ receptor type IIIA-158 polymorphism [77]. Furthermore, Genome-Wide Association Study (GWAS) in rheumatoid arthritis have identified additional proposed markers for anti-TNF response including genes encoding transcription factors (AFF3) and cell surface membrane proteins (CD226, CD45/PTPRC) [40,83,84]. Recognition of the polymorphisms may allow practitioners to better optimize the therapeutic approach in order to maximize patient response and limit adverse effects and unnecessary costs.

Anti-Interleukin-12/-23

IL-12 and IL-23 are new targets for psoriasis therapy [85]. Ustekinumb is currently the only monoclonal antibody targeting IL-12 and IL-23 on the market for the treatment of psoriasis. Ustekinumab is highly effective; about 67% of patients receiving ustekinumab achieved Psoriasis Area and Severity Index (PASI) 75 at week 12 in the pivotal phase III study [86]. *IL-12B* encodes a component of IL-12 and IL-23, two heterodimeric cytokines produced by activated dendritic cells and macrophages. IL-12 and IL-23 are involved in the production of IFN-γ and appear to play a significant role in the pathogenesis of psoriasis [87]. IL-12 drives the development of Th1 cells, leading to the production of interferon-γ (IFN-γ), while IL-23 drives the expansion of Th17 T cells [85]. Alterations in the IL-23 receptor have been associated with psoriasis. In addition, a noteworthy association between the SNPs (rs3212227) in the 3' UTR of IL-12B and psoriasis has been observed [23]. Individuals with one A allele at the rs3212227 position have a slightly increased risk of psoriasis, and individuals with two A alleles have a significantly increased risk [23]. Research on the exact functional consequences of the A allele has led to conflicting results.

Recently, Talamonti et al. investigated three different psoriasis susceptibility genetic variations (HLA-Cw6, TNFAIP3 rs610604 polymorphism, and LCE3B/3C genes deletion) and their association with therapy response to ustekinumab in 51 psoriasis patients. The authors found a significant correlation between the presence of the HLA-Cw6 allele (also implicated in response to efalizumab, and alefacept) and good clinical response with ustekinumab. The authors did not find a significant association between TNFAIP3 polymorphism (previously observed to correlate with the response to TNF antagonists) or Late Cornified Envelope 3B/3C (LCE3B/3C) genes' deletion and clinical response with ustekinumab [88].

Though ustekinumab has an excellent therapeutic effect on psoriasis, the medication is extremely expensive. Further investigation into the pharmacogenetic association and the response to therapy with ustekinumab can help reduce the cost of treating a patient with psoriasis and result in improved clinical outcomes.

There are many new biologics currently in development for the treatment of moderate to severe plaque psoriasis [85]. The new proposed target for many of the biologics is the IL-17 cytokine pathway. Preliminary data have confirmed the importance of the dysregulation of the TH-17 and IL-17 balance for the pathogenesis of psoriasis [85]. A majority of clinical trials incorporate pharmacogenetic and biomarker collection to analyze the correlation with treatment responses. It will be interesting to see if the trials reveal further information about the pharmacogenetics in psoriasis therapy and their hopeful application in clinical practice.

CONCLUSION

The ability to develop the effective therapeutic agents individualized for a specific genetic composition would truly revolutionize the practice of medicine. To rationally design a treatment regimen based on a patient's phenotype would allow the practitioners to avoid using drugs with no or little expected therapeutic response and to decrease the incidence of adverse effects. Pharmacogenetics also holds the promise of optimizing drug dosing based on drug metabolism phenotype. Furthermore, a targeted therapeutic approach will also decrease the inherent expenditure of time and finances in failed treatment regimens.

There were no funding sources for this paper.

Dr. Wu received research grants from Abbott Laboratories, AbbVie, Amgen, and Pfizer, which were not directly related to this study.

Dr. John Koo is a speaker for AbbVie, Leo, and Stiefel-GSK. Dr. Koo conducts research for Amgen, Janssen, Novartis, Photomedex, Galderma, and Pfizer. Dr. Koo has no stocks, employment, or board memberships with any pharmaceutical company. None of the grants were directly related to this study.

W.L. is supported by a grant from the National Institutes of Health (K08AR057763), which was not directly related to this study.

REFERENCES

1. Parisi R, Symmons DP, Griffiths CE, et al. Global epidemiology of psoriasis: a systematic review of incidence and prevalence. *J Invest Dermatol* 2013; 133: 377–385.
2. Staidle JP, Dabade TS, Feldman SR. A pharmacoeconomic analysis of severe psoriasis therapy: a review of treatment choices and cost efficiency. *Expert Opin Pharmacother* 2011; 12(13): 2041–2054.
3. Raut AS, Prabhu RH, Patravale VB. Psoriasis clinical implications and treatment: a review. *Crit Rev Ther Drug Carrier Syst* 2013; 30(3): 183–216.
4. Fry L, Baker BS. Triggering psoriasis: the role of infections and medications. *Clin Dermatol* 2007; 25(6): 606–615.
5. Oestreicher JL, Walters IB, Kikuchi T, et al. Molecular classification of psoriasis disease-associated genes through pharmacogenomic expression profiling. *Pharmacogenomics J* 2001; 1(4): 272–287.
6. Farber EM, Nall ML, Watson W. Natural history of psoriasis in 61 twin pairs. *Arch Dermatol* 1974; 109(2): 207–211.

7. Zippin JH. The genetics of psoriasis. *J Drugs Dermatol* 2009; 8(4): 414–417.
8. Sagoo GS, Tazi-Ahnini R, Barker JW, et al. Meta-analysis of genome-wide studies of psoriasis susceptibility reveals linkage to chromosomes 6p21 and 4q28-q31 in Caucasian and Chinese Hans population. *J Invest Dermatol* 2004; 122(6): 1401–1405.
9. Tsoi LC, Spain SL, Knight J, et al. Identification of 15 new psoriasis susceptibility loci highlights the role of innate immunity. *Nat Genet* 2012; 44(12): 1341–1348.
10. Bowcock AM, Krueger JG. Getting under the skin: the immunogenetics of psoriasis. *Nat Rev Immunol* 2005; 5(9): 699–711.
11. Enerback C, Martinsson T, Inerot A, et al. Evidence that HLA-Cw6 determines early onset of psoriasis, obtained using sequence-specific primers (PCR-SSP). *Acta Derm Venereol* 1997; 77(4): 273–276.
12. Nair RP, Stuart PE, Nistor I, et al. Sequence and haplotype analysis supports HLA-C as the psoriasis susceptibility 1 gene. *Am J Hum Genet* 2006; 78(5): 827–851.
13. Elder JT. PSORS1: linking genetics and immunology. *J Invest Dermatol* 2006; 126(6): 1205–1206.
14. Mallon E, Bunce M, Savoie H, et al. HLA-C and guttate psoriasis. *Br J Dermatol* 2000; 143(6): 1177–1182.
15. Holm SJ, Sakuraba K, Mallbris L, et al. Distinct HLA-C/KIR genotype profile associates with guttate psoriasis. *J Invest Dermatol* 2005; 125(4): 721–730.
16. Onoufriadis A, Simpson MA, Pink AE, et al. Mutations in IL36RN/IL1F5 are associated with the severe episodic inflammatory skin disease known as generalized pustular psoriasis. *Am J Hum Genet* 2011; 89(3): 432–437.
17. Marrakchi S, Guigue P, Renshaw BR, et al. Interleukin-36-receptor antagonist deficiency and generalized pustular psoriasis. *N Engl J Med* 2011; 365(7): 620–628.
18. Tomfohrde J, Silverman A, Barnes R, et al. Gene for familial psoriasis susceptibility mapped to the distal end of human chromosome 17q. *Science* 1994; 264(5162): 1141–1145.
19. Hwu WL, Yang CF, Fann CS, et al. Mapping of psoriasis to 17q terminus. *J Med Genet* 2005; 42(2): 152–158.
20. Yang CF, Hwu WL, Yang LC, et al. A promoter sequence variant of ZNF750 is linked with familial psoriasis. *J Invest Dermatol* 2008; 128(7): 1662–1668.
21. Jordan CT, Cao L, Roberson ED, et al. PSORS2 is due to mutations in CARD14. *Am J Hum Genet* 2012; 90(5): 784–795.
22. Jordan CT, Cao L, Roberson ED, et al. Rare and common variants in CARD14, encoding an epidermal regulator of NF-kappaB, in psoriasis. *Am J Hum Genet* 2012; 90(5): 796–808.
23. Nair RP, Ruether A, Stuart PE, et al. Polymorphisms of the IL12B and IL23R genes are associated with psoriasis. *J Invest Dermatol* 2008; 128(7): 1653–1661.
24. Cargill M, Schrodi SJ, Chang M, et al. A large-scale genetic association study confirms IL12B and leads to the identification of IL23R as psoriasis-risk genes. *Am J Hum Genet* 2007; 80(2): 273–290.
25. Martin DA, Towne JE, Kricorian G, et al. The emerging role of IL-17 in the pathogenesis of psoriasis: preclinical and clinical findings. *J Invest Dermatol* 2013; 133(1): 17–26.
26. Hollox EJ, Huffmeier U, Zeeuwen PL, et al. Psoriasis is associated with increased beta-defensin genomic copy number. *Nat Genet* 2008; 40(1): 23–25.
27. Lesueur F, Oudot T, Heath S, et al. ADAM33, a new candidate for psoriasis susceptibility. *PLoS One* 2007; 2(9): e906.
28. Capon F, Bijlmakers MJ, Wolf N, et al. Identification of ZNF313/RNF114 as a novel psoriasis susceptibility gene. *Hum Mol Genet* 2008; 17(13): 1938–1945.
29. Smith RL, Warren RB, Eyre S, et al. Polymorphisms in the PTPN22 region are associated with psoriasis of early onset. *Br J Dermatol* 2008; 158(5): 962–968.
30. Gabbani G, Pavanello S, Nardini B, et al. Influence of metabolic genotype GSTM1 on levels of urinary mutagens in patients treated topically with coal tar. *Mutat Res* 1999; 440(1): 27–33.
31. Godschalk RW, Ostertag JU, Zandsteeg AM, et al. Impact of GSTM1 on aromatic-DNA adducts and p53 accumulation in human skin and lymphocytes. *Pharmacogenetics* 2001; 11(6): 537–543.
32. Rojas M, Godschalk R, Alexandrov K, et al. Myeloperoxidase—463A variant reduces benzo[a] pyrene diol epoxide DNA adducts in skin of coal tar treated patients. *Carcinogenesis* 2001; 22(7): 1015–1018.
33. Roelofzen JH, Aben KK, van der Valk PG, et al. Coal tar in dermatology. *J Dermatol Treat* 2007; 18(6): 329–334.

34. Roelofzen JH, Aben KK, Oldenhof UT, et al. No increased risk of cancer after coal tar treatment in patients with psoriasis or eczema. *J Invest Dermatol* 2010; 130(4): 953–961.
35. Roelofzen JH, van der Valk PG, Godschalk R, et al. DNA adducts in skin biopsies and 1-hydroxypyrene in urine of psoriasis patients and healthy volunteers following treatment with coal tar. *Toxicol Lett* 2012; 213(1): 39–44.
36. Kragballe K, Gjertsen BT, De Hoop D, et al. Double-blind, right/left comparison of calcipotriol and betamethasone valerate in treatment of psoriasis vulgaris. *Lancet* 1991; 337(8735): 193–196.
37. Mathieu C, Adorini L. The coming of age of 1,25-dihydroxyvitamin D(3) analogs as immunomodulatory agents. *Trends Mol Med* 2002; 8(4): 174–179.
38. Chen ML, Perez A, Sanan DK, et al. Induction of vitamin D receptor mRNA expression in psoriatic plaques correlates with clinical response to 1,25-dihydroxyvitamin D3. *J Invest Dermatol* 1996; 106(4): 637–641.
39. Lee DY, Park BS, Choi KH, et al. Vitamin D receptor genotypes are not associated with clinical response to calcipotriol in Korean psoriasis patients. *Arch Dermatol Res* 2002; 294(1–2): 1–5.
40. Woolf RT, Smith CH. How genetic variation affects patient response and outcome to therapy for psoriasis. *Expert Rev Clin Immunol* 2010; 6(6): 957–966.
41. Halsall JA, Osborne JE, Pringle JH, et al. Vitamin D receptor gene polymorphisms, particularly the novel A-1012G promoter polymorphism, are associated with vitamin D3 responsiveness and non-familial susceptibility in psoriasis. *Pharmacogenet Genomics* 2005; 15(5): 349–355.
42. Saeki H, Asano N, Tsunemi Y, et al. Polymorphisms of vitamin D receptor gene in Japanese patients with psoriasis vulgaris. *J Dermatol Sci* 2002; 30(2): 167–171.
43. Li C, Liu Z, Zhang Z, et al. Genetic variants of the vitamin D receptor gene alter risk of cutaneous melanoma. *J Invest Dermatol* 2007; 127(2): 276–280.
44. Ryan C, Renfro L, Collins P, et al. Clinical and genetic predictors of response to narrowband ultraviolet B for the treatment of chronic plaque psoriasis. *Br J Dermatol* 2010; 163(5): 1056–1063.
45. Smith G, Wilkie MJ, Deeni YY, et al. Melanocortin 1 receptor (MC1R) genotype influences erythemal sensitivity to psoralen-ultraviolet A photochemotherapy. *Br J Dermatol* 2007; 157(6): 1230–1234.
46. Smith G, Weidlich S, Dawe RS, et al. Glutathione S-transferase M1 (GSTM1) genotype but not GSTT1 or MC1R genotype influences erythemal sensitivity to narrow band (TL-01) UVB phototherapy. *Pharmacogenetics Genomics* 2011; 21(4): 217–224.
47. Duffy DL, Zhao ZZ, Sturm RA, et al. Multiple pigmentation gene polymorphisms account for a substantial proportion of risk of cutaneous malignant melanoma. *J Invest Dermatol* 2010; 130(2): 520–528.
48. Fryer AA, Ramsay HM, Lovatt TJ, et al. Polymorphisms in glutathione S-transferases and non-melanoma skin cancer risk in Australian renal transplant recipients. *Carcinogenesis* 2005; 26(1): 185–191.
49. Bishop DT, Demenais F, Iles MM, et al. Genome-wide association study identifies three loci associated with melanoma risk. *Nat Genet* 2009; 41(8): 920–925.
50. Van Dooren-Greebe RJ, Kuijpers AL, Mulder J, et al. Methotrexate revisited: effects of long-term treatment in psoriasis. *Br J Dermatol* 1994; 130(2): 204–210.
51. Al-Dabagh A, Davis SA, Kinney MA, et al. The effect of folate supplementation on methotrexate efficacy and toxicity in psoriasis patients and folic acid use by dermatologists in the USA. *Am J Clin Dermatol* 2013; 14: 155–161.
52. Goldman ID, Matherly LH. The cellular pharmacology of methotrexate. *Pharmacol Ther* 1985; 28(1): 77–102.
53. Wilcken B, Bamforth F, Li Z, et al. Geographical and ethnic variation of the 677C>T allele of 5,10 methylenetetrahydrofolate reductase (MTHFR): findings from over 7000 newborns from 16 areas world wide. *J Med Genet* 2003; 40(8): 619–625.
54. van Ede AE, Laan RF, Blom HJ, et al. The C677T mutation in the methylenetetrahydrofolate reductase gene: a genetic risk factor for methotrexate-related elevation of liver enzymes in rheumatoid arthritis patients. *Arthritis Rheum* 2001; 44(11): 2525–2530.
55. Weisberg I, Tran P, Christensen B, et al. A second genetic polymorphism in methylenetetrahydrofolate reductase (MTHFR) associated with decreased enzyme activity. *Mol Genet Metab* 1998; 64(3): 169–172.
56. Bohanec Grabar P, Leandro-Garcia LJ, Inglada-Perez L, et al. Genetic variation in the SLC19A1 gene and methotrexate toxicity in rheumatoid arthritis patients. *Pharmacogenomics* 2012; 13(14): 1583–1594.

57. Kumagai K, Hiyama K, Oyama T, et al. Polymorphisms in the thymidylate synthase and methylenetetrahydrofolate reductase genes and sensitivity to the low-dose methotrexate therapy in patients with rheumatoid arthritis. *Int J Mol Med* 2003; 11(5): 593–600.
58. Campalani E, Arenas M, Marinaki AM, et al. Polymorphisms in folate, pyrimidine, and purine metabolism are associated with efficacy and toxicity of methotrexate in psoriasis. *J Invest Dermatol* 2007; 127(8): 1860–1867.
59. Warren RB, Smith RL, Campalani E, et al. Genetic variation in efflux transporters influences outcome to methotrexate therapy in patients with psoriasis. *J Invest Dermatol* 2008; 128(8): 1925–1929.
60. Wessels JA, van der Kooij SM, le Cessie S, et al. A clinical pharmacogenetic model to predict the efficacy of methotrexate monotherapy in recent-onset rheumatoid arthritis. *Arthritis Rheum* 2007; 56(6): 1765–1775.
61. Fernandes IC, Torres T, Selores M. Maintenance treatment of psoriasis with cyclosporine A: comparison between continuous and weekend therapy. *J Am Acad Dermatol* 2013; 68(2): 341–342.
62. Hu YF, Qiu W, Liu ZQ, et al. Effects of genetic polymorphisms of CYP3A4, CYP3A5 and MDR1 on cyclosporine pharmacokinetics after renal transplantation. *Clin Exp Pharmacol Physiol* 2006; 33(11): 1093–1098.
63. Ozdemir V, Kalow W, Tang BK, et al. Evaluation of the genetic component of variability in CYP3A4 activity: a repeated drug administration method. *Pharmacogenetics* 2000; 10(5): 373–388.
64. Zheng S, Tasnif Y, Hebert MF, et al. CYP3A5 gene variation influences cyclosporine A metabolite formation and renal cyclosporine disposition. *Transplantation* 2013; 95(6): 821–827.
65. Meng XG, Guo CX, Feng GQ, et al. Association of CYP3A polymorphisms with the pharmacokinetics of cyclosporine A in early post-renal transplant recipients in China. *Acta Pharmacol Sin* 2012; 33(12): 1563–1570.
66. Jordan de Luna C, Herrero Cervera MJ, Sanchez Lazaro I, et al. Pharmacogenetic study of ABCB1 and CYP3A5 genes during the first year following heart transplantation regarding tacrolimus or cyclosporine levels. *Transplant Proc* 2011; 43(6): 2241–2243.
67. Coto E, Tavira B. Pharmacogenetics of calcineurin inhibitors in renal transplantation. *Transplantation* 2009; 88(3 Suppl): S62–67.
68. Foote CJ, Greer W, Kiberd BA, et al. MDR1 C3435T polymorphisms correlate with cyclosporine levels in de novo renal recipients. *Transplant Proc* 2006; 38(9): 2847–2849.
69. Hesselink DA, van Schaik RH, van der Heiden IP, et al. Genetic polymorphisms of the CYP3A4, CYP3A5, and MDR-1 genes and pharmacokinetics of the calcineurin inhibitors cyclosporine and tacrolimus. *Clin Pharmacol Ther* 2003; 74(3): 245–254.
70. Diaz BV, Lenoir MC, Ladoux A, et al. Regulation of vascular endothelial growth factor expression in human keratinocytes by retinoids. *J Biol Chem* 2000; 275(1): 642–650.
71. Lowes MA, Bowcock AM, Krueger JG. Pathogenesis and therapy of psoriasis. *Nature* 2007; 445(7130): 866–873.
72. Brenchley PE. Angiogenesis in inflammatory joint disease: a target for therapeutic intervention. *Clin Exp Immunol* 2000; 121(3): 426–429.
73. Man XY, Yang XH, Cai SQ, et al. Overexpression of vascular endothelial growth factor (VEGF) receptors on keratinocytes in psoriasis: regulated by calcium independent of VEGF. *J Cell Mol Med* 2008; 12(2): 649–660.
74. Young HS, Summers AM, Read IR, et al. Interaction between genetic control of vascular endothelial growth factor production and retinoid responsiveness in psoriasis. *J Invest Dermatol* 2006; 126(2): 453–459.
75. Campalani E, Allen MH, Fairhurst D, et al. Apolipoprotein E gene polymorphisms are associated with psoriasis but do not determine disease response to acitretin. *Br J Dermatol* 2006; 154(2): 345–352.
76. Vasku V, Bienertova Vasku J, Pavkova Goldbergova M, et al. Three retinoid X receptor gene polymorphisms in plaque psoriasis and psoriasis guttata. *Dermatology* 2007; 214(2): 118–124.
77. Tutuncu Z, Kavanaugh A, Zvaifler N, et al. Fcgamma receptor type IIIA polymorphisms influence treatment outcomes in patients with inflammatory arthritis treated with tumor necrosis factor alpha-blocking agents. *Arthritis Rheum* 2005; 52(9): 2693–2696.
78. Seitz M, Wirthmuller U, Moller B, et al. The -308 tumour necrosis factor-alpha gene polymorphism predicts therapeutic response to TNFalpha-blockers in rheumatoid arthritis and spondyloarthritis patients. *Rheumatology (Oxford)* 2007; 46(1): 93–96.

79. Miceli-Richard C, Comets E, Verstuyft C, et al. A single tumour necrosis factor haplotype influences the response to adalimumab in rheumatoid arthritis. *Ann Rheum Dis* 2008; 67(4): 478–484.
80. Nair RP, Duffin KC, Helms C, et al. Genome-wide scan reveals association of psoriasis with IL-23 and NF-kappaB pathways. *Nat Genet* 2009; 41(2): 199–204.
81. Strange A, Capon F, Spencer CC, et al. A genome-wide association study identifies new psoriasis susceptibility loci and an interaction between HLA-C and ERAP1. *Nat Genet* 2010; 42(11): 985–990.
82. Tejasvi T, Stuart PE, Chandran V, et al. TNFAIP3 gene polymorphisms are associated with response to TNF blockade in psoriasis. *J Invest Dermatol* 2012; 132(3 Pt 1): 593–600.
83. Tan RJ, Gibbons LJ, Potter C, et al. Investigation of rheumatoid arthritis susceptibility genes identifies association of AFF3 and CD226 variants with response to anti-tumour necrosis factor treatment. *Ann Rheum Dis* 2010; 69(6): 1029–1035.
84. Cui J, Saevarsdottir S, Thomson B, et al. Rheumatoid arthritis risk allele PTPRC is also associated with response to anti-tumor necrosis factor alpha therapy. *Arthritis Rheum* 2010; 62(7): 1849–1861.
85. Toussirot E. The IL23/Th17 pathway as a therapeutic target in chronic inflammatory diseases. *Inflamm Allergy Drug Targets* 2012; 11(2): 159–168.
86. Leonardi CL, Kimball AB, Papp KA, et al. Efficacy and safety of ustekinumab, a human interleukin-12/23 monoclonal antibody, in patients with psoriasis: 76-week results from a randomised, double-blind, placebo-controlled trial (PHOENIX 1). *Lancet* 2008; 371(9625): 1665–1674.
87. Lee E, Trepicchio WL, Oestreicher JL, et al. Increased expression of interleukin 23 p19 and p40 in lesional skin of patients with psoriasis vulgaris. *J Exp Med* 2004; 199(1): 125–130.
88. Talamonti M, Botti E, Galluzzo M, et al. Pharmacogenetics of psoriasis: HLACw6 but not LCE3B/3C deletion nor TNFAIP3 polymorphism predisposes to clinical response to IL12/23 blocker ustekinumab. *Br J Dermatol* 2013; 169: 458–463.

Chapter 22

The Immunomodulatory/Immunosuppressive Classification System

John Y. M. Koo

INTRODUCTION

In the United States, patients suffering from psoriasis face two dilemmas. First, they have a disease that negatively impacts quality of life on a scale that is comparable to other serious conditions (e.g., cancer, diabetes, arthritis, and heart disease) [1]. Second, there is a real potential for being undertreated by their dermatologists. Although topical therapies may be adequate for mild cases of psoriasis, many cases of more generalized disease require systemic therapy or phototherapy [2,3]. According to data from Intercontinental Marketing Services (IMS), before the advent of the biologic agents, at least one-third of all practicing U.S. dermatologists had not prescribed a single systemic agent for psoriasis treatment in the two-year span examined. Another third only used systemic agents when they felt "pushed against the wall," and they account for only a miniscule proportion of systemic agents used. Only the last third used systemic agents on a regular basis. In fact, 11% of the U.S. dermatologists accounted for more than half of the systemic prescriptions written for psoriasis.

Results of the 1998 National Psoriasis Foundation Survey reflect this finding by showing that the majority of U.S. patients with severe generalized psoriasis were only treated with topical medications. Topical drugs were reported by these patients as generally inadequate, leading to high dissatisfaction rates among those surveyed [4]. Only 21% of generalized psoriasis patients surveyed received treatment with phototherapy, and only 18% received systemic treatments. Too frequently, a patient with generalized psoriasis leaves the dermatologist's office with only a tube of topical medication, which could be used up in a few days. Such undertreatment of moderate to severe psoriasis leads to patient frustration, to poor clinical outcome expectations, and often to treatment abandonment by the patient. Dermatology as a field loses credibility among patients when so many of us shy away from providing care that is adequate for those with moderate to severe psoriasis or other cases of widespread inflammatory skin disorders, such as eczema.

One of the major reasons behind the reluctance of dermatologists to embrace traditional systemic therapies, such as cyclosporine or methotrexate, relates to the fear of major organ toxicity associated with these agents (e.g., hepatotoxicity, nephrotoxicity, bone marrow suppression, etc.). The advent of biologic agents for the treatment of psoriasis aims to alleviate these concerns. Although some biologic agents have indeed reduced the risk of major organ system toxicities, they uniformly work by downregulating the immune system. Therefore, technically the biologics are all classified as "immunosuppressive agents," a term that makes many dermatologists uncomfortable. The average practitioner does not have the time to perform detailed literature reviews to elucidate independently the immunosuppressive potency of these agents. Many erroneously assume that the use of an immunosuppressant agent is automatically associated with increased risks of lymphomas, opportunistic infections, and so on. Thus, the perception of fearful side effects is often blown out of proportion, whereas in reality some biologics (such as etanercept) with more than a decade of human experience have not been shown to have convincing evidence for increased risk of malignancies or infections. Still, such blanket fear of immunosuppression prevents many dermatologists from making use of these agents to adequately treat their patients.

Similar concerns lead to underutilization of prebiologic agents such as cyclosporine or methotrexate. One reason for confusion in their area is the fact that, in the medical literature, one finds multiple and conflicting definitions for the terms *immunosuppression* and *immunomodulation* depending on the author, publication, or agency defining these terms. In fact, publications such as the U.S. Food and Drug Administration (FDA) Guideline for Industry do not even offer a definition for *immunomodulation* or *immunosuppression*, while others define these terms as being essentially interchangeable.

Faced with confusing information, it is not surprising that a significant proportion of dermatologists underutilize biologic and prebiologic agents. Even the FDA demonstrated the erroneous and greatly simplistic "on–off" idea of immune function and consequent fearfulness when it placed a black box warning regarding internal and skin cancer on topical pimecrolimus (Elidel® Novartis, East Hanover, NJ, USA) and topical tacrolimus (Protopic®, Astellas, Deerfield, IL USA) despite lack of human topical data convincingly demonstrating such a risk. This is a shame because in reality, downregulation of the immune system is a graduated phenomenon and not an "on–off" event. In fact, because these agents are used to treat disease states where inflammation is primary, it may be impossible to provide adequate therapy for the majority of these patients without downregulating the immune system.

There is an urgent need for these nervous practitioners and the FDA to embrace a more scientifically sophisticated understanding regarding the agents that downregulate the immune system; an understanding that includes (i) the clinical reality that downregulation of the immune system is not a "black or white" phenomenon—there is a gradient of effects involved—and (ii) there appears to be a "critical threshold" regarding the degree of immunosuppression involved that determines whether any clinically relevant consequence will occur or not.

We would like to propose a classification system that we hope will bring more clarity to the understanding of immunosuppressive effect and also offer more clinically relevant definitions for the terms "immunomodulators" and "immunosuppressors." The authors are aware that the immune mechanisms constitute a complex system where different agents work on different aspects of this system. However, we purposely refrained from creating a classification system based on the speculated impact of different agents on different aspects of immune mechanisms because doing so is likely to create endless speculation and more confusion.

In our view, the actual occurrence of immune-mediated side effects such as lymphoma or serious infection represents the "final common pathway" that can be used to compare different agents on a "level playing field." Therefore, this classification system categorizes agents based on the most clinically relevant data, which are the documented occurrences of immune-mediated, clinically relevant complications that are compiled from the actual human data.

THE PROPOSED IMMUNOMODULATORY CLASSIFICATION SYSTEM—DEFINITIONS, PARAMETERS, AND LIMITATIONS

The following is the method and logic by which we proposed this new classification system. We first defined two categories—immunomodulators and immunosuppressors (Table 22.1). Immunomodulators refer to those agents that modulate the immune response to control inflammatory disease activity without being associated with a statistically significant increased risk of clinically manifested immune-mediated complications. In other words, based on evidence-based reports rather than anecdotes, these agents are "clean" with respect to immune-mediated side effects. Immunosuppressors are those drugs that downregulate the immune function to such a degree that they can be documented in an evidence-based way to induce adverse immune-mediated side effects in humans, such as neoplasms or increased risk of infections. With regard to the immunomodulator category, we also realized that there are certain drugs that, so far, demonstrate no clinically evident immune-mediated side effects in an evidence-based (rather than just anecdotal) way, yet they have insufficient cumulative patient-years data. In addition, we also realized that, beyond the clinical trials, often even more patient-years of experience are necessary to adequately capture an increased rate of immune-mediated side effects. Consequently, we divided the immunomodulator category into two—immunomodulators (M_0) and possible immunomodulators (M_1). M_0 refers to those drugs that have greater than 100,000 cumulative patient-years and 10 or more years of human use encompassing human clinical trial and postmarketing data and have not been shown in an evidence-based way to pose an increased risk of immune-mediated clinically manifested side effects in humans. M_1 are the drugs that also lack the evidence of increasing the risk of immune-mediated side effects; but these agents have less than 100,000 cumulative patient-years of data or less than a 10-year record of human use. Basically, the M_1 category is the "gray zone" from which drugs can be moved to either the M_0 category or the immunosuppressor category based upon additional clinical data. Those agents in the M_1 group can be moved to the M_0 status when their use exceeds 100,000 cumulative patient-years and they have been in use for at least ten years without any increased rate of immune-mediated adverse events.

The rationale for using 100,000 patient-years as a threshold for defining "extensive" human data is as follows [22]. Two of the better-characterized diseases resulting from suppression of the immune system are lymphoma and tuberculosis (TB). Among lymphomas, the rare lymphoma is Hodgkin lymphoma. Tuberculosis is also rare. The baseline rate for Hodgkin lymphoma in the U.S. population is 3/100,000, and for tuberculosis it is 5 to 10/100,000 (U.S. Cancer Statistics Working Group and Centers for Disease Control and Prevention).

TABLE 22.1 The Immunomodulatory Classification System: A Proposed Prototype

Category	Definition	Hypothetical Examples of Agents That Might Belong in This Category	Examples of What Those Agents Are Used For
M_0	The agent has extensive human data (≥100,000 cumulative patient-years and ≥10 years of human experience)[a] based on both in clinical trial and postmarketing surveillance studies with no convincing[b] evidence of significantly increased risk of inducing immune-mediated complications.	NSAIDs Inhaled corticosteroids Topical corticosteroids Antibiotics	Osteoarthritis [5–7] Asthma [8] Atopic dermatitis [9–11] Rosacea [12]
M_1	The agent has extensive clinical trial but real-world data are lacking greater than100,000 cumulative patient-years and/or equal or greater than10 years of human experience yet with no convincing evidence so far of significantly increased risk of inducing immune-mediated clinically evident complications. This is the gray zone from which drugs can be moved to other categories based upon additional clinical data to be accumulated.	Topical tacrolimus Topical pimecrolimus	Atopic dermatitis [11,13,14]
S_0	The agent shows convincing evidence for immune-mediated clinical complications regardless of the number of patients exposed or duration of its usage. However, the clinical complications demonstrated are limited to relatively minor, not life threatening, and manageable conditions, such as nonmelanoma skin cancer.	Cyclosporine (dermatologic use[c])	Psoriasis [15,16]

TABLE 22.1 (*Continued*) The Immunomodulatory Classification System: A Proposed Prototype

Category	Definition	Hypothetical Examples of Agents That Might Belong in This Category	Examples of What Those Agents Are Used For
S_1	The agent causes immunosuppressive adverse events that may be life threatening, such as internal malignancies, melanoma, opportunistic infections,[e] or serious infections (e.g., sepsis or infections often requiring hospitalization or IV antibiotics). Measures should be taken to reduce the risk (e.g., PPD screening), and the potential benefit of use should justify the potential risk.	Doxorubicin Cyclosporine (transplant use[d]) Azathioprine	Acute leukemia [17,18] Transplant [19,20] Rheumatoid arthritis [21]

[a] Extensive human data: 100,000 cumulative patient-years (sufficient to capture even the smallest statistically significant increase of rare immune-mediated side effects, such as Hodgkin lymphoma and tuberculosis).

[b] "Convincing" refers to the existence of high level data according to evidence-based medicine (EBM) rather than only anecdotal cases.

[c] 3–5 mg/kg/day, healthy patients without major medical problems, short duration.

[d] >5 mg/kg/day, systemically ill patients, long duration.

[e] Opportunistic infections: clinical infections that result from immunosuppression that leads to reactivation of latent infections, including but not limited to tuberculosis, pneumocystis, cytomegalovirus, histoplasmosis, listeriosis, aspergillosis, cryptococcus, nocardia.

We performed calculations to estimate the number of patient-years required to measure a statistically significant increase of these rare adverse events. For Hodgkin lymphoma, the smallest clinically significant change is a doubling of the baseline rate (e.g., 3/100,000 to 6/100,000) because changes smaller than that would be based upon a single case. We conducted a one-sided Z-test and considered statistical significance (at $p < 0.05$). We determined that the amount of "person-time" required to measure such an increase is 100,000 person-years. This same amount of data (100,000 person-years) will allow one to measure a 50% increase in adverse events with a baseline prevalence of 10/100,000 (e.g., tuberculosis) with the same degree of statistical power. Because 100,000 patient-years are sufficient to capture a significant increase in such rare immune-mediated adverse events, it is also sufficient to capture the more common side effects, such as other types of lymphomas.

A required human experience time period of 10 years was chosen for the following reason. Not all adverse events may sprout immediately after use. It may take years before a side effect appears. A "hot" drug that may be promoted extravagantly and used massively by the public may quickly reach 100,000 patient-years of use within the first few years, but its side effects may not appear until later. Thus, in order to be moved up from the gray zone (the M_1 category), we believe that a minimum time period of 10 years is a reasonable requirement to recognize whether adverse side effects have occurred or not. If we made it 20 years, most practitioners will be contemplating retirement before the M_0 category can be decided, which greatly diminishes the utility of any classification system proposed to clarify this confusing area. However, even after being officially categorized as an "immunomodulator," any additional future data convincingly demonstrating that this particular agent increases the risk for immune-mediated complications will result in reclassification of the agent as an immunosuppressor.

With regard to the immunosuppressor category, the precise extent of patient-years becomes less critical. These are agents that have been documented to convincingly cause the immune-mediated side effects in human whether such documentation occurs early or late in its history of human usage. A distinction is proposed with regard to the degree of immune suppression induced, either minor immunosuppressors (S_0) or major immunosuppressors (S_1). S_0 is defined as those agents that show a convincing evidence for minor, manageable, and non-life-threatening immune-mediated clinical complications, such as nonmelanoma skin cancer. S_1 is defined as those agents that increase the risk for major complications, such as possible life-threatening adverse effects (e.g., internal cancers including lymphoma, opportunistic/serious infections including sepsis, or infections requiring hospitalization or antibiotics). For patients on these agents, measures should be taken to reduce the risk (e.g., purified protein derivative [PPD] screening for TB), and the potential benefit of use must justify the potential risk. A single drug may be categorized into the S_0 and S_1 categories depending upon the particular usage in question vis-à-vis *critical immunosuppressive threshold,* which, among others, depends upon the clinical setting, dose, duration, and health status of the patient population. Cyclosporine is a good example of such an agent whose immune-mediated risks depend upon the particular usage involved, as will be discussed in detail later in this chapter.

APPLYING THE IMMUNOMODULATORY CLASSIFICATION SYSTEM

Our examples are meant to hypothetically illustrate this approach and not to provide a definitive classification for the agents used as examples. A possible example of a therapy in the M_0 category would be nonsteroidal anti-inflammatory drugs (NSAIDs) (Table 22.1). NSAIDs effectively reduce inflammation and are the mainstays in the treatment of various conditions such as arthritis and headache. Although NSAIDs have associated risks of gastrointestinal bleeding, there are extensive clinical trial and posttrial surveillance data demonstrating no significant increased rates of major or even minor immunosuppressive adverse events [5,6]. A similar example is the use of oral antibiotics for the treatment of rosacea. Antibiotics such as tetracycline, minocycline, and doxycycline have been used for decades to control inflammatory skin conditions. It is believed that these antibiotics achieve their therapeutic effect primarily by downregulating immune function (i.e., anti-inflammatory effect) rather than by the killing of organisms. Yet, dermatologists frequently prescribe very long courses of antibiotics without concern for immune-mediated adverse effects [23–25].

Recently, the FDA placed a black box warning for internal and skin cancer on topical pimecrolimus (Elidel) cream and topical tacrolimus (Protopic) ointment despite the fact that clinical trial data (e.g., as compared to the placebo arm) and the postmarketing survey offer no convincing evidence for increased risk of internal or skin cancer associated with their use. Without any convincing topical application-based human data, the proposed placement of the black box warnings was justified by the FDA primarily on the basis that these two topical agents help improve eczema by downregulating the immune system. Had a classification system like this been available to the FDA, these two topical agents would have been, at worst, qualified to be in the M_1 category. Most likely, once 10 years of human experience is gained, both may qualify for the M_0 category. A few anecdotal cases of cancer associated with the use of these topical agents and extrapolation from systemic and/or animal data do not qualify as "convincing evidence" in the system proposed here. With the availability of a more rational classification system, it will be much more difficult for an agency such as the FDA to place black box warnings on a more arbitrary basis.

Cyclosporine can be classified into two categories, either as an S_0 or an S_1, depending on its use. S_0 refers to those agents that lead to immunosuppressive side effects that are nonfatal and are manageable. For example, cyclosporine used in the dermatologic setting (3–5 mg/kg/day, short duration, in systemically healthy patients, and not combined with any other immunosuppressive agents) has not been convincingly demonstrated to cause a significant increase in opportunistic infections, including tuberculosis, lymphoma, melanoma, or other internal solid tumors. Although the data from the five-year cohort have demonstrated increased risk for nonmelanoma skin malignancies, mainly in those who had extensive previous exposure to psoralen ultraviolet A (PUVA) photochemotherapy, this can easily be managed [15]. Thus, cyclosporine's use in this type of setting is considered to be barely above the immunosuppressive threshold, and thus would possibly be classified as an S_0.

In contrast, cyclosporine in transplant use (with higher dosage, for longer duration, in ill patients, and usually combined with other chemotherapy agents) is known to induce a full spectrum of serious immune-mediated complications [19,21,26]. Thus, its use in this type of setting would probably be classified as an S_1. Other examples of S_1 include chemotherapy agents, such as doxorubicin, daunorubicin, or epirubicin, which are used to treat acute leukemia, high-grade lymphoma, breast cancer, and bladder cancer. These drugs profoundly impair the immune system and are clearly associated with opportunistic infections and increased rates of tumor appearance [17,18].

For selected agents, their doses, durations, routes of delivery, clinical setting, patient population, and so on will determine whether they are deemed M_0, S_1, or somewhere in between. Other examples besides cyclosporine include topical corticosteroids and methotrexate. Topical corticosteroids for dermatologic conditions (and inhaled corticosteroids for asthma) [8] have not been demonstrated to increase risk for TB or other systemic infections. However, when corticosteroids are taken orally (or parenterally) at high doses for long periods of time (e.g., for treatment of systemic lupus erythematosus, chronic myelogenous leukemia), clinically significant immunosuppression can and does occur, along with substantial risk of serious adverse events [21]. Similarly, methotrexate is typically used in lower doses for psoriasis, rheumatoid arthritis, and inflammatory bowel disease and has a relatively safe immunoactive profile (not withstanding its potential for nonimmunologic-based hepatotoxicity, etc.) [27,28]. However, at higher doses (e.g., for breast cancer or osteogenic sarcoma), methotrexate is likely to be categorized as an S_1. Likewise, tacrolimus has similar characteristics: M_1 for topical use and an S_1 for oral high dose use for transplant patients [13,29].

Finally, a drug's immunologic category may change over time with the availability of additional data. To assess the risk of immune-mediated complications for potentially chronic therapy, sufficient exposure data (numbers of patients and chronicity of exposure) need to be considered. Recent experiences with marketing withdrawals of newer drugs prove the concept that the real-world clinical data are of paramount importance. When Baycol® (Bayer Healthcare Pharmaceuticals, Wayne, NJ, USA) (cerivastatin) was initially released, it appeared safe—based upon clinical trials. However, broader use showed a risk of fatal rhabdomyolysis [30,31]. Similarly, the safety profile of Rezulin® (Parke-Davis/Warner-Lambert now Pfizer, New York, NY, USA) (troglitazone) and Vioxx® (Merck, Whitehouse Station, NJ, USA) (rofecoxib) changed with the growing number of cases of severe hepatotoxicity and cardiovascular accidents, respectively [32]. Even though these examples involve non-immune-mediated adverse events, similar caution applies to immune-mediated risks. Therefore, as stated earlier, even after a particular agent earns classification as M_0 by raising no immune-mediated safety concerns in greater than 100,000 cumulative patient-years of use and equal or greater than 10 years of human experience, the possibility of being reclassified based on longer-term data and experience always exists.

DISCUSSION

Several valid concerns can be raised with regard to this proposed classification system. One may raise a concern regarding whether changes or aberrancies in laboratory values should be taken into consideration when categorizing drugs within this classification scheme. Examples include a drop in cluster of differentiation 8 (CD8) count by a drug that mainly suppresses CD4 levels such alefacept (Amevive,® Astellas, Deerfield, IL USA). Although we recognize there may be changes to some laboratory values, they should not be counted unless they are clinically relevant and have been demonstrated to occur as a result of immunosuppression. For this classification system, it is most important to maintain focus on the most clinically relevant basis for classification. For this reason, we purposely focus on the clinical end points rather than laboratory values per se. This means that aberrancies in laboratory values are not taken into account unless there is a clinical manifestation(s) associated with them.

Some may argue that the other methods of classification are better, for example, categorizing drugs as "safe," "probably safe," "potentially unsafe," and "unsafe." However, we purposely chose to propose a classification system that is more objective and defines a region but that does not draw sharp borders. Our concern is that in the aforementioned scheme, "unsafe" implies therapies that are fatal or harmful and therefore would deter physicians and patients from ever considering such therapies. However, we need to create a classification system that is not judgmental; even S_1 with significant risks can be indicated in certain groups of seriously ill patients. Thus, it is better to provide physicians with the freedom to make decisions on an individual case basis, weighing the risks and benefits. For example, infliximab has been demonstrated to increase the risk for certain serious infections and would therefore possibly be categorized as an S_1 (or "unsafe" if the "safe-unsafe" classification was used). However, there is a significant difference between the terms major immunosuppressor and "unsafe." The word "unsafe" clearly has a negative connotation, whereas major immunosuppressor states where this agent lies within the spectrum defined. Infliximab can be reasonably used in selected patient populations or even in a more vulnerable population if the risk:benefit ratio can be justified and if adequate precaution is taken. For example, PPD screening and chest X-ray can identify the at-risk patient population and can greatly eliminate the concern. A Centocor-sponsored tuberculosis education program aimed at educating 5000 U.S. physicians on tuberculosis screening and prophylaxis showed that spontaneous reports of active tuberculosis sharply declined after the initiation of such a program [33].

Another concern that can be raised may be a criticism that this classification system is incomplete because it focuses only on the immune-mediated, but not on the non-immune-mediated complications of drugs; therefore, there might be some risk that a clinician may make decisions based only on this important but partial information regarding an agent. As clinicians, we all know the importance of comprehensively appraising all aspects of medication choices before making a decision on which therapy to select. Having a classification system that specifically informs the clinician of the immunosuppressive risks is essentially no different than the current availability of the pregnancy category system to help us make a more optimal therapeutic selection. The pregnancy categories A, B, C, D, and X inform us instantly what is known so far about the risk (or lack of risk) a particular agent possesses with regard to teratogenicity. This is exceedingly helpful for a practicing physician. On the other hand, it would be ridiculous to assume that any responsible and competent clinician would make a final decision regarding therapeutic choice solely based on pregnancy category while ignoring every other aspect that is relevant with regard to that agent. It would be absurd to propose banning the pregnancy category system out of fear that some clinicians may thus misuse it. Our proposed classification system for the immune-mediated risks clearly parallels the pregnancy classification system in its proposed usage. Therefore, we feel that this fear is unfounded.

It is important to keep out commercial interference with scientific-based judgment regarding the categorization of each agent. There is a valid concern that, if a classification system like this is adopted, pharmaceutical companies may try to influence how their product is categorized. However, such concern need not discourage us from proposing a classification system like this. The fact that commercial interest tries to distort characterization of medications is nothing new.

The FDA and academic institutions have protocols and criterions to keep out such influences (for example, barring experts with conflicts from being part of a committee that makes judgments regarding the classification of a particular agent).

Lastly, we acknowledge that with any new classification, not all drugs fit neatly within one of the categories; there is always a gray zone of unclear areas. There exist clinical side effects where it is not clear whether they are immune-mediated or not, such as clinical lupus, demyelinating disorders, and the emergence of eczema when psoriasis is more effectively treated—possibly due to the shifting of Th1 to Th2, and so on, and, therefore, they do not fit neatly into the traditional concept of immunosuppression. Is efalizumab (Raptiva®, Genentech, San Francisco, CA, USA) induced thrombocytopenia a consequence of immunosuppression or a consequence of a totally unrelated and separate pathway? Do TNF-α inhibitor induced demyelinating disorders constitute immune-mediated side effects? Even if lupus is immune-mediated, the next question then becomes whether it should be classified as an S_0 or as a major immunosuppressor (S_1) (Is it manageable or life threatening?). However, the lack of any classification system also leads to a situation where a clinician or even the FDA might deviate from an evidence-based approach and resort to a fear-based approach due to confusion, ignorance, political pressure, and so on. These are the challenges that need to be addressed in the future. However, we should not be deterred by the fact that not every drug fits perfectly in its category but recognize the value of this new classification that will *generally* be applicable for a majority of drugs that downregulate the immune function. It needs to be stressed once more that we are proposing only the most basic conceptual framework as a better alternative to the current state of affairs where confusion reigns. It has been said that no new idea ever comes from pessimists. Although being a scientist requires certain healthy skepticism, if we all have the mentality of a "naysayer," nothing innovative and potentially useful can ever have a chance of becoming a reality. We should not allow examples that do not yet fit perfectly into this classification system to inhibit us from proposing a system that may prove in the long run to be beneficial for the medical field and for patient care.

It should be reiterated once again that, at this point, we are only proposing a concept. This is a chapter on an idea, not a review article or clinical trial data. There is reason to believe that a clinically oriented, human evidence-based classification for the immune-mediated side effect profile of therapeutic agents can facilitate optimal decision-making. This system is applicable to all medications, topical or systemic, in all fields of medical practice. We believe that the benefit of this proposed classification system can go far beyond enabling more dermatologists to avoid perceiving all immunoactive agents as fearful. It is the hope of the authors that this classification system will help upgrade physicians' conceptualization to a more sophisticated and more realistic model. By providing this conceptual framework, the authors hope to bring some order and clarity to this currently highly confusing area. However, the actual placement of any agent within this type of classification system is best left to the judgment of interest-free experts who are most knowledgeable about each of the agents in question.

REFERENCES

1. Rapp SR, Feldman SR, Exum ML, et al. Psoriasis causes as much disability as other major medical diseases. *J Am Acad Dermatol* 1999; 41: 401–407.
2. Callen JP, Krueger GG, Lebwohl M, et al. AAD consensus statement on psoriasis therapies. *J Am Acad Dermatol* 2003; 49: 897–899.
3. Lebwohl M, Ali S. Treatment of psoriasis. Part 2. Systemic therapies. *J Am Acad Dermatol* 2001; 45: 649–661.
4. Krueger G, Koo J, Lebwohl M, et al. The impact of psoriasis on quality of life: results of a 1998 National Psoriasis Foundation patient-membership survey. *Arch Dermatol* 2001; 137: 280–284.
5. Merck & Co, Inc. VIOXX® (rofecoxib tablets and oral suspension) [package insert]. Available at: http://www.fda.gov/cder/foi/label/1999/21042lbl.pdf (Accessed August 27, 2004).

6. Pharmacia and Pfizer. Celebrex (celecoxib capsules). Available at: http://www.celebrex.com/pdf/Celebrex PI.pdf (Accessed August 27, 2004).
7. U.S. Food and Drug Administration. Safety concerns associated with over-the-counter drug products containing analgesic/antipyretic active ingredients for internal use. Available at: http://www.fda.gov/cder/drug/analgesics/SciencePaper.pdf (Accessed August 27, 2004).
8. AstraZeneca. Pulmicort (budesonide inhalation suspension) package insert. Available at: http://www. astrazeneca-us.com/cgibin/azpi.asp?product = pulmicort resp (Accessed August 27, 2004).
9. American Academy of Dermatology Association. Guidelines of care for the use of topical glucocorticosteroids. *J Am Acad Dermatol* 1996; 35: 615–619.
10. Sarkar R, Kanwar A. Atopic dermatitis. *Indian Pediatr* 2002; 39: 922–930.
11. Krafchic B. Atopic dermatitis. Available at: http://www.emedicine.com/derm/topic38.htm (Accessed August 27, 2004).
12. Immunex Corp and Amgen Corp. Enbrel (etanercept) [package insert]. Available at: http://www.fda.gov/cder/foi/label/2003/etanimm060503LB.pdf (Accessed August 27, 2004).
13. Fujisawa Healthcare, Inc. Protopic (tacrolimus) [package insert]. Available at: http://www.fda.gov/cder/foi/label/2000/50777lbl.pdf (Accessed August 27, 2004).
14. Russell J. Topical tacrolimus: a new therapy for atopic dermatitis. *Am Fam Physician* 2002; 66: 1899–1902.
15. Paul CF, Ho VC, McGeown C, et al. Risk of malignancies in psoriasis patients treated with cyclosporine: a 5 y cohort study. *J Invest Dermatol* 2003; 120: 211–216.
16. Koo J, Kochavi G, Kwan J. *Contemporary Diagnosis and Management of Psoriasis*, 1st ed. Newtown, PA: Handbooks in Health Care Co; 2004, pp. 45–51.
17. DaunoXome (daunorubicin citrate) [package insert]. Available at: http://www.icon.co.za/~key/daunoxome/pres/prescribinginfo.htm (Accessed August 27, 2004).
18. Pharmacia, Inc. Adriamycin (doxorubicin hydrochloride) [package insert]. Available at: http://www. meds.com/leukemia/idamycin/adriamycin.html (Accessed August 27, 2004).
19. Penn I. Overview of the problem of cancer in organ transplant recipients. *Ann Transplant* 1997; 2: 5–6.
20. Kurki PT. Safety aspects of the long term cyclosporin A therapy. *Scand J Rheumatol Suppl* 1992; 95: 35–38.
21. Nelson RP, Jr, Ballow M. 26. Immunomodulation and immunotherapy: drugs, cytokines, cytokine receptors, and antibodies. *J Allergy Clin Immunol* 2003; 111: S720–S743.
22. Hoog R, Tanis E. *Probability and Statistical Inference*, 4th ed. New York: Macmillan; 1993.
23. Zouboulis CC, Piquero-Martin J. Update and future of systemic acne treatment. *Dermatology* 2003; 206: 37–53.
24. Jain A, Sangal L, Basal E. Anti-inflammatory effects of erythromycin and tetracycline on *Propionibacterium acnes* induced production of chemotactic factors and reactive oxygen species by human neutrophils. *Dermatol Online J* 2002; 8: 2.
25. American Osteopathic College of Dermatology. Minocycline. Dermatologic disease database. Available at: http://www.aocd.org/skin/dermatologicdiseases/minocycline.html (Accessed August 24, 2004).
26. Penn I. Post-transplant malignancy: the role of immunosuppression. *Drug Saf* 2000; 23: 101–113.
27. Aithal GP, Haugk B, Das S, et al. Monitoring methotrexate-induced hepatic fibrosis in patients with psoriasis: are serial liver biopsies justified? *Aliment Pharmacol Ther* 2004; 19: 391–399.
28. Polo Romero FJ, Blasco Colmenarejo MM, Tirado MR, et al. Advanced liver fibrosis secondary to methotrexate treatment. *Gastroenterol Hepatol* 2003; 26: 617–618.
29. Fung JJ. Tacrolimus and transplantation: a decade in review. *Transplantation* 2004; 77: S41–S43.
30. Schosser R. Risk/benefit evaluation of drugs: the role of the pharmaceutical industry in Germany. *Eur Surg Res* 2002; 34: 203–207.
31. Sparing R, Sellhaus B, Noth J, et al. Rhabdomyolysis following cerivastatin monotherapy—implications for therapy with HMG-CoA reductase inhibitors. *Nervenarzt* 2003; 74: 167–171.
32. Lee WM. Drug-induced hepatotoxicity. *N Engl J Med* 2003; 349: 474–485.
33. Centocor Corporation. Remicade (infliximab) FDA Arthritis Advisory Committee Briefing Document. Available at: http://www.fda.gov/ohrms/dockets/ac/03/briefing/3930b1.htm (Accessed August 27, 2004).

Chapter 23

Biologic Therapy and the Risk of Systemic Immunosuppression

Whitney A. Fisk, Ethan C. Levin, Judith Hong, and John Y. M. Koo

INTRODUCTION

Many psoriasis patients delay starting biologic therapy or may not be offered it when clinically indicated [1]. This may be partially due to concerns about the immunomodulating effects of these medications. These concerns are reinforced because biologics are often labeled by physicians as "immunosuppressants."

In contrast to the oral immunosuppressants used to treat psoriasis, biologic medications target specific components of the immune system. The effect of biologic medications on systemic immunity can be measured by examining the number of immune cells and the quantity of cytokines that they produce before and after treatment. These data can help to clarify the effect of biologics on immune function and may be helpful for physicians counseling patients who fear global immunosuppression. This chapter will review the effect on immune function in patients treated with adalimumab, etanercept, and ustekinumab.

Evaluating Systemic Immunity

One clinical method of evaluating immunocompetence is monitoring infection rates [2]. For this strategy to adequately evaluate rare infections, large populations of patients need to be followed over many years, which is unrealistic for many disease populations—especially with new medications. An alternate approach is to use *in vivo* and *in vitro* assays to assess cellular and innate immunity. These include, for example, assays that quantify immune cell populations and antigen-specific assays that assess immune cell function.

Clinical Studies Demonstrating Preservation of Global Immune Function

Immune Cell Populations and Cytokine Assays Several studies measured changes in leukocyte subpopulations during therapy with adalimumab, etanercept, and ustekinumab (Tables 23.1 and 23.2). In all studies, post treatment T-cell counts and cytokine levels were *not different* from healthy controls. Serum concentrations of cytokines, including those secreted by T-helper cell type 1 (Th1), Th2, and innate immune cells, were not altered in these studies. These cytokines include interleukin-2 (IL-2), IL-8, IL-10, tumor necrosis factor-α (TNF-α), and interferon (IFNγ) [3,7,8].

Both T cells and cytokines characteristic of the Th17 pathway were normalized after treatment with biologic medications to levels that were *not different* from those measured in healthy controls (Table 23.2). T regulatory cells, which increased after therapy, are responsible for suppressing the Th17 response.

TABLE 23.1 T-Cell Counts after Biologic Therapy for Psoriasis

Intervention and Participants	Outcome Measure	T-Cell Type	Before Treatment	After Treatment	Healthy Controls
Anti-TNF therapy for 4 weeks and 12 weeks [3] Pretreatment psoriasis (n = 11) Three months posttreatment (n = 5) Healthy controls (n = 31)	Subpopulations presented as percent of peripheral blood mononuclear cells	CD3 + cells	72.8 ± 12.3	77.2 ± 6.3	72.1 ± 6.8
		CD4 + cells	35.8 ± 9.1	42.4 ± 8.9	35.5 ± 10.2
		CD8 + cells	29.9 ± 8.2	28.4 ± 4.4	26.9 ± 7.2
		CD56 + cells	14.0 ± 7.4	14.6 ± 6.2	11.2 ± 4.5
		CD19 + cells	10.7 ± 4.0	9.08 ± 2.7	11.9 ± 4.8
		CD69 + cells (T-cell activation marker)	0.7 ± 0.5*	0.41 ± 0.4	0.4 ± 0.5
		CD25+ cells (T-cell activation marker)	4.0 ± 2.5*	2.08 ± 0.9	2.6 ± 2.2
		CD71+ cells (B-cell activation marker)	4.2 ± 1.7	4.02 ± 2.2 (after one month of therapy)	4.2 ± 2.7
Etanercept for 12 weeks [4] Psoriasis (n = 15) Healthy controls (n = 10)	Subpopulations presented as percent of total peripheral CD4+ cells	Th1 cells	20.0 ± 11.0	27.7 ± 6.5	32.7 ± 7.0
		Th2 cells	1.1 ± 0.5	1.2 ± 0.6	1.6 ± 0.3
Ustekinumab for 12 weeks [5] Psoriasis (n = 3–4)	Subpopulations presented as percent of total peripheral CD4+ cells	Natural regulatory T cells	Not supplied	1.9%–3.5% (n = 4)	0.97%–4.4% (n = 3)

Note: Studies that did not show a difference in comparison to healthy controls.
*p value < 0.05 for comparison with healthy controls. All other comparisons not statistically significant.

Immune Cell Function To assess cell function, immune cells are isolated from the serum of treated psoriasis patients and then cultured in the presence of cytokines, antigens, or stimulatory molecules. Cytokine secretion and cell surface markers of activation can then be measured with immunoflow cytometry. After treatment with biologic therapies, T-cell function was *not decreased* when compared to untreated controls (Table 23.3).

Are Immune Parameters Suppressed below Levels of Healthy Controls? Serum levels of Th17 cells [4], IL-17 [7], and IL-22 [9] are increased and regulatory T cells are decreased [6] in untreated psoriasis patients when compared to healthy controls (Table 23.2). This is consistent with a hyperactive Th17 pathway characteristic of psoriasis. After treating these patients with biologic therapy, serum levels of these cells and cytokines normalize toward, but not beyond, levels measured in healthy controls. Further, these laboratory changes correlate with clinical improvement in psoriasis.

TABLE 23.2 T-Cell Counts and Cytokine Levels of Th17 Pathway after Biologic Therapy

Intervention	Immune Parameter	Before Treatment	After Treatment	Healthy Controls	Clinical Considerations
Etanercept for 12 weeks [4] Psoriasis (n = 15) Healthy controls (n = 10)	Th17 cells (percent of serum IL-17 + IFNγ-T cells)	2.8% ± 1.8*	Depicted graphically, similar to but not less than controls	0.9% ± 0.5	Change correlated with treatment based on PASI score
	IL-8 + T cells (percent of serum T cells expressing IL-8)	12.1% ± 6.7*	Depicted graphically, similar to but not less than controls	3.7% ± 2.7	Change correlated with treatment based on PASI score
Anti-TNF (etanercept and infliximab) for 6 Months [6] Psoriasis (n = 28) Healthy controls (n = 30)	Natural regulatory T cells (percent of serum T cells expressing CD25 + FoxP3+)	2.4%*	3.4%	3.5%	Increase seen only in responding patients
Anti-TNF for 12 weeks [7] Psoriasis (n = 30) Healthy controls (n = 10)	Serum IL-17 (pg/mL)	52.9 ± 27.6*	21.5 ± 14.0	19.7 ± 9.8	Change correlated with treatment based on PASI score
	Serum IL-22 (pg/mL)	50.6 ± 46.2*	22.0 ± 25.4	6.5 ± 2.3	

Note: *$p < 0.05$ for the comparison between before treatment psoriasis patients and healthy controls.

Other than suppression of Th17 pathway, there is a decrease in IL-8-producing CD4+ and CD8+ cells [4] after etanercept treatment. Levels of IL-8-producing CD4+ and CD8+ T cells are shown to be elevated in untreated psoriasis patients. After biologic therapy, these cells are decreased to levels that are not significantly different from healthy controls [4]. The authors point out that IL-8 production is enhanced by IL-17 and suggest that the reduction in IL-8-producing cells is likely secondary to suppression of Th17 cells.

SUMMARY

Many laboratory parameters of systemic immunity appear not to be suppressed by biologic therapy, including various serum immune cell populations and T-cell response to antigen stimulation. Biologic therapy decreases the cell populations and cytokines characteristic of the Th17 pathway close to, but not below, levels of healthy controls. Thus, the Th17 pathway appears to "normalize" with biologic therapy.

TABLE 23.3 Immune Cell Function in Psoriasis Patients Treated with Biologic Therapy

Intervention and Participants	Immune Function Studied	Outcome Measure	*p*-Values: Treated Psoriasis Patients versus Healthy Controls	*p*-Values: Pretreatment versus Posttreatment Psoriasis Patients
Ustekinumab for 4 weeks [5] Psoriasis ($n = 5$) Healthy controls ($n = 5$)	Cytokine secretion by memory T-cell subsets	Th1 cells cytokine secretion	$p = 0.48$	Not reported
		Th2 cells cytokine secretion	$p = 0.84$	Not reported
		IL-17+ cells cytokine secretion	$p = 0.55$	Not reported
	Naïve T-cell differentiation	Differentiation into Th1 cells	$p = 0.42$	Not reported
		Differentiation into Th2 cells	$p = 0.99$	Not reported
		Differentiation into Th17 cells	$p = 0.99$	Not reported
Ustekinumab therapy for 12 weeks [8] Psoriasis ($n = 38$)	Ability to generate Th1 and Th2 responses	IFNγ production from stimulated PBMC	Not reported	$p > 0.05$
		IL-5 production from stimulated PBMC	Not reported	$p > 0.05$
Anti-TNF therapy for 4 weeks and 12 weeks [3]	Pathogen response	IFNγ secretion from $CD4^+$ T cells after stimulated with TSST-1 or recall antigen	Not reported	$p > 0.05$
Psoriasis ($n = 16$) Healthy controls ($n = 19$)	Cytokine secretion induced by TCR stimulation	IL-2, IL-10, IL-17 secretion from PBMC	Enhanced secretion $p < 0.05$	Enhanced secretion $p < 0.05$

Note: TCR, T-cell receptor; PBMC, peripheral blood mononuclear cell; TSST, toxic shock syndrome toxin.

Given that biologic medications in psoriasis target a specific pathway (i.e., Th17) that is hyperactive at baseline, use of the term "immunosuppressant" may be misleading. When used to treat psoriasis, alternative terms, such as "anti-inflammatory" can be considered to describe these agents.

There is one obvious exception and that is a proven increased risk for tuberculosis, especially from adalimumab and infliximab. This may be mediated through a specific effect on granuloma cells, which are involved in host defense against tuberculosis and other indolent fungal organisms such as histoplasmosis and coccidiomycosis. Therefore, the clearly increased risk associated with anti-TNF agents appears to be limited to granulomatous disease.

The patients represented by these studies were all considered appropriate candidates for biologic therapy and did not have comorbid immunosuppressive conditions (e.g., human immunodeficiency virus [HIV], hepatitis), were not on concurrent immunosuppressive medications, and did not have a history of malignancy. Thus, the results should be interpreted with caution with respect to patients who are immunocompromised, have active malignancy, or have a history of malignancy.

From a big picture perspective, the data reviewed in this chapter may indicate that biologic medications "normalize" immune function in psoriatic patients. The only evidence-based effect of biologic agents in decreasing immune function below that of untreated controls appears to be limited to granulomatous disease. The results reported in this review have not yet been reproduced and the study methodology is not standardized, making comparison among trials difficult. Further studies are needed to validate these preliminary findings.

REFERENCES

1. Nast A, Mrowietz U, Kragballe K, de Jong EM, Puig L, Reich K, et al. Barriers to the prescription of systemic therapies for moderate-to-severe psoriasis – a multinational cross-sectional study. *Arch Dermatol Res* 2013. [Epub ahead of print].
2. Looney RJ, Diamond B, Holers VM, Levesque MC, Moreland L, Nahm MH, et al. Guidelines for assessing immunocompetency in clinical trials for autoimmune diseases. *Clin Immunol* 2007;123:235–43.
3. Bose F, Raeli L, Garutti C, Frigerio E, Cozzi A, Crimi M, et al. Dual role of anti-TNF therapy: enhancement of TCR-mediated T cell activation in peripheral blood and inhibition of inflammation in target tissues. *Clin Immunol* 2011;139:164–76.
4. Antiga E, Volpi W, Cardilicchia E, Maggi L, Fili L, Manuelli C, et al. Etanercept downregulates the Th17 pathway and decreases the IL-17+/IL-10+ cell ratio in patients with psoriasis vulgaris. *J Clin Immunol* 2012;32:1221–32.
5. Tsuda K, Yamanaka K, Kondo M, Matsubara K, Sasaki R, Tomimoto H, et al. Ustekinumab improves psoriasis without altering T cell cytokine production, differentiation, and T cell receptor repertoire diversity. *PLoS One* 2012;7:e51819.
6. Quaglino P, Ortoncelli M, Comessatti A, Ponti R, Novelli M, Bergallo M, et al. Circulating CD4+CD25 bright FOXP3+ T cells are up-regulated by biological therapies and correlate with the clinical response in psoriasis patients. *Dermatology* 2009;219:250–8.
7. Caproni M, Antiga E, Melani L, Volpi W, Del Bianco E , Fabbri P. Serum levels of IL-17 and IL-22 are reduced by etanercept, but not by acitretin, in patients with psoriasis: a randomized-controlled trial. *J Clin Immunol* 2009;29:210–14.
8. Reddy M, Torres G, McCormick T, Marano C, Cooper K, Yeilding N, et al. Positive treatment effects of ustekinumab in psoriasis: analysis of lesional and systemic parameters. *J Dermatol* 2010;37:413–25.
9. Shimauchi T, Hirakawa S, Suzuki T, Yasuma A, Majima Y, Tatsuno K, et al. Serum interleukin-22 and vascular endothelial growth factor serve as sensitive biomarkers but not as predictors of therapeutic response to biologics in patients with psoriasis. *J Dermatol* 2013;40:805–12.

INDEX

D

W

X

Z